Register Now for On~~line Access~~
to Your Bo~~ok~~

SPRINGER PUBLISHING
C**O**NNECT™

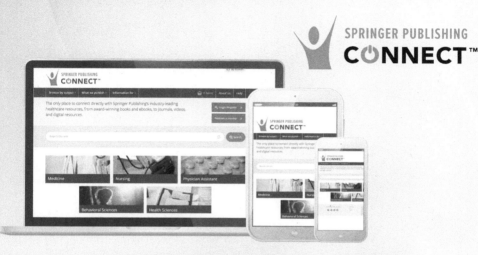

Your print purchase of *Manual of Traumatic Brain Injury: Assessment and Management, Third Edition* **includes online access to the contents of your book**—increasing accessibility, portability, and searchability!

Access today at:

WITHDRAWN

http://connect.springerpub.com/content/book/978-0-8261-4768-4
or scan the QR code at the right with your smartphone. Log in or register, then click "Redeem a voucher" and use the code below.

TXAKAJHX

Scan here for quick access.

Having trouble redeeming a voucher code?
Go to https://connect.springerpub.com/redeeming-voucher-code

If you are experiencing problems accessing the digital component of this product, please contact our customer service department at cs@springerpub.com

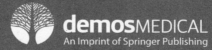

demosMEDICAL
An Imprint of Springer Publishing

View all our products at springerpub.com/demosmedical

Manual of Traumatic Brain Injury

Manual of Traumatic Brain Injury

Assessment and Management

Third Edition

Editor

Felise S. Zollman, MD, FAAN, FAAMA
Voluntary Associate Clinical Professor
Department of Neurosciences
University of California San Diego, Health Sciences
San Diego, California

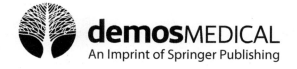

demosMEDICAL
An Imprint of Springer Publishing

Springer Publishing Company, LLC
11 West 42nd Street, New York, NY 10036
www.springerpub.com
connect.springerpub.com/

Acquisitions Editor: Beth Barry
Compositor: Exeter Premedia Services Private Ltd.

ISBN: 978-0-8261-4767-7
ebook ISBN: 978-0-8261-4768-4
DOI: 10.1891/9780826147684

21 22 23 24 25 / 5 4 3 2 1

Medicine is an ever-changing science. Research and clinical experience are continually expanding our knowledge, in particular our understanding of proper treatment and drug therapy. The authors, editors, and publisher have made every effort to ensure that all information in this book is in accordance with the state of knowledge at the time of production of the book. Nevertheless, the authors, editors, and publisher are not responsible for any errors or omissions or for any consequence from application of the information in this book and make no warranty, expressed or implied, with respect to the content of this publication. Every reader should examine carefully the package inserts accompanying each drug and should carefully check whether the dosage schedules therein or the contraindications stated by the manufacturer differ from the statements made in this book. Such examination is particularly important with drugs that are either rarely used or have been newly released on the market.

Library of Congress Control Number: 2021937070

Contact sales@springerpub.com to receive discount rates on bulk purchases.

Publisher's Note: **New and used products purchased from third-party sellers are not guaranteed for quality, authenticity, or access to any included digital components.**

Printed in the United States of America.

CONTENTS

PART III: MODERATE TO SEVERE TRAUMATIC BRAIN INJURY

PART V: SPECIAL CONSIDERATIONS AND TRAUMATIC BRAIN INJURY RESOURCES

CONTRIBUTORS

Rugaieh Abaza, MD, Resident, General Surgery, University of Florida College of Medicine Jacksonville, Jacksonville, Florida

Amar Agha, MD, Endocrinologist, Department of Endocrinology, Beaumont Hospital and RCSI Medical School, Dublin, Ireland

David N. Alexander, MD, Susan and David Wilstein Endowed Chair in Rehabilitation Medicine, Professor, Department of Neurology, David Geffen School of Medicine at UCLA, Los Angeles, California

Yazeed Alolayan, MD, Neurocritical Care Fellow, Department of Neurology, University of Miami, Miami, Florida

Cynthia L. Beaulieu, PhD, ABPP-CN, Associate Professor, Division of Rehabilitation Psychology, Department of Physical Medicine and Rehabilitation, The Ohio State University, Columbus, Ohio

Lucy-Ann Behan, MD, Consultant Endocrinologist, Department of Endocrinology, Tallaght University Hospital, Dublin, Ireland

Heather G. Belanger, PhD, ABPP, Senior Researcher, United States Special Operations Command (USSOCOM); Professor, Department of Psychiatry & Behavioral Neurosciences, University of South Florida, Tampa, Florida

Erica Bellamkonda, MD, Consultant, Department of Physical Medicine and Rehabilitation, Mayo Clinic, Rochester, Minnesota

Laura M. Benson, PhD, Clinician Educator, Department of Psychiatry and Behavioral Sciences, NorthShore University HealthSystem, Evanston, Illinois

Debra E. Berens, PhD, President, Foundation for Life Care Planning Research; Clinical Assistant Professor, Department of Counseling and Psychological Services, Georgia State University, Atlanta, Georgia

Thomas Bergquist, PhD, Associate Professor, Department of Physical Medicine and Rehabilitation, Department of Psychiatry and Psychology, Mayo Clinic, Rochester, Minnesota

Ann S. Bines, MS, RN, CCRN, Nurse Manager, Brain Innovation Center, Shirley Ryan AbilityLab, Chicago, Illinois

Jennifer Bogner, PhD, Bert C. Wiley Professor, Chair in Physical Medicine and Rehabilitation, Vice-Chair of Research and Academic Affairs, Director, Division of Rehabilitation Psychology, Department of Physical Medicine and Rehabilitation, The Ohio State University, Columbus, Ohio

Amy O. Bowles, MD, Chief, Brain Injury Rehabilitation Service, Department of Rehabilitation Medicine, Brooke Army Medical Center, Fort Sam Houston, San Antonio, Texas

Matthew Breiding, PhD, Traumatic Brain Injury Lead, Division of Injury Prevention, National Center for Injury Prevention and Control, Centers for Disease Control and Prevention, Atlanta, Georgia

Catherine Burress Kestner, PT, DPT, Physical Therapist, Shirley Ryan AbilityLab, Chicago, Illinois

Robert C. Cantu, MA, MD, FACS, FAANS, FACSM, Chair, Neurosurgery Section, Medical Director and Director of Clinical Research, Dr. Robert C. Cantu Concussion Center, Emerson Hospital, Concord, Massachusetts

David X. Cifu, MD, Associate Dean for Innovation and System Integration, Virginia Commonwealth University School of Medicine; Senior TBI Specialist, U.S. Department of Veterans Affairs, Richmond, Virginia

John D. Corrigan, PhD, Professor, Department of Physical Medicine and Rehabilitation, The Ohio State University, Columbus, Ohio

Marie Crandall, MD, MPH, FACS, Professor of Surgery, Associate Chair for Research, Department of Surgery, Program Director, General Surgery Residency, University of Florida College of Medicine Jacksonville, Jacksonville, Florida

Nora Cullen, MD, MSc, Professor, Department of Medicine, McMaster University, Hamilton, Ontario, Canada

Cherina Cyborski, MD, Chief of Physical Medicine and Rehabilitation, Washington DC VA Medical Center, Washington, DC

Ramon Diaz-Arrastia, MD, PhD, Presidential Professor, Director of Clinical Traumatic Brain Injury Research, University of Pennsylvania Perelman School of Medicine, Philadelphia, Pennsylvania

Kan Ding, MD, Assistant Professor, Department of Neurology and Neurotherapeutics, UT Southwestern Medical Center at Dallas, Dallas, Texas

Randi Dubiel, DO, Medical Director of Traumatic Brain Injury, Department of Physical Medicine and Rehabilitation, Baylor Scott & White Institute for Rehabilitation, Dallas, Texas

Blessen C. Eapen, MD, Chief, Physical Medicine and Rehabilitation, VA Greater Los Angeles Health Care System; Associate Clinical Professor, Division of Physical Medicine and Rehabilitation, Department of Medicine, David Geffen School of Medicine at UCLA, Los Angeles, California

Elie P. Elovic, MD, Clinical Professor, Department of Medicine, University of Nevada at Reno, Reno, Nevada

Dmitry Esterov, DO, Instructor, Department of Physical Medicine and Rehabilitation, Mayo Clinic, Rochester, Minnesota

Jennifer Field, Peterborough, New Hampshire

Jennifer Fleming, PhD, BOccThy (Hons), FOTARA, Professor and Head of Occupational Therapy, School of Health and Rehabilitation Sciences, The University of Queensland, Brisbane, Australia

Brandon A. Francis, MD, MPH, Assistant Professor, Department of Neurology, Michigan State University, East Lansing, Michigan

Joshua B. Gaither, MD, Associate Professor, Department of Emergency Medicine, College of Medicine, The University of Arizona–Tucson, Tucson, Arizona

Mina Gayed, DO, Resident Physician, Department of Physical Medicine and Rehabilitation, JFK Johnson Rehabilitation Institute, Hackensack Meridian Health, Edison, New Jersey

Nigel Glynn, MD, Consultant Endocrinologist, Department of Endocrinology, St. Bartholomew's Hospital, London, United Kingdom

Gary Goldberg, BASc, MD, FABPMR(BIM), Adjunct Clinical Professor, Department of Physical Medicine and Rehabilitation, Medical College of Virginia/VCU Healthcare System, Richmond, Virginia

Arlene I. Greenspan, DrPH, MPH, PT, Associate Director for Science, National Center for Injury Prevention and Control, Centers for Disease Control and Prevention, Atlanta, Georgia

Brian D. Greenwald, MD, Medical Director, Center for Brain Injuries, Department of Physical Medicine and Rehabilitation, JFK Johnson Rehabilitation Institute, Hackensack Meridian Health, Edison, New Jersey

Christine Greiss, DO, FAAPMR, Director, The Concussion Program, Department of Physical Medicine and Rehabilitation, JFK Johnson Rehabilitation Institute, Hackensack Meridian Health, Edison, New Jersey

Flora M. Hammond, MD, FACRM, BIM, Professor and Chair, Department of Physical Medicine and Rehabilitation, Indiana University School of Medicine, Rehabilitation Hospital of Indiana, Indianapolis, Indiana

Amy Y. Hao, MD, Medical Director, Polytrauma Network Site, Department of Physical Medicine and Rehabilitation, VA Greater Los Angeles Health Care System, Los Angeles, California

Mark Harniss, PhD, Associate Professor, Department of Rehabilitation Medicine, School of Medicine, University of Washington, Seattle, Washington

Christopher R. Harper, PhD, Behavioral Scientist, National Center for Injury Prevention and Control, Centers for Disease Control and Prevention, Atlanta, Georgia

Hunaid Hasan, MD, Clinical Neurology Attending and President, Hasan & Hasan Neurology Group PC, Lapeer, Michigan

Micelle J. Haydel, MD, Albert J. Lauro Endowed Professorship in Emergency Medicine, Clinical Professor of Medicine/Emergency Medicine, Louisiana State University Health Science Center, New Orleans, Louisiana

Michael Henrie, DO, Assistant Professor, Division of Physical Medicine and Rehabilitation, University of Utah, Salt Lake City, Utah

Lindsay Hong, MS, RN, CRRN, Clinical Nurse Coordinator, Brain Innovation Center, Shirley Ryan AbilityLab, Chicago, Illinois

Nancy H. Hsu, PsyD, ABPP, Associate Professor, Department of Physical Medicine and Rehabilitation, Virginia Commonwealth University, Richmond, Virginia

Anne W. Hunt, PhD OT Reg. (Ont.), Assistant Professor, Teaching Stream, Department of Occupational Science & Occupational Therapy, University of Toronto, Toronto, Ontario, Canada

Mary Alexis Iaccarino, MD, Assistant Professor, Department of Physical Medicine and Rehabilitation, Harvard Medical School; Spaulding Rehabilitation Hospital, Boston, Massachusetts

Grant L. Iverson, PhD, Professor, Department of Physical Medicine and Rehabilitation, Harvard Medical School; Spaulding Rehabilitation Hospital and Spaulding Research Institute; Massachusetts General Hospital for Children Sports Concussion Program; Home Base, A Red Sox Foundation and Massachusetts General Hospital Program, Charlestown, Massachusetts

Michael S. Jaffee, MD, FAAN, FANA, Vice Chair, Department of Neurology, Director, Brain Injury, Rehabilitation, and Neuroresilience (BRAIN) Center, Bob Paul Family Professor of Neurology, University of Florida College of Medicine, McKnight Brain Institute, Gainesville, Florida

Carlos A. Jaramillo, MD, Staff Physician, Director, Clinical Research, San Antonio Polytrauma Rehabilitation Center, South Texas Veterans Health Care System, San Antonio, Texas

Jonathan Jenness, OD, Optometrist, Daniel and Davis Optometry, Carlsbad, California

Kurt L. Johnson, PhD, Professor, Department of Rehabilitation Medicine, School of Medicine, University of Washington, Seattle, Washington

Ricardo E. Jorge, MD, Professor, Department of Psychiatry and Behavioral Sciences, Baylor College of Medicine, Houston, Texas

Jacob R. Joseph, MD, Clinical Assistant Professor, Department of Neurosurgery, University of Michigan, Ann Arbor, Michigan

Sheryl D. Katta-Charles, MD, BIM, Assistant Professor, Department of Physical Medicine and Rehabilitation, Indiana University School of Medicine, Rehabilitation Hospital of Indiana, Indianapolis, Indiana

Kristi L. Kirschner, MD, Clinical Professor, Departments of Medical Education, and Neurology & Rehabilitation Medicine, University of Illinois at Chicago, Chicago, Illinois

Kristen M. Klipfel, PhD, Postdoctural Fellow, Department of Psychiatry and Behavioral Sciences, NorthShore University HealthSystem, Evanston, Illinois

Matthew Kochuba, MD, Assistant Professor of Surgery, University of Florida College of Medicine Jacksonville, Jacksonville, Florida

Sunil Kothari, MD, Attending Physician, TIRR-Memorial Hermann; Assistant Professor, H. Ben Taub Department of Physical Medicine and Rehabilitation, Baylor College of Medicine, Houston, Texas

Jason Krellman, PhD, ABPP, Assistant Professor of Neuropsychology, Department of Neurology, Columbia University Irving Medical Center, New York, New York

Richard D. Kunz, MD, Associate Professor, Department of Physical Medicine and Rehabilitation, Virginia Commonwealth University, Richmond, Virginia

Rael T. Lange, PhD, Research Director and Senior Scientist, Defense and Veterans Brain Injury Center, Walter Reed National Military Medical Center, National Intrepid Center of Excellence, Bethesda, Maryland; University of British Columbia, Vancouver, British Columbia, Canada

Michelle C. LaPlaca, PhD, Associate Professor, Wallace H. Coulter Department of Biomedical Engineering, Georgia Tech at Emory, Atlanta, Georgia

Eric B. Larson, PhD, ABPP, Director of Psychology and Brain Injury, Marianjoy Rehabilitation Hospital, Wheaton, Illinois

Jeffrey David Lewine, PhD, Adjunct Professor of Translational Neuroscience, the MIND Research Network; CEO/CSO, Center for Advanced Diagnostics, Evaluation and Therapeutics; Adjunct Associate Professor of Neurology, University of New Mexico Health Sciences Center; Adjunct Associate Professor of Psychology, University of New Mexico, Albuquerque, New Mexico

Lisa A. Lombard, MD, Medical Director, Department of Physical Medicine and Rehabilitation, Ohio Health Rehabilitation Hospital; Regional Medical Director, US Physiatry, Columbus, Ohio

David F. Long, MD, Neurologist, Brain Injury Program, Bryn Mawr Rehab Hospital, Malvern, Pennsylvania

Matthew B. Maas, MD, MS, Associate Professor, Departments of Neurology and Anesthesiology, Northwestern University, Chicago, Illinois

Barbara Magnuson-Woodward, PharmD, CNSC, Nutrition Support Program Coordinator, University of Kentucky HealthCare; Professor (Adjunct), Department of Pharmacy Practice & Science, University of Kentucky College of Pharmacy, Lexington, Kentucky

Mithra B. Maneyapanda, MD, Medical Director, Brain Injury Program, Bryn Mawr Rehab Hospital, Malvern, Pennsylvania; Assistant Professor, Department of Rehabilitation Medicine, Sidney Kimmel Medical College at Thomas Jefferson University, Philadelphia, Pennsylvania

Susan S. Margulies, PhD, Professor and Chair, Wallace H. Coulter Department of Biomedical Engineering, Georgia Tech and Emory, Atlanta, Georgia

Joshua M. Masino, PsyD, Neuropsychologist, Department of Clinical Neuropsychology, Baylor Scott & White Institute for Rehabilitation, Dallas, Texas

Philip H. Montenigro, MD, PhD, Research Faculty, Department of Neuropsychology, University of New Hampshire, Manchester, New Hampshire; Department of Anatomy and Neurobiology, Boston University, Boston, Massachusetts

Matthew D. Moore, DO, Attending Physician, Department of Physical Medicine and Rehabilitation, JFK Johnson Rehabilitation Institute, Hackensack Meridian Health, Edison, New Jersey

Debjani Mukherjee, PhD, HEC-C, Interim Assistant Professor, Department of Medical Ethics in Clinical Medicine and in Clinical Rehabilitation Medicine, Division of Medical Ethics, Weill Cornell Medical College, New York, New York

Melissa A. Nestor, PharmD, Clinical Pharmacist, University of Kentucky HealthCare; Assistant Professor (Adjunct), Department of Pharmacy Practice & Science, University of Kentucky College of Pharmacy, Lexington, Kentucky

Kristine O'Phelan, MD, FNCS, Director, Neurocritical Care, Professor of Clinical Neurology, University of Miami Miller School of Medicine, Miami, Florida

David O. Okonkwo, MD, PhD, Professor, Department of Neurosurgery, University of Pittsburgh, Pittsburgh, Pennsylvania

William V. Padula, OD, SFNAP, FAAO, FNORA, Associate Professor, Department of Optometry, Salus University College of Optometry, Guilford, Connecticut

Rachel Pearson, MD, DABPN, FAAP, Staff Neurologist, Department of Pediatrics, CHOC Children's, University of California–Los Angeles, School of Medicine, Los Angeles, California

Vani A. Rao, MD, Associate Professor, Department of Psychiatry and Behavioral Sciences, The Johns Hopkins University, Baltimore, Maryland

William A. Robbins, MD, FABPMR(BIM), Medical Director, Service Member Transitional Advanced Rehabilitation Program; Medical Director, Polytrauma Transitional Rehabilitation Unit; PNS Outpatient Clinic Service Provider, Department of Physical Medicine and Rehabilitation, Central Virginia VA Health Care System; Adjunct Clinical Professor, Department of Physical Medicine and Rehabilitation, Medical College of Virginia/VCU Healthcare System, Richmond, Virginia

Jonathan Romain, PhD, MS, ABPP, Staff Physician, Department of Pediatrics, CHOC Children's, University of California–Irvine, School of Medicine, Orange, California

Joshua M. Rosenow, MD, FAANS, FACS, Director of Functional Neurosurgery, Professor of Neurosurgery, Neurology and Physical Medicine and Rehabilitation, Northwestern University Feinberg School of Medicine, Chicago, Illinois

Durga Roy, MD, Assistant Professor, Department of Psychiatry and Behavioral Sciences, The Johns Hopkins University School of Medicine, Baltimore, Maryland

Angelle M. Sander, PhD, Associate Professor, H. Ben Taub Department of Physical Medicine and Rehabilitation, Baylor College of Medicine, Houston, Texas

Teresa A. Savage, PhD, RN, Clinical Associate Professor, Emerita, Department of Human Development Nursing Science, College of Nursing, University of Illinois Chicago; Consultant, Shirley Ryan AbilityLab; Adjunct Clinical Associate Professor, Department of Physical Medicine and Rehabilitation, Northwestern University Feinberg School of Medicine, Chicago, Illinois

Billie A. Schultz, MD, Assistant Professor, Department of Physical Medicine and Rehabilitation, Mayo Clinic, Rochester, Minnesota

Hazem Shahin, MD, Resident, Department of Psychiatry and Behavioral Sciences, Baylor College of Medicine, Houston, Texas

Tracy Shannon, PsyD, ABPP-CN, RP, Assistant Professor, Division of Rehabilitation Psychology, Department of Physical Medicine and Rehabilitation, The Ohio State University, Columbus, Ohio

Noah D. Silverberg, PhD, Assistant Professor, Department of Psychology, University of British Columbia; Rehabilitation Research Program, Vancouver Coastal Health Research Institute, Vancouver, British Columbia, Canada

Caroline Sizer, MD, Attending Physician, Department of Physical Medicine and Rehabilitation, Lifespan Physician Group; Assistant Professor, Warren Alpert Medical School of Brown University, Providence, Rhode Island

Bruno S. Subbarao, DO, Medical Director, Polytrauma Network Site, Department of Physical Medicine and Rehabilitation, Phoenix VA Health Care System, Phoenix, Arizona

Jerry J. Sweet, PhD, Head, Psychology Division, Director, Neuropsychology Service, Department of Psychiatry and Behavioral Sciences, NorthShore University HealthSystem, Evanston, Illinois

Eric S. Swirsky, JD, MA, Clinical Assistant Professor, Director of Graduate Studies; PhD Program Director, Department of Biomedical and Health Information Sciences, University of Illinois at Chicago, Chicago, Illinois

Sharief Taraman, MD, DABPN, DABPM, FAAP, Division Chief, Department of Pediatric Neurology, CHOC Children's, University of California–Irvine, School of Medicine, Orange, California

Sarah Taylor, MS, CCC-SLP, MBA, BCS-S, CBIS, Speech Pathology Chief, Communication Disorders Department, Rancho Los Amigos National Rehabilitation Center, Downey, California

Douglas P. Terry, PhD, Assistant Professor, Department of Physical Medicine and Rehabilitation, Harvard Medical School; Spaulding Rehabilitation Hospital; Massachusetts General Hospital for Children Sports Concussion Program; Home Base, A Red Sox Foundation and Massachusetts General Hospital Program, Charlestown, Massachusetts

Theodore Tsaousides, PhD, ABPP, Assistant Clinical Professor, Department of Rehabilitation Medicine, Mount Sinai Health System, New York, New York

Sandeep Vaishnavi, MD, PhD, Medical Director, MindPath Care Centers Clinical Trials Institute; Medical Director, MindPath Care Centers Brain Stimulation Program, Raleigh, North Carolina

William C. Walker, MD, Endowed Professor and Associate Chairman of Clinical Care, Virginia Commonwealth University; Department of Physical Medicine and Rehabilitation, Medical College of Virginia/VCU Healthcare System, Richmond, Virginia

Thomas K. Watanabe, MD, Clinical Director, Drucker Brain Injury Center, Moss Rehab at Elkins Park/Einstein Healthcare Network, Elkins Park, Pennsylvania

Roger O. Weed, PhD, Professor Emeritus, College of Education and Human Development, Georgia State University; Fellow Emeritus, International Academy of Life Care Planners; Board Member Emeritus, Foundation for Life Care Planning Research, Mount Dora, Florida

F. Scott Winstanley, PhD, Staff Neuropsychologist, Department of Neuropsychology, Ohio Health Rehabilitation Hospital, Columbus, Ohio

Julie Witkowski, MD, Brain Injury Rehabilitation Fellow, Department of Physical Medicine and Rehabilitation, Mayo Clinic, Rochester, Minnesota

Bonny S. Wong, MD, Medical Director of Brain Injury Rehabilitation, St. David's Medical Center and St. David's Rehabilitation Hospital, Austin, Texas

Ellen C. Wong, MD, Faculty Fellow, Department of Neurology, Keck School of Medicine at University of Southern California, Los Angeles, California

David W. Wright, MD, Professor and Chair, Department of Emergency Medicine, Emory University School of Medicine, Atlanta, Georgia

Ross Zafonte, DO, Earle P. and Ida S. Charlton Professor and Chair, Department of Physical Medicine and Rehabilitation, Harvard Medical School; Spaulding Rehabilitation Hospital, Boston, Massachusetts

Nathan D. Zasler, MD, DABPM&R, FAAPM&R, FACRM, BIM-C, CBIST, Affiliate Professor, Department of Physical Medicine and Rehabilitation, Virginia Commonwealth University; Associate Professor, Adjunct, Department of Physical Medicine and Rehabilitation, University of Virginia, Charlottesville, Virginia

Bei Zhang, MD, MSc, Resident Physician, Department of Physical Medicine and Rehabilitation, McGovern Medical School, University of Texas Health Science Center at Houston, Houston, Texas

Felise S. Zollman, MD, FAAN, FAAMA, Voluntary Associate Clinical Professor, Department of Neurosciences, University of California San Diego, Health Sciences, San Diego, California

PREFACE

The first edition of the *Manual of Traumatic Brain Injury Management*, published in 2011, was designed to fill a unique niche: to provide relevant clinical information about management of traumatic brain injury (TBI) in a succinct, readily accessible format while at the same time offering readers specific chapter-by-chapter recommendations for those who wished to delve into any particular topic more deeply. The second edition introduced additional content areas and added a Key Points section to each chapter.

This third edition introduces another new feature: Each chapter has a Study Question section that offers four to five questions in multiple choice format, designed to further reinforce core chapter concepts. Further, as with the second edition, chapter content has been updated throughout on the basis of knowledge developed over the intervening period in this rapidly growing field. For many topics, chapter material was comprehensively overhauled (e.g., neuropathology, chronic traumatic encephalopathy, TBI in the military/blast injury). In addition, a new chapter has been added to this third edition, dedicated to substance abuse and TBI, situated alongside the existing chapter addressing alcohol misuse.

This edition is once again divided into five parts. Part I, Core Concepts, acquaints the reader with the basic essentials needed to provide a context for clinical decision-making. Part II, Mild Traumatic Brain Injury, offers a comprehensive treatment of this topic, including natural history, initial management, persistent postconcussive symptomatology, and sport-related concussion. Part III, Moderate to Severe Traumatic Brain Injury, covers prehospital and intensive care management, rehabilitation care, community reintegration, and management of selected associated impairments, including cognitive and behavioral impairments, challenges with sexuality, and decision-making capacity. The chapter on prognosis in TBI has been updated to reflect the most current evidence-based approach to understanding post-injury outcomes. Part IV, Complications and Long-Term Sequelae, covers a variety of topics from posttraumatic epilepsy and hydrocephalus to chronic cognitive, behavioral, and motor sequelae, including spasticity and movement disorders. Part V, Special Considerations and Traumatic Brain Injury Resources, addresses selected populations based on age (pediatrics and geriatrics) or injury environment (military, workers' compensation), as well as return to work, complementary and alternative treatment modalities, and ethical and medicolegal issues associated with TBI, and offers a unique perspective on life after TBI from a patient's perspective. For all chapters, to keep the print version as concise in format as feasible, chapter references have been moved online with publication of this third edition.

The content of this book can be digested at several levels of complexity: as a succinct introduction to TBI, reliant on the Key Points and Study Questions provided in each chapter to focus in on core content; as a concise but thorough chapter-by-chapter treatment of each topic relevant to TBI; or as a springboard to more comprehensive learning based on the directed Additional Reading recommendations of each chapter author. For those using the electronic version, hyperlinks to many of these Additional Reading recommendations are provided. There is truly something meaningful in the pages which follow for everyone interested in understanding the management of TBI.

ACKNOWLEDGMENTS

This project would not have been possible without the assistance of a few key individuals. Thank you to my editor at Demos Medical Publishing/Springer Publishing Company, Beth Barry, who has shepherded all three editions through from conception to production with a steady hand and deep understanding of the world of medical publishing, without which this project would have never gotten off the ground. Thank you also to my associate editor, Jaclyn Shultz, who helped keep the train running on the tracks throughout the production process. A big thank you is also due to Dr. Frances Daly, who has been my sounding board through the editing process for each edition of this textbook.

This third edition came into form during a taxing year. 2020 brought many challenges our way, not the least of which was a global pandemic the magnitude of which has not been seen in over 100 years. This year also marked the loss of a personal hero, Justice Ruth Bader Ginsberg. This edition is dedicated to the memory of Justice Ginsberg, for all she did to pave the way for equality for women in the workforce, and is also dedicated to my daughter Erin…from generation to generation….

I CORE CONCEPTS

TRAUMATIC BRAIN INJURY: DEFINITIONS AND NOMENCLATURE

KRISTINE O'PHELAN AND YAZEED ALOLAYAN

INTRODUCTION

Traumatic brain injury (TBI) has a broad spectrum of severity, pathology, physiology, and sequelae. This chapter will present pertinent definitions, nomenclature, and concepts relevant to the discussion of TBI.

CLASSIFICATION OF TRAUMATIC BRAIN INJURIES

TBI classification has evolved over the past decades. Historically, the classification started as a quantified bedside assessment described in Teasdale and Jennett's exemplary paper that described the Glasgow Coma Scale (GCS).[1] With the advancement of brain imaging, TBI classification has evolved to a more nuanced approach incorporating not only clinical presentation, but also primary versus secondary effects of injury, mechanism of injury, and anatomic/structural manifestations.

PRIMARY VERSUS SECONDARY INJURY

Primary injury alludes to the unavoidable, immediate parenchymal or calvarial damage that occurs at the moment of and as a direct consequence of the injurious event. Secondary injury alludes to conceivably avoidable damage that happens after injury. The distinction is somewhat arbitrary and the specific combination and magnitude of secondary injury is, to a great extent, determined by the nature of the primary injury. This description is useful, however, in order to aid clinicians in identifying potential preventable or reversible causes of secondary brain injury. (See Chapter 2 for further details.)

- **Primary injury**—The physiological or anatomical insult, often but not exclusively the result of direct trauma to head. The primary injury may be associated with structural changes resulting from mechanical forces initially applied during injury. These forces may cause tissue distortion, shearing, and vascular injury as well as destabilization of cell membranes and frank membrane destruction.
- **Secondary injury**—Systemic or local changes, which increase tissue damage. Many secondary insults result directly from the primary injury and some are caused by

---

The full reference list appears in the digital product found on http://connect.springerpub.com/content/book/978-0-8261-4768-4/part/part01/chapter/ch01

discrete systemic or local phenomena. Secondary injury mechanisms include generation of free radicals, excitotoxicity, disturbance of ionic homeostasis, disruption of the blood–brain barrier, generation of nitric oxide, lipid peroxidation, mitochondrial dysfunction and energy failure, inflammation, secondary hemorrhage, axonal disruption, apoptotic cell death, and ischemia. Ischemia may be due to microvascular changes, systemic hypotension or hypoxia, or elevated intracranial pressure.

CLASSIFICATION OF TRAUMATIC BRAIN INJURY BY MECHANISM

This classification is useful because injuries produced by different mechanisms are distinct in their pathophysiologies and natural courses.

- **Closed/blunt force**—Injury caused by direct force to the head, acceleration–deceleration, or rotational forces. Common causes include falls, assaults, and motor vehicle collisions.
- **Blast injury**—Injury caused by overpressure waves generated from high-grade explosives. A large amount of thermal, mechanical, and electromagnetic energy is transferred to the brain. Energy can come directly through the cranium or be transmitted indirectly through oscillating pressures in fluid-filled large blood vessels. This may cause damage to the blood–brain barrier or gray–white matter junction, and can cause cerebral edema, axonal injury, apoptosis, and tissue degeneration.
- **Penetrating injury**—Injury induced by an object that penetrates the cranial vault. Common causes include gunshot wounds, shrapnel, and knife wounds.

CLINICAL CLASSIFICATION OF TRAUMATIC BRAIN INJURY

The GCS[1] (Table 1.1) is central to clinical classification of TBI. Clinical/injury severity classification is the most commonly used classification system in the clinical care of patients with TBI as well as in clinical neurotrauma research. (See Chapter 3 for further discussion of this topic.)

- **Mild TBI (MTBI)**—GCS 13 to 15; the majority of patients with cranial trauma fall in this group. Patients are awake, and may be confused but can communicate and follow commands.

TABLE 1.1   Glasgow Coma Scale

Eye Opening	Best Verbal Response	Best Motor Response
Spontaneous 4	Oriented 5	Obeys commands 6
To speech 3	Confused conversation 4	Localizes pain 5
To pain 2	Inappropriate words 3	Withdrawal 4
None 1	Incomprehensible sounds 2	Abnormal flexion (decorticate) 3
	None 1	Extension (decerebrate) 2
		None 1

■ **Moderate TBI**—GCS 9 to 12; these patients are generally drowsy to obtunded but not comatose. They can open their eyes and localize painful stimuli. They are at high risk of clinical deterioration and must be monitored carefully.

■ **Severe TBI**—GCS 3 to 8; these patients are obtunded to comatose. They do not follow commands and may exhibit decerebrate or decorticate posturing. They have significant structural and metabolic brain dysfunction and are at high risk of secondary brain injury and deterioration.

TRAUMATIC BRAIN INJURY IMAGING CLASSIFICATION

A number of classifications have been proposed based on imaging findings, and patho-anatomic description. A commonly used scale is the Marshall score for computed tomography (CT) findings.[2]

The Marshall score aims to stratify patients' risk of morbidity and mortality based on the status of the basilar cisterns, presence/degree of midline shift, and different density mass lesions. Some reported limitations to this score are that it doesn't take into account the location of hemorrhage, presence of axonal injury, or different variants of herniation.

STRUCTURALLY BASED DESCRIPTIONS OF TRAUMATIC BRAIN INJURY

Structural descriptions incorporate information from imaging studies. They often aid in selection of patients who may benefit from a specific therapy such as surgical evacuation of a hematoma.

■ **Epidural hematoma (EDH;** Figure 1.1)—An extradural collection of blood. It is often associated with a skull fracture and typically has an arterial origin. Margins of the

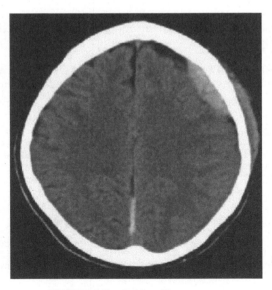

FIGURE 1.1   Epidural hematoma.

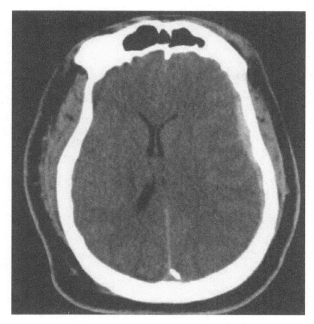

FIGURE 1.2   Subdural hematoma.

hematoma do not cross the skull suture lines and often appear convex on imaging studies. If an EDH is evacuated in a timely fashion to reverse mass effect or if the hematoma is small in size, patient outcomes are usually good.

- **Subdural hematoma (SDH;** Figure 1.2)—A collection of blood in the subdural space. SDHs may be chronic or acute, and are caused by venous bleeding from cortical bridging veins. Bleeding may extend over the entire hemisphere. Acute SDHs are significantly associated with seizures. Acute SDHs are also associated with significant alteration of cerebral blood flow and metabolism of the underlying hemisphere and generally have a worse outcome than EDHs.
- **Traumatic axonal injury** (TAI, also referred to as diffuse axonal injury [DAI])—Injury to axonal connections triggered by inertial forces, predominantly acceleration–deceleration, with subsequent structural and metabolic consequences of mechanical deformation.
- **Traumatic subarachnoid hemorrhage (TSAH or SAH;** Figure 1.3)—Hemorrhage in the subarachnoid space that is not associated with significant mass effect. It often accompanies other types of traumatic hemorrhage. The presence of TSAH has been associated with an increased risk of an unfavorable 6-month outcome in patients with moderate to severe TBI.[3]
- **Intraventricular hemorrhage (IVH)**—Bleeding into the ventricular system after trauma. It may be associated with acute hydrocephalous and is a risk factor for development of delayed hydrocephalous. IVH is typically seen in conjunction with TSAH.
- **Contusion** (Figure 1.4)—Parenchymal hemorrhage, typically in frontal or temporal lobes. Contusions may be "coup" or "contre coup."
  - **Coup injury**—Results from direct transmission of force to brain tissue underlying the region of impact.
  - **Contre coup injury**—Results from the indirect forces acting in a region contralateral to the region of impact.

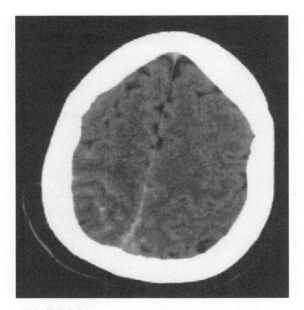

FIGURE 1.3   Traumatic subarachnoid hemorrhage.

- **Skull fractures**—Skull fractures may occur after trauma because of blunt or penetrating injury. They may involve the convexity or the skull base and may be open or closed depending on the presence of an overlying scalp laceration. Large depressed skull fractures may need to be surgically elevated. Depressed skull fractures are associated with an increased risk of seizures.[4]

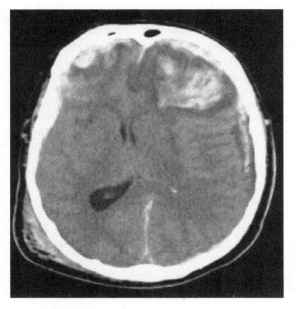

FIGURE 1.4   Cerebral contusion.

CONCUSSION

The term "concussion" has been used as a synonym for mild TBI (MTBI). The American Academy of Neurology (AAN) has defined it as "a clinical syndrome of biomechanically induced alteration of brain function, typically affecting memory and orientation, which may involve loss of consciousness."[3] Symptoms reflect a functional disturbance rather than structural injury. There are several diagnostic tools that can be used to aid in identifying those with concussion after head injury. Several of these are listed in Table 1.2; however, they are not meant to be used to "rule out" concussion. See, for example, the AAN 2013 guideline on the management of concussion in sports[5] and the 2017 Berlin Concussion in Sport Group Consensus Statement in contact and collision sports.[6,7] (See also Chapter 6 for a more detailed discussion of concussion vs. MTBI.)

POSTTRAUMATIC AMNESIA

Posttraumatic amnesia (PTA) is the impaired recall of events surrounding the injury. Retrograde PTA involves impaired recollection of events immediately preceding the injury and anterograde PTA is a deficit in forming new memories after the injury.[8]

POSTCONCUSSION DISORDER

Also known as postconcussion syndrome, this term refers to postconcussive symptoms that persist for 3 or more months post injury. Symptoms are quite variable and are not unique to this diagnosis.[5-7] (See Table 1.3; see Chapters 15–17 for further discussion of this topic.)

TABLE 1.2   Commonly Used Tools to Identify Those Individuals with Concussion after Sport-Related Head Trauma

PCSS: Postconcussion symptom scale
GSC: Graded symptom checklist
SAC: Standardized assessment of concussion
Neuropsychological testing
BESS: Balance error scoring system
SOT: Sensory organization test
Video technology used to identify concussion

Source: From Giza CC, Kutcher JS, Ashwal S, et al. Summary of evidence-based guideline update: evaluation and management of concussion in sports: report of the Guideline Development Subcommittee of the American Academy of Neurology, *Neurology.* 2013;80(24):2250–2257. doi:10.1212/WNL.0b013e31828d57dd; Patricios JS, Ardern CL, Hislop MD, et al. Implementation of the 2017 Berlin Concussion in Sport Group Consensus Statement in contact and collision sports: a joint position statement from 11 national and international sports organisations. *Br J Sports Med.* 2018;52(10):635–641. doi:10.1136/bjsports-2018-099079; McCrory P, Meeuwisse W, Dvořák J, et al. Consensus statement on concussion in spor—the 5th international conference on concussion in sport held in Berlin, October 2016. *Br J Sports Med.* 2017;51(11):838–847. doi:10.1136/bjsports-2017-097699

TABLE 1.3 Signs of Concussion

Loss of consciousness
Lying motionless for >5 seconds
Confusion/disorientation
Amnesia
Vacant look
Motor incoordination
Tonic posturing
Impact seizure
Ataxia

Source: Reproduced with permission from Temkin NR. Antiepileptogenesis and seizure prevention trials with antiepileptic drugs: meta-analysis of controlled trials. *Epilepsia*. 2001;42(4):515–524.

SECOND IMPACT SYNDROME

A second MTBI occurring while an individual remains symptomatic from the first MTBI may cause the "Second Impact Syndrome." This rare phenomenon involves acute cerebro-vascular congestion and loss of cerebrovascular autoregulation resulting in malignant brain swelling, which is life-threatening.[7] (See Chapter 11 for further discussion of this topic.)

RECOVERY AND SEQUELAE

Definitions

- **Diaschisis**—Dysfunction in an area of the brain that is remote from an area with structural damage but is connected to the damaged area via neuronal pathways.
- **Neuroprotection**—Therapies or management strategies that prevent or limit secondary injury and lead to improved survival of neurons, microglia, or the supporting microvasculature.
- **Neuroplasticity**—Changes in brain structure (neuronal and glial connectivity) and function due to experience. This is a major mechanism for recovery of function after traumatic injury.
- **Gliosis**—Formation of a dense network of glial cells in areas of brain injury that do not contribute to functional recovery. This can occur after trauma, stroke, or demyelination.
- **Atrophy**—Loss of neurons and glia and their connections. This can occur after TBI and is usually related to the severity of the initial injury.

KEY POINTS

- Primary injury refers to the unavoidable, immediate parenchymal or calvarial damage that occurs at the moment of and as a direct consequence of an external biomechanical event.
- Secondary injury refers to further damage resulting from a complex cascade of cellular, metabolic, and inflammatory events triggered by the initial traumatic event.
- TBI can be classified based on a number of different criteria or parameters, including clinical presentation, imaging findings, and injury mechanism.

STUDY QUESTIONS

A 25-year-old man presented to the emergency department (ED) after a motor vehicle collision. Per EMS report the patient was found in the car nonresponsive, gasping for air and was emergently pulled out of the vehicle and intubated in the field; GCS was 3, E(1) V(1) M(1). The patient was rushed to the ED.

1. On arrival to the ED his vitals were T 37, R 16, BP 120/80, HR 80 sating 100% on a ventilator. He was placed on a fentanyl drip for intubation. Initial labs showed mild leukocytosis, normal hemoglobin, and normal clotting and renal function. CT scan of the head did not show any signs of loss of gray–white matter differentiation, no hemorrhage appreciated. CT spine did not show any fracture, patient was placed on Miami J cervical collar. After assessing and stabilizing the patient what would you do next?
   a. Consult neurosurgery for placement of an intracranial pressure (ICP) monitor
   b. Repeat head CT in 6 hours
   c. Hold sedation to assess a post resuscitation neurological exam
   d. Order brain magnetic resonance imaging (MRI) to rule out traumatic axonal injury

2. Based on the vignette, what is the likely mechanism of injury?
   a. Traumatic subarachnoid hemorrhage (TSAH)
   b. Traumatic axonal injury (TAI)
   c. Coup contrecoup
   d. Traumatic subdural hematoma

3. Which of the following is a correct statement?
   a. Skull fracture is an example of secondary injury
   b. Secondary injury usually occurs as a direct result of and at the time of the initial insult
   c. The primary injury alludes to the unavoidable, immediate structural damage happening at the time of injury
   d. Increased intracranial pressure a week after the initial injury is an example of primary injury

4. What are the components of the Marshall score?
   a. Thickness of blood clot around the basal cisterns and midline shift
   b. Basal cistern visibility and midline shift
   c. Different density lesions and thickness of subdural blood
   d. Midline shift, basal cistern visibility, and different density mass lesions

ADDITIONAL READING

CDC definition of TBI: https://www.cdc.gov/traumaticbraininjury/get_the_facts.html
Brain Trauma Foundation Website. www.braintrauma.org
Puderbaugh M, Emmady PD. Neuroplasticity. In: *StatPearls* [Internet]. StatPearls Publishing; 2020.

ANSWERS TO STUDY QUESTIONS

1. Correct Answer: c
Reassessing GCS is crucial on admission; for that reason the correct answer would be holding sedation for a post resuscitation exam.[9]

Further Reading:
Marklund N. The Neurological Wake-up Test—A Role in Neurocritical Care Monitoring of Traumatic Brain Injury Patients? *Front Neurol*. 2017;8:540. Published 2017 Oct 17. doi:10.3389/fneur.2017.00540

2. Correct Answer: b
TAI—an injury to axonal connections triggered by inertial forces, predominantly acceleration–deceleration, with subsequent structural and metabolic consequences of mechanical deformation.[10]

Further Reading:
Ravindra VM, Hawryluk, GWJ, Classification of traumatic brain injury. Ch 3 in *Neurotrauma and Critical Care of the Brain*. 2nd ed. Thieme Verlagsgruppe; 2018.

3. Correct Answer: c
The primary injury alludes to the unavoidable, immediate structural damage happening at the time of injury.[11]

Further Reading:
Abou El Fadl MH, O'Phelan KH. Management of traumatic brain injury: an update. *Neurosurg Clin N Am*. 2018;29(2):213–221. PMID:29502712. doi:10.1016/j.nec.2017.11.002

4. Correct Answer: d
Midline shift, basal cistern visibility, and different density mass lesions.[2]

Further Reading:
Marshall LF, Marshall SB, et al. The diagnosis of head injury requires a classification based on computed axial tomography. *J Neurotrauma*. 1992;9(Suppl 1):S287–292.

REFERENCES

The full reference list appears in the digital product found on http://connect.springerpub.com/content/book/978-0-8261-4768-4/part/part01/chapter/ch01

2 ESSENTIAL CONCEPTS IN TRAUMATIC BRAIN INJURY BIOMECHANICS AND NEUROPATHOLOGY

MICHELLE C. LAPLACA, SUSAN S. MARGULIES, AND DAVID W. WRIGHT

GENERAL PRINCIPLES

Traumatic Brain Injury as a Continuum

Traumatic brain injury (TBI) can be defined as transient or persistent brain dysfunction, occurring as the result of a biomechanical event that causes suprathreshold loading to the brain. The TBI response is the result of numerous interrelated processes that have inherent heterogeneity and complexity across time scales (the continuum) and system levels (subcellular [nano], cellular [micro], tissue/organ [meso], and systemic/organism [macro]). Biomechanics plays a critical role in understanding the TBI continuum, from the traumatic event to patient outcome:

- *Traumatic insult*: The external cause itself is a physical event described by the biomechanical concepts described in the following section Biomechanics and Primary Injury, and further categorized by the *mechanism* (e.g., motor vehicle collision, fall, being struck by an object) and the *intent* (e.g., unintentional).[1,2] Injurious loading to the head typically occurs due to impact and head movement, and is on the order of milliseconds to seconds. The physical event may also occur without impact or head movement (e.g., crush, blast).
- *Primary injury*: The immediate (milliseconds to seconds) *mechanically induced* cell and tissue damage; the resulting brain pathology may be grossly apparent upon physical examination or imaging (e.g., epidural or subdural hemorrhage as a result of direct vessel damage), microscopic only (e.g., cell and axonal stretch), or subcellular (e.g., microtubule disruption). The initiation of secondary processes does not require visible damage.
- *Secondary cascade:* The cascade of changing biochemical and molecular events (seconds to weeks) that result from the primary injury and may occur clinically or subclinically. Neuroprotective strategies aim to curb secondary cascades and improve outcome, but clinical translation of such interventions is extremely challenging.[3]
- *Secondary injury*: The acute to subacute (seconds to weeks) systemic response to the secondary injury cascade. Manifests as intracranial hypertension, delayed intracranial hemorrhage, hypotension, hypoxia, edema, and so forth. The focus of clinical management during this phase is to reduce further brain damage and preserve function.
- *Injury outcome (seconds to years)*: Consequences of the primary and secondary injury, combined with repair and compensation of the brain, manifesting as sensory, motor, cognitive, behavioral, affective, systemic, and/or somatic conditions. The ability to recover depends on many factors, including sex, age, underlying health status, genetic constellation, resilience, metabolic state, endogenous repair capacity, plasticity (see TBI Heterogeneity).

The full reference list appears in the digital product found on http://connect.springerpub.com/content/book/978-0-8261-4768-4/part/part01/chapter/ch02

BIOMECHANICS AND PRIMARY INJURY

The biomechanics of the physical event (external load and resulting head movement) and the mechanical response (primary injury to the brain) are linked.

- *Types of external loads. Loading conditions* refer to the force magnitude, rate, and other parameters of the load.
  - *Impact load*: Force resulting from the head striking a mass or obstruction, or a moving object or obstruction striking the head. The collision transfers energy and produces contact phenomenon *(focal injury)*.
  - *Inertial or impulsive load*: Load resulting when a person is put in motion by an applied force. Unless there is rigid support, the head will rotate, with the neck as a pivot. Energy transduced to the brain is *diffuse*.
  - *Penetrating load (e.g., bullet)*: An object with a small surface area penetrates the brain with high velocity and transfers energy over a limited impact area.
  - *Crush load* (e.g., *building collapse)*: Variable loading types, sustained load.
  - *Blast*: Explosion releases energy to surrounding environment, causing rapid propagation of pressure waves in the brain (typically low strain, high frequency). Can cause objects to strike head or head to impact surface[4] (see also Chapter 66).
  - *Combination load:* Loads are usually a combination (e.g., inertial followed by impact, such as motor vehicle collision with subsequent head to windshield impact; or impact followed by head movement, such as baseball bat to motionless cranium). Trauma may involve multiple loading events (e.g., head to head collision in sports followed by ground impact, vehicular rollover).
- *Acceleration and temporal considerations.*
  - *Acceleration = Velocity/Time. Linear or translational acceleration* occurs when movement is directly through the center of gravity. *Rotational acceleration* occurs when movement is around the center of gravity. Real-world loading of the head is a combination of translational and rotational acceleration (i.e., angular acceleration).
  - *Deceleration.* Occurs when a head in motion comes to a sudden stop; the relatively soft brain collides with the interior of the hard cranium and dural septa, rapidly deforming tissue.
  - *Force = Mass × Acceleration.* The lower the mass, the higher the acceleration must be to keep the force constant. Force transduction to the tissue and cells is complex because of nonuniform cell arrangement and variable loading conditions from injury to injury. Protective gear and safety measures aim to distribute and dissipate force.
  - *Loading rate is important.* Slowly applied force will result in lower stress than rapidly applied force.
- *The primary injury: Stress and strain.* For a TBI to occur, the external load to the head must be transduced to the brain and surpass structural and functional thresholds. The biomechanical response manifests as *stress* and *strain* in the tissue and cells, and is a function of the force, the surface area over which the force occurs, and the material properties.
  - *Material properties* across brain regions vary.[5] The brain is a compliant, soft tissue. Cell orientation and tissue composition (e.g., blood vessels, white matter tracts) contribute to differences in properties.[6]
  - *Deformation* (or *strain*) can be *tensile* (stretch), *compressive*, and/or *shear* (note: the brain is especially vulnerable to shear strain); more force + softer tissue = more strain; suprathreshold force will deform tissue to the point of functional or structural damage.
  - Higher *strain rate* is more damaging than lower strain rate. For example, high-velocity impacts typically result in more widespread damage including diffuse axonal injury (DAI).

- *Plane of motion*. The plane of brain motion during an impact may be associated with characteristic pathology. In general, structures with the same directionality as the motion will undergo higher strains and stresses (e.g., loading in the coronal plane may be associated with corpus callosum stretching, which sagittal loading may result in more stretching of anterior to posterior bridging veins).[7]
- Structural failure of the brain (macro- and mesoscale) includes microtears, macrotears, stretching, and/or shearing within and between brain regions (e.g., gray/white matter), vascular damage (e.g., acute hemorrhage).
- Immediate damage to neurons, glia, and vascular cells (micro- and nanoscale) may manifest as axonal stretching, membrane disruption, rapid ion flux, blood–brain barrier (BBB) disruption, bleeding, or conduction interruption.
- Skull fracture may or may not be involved in primary damage to the brain.
- *Injury threshold*. The loading conditions at which structural and functional compromise or failure takes place; described using *injury tolerance criteria*. Development of tolerance criteria requires understanding of the multiscale relationships among *traumatic insult*, *mechanical response*, and the resulting *injury cascades* and *neuropathology*. Injury risk curves are developed experimentally and guide preventive measures (e.g., helmet use, playground surfaces).
- *Clinical management and biomechanics*. Specific quantitative details of the biomechanical conditions around a traumatic insult are typically not known in most clinical scenarios.
  - Information about the injury mechanism and loading conditions can guide clinical inquiry (e.g., location and nature of lesion, multifocal contusions, functional tests) and likelihood of injury severity (e.g., high acceleration and impact raises suspicion of intracranial hemorrhage).
  - Known injury mechanism and intent can guide prevention and discharge messaging to the patient and caregiver (e.g., when to avoid or mitigate injury risk), inform likelihood for continued risk (e.g., athletic exposure), and guide referral decisions (e.g., suspected substance abuse or domestic violence).

SECONDARY INJURY CASCADES

Primary structural damage (membrane and axonal stretching, tissue shearing, frank cellular disruption) initiates secondary cascades, which manifest clinically as secondary injury. Variability in secondary cascades contributes to clinical heterogeneity in secondary injury manifestations,[8] which is evident during the acute monitoring phase of injury.[9] The relationship between biomechanics and specific secondary pathways is complex due to heterogeneity in the insults and individual responses, interrelated cellular signaling pathways, and constantly changing cellular activities and systemic adaptations.[10]

Major Categories of Secondary Cascades

- *Neurochemical and electrochemical imbalances* (ions, neurotransmitters, cell signaling)
  - Mechanical loading disrupts ion homeostasis (Ca^{2+}/Na^+ influx);[11] ion channel dysfunction[12] can cause hyperexcitability and mass depolarization[13] as well as cessation of normal action potential conduction; mechanosensitive channels and receptors[14] contribute to hyperexcitability, neurotransmitter imbalance, and excitotoxicity.
  - Mechanical loading can lead directly to nonspecific membrane damage, termed mechanoporation, directly affecting membrane permeability,[15] exacerbating ion imbalance, and causing fluid and solute flux in and out of the cell body and axon.

- *Excitotoxicity:* Excess glutamate activates NMDA and AMPA receptors, exacerbates calcium influx and calcium-mediated proteolytic activity
- Patho-mechanotransduction[16]: Force transduction through the extracellular matrix and aberrant cell signaling lead to abnormal action at downstream intracellular targets.

■ *Impaired brain metabolism* (oxygen and glucose availability and use)[17]
- Periods of hyperactivity and hypoactivity; mismatch of metabolic demand and availability of energy substrates; different brain regions may have varying metabolic crises.
- Changes in cerebral perfusion result in hypoxia due to fluctuations in oxygen delivery.[18]
- Impaired mitochondrial function[19] and diminished glucose substrates lead to reduced cellular respiration and less ATP production, increases in CO_2 (hypercapnia) and H^+ (acidosis).

■ *Biomolecular degradation* (enzyme activation, free-radical attack); biomolecular degradation processes are initiated as a result of aberrant cellular signaling and activation of proteases, lipases and endonucleases, as well as production of free radicals:
- Proteases attack the cytoskeleton (e.g., calcium-mediated calpain activation), lipases disrupt lipid metabolism (e.g., phospholipase A_2), endonucleases initiate nucleic acid damage.[20]
- *Free-radical production* (reactive oxygen species [ROS]; reactive nitrogen species [RNS]): An increase in hydroxyl radicals causes lipid peroxidation and exacerbates degradative processes.[21]
- Secondary membrane damage (e.g., lipid peroxidation) impairs axonal transport and signaling, as well as stability of membrane phospholipids.[22]

■ *Axonal damage and diffuse axonal injury (DAI)*[23,24]
- Axonal stretch causes loss of elasticity,[25] transient axolemmal permeability, and impaired axonal transport.[26]
- Axonal and myelin degradation affect white matter tracts and contribute to disrupted network activity.[27]

■ *Vascular dysfunction* (permeability, hemorrhage, reactivity)[28,29]
- BBB disruption causes infiltration of blood-borne proteins, cells.[30]
- Vascular leakage and microbleeding cause brain toxicity, hypoxia, coagulation, and hematoma formation or contusion. Macroscopic bleeding or hemorrhage can compress and shift the brain, and cause extrusion.
- Uncoupling of cerebral blood flow and metabolism, hyperemia, uncontrolled cerebral perfusion pressure, vasospasm, contribute to edema and increased intracranial pressure.

■ *Inflammation* (central and peripheral contribution)[31,32]
- Acute inflammatory response (e.g., release of cytokines, arachidonic acid, nitric oxide) can become chronic and contribute to degenerative processes
- Activation of microglia triggered by cell damage and related signals (e.g., damage-associated molecule patterns [DAMPs]) results in further increase in pro-inflammatory cytokines; that is, IL-1-β, IL-6, TNF-α).[33] Opening of the BBB or overt bleeding will exacerbate the inflammatory response due to infiltration of blood-borne immune cells (e.g., T-cells, monocytes).
- Pro-inflammatory and anti-inflammatory processes both contribute to the overall response[34,35] (e.g., microglia serve to isolate damage as well as to release chemokines to support neighboring cells).

■ *Cerebral edema*[36]
- Brain tissue edema can occur when osmolality changes, resulting in fluid movement between fluid compartments (e.g., capillary leak, cell swelling), contributing to intracranial pressure (ICP) increases and fluid dysregulation.

- Underlying causes are increased intravascular hydrostatic pressure, disrupted BBB, protein leakage/abnormal oncotic pressures (vasogenic edema), leading to increased interstitial/extracellular fluid, and cellular swelling due to ionic imbalance and osmosis (cytotoxic edema).
- Management centers around ICP control (e.g., decompressive craniectomy, hyperosmotic therapy in acute cerebral edema), with emerging novel therapies focused on edema source (e.g., aquaporins, Na^+-K^+-$2Cl^-$ cotransporter (NKCC1).[37]
- *Cell death and cytotoxicity*[38] can occur as a result of the biomolecular cascades just described, as the balance of damage outweighs the ability to recover. While specific cell death pathways are promising therapeutic targets, TBI-induced cell death may result from multiple cell death mechanisms.
  - *Apoptosis:* Programmed cell death characterized by caspase activation and shrunken cells with DNA fragmentation
  - *Necroptosis:* Programmed cell death in the absence of apoptotic pathway activation characterized by loss of membrane integrity and cell lysis
  - *Necrosis:* Passive cell death, enzymatically propagated, exacerbated by inflammation
  - *Autophagy:* Cell death through phagocytic processes[39]
- *Genetic and epigenetic changes*[40,41] can alter secondary cascades and influence secondary injury manifestation.
  - Genetic predisposition can render some individuals more vulnerable to TBI.[42]
  - Polymorphisms can emerge and affect inflammation, ion channel regulation, cell death pathways, repair capacity, and many other processes.
  - Epigenetic changes influence gene expression without changing DNA sequence.
  - Cognitive and behavioral outcomes are under polygenic control.

Secondary Injury Mitigation (See Also Chapter 25)

- Clinical symptoms and presentation of secondary injury are caused by numerous changing secondary cascades, necessitating frequent evaluation of clinical management strategies.
- It is difficult to narrow down dominant secondary pathways at the cell level as they relate to clinically significant features and injury mitigation.[43]
- *Combination therapeutics*: Neuroprotective strategies will likely need to target multiple pathways.[3,44]

TRAUMATIC BRAIN INJURY HETEROGENEITY

Heterogeneity stems from the variation in the inherent nature of a system and/or in the response to a changing state. TBI is extremely heterogeneous, spanning a spectrum of phenotypes.[45] TBI heterogeneity necessitates personalized diagnostic and treatment strategies.

- *Pre-injury heterogeneity* (innate, premorbid):
  - *Innate heterogeneity (nonchangeable):* Individual characteristics such as sex, age, stature, genetic and epigenetic factors, resilience, and neuroanatomic and musculoskeletal variations[46]
  - *Premorbid factors (potentially changeable):* Individual preexisting medical conditions or disease (e.g., previous head injury exposure, cardiovascular disease); health state at time of injury (e.g., hydration, nutritional status, recent sleep pattern, stress state)

- *Event heterogeneity* (biomechanics, environmental):
  - *Biomechanics of the causative event* (i.e., injury mechanism): Magnitude and direction of force and acceleration (e.g., height of fall; vehicle velocity), surface area of impact (i.e., force distribution), loading duration (e.g., deceleration time after impact), location of injury in the brain (e.g., prefrontal vs. occipital cortex)
  - Environmental heterogeneity at the time of the event (e.g., temperature)
  - *Injury mitigation strategies*: Head protection (e.g., helmets), modifying impact surface, use of occupant restraints, degree of anticipation (e.g., neck muscle tension pre-impact)
- *Peri-injury heterogeneity* (early injury response, clinical intervention):
  - Primary injury (e.g., tissue and vessel stretching, tearing) is dependent on tissue mechanical properties, tissue orientation, and loading direction.
  - Early secondary injury (e.g., edema) and early secondary cascades (e.g., ion imbalance) are dependent on type and number of cells affected, intrinsic cellular characteristics.
  - *Clinical intervention*: Variations in the time window to care and prehospital protocols
- *Post-injury heterogeneity* (secondary injury, repair capacity, clinical management):
  - *Secondary injury* (e.g., reduced oxygen tension): Overlapping signaling cascades (e.g., excitotoxicity), systemic influences (e.g., inflammation, cardiovascular response)
  - *Repair capacity*: Innate and premorbid factors superimposed with the injury response and ability to stably repair (i.e., neuroplasticity, compensatory capacity)
  - *Clinical management*: Variable stabilization protocols, treatment options, and rehabilitation strategies[47]

KEY POINTS

- The full spectrum of TBI (from biomechanics to outcome) is complex and heterogeneous across both time scales and system levels.
- *Biomechanical sequence*: External force (load) → Dynamic head response (velocity, acceleration) → Transduction to brain (stress, strain) → Brain response (compression, shearing, stretching, tearing).
- The traumatic insult initiates the propagation of secondary cascades, which manifest as physiological and neurological secondary injuries.
- Knowing the biomechanical circumstances of the injury can inform the clinician about severity and potential complications.
- Heterogeneity, from the injurious event to individual characteristics and clinical intervention, manifests as different injury phenotypes/outcomes.

STUDY QUESTIONS

1. An 18-year-old female restrained passenger presents to the emergency department (ED) after a high-speed head-on motor vehicle collision (MVC). EMS reported brief loss of consciousness (LOC) and a Glasgow Coma Scale (GCS) of 9 on arrival to the ED, contusions across her chest, and no head or face lacerations or contusions. A head computed tomography (CT) is performed. Given the mechanism and clinical findings, which of these imaging scenarios is the most likely finding?

  a. Negative CT findings, as she was wearing a seatbelt and had no head or face lacerations
  b. Subdual hemorrhage due to the sagittal plane rapid deceleration
  c. Skull fracture and epidural hemorrhage
  d. Negative CT findings because edema would not appear until secondary injury was more developed

2. A 45-year-old unrestrained driver in a 70-mph head-on MVC presents to the emergency department by EMS on a backboard with a C-collar in place. He is awake and mildly confused, and smells of alcohol. EMS reports multiple facial and extremity contusions. Patient reports being knocked out for an unknown period of time but was awake on EMS arrival. Initial vital signs are unremarkable. What elements of this history are the most concerning for a life-threatening injury?
  a. The patient is awake but mildly confused
  b. The fact that EMS put the patient on a backboard with C-collar
  c. The patient reports loss of consciousness
  d. The patient was an unrestrained driver in high-speed MVC
  e. Multiple contusions with unremarkable initial vital signs

3. A mechanical load on neurons can activate a secondary cascade of events that contributes to neurological dysfunction. Initial rapid stretching of cell bodies and axons directly leads to membrane damage and increased membrane permeability. How does this affect neuronal function acutely following TBI?
  a. Ions such as Na^+, K^+, and Ca^{2+} will cross the membrane through nonspecific membrane defects and faulty channels, contributing to an inability to send action potentials
  b. It causes the axons to immediately break and prevent signal transmission down the axon
  c. Only myelinated axons will be affected, preventing normal network communication, but most cortical neurons would not be affected
  d. Membrane permeability will be temporary and not significantly affect function

4. Force from a head impact is transduced to the brain and causes tissue stress and deformation. What best describes the biomechanics between loading to the skull and loading to the brain?
  a. The skull is going to protect the brain by absorbing energy except in the most severe trauma, when energy will be dissipated and absorbed by the skull and the brain
  b. The skull is relatively hard compared to the soft tissue of the brain and therefore brain tissue will only deform when it hits the skull
  c. Because the brain is encapsulated in the skull they will always move and deform the same unless there is a skull fracture
  d. Rotational loading must occur to deform the brain; translational loading will cause more stress to the skull than the brain
  e. Rotational acceleration and impact will cause the soft tissue of the brain to keep moving after the relatively hard skull stops at impact (deceleration), leading to higher deformation of the brain compared to the skull

5. Pre-clinical researchers have discovered a very promising treatment (Drug X) for severe TBI. It has been tested in multiple animal species, including gyrencephalic animals (i.e., pig) and a robust treatment effect is maintained. It appears safe in single-center Phase I and II clinical trials. You have been selected to design a Phase III multicenter clinical trial to determine if Drug X improves outcome (Glasgow Outcome Scale) at 6 months

post-injury for patients with severe TBI. You design a double blind randomized pla-cebo control pragmatic (very few to no exclusion criteria) trial. The study successfully enrolled 1200 subjects (per protocol). The trial failed to show efficacy of Drug X. What is likely the most important contributing factor to the trial's failure?

a. Focusing on severe TBI because these patients are unlikely to survive their injury
b. The heterogeneity of the patient's enrolled and multiple non-study treatments received
c. The fact that pre-clinical studies are not relevant to human disease; therefore, the robust effect found did not translate to humans
d. The lack of adequate blinding of the investigators in the trial
e. The inexperience of the clinical teams managing the study patients

ADDITIONAL READING

National Highway Traffic Safety Administration https://one.nhtsa.gov/Research/Biomechanics-&-Trauma

Rowson, B, Rowson, S, Duma SM. Biomechanical forces involved in brain injury. In: McAllister M, Silver JM, Arciniegas DB, eds. *Textbook of Traumatic Brain Injury*. American Psychiatric Association Publishing; 2019:78–103.

Meaney, DF, Morrison, B, Bass, CD. The mechanics of traumatic brain injury: a review of what we know and what we need to know for reducing its societal burden. *J Biomech Eng*. 2014;136(2):021008. doi:10.1115/1.4026364

McGinn, MJ Povlishock, JT. Pathophysiology of traumatic brain injury. *Neurosurg Clin N Am*. 2016;27(4):397–407. doi:10.1016/j.nec.2016.06.002

ANSWERS TO STUDY QUESTIONS

1. Correct Answer: b
   A front end collision is associated with sagittal plan motion and anterior-posterior bridging vein hemorrhage. The patient was wearing a seatbelt, and there was no evi-dence of head impact. A high-speed impact with seatbelt use will still produce angular acceleration of the head.

   Further Reading:
   Post A, Hoshizaki TB, Gilchrist MD, et al. Traumatic brain injuries: the influence of the direc-tion of impact. *Neurosurgery*. 2015;76(1):81–91. doi:10.1227/NEU.0000000000000554

2. Correct Answer: d
   Unrestrained motor vehicle occupants are more likely to sustain serious injuries due to higher impact forces with vehicle interior elements.

   Further Reading:
   Mbarga, NF, Abubakari, A-R, Aminde, LN, Morgan, AR. Seatbelt use and risk of major injuries sustained by vehicle occupants during motor-vehicle crashes: a systematic review and meta-analysis of cohort studies. *BMC Pub Health*. 2018;18(1):1–11. doi:10.1186/s12889-018-6280-1
   Meaney, DF, Morrison, B, Bass, CD. The mechanics of traumatic brain injury: a review of what we know and what we need to know for reducing its societal burden. *J Biomech Eng*. 2014;136(2):021008. doi:10.1115/1.4026364

3. Correct Answer: a
Membrane defects will cause ion imbalance, overwhelming sodium and potassium pumps, causing membrane potential fluctuations that affect normal electrophysiological conduction. Delayed signal transduction leads to asynchronous and disharmonious signal processing which clinically presents as delayed reaction time, cognitive impairment, and other clinical findings.

Further Reading:
LaPlaca MC, Lessing MC, Prado GR, et al. Mechanoporation is a potential indicator of tissue strain and subsequent degeneration following experimental traumatic brain injury. *Clin Biomech*. 2019;64:2–13. doi:10.1016/j.clinbiomech.2018.05.01615
McGinn, MJ, Povlishock, JT. Pathophysiology of traumatic brain injury. *Neurosurg Clin N Am*. 2016;27(4):397–407. doi:10.1016/j.nec.2016.06.002

4. Correct Answer: e
The brain will move differently than the skull in response to head loading and will deform more because it is more pliable than bone. Rotational acceleration and deceleration (with or without) impact will cause higher deformation in the brain versus the skull and typically is associated with shear strain—deformation in two different directions—which is thought to be more damaging that pure compression or tensile (stretching) strain.

Further Reading:
Meaney, DF, Morrison, B, Bass, CD. The mechanics of traumatic brain injury: a review of what we know and what we need to know for reducing its societal burden. *J Biomech Eng*. 2014;136(2):021008. doi:10.1115/1.4026364
Rowson, B, Rowson, S, Duma SM. Biomechanical forces involved in brain injury, in: McAllister M, Silver JM, Arciniegas DB, eds. *Textbook of Traumatic Brain Injury*. American Psychiatric Association Publishing; 2019:78–103.

5. Correct Answer: b
Each TBI is slightly different and the heterogeneity of secondary injury cascades means that multiple, sometimes overlapping cell and molecular events are initiated. This is a major challenge in translating neuroprotective or neuroreparative pharmaceuticals for TBI.

Further Reading:
Somayaji, MR, Przekwas, AJ, Gupta RK. Combination therapy for multi-target manipulation of secondary brain injury mechanisms. *Curr Neuropharmacol*. 2018;16(4):484–504. doi:10.2174/1570159X15666170828165711
Margulies S, Anderson G, Atif F, et al. Combination therapies for traumatic brain injury: retrospective considerations. *J Neurotrauma*. 2016;33(1):101–112. doi:10.1089/neu.2014.3855

REFERENCES

The full reference list appears in the digital product found on http://connect.springer-pub.com/content/book/978-0-8261-4768-4/part/part01/chapter/ch02

CHARACTERIZATION OF TRAUMATIC BRAIN INJURY SEVERITY

LISA A. LOMBARD AND F. SCOTT WINSTANLEY

OVERVIEW: CHALLENGES IN CLASSIFICATION OF TRAUMATIC BRAIN INJURY

- No universally accepted classification system exists for all stages of traumatic brain injury (TBI).
- Heterogeneity of characterization scales results in difficulty in interpretation and comparison of research studies and in prognostication for individual patients.
- Challenges to the creation of a scale includes difficulty in capturing the wide range of severity of persons with TBI (from concussion to coma), confounding factors on admission (intoxication, shock, etc.), other physical injuries that may limit function, and potential language deficits that may give inaccurate representation of orientation and command-following.

CHARACTERIZATION OF INJURY

Glasgow Coma Scale

- Introduced by Teasdale and Jennett[1]; the most commonly used assessment for acute TBI (see Table 1.1)
- Assessment of three domains of eye opening, motor response, and verbal response
- Glasgow Coma Scale (GCS) score 3 to 8 is defined as severe TBI, 9 to 12 moderate, and 13 to 15 mild
- Limitations:
  - Unable to assess when administered after neuromuscular blockade, and verbal score cannot be obtained when the patient is intubated and is thus recorded as a 1T; this has led to outcome data where those with GCS 4 have a better outcome than with a GCS 3.[2] These factors may lead to overestimation of brain injury severity and inability to acknowledge worsening neurological deficit.
  - Many different providers may record the GCS in a trauma patient; studies cite inaccuracies in inter-rater reliability more than one third of the time.[3]
- As a single factor, the GCS has been shown to be only a modest predictor of rehabilitation outcome.[4]

Rancho Los Amigos Levels of Cognitive Functioning

- Also known as the Levels of Cognitive Functioning Scale (LCFS), it was first outlined in 1972; it describes cognitive functioning after TBI on the basis of the interaction with the environment.[5] The original scale containing seven categories was expanded in 1997

The full reference list appears in the digital product found on http://connect.springerpub.com/content/book/978-0-8261-4768-4/part/part01/chapter/ch03

to include 10 total categories in order to better characterize recovery in patients on the higher end of the original scale[6] (Table 3.1).

▪ Commonly used as a descriptive tool between professionals or for family education, or as a tracking tool for recovery; however, it has no value in predicting outcome.

Mayo Portland Adaptability Inventory (MPAI-4)[7]

▪ Designed to be a post-hospital evaluation of the physical, cognitive, emotional, behavioral, and social issues experienced in persons with TBI
▪ Measurements in three subsets: Ability (sensory, motor, and cognitive abilities); adjustment (mood, interpersonal interactions); and participation (social contacts, initiation, money management)
▪ May identify barriers to community reintegration
▪ Can be performed by professionals, caretakers, or persons with brain injury

TABLE 3.1 Rancho Los Amigos Scale-Revised (RLAS-R) (With Associated Typical Functional Level in Parentheses)

I. *No Response* **(Total Assistance):** Unresponsive to any external stimulus

II. *Generalized Response* **(Total Assistance):** Limited, inconsistent, and non-purposeful responses—often to pain only

III. *Localized Response* **(Total Assistance):** Purposeful, inconsistent responses; may follow simple commands; may focus on presented object; responds better to familiar people (friends and family) versus strangers

IV. *Confused/Agitated* **(Maximal Assistance):** Heightened state of activity; confusion, disorientation; aggressive behavior; unable to perform self-care; unaware of present events; agitation appears as a result of internal confusion

V. *Confused/Inappropriate, Nonagitated* **(Maximal Assistance):** Appears alert; responds to commands; distractible; does not concentrate on task; agitated responses to external stimuli; verbally inappropriate; does not learn new information

VI. *Confused/Appropriate* **(Moderate Assistance):** Good directed behavior, needs cuing; can relearn old skills as activities of daily living; serious memory problems; some awareness of self and others

VII. *Automatic, Appropriate* **(Minimal Assistance for Daily Living Skills):** Appears generally oriented; frequently robot-like in daily routine; minimal or absent confusion; shallow recall; increased awareness of self and interaction in environment; lacks insight into condition; decreased judgment and problem solving; lacks realistic planning for the future

VIII. *Purposeful, Appropriate* **(Stand-By Assistance):** Consistently oriented to person, place, and time; improved memory consolidation; able to consistently carry out tasks in a non-distracting environment; emerging awareness of impairments; able to acknowledge others' emotional states; experiences emotional lability and low frustration tolerance.

IX. *Purposeful, Appropriate* **(Stand-By Assistance):** Able to shift between and to complete tasks; aware of impairments and impact on daily functioning, but unable to prospectively anticipate obstacles that may arise as a result; able to utilize compensatory strategies; continued improvement in acknowledging emotional needs of others; continued emotional lability and low frustration tolerance.

X. *Purposeful, Appropriate* **(Modified Independent):** Able to multitask in many different environments when allowed extra time or with devices to assist; able to make decisions and act appropriately but may require more time or compensatory strategies; anticipates obstacles that may occur as a result of impairments and can take corrective actions; able to create own compensatory strategies; emotional lability and low frustration tolerance emerge only when under stress.

ASSESSMENT OF OUTCOME: THE GLASGOW OUTCOME SCALE

- One of the earliest scales used to record outcomes from moderate or severe TBI (Table 3.2).
- Five categories, ranging from dead to good recovery. Some have concerns that the Glasgow Outcome Scale (GOS) oversimplifies patterns of recovery from TBI.
- The GOS-E (extended) increases the categories to eight, splitting each of the categories of severe disability, moderate disability, and good recovery into two each (upper and lower).

ASSESSMENT OF FUNCTIONAL STATUS

Disability Rating Scale

Designed to track changes through the spectrum of TBI, from coma to community re-entry[8] (Table 3.3)

- First three areas are directly from the GCS: eye opening, verbal response, and motor response
- Second section reflects cognitive ability for feeding, grooming, and toileting
- Third section is related to need for assistance and employability
- Scores range from 0 (no disability) to 29 (deep coma)
- Has been validated for self- or caregiver reporting and for telephone interviews
- Has been shown to be more sensitive than GOS in measurement of improvement during in-patient rehabilitation as well as 1 year post injury[9]

Functional Independence Measure and the Functional Assessment Measure

- Functional Independence Measure (FIM)[10] has been one of the most commonly used measurements of independence in in-patient rehabilitation, and is a frequently used tool in outcomes research.
  - Has 18 domains (13 motor/activities of daily living [ADL] and 5 cognitive/communication), all individually scored from 1 (total dependence) to 7 (complete independence)
  - Intended for all types of disabilities that lead to some complaints of it being more weighted toward motor impairments, and thus less sensitive in assessing cognitive issues in persons with TBI
- The Functional Assessment Measure (FAM) adds 12 items to assess more cognitive and psychosocial domains.
- Both the FIM and the FAM were found to have good sensitivity to change after TBI, especially in the early stages of recovery.[11]

TABLE 3.2 Glasgow Outcome Scale

1. Dead
2. Vegetative state—Unable to interact with environment; unresponsive
3. Severe disability—Able to follow commands; unable to live independently
4. Moderate disability—Able to live independently; unable to return to work or school
5. Good recovery—Able to return to work or school

TABLE 3.3   Disability Rating Scale

Eye opening 　　0—Spontaneous 　　1—To speech 　　2—To pain 　　3—None	Toileting (cognitive ability only) 　　0—Complete 　　1—Partial 　　2—Minimal 　　3—None
Communication ability 　　0—Orientated 　　1—Confused 　　2—Inappropriate 　　3—Incomprehensible 　　4—None	Grooming (cognitive ability only) 　　0—Complete 　　1—Partial 　　2—Minimal 　　3—None
Motor response 　　0—Obeying 　　1—Withdrawing 　　2—Flexing 　　3—Extending 　　4—None	Level of functioning 　　0—Completely independent 　　1—Independent in a special environment 　　2—Mildly dependent 　　3—Moderately dependent 　　4—Markedly dependent 　　5—Totally dependent
Feeding (cognitive ability only) 　　0—Complete 　　1—Partial 　　2—Minimal 　　3—None	Employability 　　0—Not restricted 　　1—Selected jobs, competitive 　　2—Sheltered workshop, noncompetitive 　　3—Not employable

- Both the FIM and the FIM + FAM require training to properly score.
- Due to changes in Center for Medicare & Medicaid Services (CMS) rules in 2019, FIM scores are no longer reported and have been replaced by the Section GG Self-Care & Mobility Activities, a 6-point functional ability rating scale, scored from 0 (dependent) to 6 (independent).

ASSESSMENT OF POSTTRAUMATIC AMNESIA

- Serves as a measure of TBI severity; objective measurement of orientation can be correlated with outcome in rehabilitation[12] and long-term outcome.[13]

Galveston Orientation and Amnesia Test

Ten question assessment, with error points subtracted from 100. Initially designed for mild TBI, critics claim that some of the questions, such as those about the mode of transport to the hospital, are of little personal significance to severely injured patients. In addition, there are various point values assigned to questions with no justification for the relative weighting of questions.

Orientation Log

The Orientation Log (O-Log) contains 10 questions focusing on domains of time, place, and condition. Scores on each question range from 0 to 3. It can be used in nonverbal patients, and allows the examiner to use logical cuing to prompt the patient for the correct answer.

ASSESSMENT OF POSTTRAUMATIC AGITATION

Agitation Behavior Scale (ABS)

The Agitation Behavior Scale (ABS) consists of fourteen items dealing with agitation, which load on three different categories (aggression, disinhibition, and lability).[14] Items are scored 1 to 4 with maximum score of 56. Developed to provide an objective assessment of the nature and severity of agitation following acquired brain injury. It can be utilized as a serial assessment and has been demonstrated to predict outcome in TBI patients.[15]

Overt Agitation Severity Scale

The Overt Agitation Severity Scale (OASS) addresses verbal and physical aggression and agitation in acute brain injury. Behaviors are charted as verbal aggression, as well as physical aggression toward self, others, and objects.[16]

ASSESSMENT OF POSTTRAUMATIC CONFUSIONAL STATE

Cognitive Log (Cog-Log)

Cog-Log is a 10-item scale (scores 0–3 for each item) that addresses Cognitive Log or orientation as well as additional cognitive abilities such as attention, memory, and executive skills. The Cog-Log was validated through correlation with a number of neuropsychological tests and found to contribute significantly to the prediction of cognitive outcomes in TBI patients.[17]

Neurobehavioral Rating Scale

The Neurobehavioral Rating Scale (NBRS) itemizes a wide variety of psychiatric symptoms including disorientation, inattention, anxiety, guilt, agitation, poor insight, depressed mood, fatigability, hallucinations, disinhibition, guilt, affect, and speech articulation deficit.[18]

The Toronto Test of Acute Recovery After Traumatic Brain Injury

The Toronto Test of Acute Recovery After TBI (TOTART) assesses orientation and retrograde and anterograde memory using items from the GOAT and Westmead scale. The TOTART also measures verbal recall and recognition, attention, vigilance, and working memory.[19]

Confusion Assessment Protocol

The CONFUSION ASSESSMENT PROTOCOL (CAP) assesses orientation and cognitive impairment (using items from the Cognitive Test for Delirium-CTD and TOTART), agitation (using full ABS), and sleep disturbance, daytime arousal, psychotic-like symptoms, and fluctuation of symptoms (from the Delirium Rating Scale Revised-98).[20]

ASSESSMENT OF DISORDERS OF CONSCIOUSNESS

■ Assessing the patient with a disorder of consciousness (DOC) can be difficult, but the ability to objectively distinguish between minimally conscious state (MCS) and unresponsive wakefulness syndrome/vegetative state (UWS/VS) may have significant importance for tracking recovery, assessing success of interventions, and establishing appropriate plans of care.

Coma/Near-Coma Scale

First described in 1982, it uses eight parameters and 11 different stimuli.[13] Scores for responses to individual stimuli range from 0 (normal) to 4 (no response); the composite score is divided by number of items tested to create an average score of 0 to 4. It requires equipment of a bell, a light, noxious olfactory stimulus, and a nasal swab.

JFK Coma Recovery Scale

Published in 1991 and later revised in 2004,[21] it is composed of 23 items and six subscales, with each subscale in order of brainstem, subcortical, and cortical functions. In a study comparing the diagnostic strengths of this scale with the disability rating scale (DRS) in 80 patients with a severe DOC, the JFK Coma Recovery Scale (CRS) was able to diagnose 10 additional patients who were in a minimally conscious state, or who were determined to be in a vegetative state by the DRS.[22]

Disorders of Consciousness Scale

A clinical bedside observation assessment tool which scores set stimuli responses in eight subscales. Patients are scored 0 (no response), 1 (general response), or 2 (localized response) in response to stimuli. Testing requires a variety of different stimuli, including spoons, pictures, juice, and a television. Some authors cite that the scoring of the DOCS allows for a better assessment of responses in comparison with the CRS, which records presence or absence of responses.[23]

KEY POINTS

■ Because of significant variation in severity and presentation of TBI, a uniform assessment tool for the characterization of injury is lacking.

■ The selection of an appropriate measurement tool is dependent on the goal: DRS, Rancho Los Amigos, FIM scores, and the Mayo Portland may be used for tracking of recovery status, while other assessments may offer measurement of a specific factor (e.g., functional status, presence of posttraumatic amnesia, severity of disorder of consciousness).

STUDY QUESTIONS

1. A 32-year-old man is brought to the emergency department after being involved in a motorcycle crash. He was not wearing a helmet. His eyes are closed, he is making groaning noises, and is not following commands, but pulls away from painful stimuli. What is his GCS score?

a. 3
b. 5
c. 8
d. 10

2. Which of the following would be the best tool to use in assessing long-term outcomes for persons with moderate TBI?
   a. Glasgow Coma Scale
   b. Disability Rating Scale
   c. JFK Coma Recovery Scale
   d. Functional Independence Measure

3. Which assessment would be the best tool to determine clearance of posttraumatic amnesia?
   a. O-Log
   b. Mayo Portland
   c. Glasgow Outcome Score
   d. Coma/Near Coma Scale

4. A 48-year-old man is undergoing inpatient rehabilitation after sustaining a brain injury after an assault. He is cooperative with staff, performs self-care with cuing, but has very poor short-term memory. Which Rancho Los Amigos scale score would be assigned to him?
   a. II
   b. IV
   c. VI
   d. VIII

5. Which of the following would be the best tool for an objective assessment of a patient demonstrating behaviors such as pulling at tubes, restraints; restlessness, pacing, excessive movement; impulsive, impatient, low tolerance for pain or frustration, and has been shown to predict outcome in brain injury patients.
   a. Mayo Portland
   b. Disorders of Consciousness
   c. Agitated Behavior Scale
   d. Functional Independence Measure

ADDITIONAL READING

Center for Outcome Measurement in Brain Injury: www.tbims.org/combi

CMS Self-Care & Mobility Activities scale: https://www.cms.gov/Medicare/Quality-Initiatives-Patient-Assessment-Instruments/HomeHealthQualityInits/Downloads/GG-Self-Care-and-Mobility-Activities-Decision-Tree.pdf

Posner JB, Saper CB, Shiff ND, Plum F. *Diagnosis of Stupor and Coma*. 4th ed. Oxford University Press; 2007. doi:10.1093/med/9780195321319.001.0001

Hall KM, Hamilton BB, Gordon WA, Zasler ND. Characteristics and comparisons of functional assessment indices: disability rating scale, functional independence measure, and functional assessment measure. *J Head Trauma Rehabil*. 1993;8(2):60–74. doi:10.1097/00001199-199308020-00008

ANSWERS TO STUDY QUESTIONS

1. Correct answer: c
   This patient demonstrates no eye opening, giving him a eye score of 1, groaning for a verbal score of 2, and localizing to stimuli for a motor score of 5.

   Further Reading:
   Teasdale G, Jennett B. Assessment of coma and impaired consciousness. A practical scale. *Lancet*. 1974;2(7872): 81–84. doi:10.1016/S0140-6736(74)91639-0

2. Correct answer: b
   Of the options listed, the Disability Rating Scale is the only one designed to measure TBI status through the continuum of hospitalization through community reentry.

   Further Reading:
   Rappaport M, Hall KM, Hopkins K, et al. Disability rating scale for severe head trauma: coma to community. *Arch Phys Med Rehabil*. 1982;63(3): 118–123. doi:10.1037/t29015-000

3. Correct answer: a
   O-log (Orientation log) is specifically designed to assess posttraumatic amnesia.

   Further Reading:
   Novack T. The orientation log. *The Center for Outcome Measurement in Brain Injury*. 2000; www.tbims.org/combi/olog

4. Correct answer: c
   Rancho Los Amigos level VI is defined as good directed behavior, needs cuing; can relearn old skills as activities of daily living; serious memory problems, some awareness of self and others.

   Further Reading:
   Hagen C, Malkmus D, Durham P. *Rancho Los Amigos Levels of Cognitive Functioning Scale*. Rancho Los Amigos Hospital; 1972.

5. Correct answer: c
   Agitated Behavior Scale (ABS) has been a validated measure for characterizing and assessing severity of a patient's agitation following TBI. ABS has also been shown to play a role in predicting outcome following TBI.

   Further Reading:
   Bogner JA, Corrigan JD, Strange M, et al. Reliability of the agitated behavior scale. *J Head Trauma Rehabil*. 1999;14:91–96. doi:10.1097/00001199-199902000-00012
   Bogner JA, Corrigan JD, Fugate L, et al. Role of agitation in prediction of outcomes after traumatic brain injury. *Am J Phys Med Rehabil*. 2001;80:636–644. doi:10.1097/00002060-200109000-00002

REFERENCES

The full reference list appears in the digital product found on http://connect.springer-pub.com/content/book/978-0-8261-4768-4/part/part01/chapter/ch03

EPIDEMIOLOGY OF TRAUMATIC BRAIN INJURY

RUGAIEH ABAZA AND MARIE CRANDALL

DEFINITION

Traumatic brain injury (TBI) occurs when there is a blow or jolt to the head due to rapid acceleration or deceleration or a direct impact. It can also be caused by direct penetrating injury of the brain. Brain function is temporarily or permanently impaired and structural damage may or may not be detectable.[1] Not all blows, bumps, or injuries cause TBI, and the severity of the injury may vary widely.

INCIDENCE AND PREVALENCE

Overview

The overall incidence of TBI is difficult to calculate because of differences in outcome measures, definitions, and reporting.[2] Estimates may include only TBI patients admitted to the hospital and may exclude patients presenting to nontrauma or non–ED practitioners and/or ED visits that do not lead to admission, and typically do not include individuals who suffer injuries but do not seek medical attention. CDC data from 2014 suggest that 2.9 million people annually suffer TBIs. This can be thought of as a pyramid, with 56,800 deaths at the top, then 288,000 hospital admissions, and 2.5 million ED visits.[3]

Mortality

Injury is the leading cause of death for all individuals aged 1 to 45, accounting for more than 200,000 deaths every year in the United States, and more than 5 million deaths worldwide.[4,5] Head injury is responsible for the largest proportion of these deaths, contributing to one third of all injury-related deaths.[1,6] The Centers for Disease Control and Prevention estimates that more than 50,000 people die from TBI every year in the United States.[7]

Many patients with TBI will die shortly after their trauma, but mortality depends on a number of factors including age, severity and mechanism of brain injury, and presence of other injuries. The overall mortality of moderate to severe TBI is 21% at 30 days,[8] and increases to 50% for severe TBI.[9] From 2006 to 2014, the death rate from TBIs decreased by 6% despite a 54% increase in TBI-related emergency department (ED) visits over the same time period.[10]

The full reference list appears in the digital product found on http://connect.springerpub.com/content/book/978-0-8261-4768-4/part/part01/chapter/ch04

DISABILITY

Mild Traumatic Brain Injury

The presentation and outcomes of TBI vary widely, from a brief loss of consciousness to permanent disability and death. Most TBIs are mild and do not cause permanent or long-term disability; however, all severity levels of TBI have the potential to cause significant, long-lasting disability.[11] Within the first 2 years after discharge from a TBI-related rehabilitation facility stay, 40% of adolescents and adults with a TBI will experience a decrease in function. Five years after rehabilitation facility discharge, 20% will have died.[12] The risk of permanent disability is low with mild TBI (MTBI), with most patients having complete resolution of posttraumatic symptoms by 3 months post injury. However, up to 10% of patients, typically with a more severely impaired presentation and often with obvious intracranial pathology on imaging, may suffer persistent symptoms.[13] By contrast, permanent disability may be experienced by up to 65% of individuals with moderate TBI, and nearly 100% with severe TBI.[14]

Approximately 75% of all brain injuries are concussions or MTBI.[15] Patients with MTBI may still suffer symptoms after the incident, including headaches, dizziness, inability to concentrate, and nausea. Up to 30% of patients will report posttraumatic symptoms, and some patients will have persistent complaints,[16] especially when the injury follows multiple prior TBIs.[17] However, most of those with persistent symptoms do report improvement by 1-year post injury.[18]

Moderate to Severe Traumatic Brain Injury

Individuals with moderate to severe TBI may have significant impairments, and prognosis depends on the severity of injury.[19] However, in the first 2 years post-injury, up to 90% of patients with moderate to severe TBI will be able to return to living in a private home (although 30% will need assistance from another person), and of those who originally lived alone, 50% will return to living alone. Fifty percent of those with a moderate to severe TBI will return to driving, and 30% will return to work in the first 2 years, although it may be a different job than the one they had prior to injury.[20] Approximately 30% to 40% of people who have suffered severe TBI will make a good recovery, similar to that of moderate TBI.[21] The remaining patients may have profound and prolonged disability, existing in a permanent vegetative state or minimally conscious state, or have significant impairments, such as limited mobility or posttraumatic epilepsy.

Prediction of outcomes early after injury is based on logistic regression models including variables such as age, socioeconomic status, injury severity, biologic markers, and comorbidities, but these predictors are imperfect. Typically, younger patients, those with commercial insurance, Caucasians, and those with less severe TBI and fewer concomitant injuries will have better outcomes.[11,22,23] Race and socioeconomic status also impact the likelihood of receiving post-TBI rehabilitation, which affects both short- and long-term outcomes.[22,23]

Costs

From a financial perspective, the costs of TBI are significant. In 2010, direct and indirect medical costs of TBIs were approximately $76.5 billion, with 90% of this cost attributed to the care of those with TBIs that were fatal or required hospitalization.[24]

DEMOGRAPHICS

Causes

Falls are the leading cause of TBI among all age groups (47.9%), followed by being struck by/ against an object (17.1%), and motor vehicle collisions or traffic accidents (13.2%).[25] However, causes of TBI fatalities are slightly different. Among all mechanisms of injury, intentional self-harm was the leading cause of TBI-related deaths (32.5%) followed by falls (28.1%), and motor vehicle collisions (18.7%).[5] The lethality of gunshot wounds to the head is approximately 90%, which could explain why intentional self-harm made up such a large portion of TBI-related deaths despite its low overall incidence. Because of this, gunshot wounds are a much higher percentage of TBI fatalities than the overall incidence would suggest.[15]

Risk Factors

The major risk factors for TBI are age, gender, and socioeconomic status. Infants and toddlers up to 4 years of age, older adolescents and young adults aged 15 to 24, and adults older than 75 years of age are the highest risk age groups for TBI.[10] This trimodal distribution has been demonstrated for most ethnic and racial groups studied, as well as in global studies of TBI.[26-28] Rates of TBI-related deaths increase with age, with those over 75 having the highest rate (78.5 per 100,000 population). However, injury and debility in young adults also carries significant morbidity, with many more years of potential life lost (YPLL) and lost productivity for injuries incurred in young people. For every age group studied, males are more likely to suffer TBI than females.[29] Among young people, males are up to seven times more likely to suffer a TBI.[30] Men are also consistently at least twice as likely as women to die from TBI. People of color and those of lower socioeconomic strata also suffer rates of TBI 30% to 50% higher than majority individuals and are more likely to suffer complications and poorer outcomes.[22,30,31] Substance use is another risk factor for TBI; 30% to 50% of those who sustain a TBI were intoxicated at the time of their injury and 50% to 66% have a history of alcohol or drug use. Concomitant substance use disorder in the TBI population has also been associated with poorer outcomes.[32,33]

SUMMARY

TBI is the leading cause of death among the injured, killing more than 50,000 people per year in the United States. Outcomes vary widely depending on mechanism of injury, age, and concomitant injuries or morbidities. Young males, people of color, and the socioeconomically disadvantaged are particularly at risk.

KEY POINTS

- TBI affects over 2 million people per year in the United States and causes 50,000 deaths.
- TBI occurs on a spectrum ranging from mild to moderate to severe, each associated with different expectations for post-injury recovery and disability.
- The major risk factors for TBI are age, gender, and socioeconomic status. Individuals at the extremes of age, young men, and those of lower socioeconomic status are at highest risk.

STUDY QUESTIONS

1. Which of the following would be expected to have the best outcomes after a mild to moderate TBI?
   a. A 25-year-old male who was involved in a motor vehicle collision also resulting in multiple long bone fractures and a small bowel injury
   b. A 65-year-old homeless male who fell off a high fence
   c. A 30-year-old female with private insurance who was assaulted
   d. A 65-year-old female with a history of poorly controlled diabetes and stroke who fell off a ladder
   e. A 75-year-old male with no past medical history who fell off of a roof

2. An intervention focused on which of the following would lead to the biggest decrease in the rate of TBI-related fatalities?
   a. Ladder safety
   b. Proper use of car seats for children and infants
   c. Use of properly fitting bike helmets in elementary school children
   d. Suicide prevention in high-risk populations

3. A 75-year-old male falls off of his ladder while hanging Christmas lights on his house. He is found to have a severe TBI on presentation to the ED and is admitted to the ICU. Which of the following measures will decrease his risk of mortality most in the early post-injury phase?
   a. Infection control measures while in the ICU
   b. Early physical therapy during acute hospital admission
   c. Ensuring placement into a rehabilitation center after discharge
   d. Ensuring adequate supervision upon returning home

4. Which of the following interventions could best improve TBI outcomes in the elderly population?
   a. Fall prevention protocols for the elderly in skilled nursing facilities and assisted living facilities
   b. Decision-making tools aimed at early detection of TBI in those with suspected head trauma
   c. Infection control protocols for those with TBI in the ICU
   d. Increasing access to post discharge rehabilitation for patients with TBI

5. Which of the following statements regarding incidence and mortality of TBI is false?
   a. TBI is responsible for approximately one third of all injury-related deaths
   b. Despite public health interventions, TBI mortality continues to increase in recent years
   c. Early recognition and intervention in TBI cases has improved outcomes in especially vulnerable populations
   d. Among the most vulnerable populations are infants and toddlers, older adolescents and young adults, the elderly, and those with concomitant substance use disorders

ADDITIONAL READING

Centers for Disease Control and Prevention. www.cdc.gov/ncipc/factsheets/tbi.htm and www.cdc.gov/
traumaticbraininjury/data/rates.html

Bruns J, Hauser WA. The epidemiology of traumatic brain injury: a review. *Epilepsia*. 2003;44(s10):2–10.
doi:10.1046/j.1528-1157.44.s10.3.x

Greenwald BD, Burnett DM, Miller MA. Brain injury: epidemiology and pathophysiology. *Arch Phys Med
Rehabil*. 2003;84(3 suppl 1):S3–S7. doi:10.1053/ampr.2003.50052

ANSWERS TO STUDY QUESTIONS

1. Correct answer: c
Positive prognostic factors for TBI include young age, female gender, commercial insurance, higher socioeconomic status, Caucasian race, and absence of comorbidities or
concomitant injuries from the same event.

Further Reading:
Bowman SM, Martin DP, Sharar SR, Zimmerman FJ. Racial disparities in outcomes of
persons with moderate to severe traumatic brain injury. *Med. Care*. 2007;45(7):686–690.
doi:10.1097/MLR.0b013e31803dcdf3

2. Correct answer: d
While the incidence of TBI due to self-harm is relatively low, it is the leading cause of
TBI-related death. This is likely due to the high fatality of gunshot wounds to the head
(90%).
Further Reading:
Centers for Disease Control and Prevention. CDC-Traumatic Brain Injury and Concussions
- TBI-Related Deaths. 2019. https://www.cdc.gov/traumaticbraininjury/data/tbi-deaths.
html

3. Correct answer: a
While early mobility, adequate supervision after discharge, and rehabilitation can
improve outcomes in those with TBI, in the immediate post-injury phase infectious
complications confer the highest mortality risk in those with severe TBI.
Further Reading:
Centers for Disease Control and Prevention. National Center for Injury Prevention and
Control; Division of Unintentional Injury Prevention. *Report to Congress on Traumatic
Brain Injury in the United States: Epidemiology and Rehabilitation*. Centers for Disease
Control and Prevention; 2015.

4. Correct answer: a
As with most injuries, prevention is most effective when it comes to improving outcomes. In the elderly population, falls are the most common mechanism of injury
leading to TBI, and protocols aimed at preventing these injuries could decrease the
incidence of falls in this population
Further Reading:
Centers for Disease Control and Prevention. *Traumatic Brain Injury and Concussion—
Data and Statistics—TBI-related Emergency Department (ED) Visits*. 2019. https://www.
cdc.gov/traumaticbraininjury/data/tbi-ed-visits.html

5. Correct answer: b

Despite a 54% increase in incidence of TBI presenting to the ED, TBI mortality has decreased by 6% in recent years. This is thought to be related to better imaging, earlier recognition of TBIs, and better treatment for those with TBI of all levels of severity.

Further Reading:
Centers for Disease Control and Prevention. Traumatic Brain Injury and Concussion—Data and Statistics—TBI-related Emergency Department (ED) Visits. 2019. https://www.cdc.gov/traumaticbraininjury/data/tbi-ed-visits.html

REFERENCES

The full reference list appears in the digital product found on http://connect.springer-pub.com/content/book/978-0-8261-4768-4/part/part01/chapter/ch04

5 INJURY PREVENTION

ARLENE I. GREENSPAN, MATTHEW BREIDING, AND
CHRISTOPHER R. HARPER

OVERVIEW

Traumatic brain injury (TBI) is a major cause of death and disability. In 2017 the Centers for Disease Control and Prevention reported more than 61,000 TBI-related deaths, representing just over 2% of all U.S. deaths for that year.[1] Trends in TBI suggest an overall increase in incidence, with a 53% increase in the total number of emergency department (ED) visits, hospitalizations, and deaths from 2006 to 2014.[2] This translates to 2.87 million deaths, hospitalizations, and ED visits in 2014.[2] TBI may be unintentional, due to assault, or self-inflicted. The distribution of causes for TBI varies by demographic characteristics (e.g., age). Prevention strategies should target those at greatest risk. For example, among children aged 0 to 4 years, assault accounts for 45% of all TBI-related deaths, followed by motor vehicle crashes (26%); for youth and young adults, motor vehicle crashes are the main cause of TBI-related death and account for 54% of TBI deaths in 5- to 14-year-olds and 38% of TBI deaths for those aged 15 to 24 years; for adults 65 years and older, falls are the leading cause of TBI-related death.[2] This chapter focuses on evidence-based prevention strategies for TBI due to transportation crashes, falls, and assault, though epidemiology will also be touched upon as it relates to the rationale for selected preventive strategies.

TRANSPORTATION-RELATED TRAUMATIC BRAIN INJURY

Definition/Mechanism

The broad term *transportation injuries* typically includes injuries that involve single or multiple vehicle motor vehicle crashes and motorcycle crashes, as well as other modes of transportation including bicycles, and pedestrian injuries involving a motor vehicle or other mode of transportation. During a transportation crash, brain injury can occur through direct contact with a hard surface such as the steering wheel or the ground, or by rapid rotation of the brain inside the skull. The severity of TBI may vary from minor concussions to severe intracranial injury or death.

Epidemiology

Motor vehicle crashes are a leading cause of TBI-related death. This translates to more than 10,600 motor vehicle-related TBI deaths in 2017.[1] Motor vehicle-related deaths due to TBI disproportionately affect children and young adults, with more than half of all

---

The full reference list appears in the digital product found on http://connect.springerpub.com/content/book/978-0-8261-4768-4/part/part01/chapter/ch05

TBI-related deaths in children aged 5 to 14 years (54%) and 38% of TBI-related deaths in adolescents and young adults aged 15 to 24 years due to a motor vehicle crash.[2] Among adults, motor vehicle crashes account for 29% of TBI-related deaths in those aged 25 to 44 years, 19% of TBI-related deaths for those aged 45 to 64 years, and 7% of TBI-related deaths among adults 65 years and older.[2] The risk for sustaining a TBI for occupants in a motor vehicle crash increases for older adults, who are at greater risk for intracranial bleeding and increased morbidity and mortality compared to their younger counterparts.[3–6] Motor vehicle crashes also result in a substantial number of nonfatal TBIs each year.

Etiology

Risk factors that increase the probability of sustaining a TBI following a motor vehicle crash include the type of road user (e.g., motor vehicle occupant, motorcyclist, bicyclist, pedestrian), crash severity, type of crash (e.g., frontal, side, rollover crash), protective equipment used (e.g., seat belts, airbags, helmets), and individual factors (e.g., age).

Studies have demonstrated that vulnerable road users such as pedestrians, bicyclists, and motorcyclists have a higher probability of sustaining a TBI compared with vehicle occupants.[7,8] Vulnerable road users lack the protection of the vehicle and often collide with an object of greater mass that may be traveling at greater speed (e.g., pedestrian or cyclists colliding with a moving car). Pedestrians are at greatest risk for severe TBI, followed by moped riders and cyclists.[8]

Among motor vehicle occupants, two factors that influence the risk of sustaining a TBI following a motor vehicle crash are the type and severity of the crash. TBIs are most frequently seen following side impact and frontal crashes.[9,10] A study which compared TBI risk for frontal and side impact crashes with specific TBI diagnosis (e.g., concussion, parenchymal contusion, hematoma, diffuse axonal injury) found that, with the exception of contusion, side impact crashes are associated with greater risk for TBI, while risk for contusion is greater with frontal crashes.[10] Another study addressing the impact of motor vehicle crashes on severe TBI found that, while representing a smaller proportion of overall crashes, the risk for sustaining a severe TBI or skull fracture is greatest for persons involved in rollover crashes.[9] Rear impact crashes are associated with the lowest risk for severe TBI.[9]

Change in velocity (Delta V) is often used as a measure of crash severity. It is calculated as the change in vehicle velocity for the duration of the crash event. As Delta V increases, so does the risk for TBI. Although the risk for severe TBI increases with increasing Delta V, concussions can occur at speeds as low as 10 miles per hour (mph) with risk increasing to 10% at speeds of 34 mph.[9]

Older adults are at increased risk for morbidity and mortality compared to their younger counterparts from all causes of TBI, including motor vehicle injury.[5,6] Physiologic changes to the brain as individuals age result in increased risk for intracranial bleeding, especially subdural hematoma.[11] Older adults therefore have increased risk for developing intracranial bleeding if involved in an occupant-related[3–6] or pedestrian[12] motor vehicle crash. Older adults are at increased risk for intracranial bleeding for crashes even with relatively low Delta V.[4] Among pedestrian injuries, greater risk for subdural hematoma is seen with increasing age, although the overall number of pedestrian injuries was greater for children and young adults, aged 12 to 25.[12]

Little research exists regarding the influence of gender on TBI risk following a motor vehicle crash. One study that examined the influence of gender on motor vehicle-related TBI risk found females were one and one-half times more likely to sustain a concussion following a frontal collision; however, no differences were found with respect to side impact collisions.[10] Structural differences in the corpus callosum between male and female brains[13] as well as reduction in cortical thickness of female, but not male, brains with aging[14] suggest that females may be more vulnerable to brain injury than males. In addition, research on sport-related concussion suggests that females may be at greater risk for concussion than their male counterparts.[15] More research is needed to confirm whether and under what circumstances gender may play a role in risk for TBI following motor vehicle crashes.

Prevention Strategies

Seat belt use is the most effective means for reducing deaths and injuries from a motor vehicle crash.[16] The National Highway Traffic Safety Administration (NHTSA) reports that use of seat belts reduces risk of death by 45% for front seat occupants of passenger vehicles and by 60% for occupants of light trucks and reduces risk of moderate to critical injury by 50% for front seat occupants of passenger vehicles and by 65% for light truck occupants.[16] In 2016, NHTSA estimates that almost 15,000 lives were saved by wearing seat belts and that an additional 2,500 more lives could have been saved if everyone wore seat belts.[17] Although many studies have found that seat belt use reduces the risk of TBI due to a motor vehicle crash,[7,9,10,18] a recent meta-analysis did not find a statistically significant difference in risk of head injuries between belted and unbelted occupants.[19] Examination of the 11 studies included in this analysis found significant heterogeneity among the studies, suggesting that risk for head injury in restrained occupants may also vary by other crash characteristics. For example, one study found that seat belts were least effective in preventing concussions in rollover crashes and most effective in preventing diffuse axonal injuries in frontal crashes.[9] Despite the equivocal findings from this one meta-analysis, the multiple studies that have found seat belt users less likely than nonusers to sustain TBI support the use of seat belts to prevent and reduce morbidity and mortality due to TBI.[7,9,10,18]

Seat belt laws have increased seat belt use, and primary laws are more effective than secondary laws.[20] Primary laws allow police officers to issue citations for occupants who are not wearing a seat belt. Secondary laws only allow police officers to issue a citation for not wearing a seat belt if the driver is pulled over for another infraction. States with primary laws have seat belt use rates that on average are 9% higher than states with secondary laws.[20] Currently 34 states and the District of Columbia have primary seat belt laws. New Hampshire is currently the only state without either a primary or a secondary seat belt law (www.iihs.org/topics/seat-belts/seat-belt-law-table).

Among infants and children, age- and size-appropriate car seats reduce the risk of death or injury, including TBI. One study that examined the factors associated with TBI among children involved in motor vehicle crashes found that unrestrained children were three times more likely to sustain a TBI than children who were in age-appropriate car seats.[21] Another study[22] found that 4- to 8-year-old children restrained in adult seat belts were twice as likely to sustain a TBI as children restrained in appropriate child car seats. Use of car seats reduces risk of death by 71% for infants less than 1 year of age and by 54% among toddlers aged 1 to 4 years.[23] In addition, compared to adult seat belts, use of booster seats among children aged 4 to 8 years reduces the risk of serious injury by 45%.[15] In 2018, the American Academy of Pediatrics (AAP) updated their recommendations regarding the use of infant and child car seats.[24] The AAP recommends that infants and young children remain in rear-facing infant/car seats until 2 years of age or until they reach the height and weight limit of their car seat. From age 2 or until they reach the height and weight limit on their rear-facing seat, children should be restrained in forward-facing car seats with harness straps for as long as possible. Young children should remain in forward-facing car seats until they reach the height and weight limit of the seat. Once children outgrow their child safety seats, they should next transition to a belt-positioning booster seat until they can appropriately fit into an adult seat belt. Children can usually fit into an adult seat belt when they are approximately 57 inches tall.[24] For most children, this is between the ages of 8 and 12 years. Results from a Community Guide systematic review on interventions to increase child safety seat use found strong evidence for the effectiveness of child safety seat laws.[25] Although the Community Guide found insufficient evidence that education programs alone increased child safety seat use, education programs paired with car seat distribution or incentives to buy car seats resulted in increased car seat use.[25]

Airbags, when used in combination with seat belts, provide added protection compared to seat belts alone.[26] Head-protecting side airbags reduce the risk of TBI by 30% to 37%.[27,28] Note that, while frontal airbags protect adults from injury when deployed in a crash, a deployed frontal airbag can kill infants and children if seated in front of an airbag; they are especially harmful for infants/children in rear-facing infant/car seats. Children 12 years old and younger should always be restrained in the back seat.[24]

Per vehicle mile traveled, motorcycle riders are 27 times more likely to die in a traffic crash than occupants of passenger vehicles.[29] Motorcycle helmets help protect the brain during a crash. Wearing a motorcycle helmet reduces the risk of death by 37% and reduces the risk of nonfatal TBI by 69%.[29] However, wearing a motorcycle helmet may not provide equal protection for all types of brain injury. Results from a systematic review found that wearing a motorcycle helmet reduced the risk of death from TBI by 42% and reduced the risk of nonfatal TBI by 69%.[30] However, another recent study found that while wearing a motorcycle helmet reduced skull fractures by 69%, cerebral contusion by 71%, and intracranial hemorrhage by 53%, motorcycle helmet use did not demonstrate a significant protective effect for concussions,[31] suggesting that further research is needed to improve protection from the rotational forces that lead to concussion. Laws that require use of motorcycle helmets are an effective means for increasing helmet use.[29] Currently 19 states have motorcycle helmet laws that require all riders to be helmeted. An additional 28 states have laws that require some riders to be helmeted, and three states (Illinois, New Hampshire, and Iowa) do not have any laws governing helmet use.[29] Riders are more likely to wear helmets in states that have universal helmet laws (87% versus 44%).[29] Injuries to the face and head, including TBI, are more common in states with partial rather than universal helmet laws.[32]

Multiple studies over the past 30 years have demonstrated the effectiveness of bicycle helmets in reducing the risk of TBI, despite some controversy regarding the magnitude of the effect.[33-36] The effectiveness of bicycle helmets has been demonstrated among all age groups, in crashes with and without motor vehicle involvement, and in various regions.[33-36] A more recent meta-analysis of 55 studies supported these previous findings and concluded that wearing a bicycle helmet reduced the odds of sustaining a TBI by 53%.[37] While helmets may be an effective method for preventing TBI in the event of a crash, other prevention strategies, such as creating bicycle paths that separate cyclists from motorists, can further reduce risk for injury.[38]

FALL-RELATED TRAUMATIC BRAIN INJURY

Definition/Mechanism

Falls are often distinguished by whether they occur from a height or at ground level. Some common scenarios in which falls from heights occur are falls from playground equipment, windows, ladders, or animals (e.g., horses), as well as falls down stairs. Ground-level falls most commonly occur as a result of stumbling, tripping, or slipping while engaged in a variety of activities ranging from standing still to normal household activities to participation in sports or recreational activities.

Epidemiology

In 2014, falls were the leading cause of TBI-related ED visits (when the cause was documented) among all age groups combined (47.9% of all TBIs), but particularly among those 75 years of age and older (85.8%), 65 to 74 years of age (72.4%), and 0 to 4 years of age (71.7%).[2] In 2014, falls accounted for 52.3% of TBI-related hospitalizations for all ages combined; among those 75 years of age and older, falls accounted for 79.3% of TBI-related hospitalizations, and for those 65 to 74 years of age and older, 65.7%.[1] Finally, in 2014 falls were the second leading cause of TBI-related deaths overall and the leading cause of TBI-related death among those 65 to 74 years of age and those 75 years of age and older.[2] There has been a marked increase over time in the number and rate of TBI-related ED visits, hospitalizations, and deaths due to falls among older adults.[39] There is concern that this will increase further in the coming years due in part to the aging of the U.S. population.

Etiology

Falls Among Older Adults

An Australian study of TBIs among those over the age of 65 found that the majority of fall-related TBIs (64.2%) were due to slipping, tripping, stumbling, or colliding with another person; 16.6% were due to falls down stairs; 10.2% were due to falls involving furniture; and 4.1% were due to falling off a ladder or scaffold.[40] A literature review identified a number of risk factors for falls among older adults including advanced age, having a gait or balance disorder, poor lower extremity strength, dizziness, impaired cognition, cardiovascular disease, dementia, and depression.[41] Finally, particular medications, home conditions (e.g., poor lighting, loose rugs), and certain types of footwear have all been shown to influence the risk of falls among older adults.

Falls Among Children and Adolescents

In a study of children aged 0– to 5 years who were hospitalized due to a fall from either furniture or stairs, those who fell from stairs were significantly more likely to sustain an injury to their head (64.3%), compared to falls from furniture (38.1%).[42] An Australian study examining TBI in children 0 to 3 years old found that the leading causes of fall-related TBI were falls from furniture, falls while standing, and falls after being dropped by an adult, with the latter cause particularly prominent among those 0 to 6 months old.[43] A recent study of TBI-related ED visits among children 0 to 4 years of age found that the leading causes were falls from a surface (24.9%), furniture (20.5%), and structures/fixtures (17.7%) and falls during sports or recreational activities (12.8%).[44] Another study examined fall-related hospitalizations among adolescents aged 10 to 19 and found that among TBI-related hospitalizations caused by falls, 28% could be classified as sports related.[45] A number of studies have examined the role of direct adult supervision and found a positive relationship between more adult supervision and reduced injury among children.[46]

Falls Among Other Age Groups

Among adults 60 and younger, 64% of falls were a result of a fall from a height, with 27% due to a fall down stairs and 15% due to a fall from a ladder; alcohol was a potential contributing factor in 30% of fall-related TBIs in this age group.[47]

Prevention Strategies

There has been a significant amount of research examining the prevention of falls in the elderly and quite a few efficacious preventive interventions have been identified.

Multicomponent physical exercise programs, particularly those that include balance retraining and muscle strengthening, have been shown to significantly reduce the risk of falls among the elderly living in the community.[48] Tai chi, which includes both strength and balance training, has been identified as a specific exercise program with beneficial effects.[48] Vitamin D supplementation has been shown to have positive benefits, but only for those with low levels of vitamin D.[48] Surgical interventions, such as pacemakers and cataract surgery, have been found to reduce the rate of falls among those that are in need of these interventions.[48] Interventions in which home hazards are reduced have been shown to be effective in reducing fall risk.[48] Finally, prevention programs focused on multiple efficacious interventions, often tailored to an individual's unique risk factor profile, have been examined and found to be helpful in reducing the rate of falls.[48]

A number of strategies have been identified for preventing childhood injuries, including injuries from falls, although they may not necessarily have been tested in relation to falls specifically. Some of these strategies include use of safety gates at the top and bottom of stairways; not allowing children under 6 years of age to sleep in the top bunk of a bunk bed; use of a seat belt in the seat of a shopping cart; use of an appropriate helmet for activities such as bicycle riding, skateboarding, and horseback riding; and age and activity-appropriate supervision by adult caregivers.[49] Finally, a number of countries have developed playground safety standards in order to reduce the risk of playground injury. Research suggests that lowering the height of play structures and using softer surfaces at ground level can reduce the risk of playground injuries.[50]

ASSAULT-RELATED TRAUMATIC BRAIN INJURY

Definition/Mechanism

Assault-related TBIs are injuries intentionally inflicted by another person. Assault-related TBI can result from firearms, sharp objects, blunt objects, pushing, or punching. A special type of assault-related TBI is pediatric abusive head trauma, which is caused by violent shaking, impact to the head, or both.[51]

Epidemiology

As of 2014, assault-related brain injury remains the leading cause of death in children with TBI aged 0 to 4.[2] In 2014, 322 brain injury deaths were attributed to homicide for children aged 0 to 4, compared to 187 for motor vehicle crashes and 136 for other unintentional, unspecified injury.

Among children younger than 2 years of age, the population rate of fatal TBI that does not meet the definition for pediatric abusive head trauma is 3.6 times higher than the rate of fatal pediatric abusive head trauma.[51] The fatal abusive head trauma rates in 2013 and 2014 were 0.41 per 100,000 children aged less than 5 years and 0.43 per 100,000, respectively.[52] Fatal assault-related TBI among young children is higher among males compared to females; Black and Hispanic/Latino children compared to White children; and the Southeast compared to other regions.[53]

Assault-related TBI is the fourth leading cause of TBI-related hospitalizations.[2] The incidence of hospitalizations attributed to assault-related TBI among children up to 3 years of age is 58 per 100,000 with the highest incidence among infants.[54] The annual incidence of hospitalizations attributed to pediatric abusive head trauma is lowest in the Northeast and highest in the Midwest.[55] The most recent estimates suggest that abusive head trauma results in nearly $70 million in medical cost annually.[56]

Etiology

There are multiple individual, family, neighborhood, and societal-level risk factors for perpetrating assault or violence. It is the cumulative and interactive impact of risk factors that lead to perpetration of violence. Perpetrators of violence, regardless of the relationship (e.g., caregiver, partner, friend, or acquaintance) or lack of relationship (i.e., stranger) to their victim, have several risk factors in common. At the individual level, perpetrators often show certain neurocognitive deficits, such as hostile attributional biases and poor impulse control.[57-59] A large and growing body of research links these deficits to exposure to chronic stressors prenatally or in early childhood affecting the volume, connectivity, and chemistry of the brain, especially in the prefrontal cortex, the hippocampus, and the amygdala.[60] Family-level stressors that may contribute to violence perpetration include experiencing child maltreatment or witnessing partner violence as a child.[60] Chronic stressors may also result from living conditions that affect children directly (e.g., poverty)[61] or through their effects on parenting behaviors[62] or parental relationships.[63] At the community level, stressors shared by different types of perpetrators include living in concentrated disadvantage[64-66] and exposure to community violence,[64-65,67] while income inequality[68-70] and country-level poverty[69-71] are societal-level stressors commonly shared.

Prevention Strategies

The widely implemented strategy of educating new parents about infant crying and the dangers of shaking has shown positive impact on pediatric abusive head trauma in some settings,[72,73] but not in others.[74-76] However, there are several evidence-based approaches to preventing overall child maltreatment (i.e., primary prevention) such as screening parents of young children for risk factors of child maltreatment[77] or for needed services,[78] home visitation,[79] child–parent centers,[80] and strengthening household economics.[81] Home visitation and strengthening household economics have also shown promise in preventing youth violence perpetration[82-85] and preventing involvement in partner violence.[86] Child–parent centers can also have preventive effects on youth violence.[83]

Focusing on preventing violence and early adversity in childhood is key to disrupting the intergenerational transmission of violence and setting children on a positive trajectory.[87] However, even when children have been exposed to early adversity, preschool and school-based interventions can help children develop socio-emotional and problem-solving skills to avoid interpersonal violence.[88] Moreover, there is growing recognition that many of the strategies that can help prevent early adversity can also prevent other types of interpersonal violence, including intimate partner violence, youth violence, and sexual violence.[89-91] Policies and programs that promote economic stability for families can help prevent adverse child experiences as well as intimate partner violence.[87,89] Creating social norms that can protect against violence and promote positive environments should impact multiple forms of violence. Given the shared risk and protective factors that underscore early adversity and other forms of interpersonal violence, interventions that address early adversity are likely to prevent violence and create safer communities for all children, families, and adults.[92]

KEY POINTS

- Seat belts and age and size-appropriate car seats for infants and young children are the most effective means for reducing deaths and injuries from a motor vehicle crash.
- Motorcycle and bicycle helmets significantly reduce risk for TBI.
- Fall prevention programs should be tailored to older adults' unique risk factor profile and may include but are not limited to exercise and home hazard reduction.
- Evidence-based strategies to reduce child maltreatment include programs that screen parents and young children for risk factors or need for services, home visitation programs, child–parent centers, and strengthening household economics.

STUDY QUESTIONS

1. All of the following are good strategies to prevent TBI due to a transportation crash, *except*
   a. Seat belt use
   b. Riding in a car with an airbag, in lieu of using a seat belt
   c. Using a motorcycle helmet when riding as a passenger on a motorcycle
   d. Placing children in an age- and size-appropriate child safety seat

2. Infants and young children less than 2 years of age should always
   a. Ride in the back seat with a forward-facing child safety seat
   b. Ride in the front seat with a forward-facing child safety seat
   c. Ride in the back seat with a rear-facing child safety seat
   d. Ride in the front seat with a rear-facing child safety seat

3. All of the following are known risk factors for falls among older adults, *except*
   a. Poor lower extremity strength
   b. Dementia
   c. Male gender
   d. Gait or balance disorder

4. All of the following interventions have been shown to reduce the likelihood of older adult falls, *except*
   a. Multicomponent physical exercise programs
   b. Evaluating and reducing home hazards
   c. Surgical interventions (e.g., pacemakers, cataracts)
   d. Vitamin A supplements

5. _____ are the leading cause of death due to TBI for children up to 4 years of age.
   a. Car crashes
   b. Falls
   c. Assaults
   d. Unknown causes

ADDITIONAL RESOURCES

Injury Prevention and Control: Motor Vehicle Safety. http://www.cdc.gov/motorvehiclesafety/
Older Adult Falls: Get the Facts: http://www.cdc.gov/HomeandRecreationalSafety/Falls/adultfalls.html
Evidence-based interventions that prevent child maltreatment: http://www.cebc4cw.org/
Doll L, Bonzo S, Sleet D, et al. (Eds.). *Handbook of Injury and Violence Prevention.* Springer; 2007.
Centers for Disease Control and Prevention (CDC). CDC grand rounds: reducing severe traumatic brain injury in the United States. *MMWR Morb Mortal Wkly Rep.* 2013;62(27):549–552.

ANSWERS TO STUDY QUESTIONS

1. Correct Answer: b
Use of an airbag without a seat belt is not protective since a seat belt will hold you in place and an airbag will soften your contact. While a seat belt alone reduces injury, an airbag alone does not confer sufficient protection to be an effective strategy.

Further Reading
Pintar FA, Yoganandan N, Gennarelli TA. Airbag effectiveness on brain trauma in frontal crashes. *Annu Proc Assoc Adv Automot Med.* 2000;44:149–169. (seat belt and airbag facts)
National Highway Traffic Safety Administration. *Traffic Safety Facts, 2017 Data: Motorcycles.* US Department of Transportation, National Highway Traffic Safety Administration; 2019. https://crashstats.nhtsa.dot.gov/Api/Public/ViewPublication/812785 (motorcycle helmets)
Durbin DR, Hoffman BD. Child passenger safety. *Pediatrics.* 2018;142(5):e20182461. doi:10.1542/peds.2018-2460

2. Correct Answer: c
Children should ride in the back seat until they are 12, and infants who have lack of head control are safest riding in a rear-facing child seat. In addition, it is dangerous for a young child to ride rear facing in a front seat.

Further Reading:
Durbin DR, Hoffman BD. Child passenger safety. *Pediatrics.* 2018;142(5):e20182461. doi:10.1542/peds.2018-2460

3. Correct Answer: c
Gender alone is not a risk factor for falls in older adults.

Further Reading:
Ambrose AF, Paul G, Hausdorff JM. Risk factors for falls among older adults: a review of the literature. *Maturitas.* 2013;75(1):51–61. doi:10.1016/j.maturitas.2013.02.009

4. Correct Answer: d
Lack of vitamin A is not a risk factor. Vitamin D is a risk factor if an older adult has vitamin D deficiency.

Further Reading:
Gillespie LD, Robertson MC, Gillespie WJ, et al. Interventions for preventing falls in older people living in the community. *Cochrane Database Syst Rev.* 2012;9:CD007146. doi:10.1002/14651858.CD007146.pub3

5. Correct Answer: c

As of 2014, the Centers for Disease Control and Prevention estimates that assault is the leading cause of death due to TBI for children up to 4 years of age, based on data from the National Vital Statistics System's 2014 multiple-cause-of-death files.

Further Reading:

Centers for Disease Control and Prevention. *Surveillance Report of Traumatic Brain Injury-related Emergency Department Visits, Hospitalizations, and Deaths—United States, 2014*. Centers for Disease Control and Prevention, U.S. Department of Health and Human Services; 2019.

REFERENCES

The full reference list appears in the digital product found on http://connect.springer-pub.com/content/book/978-0-8261-4768-4/part/part01/chapter/ch05

II   MILD TRAUMATIC BRAIN INJURY

6   CONCUSSION AND MILD TRAUMATIC BRAIN INJURY: DEFINITIONS, DISTINCTIONS, AND DIAGNOSTIC CRITERIA

NOAH D. SILVERBERG, RAEL T. LANGE, AND
GRANT L. IVERSON

INTRODUCTION

A mild traumatic brain injury (MTBI) results from a transfer of mechanical energy to the brain from an external force, causing a disturbance in brain physiology. Mechanisms of injury include the (a) head being struck with an object, (b) head striking a hard object or surface, (c) brain undergoing an acceleration/deceleration movement without direct contact between the head and an object or surface, and/or (d) forces generated from a blast or explosion. These forces result in a neurometabolic cascade of cellular and vascular changes.[1-4] (See also Chapter 2.) MTBI may or may not result in macrostructural brain damage visible on computed tomography (CT) or magnetic resonance imaging (MRI).

TERMINOLOGY

A concussion, by definition, is an MTBI. By convention, the term "MTBI" is typically used in civilian trauma and military settings, whereas "concussion" is usually the preferred term in sport. Much of the sports medicine literature uses the phrase "sport-related concussion." Concussions in sport typically fall on the milder end of the MTBI spectrum.

    MTBI can also be subclassified as uncomplicated and complicated based on neuroradiologic findings.[5,6] As originally conceptualized, a *complicated* MTBI is diagnosed if the person meets operational criteria for MTBI (see the following sections) and has some trauma-related macroscopic intracranial abnormality on acute CT.[5] MRI can detect abnormalities missed by CT.[7-13] More sophisticated experimental quantitative neuroimaging methods may identify neurometabolic, functional, and microstructural changes associated with MTBI,[11,14-20] but these changes have not been considered part of the definition of complicated MTBI. MTBI is traditionally distinguished from moderate to severe TBI on the basis of the acute clinical presentation, in particular, the duration of loss of consciousness, the level of consciousness (as measured by the Glasgow Coma Scale), and the duration of posttraumatic amnesia (see definitions in the following section).

The full reference list appears in the digital product found on http://connect.springerpub.com/content/book/978-0-8261-4768-4/part/part02/chapter/ch06

Author Note: The views expressed in this chapter are those of the authors and do not reflect the official policy of the Department of Defense or U.S. Government.

DEFINITIONS

There is no universally agreed-upon definition of MTBI. Commonly cited definitions have been proposed by the (a) Mild Traumatic Brain Injury Committee of the Head Injury Interdisciplinary Special Interest Group of the American Congress of Rehabilitation Medicine (ACRM) MTBI Committee,[21] (b) Centers for Disease Control and Prevention (CDC) working group,[22] (c) World Health Organization (WHO) Collaborating Centre Task Force on Mild Traumatic Brain Injury,[23] (d) Department of Veterans Affairs and The Department of Defense (VA/DoD),[24,25] (e) Demographics and Clinical Assessment Working Group of the International and Interagency Initiative toward Common Data Elements (CDE) for Research on Traumatic Brain Injury and Psychological Health,[26] and (f) Concussion in Sport Group (CISG).[27]

The ACRM, CDC, WHO, VA/DoD, CDE, and CISG definitions of MTBI have areas of agreement and discrepancy. All specify that MTBI is caused by a transfer of mechanical energy from an external force. All definitions require clinical evidence of brain injury but differ in how the lower threshold of this criterion is operationalized. Any one of the following constitutes sufficient evidence of MTBI, or a suspected diagnosis of sport-related concussion,[27] according to all six definitions: loss of consciousness (LOC) of any duration, posttraumatic amnesia (PTA), or a focal neurological sign (e.g., impact seizure). Five definitions also consider an immediate alteration in mental status to be sufficient, but they characterize this construct differently, and the CISG definition is unclear regarding immediate mental status changes. WHO's definition requires that altered mental status is evidenced by transient confusion or disorientation. Other definitions have a less stringent threshold, allowing for altered mental status to be demonstrated by signs and symptoms such as feeling "dazed" or having slowed thinking. In the CISG definition, even a single physical (e.g., headache), cognitive (e.g., feeling as if in a fog), or emotional (e.g., lability) symptom qualifies. Retrograde amnesia is sufficient clinical evidence of brain injury for all definitions except WHO. Note that a frank loss of consciousness is not required by any definition.

Some definitions (e.g., WHO, CDE, and CISG) require that potential confounds of altered mental status, such as psychological trauma and alcohol intoxication, be considered. For example, if a patient cannot recall aspects of the event but has no other evidence of brain injury, and responded to the event with intense fear and experienced acute traumatic stress symptoms (e.g., detachment, derealization, and/or depersonalization), psychological trauma, rather than MTBI, may explain the gap in the patient's memory.

The CDE definition is for TBI of all severities and, therefore, does not have a ceiling threshold. The ACRM and WHO definitions concur that injuries involving a reduced level of consciousness (i.e., Glasgow Coma Scale score of less than 13) or LOC greater than 30 minutes, or a period of PTA lasting more than 24 hours, should not be classified as "mild." The CDC definition is similar, but it recognizes that case ascertainment typically occurs by interview or survey where Glasgow Coma Scale scores are not available.

The clinical features that differentiate mild from moderate to severe TBI are summarized in Table 6.1. In addition to these clinical features, the VA/DoD uses neuroimaging to stratify TBI severity. Specifically, the guidelines specify that "abnormal structural imaging (e.g., magnetic resonance imaging or computed tomography scanning) attributed to the injury will result in the individual being considered clinically to have greater than mild injury"[24] (pg. 19). The CISG definition excludes cases with trauma-related intracranial abnormalities on structural imaging, whereas the ACRM and WHO do not. Regardless of the definition, the MTBI classification range includes an extraordinarily broad spectrum of

TABLE 6.1 Clinical Features that Differentiate Mild From Moderate to Severe Traumatic Brain Injury

	Loss of Consciousness	Posttraumatic Amnesia	Glasgow Coma Scale
ACRM[21]	30 min or less	24 hours or less	13–15 by 30 min after the injury
CDC[22]	N/A	N/A	N/A
WHO[23]	30 min or less	24 hours or less	13–15 by 30 min after the injury
VA/DoD[24,25]	30 min or less	24 hours or less**	Best available score between 13 and 15 within 24 hours of the injury
CDE[26]	N/A	N/A	N/A
CISG[27]	N/A	N/A	N/A

injury severity. Injuries characterized by seconds of confusion to injuries involving several minutes of traumatic coma and several hours of PTA all qualify as MTBI.

Integrating the ACRM, CDC, WHO, VA/DoD, CDE, and CISG definitions, a diagnosis of MTBI is likely when a person has (a) accompanied by LOC immediately following a head trauma event, and/or (b) amnesia for a period that includes or abuts the moment of head impact, and/or (c) an alteration in mental status immediately following a head trauma event; where (a), (b), and (c) cannot be fully explained by factors other than brain injury (e.g., psychological trauma, drug or alcohol intoxication, sedation for pain or intubation, or massive blood loss).

When a patient remembers the moment of head impact and surrounding events, altered mental status is most compellingly demonstrated by confusion (e.g., inability to follow commands or answer orientation questions). Clinical judgment is necessary to differentiate confusion induced by brain injury from being startled by an unexpected event. If the alteration in mental status is equivocal and not accompanied by LOC or amnesia, contextual factors such as head impact velocity and acute signs (e.g., vomiting) will factor into the determination.

Clinical and laboratory findings may play an important role in identifying MTBI. There is considerable evidence that cognitive impairment, balance impairment, and/or oculomotor impairment on acute clinical examination differentiate patients with versus patients without MTBI, although classification accuracy varies across studies, likely based on the specific test/procedure used, the timing of administration (sensitivity tends to diminish over the hours to days following injury), and the nature of the comparison group (accuracy rates are highest when patients with MTBI are compared to healthy control subjects). An early focus of research with blood biomarkers was on their utility for predicting the presence of clinically important intracranial abnormalities visible on CT.[28] More recently, blood biomarkers such as glial fibrillary acidic protein (GFAP)[28,29] have been shown to be sensitive to TBI even in cases with normal CT. Such biomarkers may, therefore, contribute to MTBI diagnosis.

APPLICATION TO CLINICAL PRACTICE

Patients with suspected MTBI may present for medical attention shortly after (e.g., in the emergency department) or long after (e.g., in a clinic) any observable clinical signs have

TABLE 6.2 Diagnosing a Mild Traumatic Brain Injury in Clinical Practice and Research

Mechanism of Injury: A biomechanically plausible mechanism of injury is required (e.g., head being struck with an object, head striking a hard object or surface, brain undergoing an acceleration/deceleration movement in a motor vehicle crash, and/or forces generated from a blast or explosion).

Clinical Signs: An acute physiological disruption in brain functioning illustrated by *one or more clinical signs*. Intoxication, polytrauma, severe psychological trauma, and/or general anesthesia can confound or preclude the reliable assessment and documentation of these clinical signs. In the very mildest form of injury, it can be difficult to reliably detect and document these clinical signs.

1. Loss of Consciousness: LOC of any duration up to a maximum of 30 minutes. Traumatic LOC greater than 30 minutes indicates a moderate or greater TBI. If a patient is conscious when first medically evaluated, it is usually only possible to establish LOC with witness or bystander observations.
2. Amnesia: Complete or partial amnesia for events immediately following the injury (or after regaining consciousness), for any duration up to a maximum of 24 hours. It is usually not feasible to reliably document amnesia of only a few seconds duration. PTA greater than 24 hours indicates a moderate or greater TBI.
3. Mental Status and Behavioral Changes: Immediate changes in mental status or behavior illustrated by reduced responsiveness or inappropriate responses to the environment or external stimuli immediately following the injury (e.g., slowness to respond to questions or instructions; indifferent, uncooperative, agitated, or aggressive behavior; inability to follow two-step commands; or disorientation to place or situation).
4. Neurological Signs: Neurological signs include a brief seizure immediately following injury, motor incoordination upon standing or ataxia (e.g., viewed during a sporting event), cranial nerve palsy, and paresis.

Symptoms: Acute symptoms, emerging within seconds to hours following injury, include a combination of (a) subjective alteration in mental status (e.g., feeling confused, feeling disoriented, feeling dazed), (b) physical symptoms (e.g., headache, nausea, dizziness, balance problems, vision problems, sensitivity to light, sensitivity to noise), (c) cognitive symptoms (e.g., feeling slowed down, "mental fog," difficulty concentrating, memory problems), and/or (d) acute emotional reactivity or lability. These acute symptoms increase confidence in the diagnosis of mild TBI, but they can also be caused or worsened by other factors (e.g., orthopedic injury or psychological distress). A plausible injury event and the presence of acute symptoms in the absence of clear evidence of the above clinical signs can raise suspicion for an MTBI diagnosis, but the clinician should have considerably less confidence in the accuracy of the diagnosis if none of the clinical signs were likely present.

resolved. Establishing the diagnosis then rests on a clinical interview, and when possible, an interview of people who observed the head trauma event and a review of medical records from the first medical contacts (e.g., ambulance crew report). Some considerations for clinicians are provided in the following list and in Table 6.2.

■ A careful and deliberate approach should be used that retrospectively assesses for altered consciousness or gaps in memory (retrograde and posttraumatic). One cannot assume that a very careful and thorough approach was taken by healthcare providers at the scene or in the emergency department. A diagnosis of MTBI can be missed initially, especially in the presence of traumatic bodily injuries that require urgent care. Alternatively, MTBI may be misdiagnosed based on inaccurate history and an inadequate differential diagnosis.

- Clinicians should be careful not to misinterpret PTA for LOC (e.g., a patient who is experiencing PTA and who was walking and talking following injury often incorrectly states that "I woke up in the emergency room"). Patients cannot give a first-person account of the presence and duration of LOC because, by definition, they will be amnestic for that period. It is best to clarify when a patient is (a) making an inference rather than providing an experiential account, and (b) relaying information that they were told.
- A substantial percentage of patients evaluated in the emergency department (ED) are intoxicated with alcohol when they sustain an MTBI. The best available evidence suggests that alcohol intoxication has a modest impact on Glasgow Coma Scale scores[30,31]; severe intoxication must be considered as a potential explanation for confusion and amnesia. Traumatic bodily injuries disrupting hemodynamic or respiratory function can also complicate the identification of mental status changes associated with TBI. Finally, acute medical interventions (e.g., intubation or administration of sedating medications) can make it difficult to estimate the duration of TBI-related mental status changes.
- Reduced awareness of one's surroundings at the scene of the event and an inability to later remember parts of the traumatic event are diagnostic criteria for acute stress disorder.[32] In other words, these symptoms are characteristic of psychological "shock" and not necessarily caused by TBI. Amnesia for the impact and the following moments, minutes, or hours is much more likely attributable to brain injury when it is (a) preceded by a temporally graded retrograde amnesia, (b) associated with confusion and disorientation, (c) initially dense but then resolves gradually (i.e., becomes less and less patchy), and (d) not preceded by intense fear and related symptoms (e.g., rapid heart rate, muscle tension, depersonalization).
- Confusion due to chaotic or traumatic events might not reflect the effects of neurotrauma. In combat situations involving explosions and firefights, a military service member might feel confused for a brief period due to the chaotic and overwhelming situation and not because of injury to the brain. Similarly, confusion is commonly experienced by civilians during or immediately after a traumatic event.
- Neuroimaging is adjunctive. An urgent CT scan may be indicated to rule out the need for neurosurgical intervention. When trying to identify MTBI in the presence of confounds (e.g., polytrauma, alcohol intoxication), imaging or other neurodiagnostic techniques may be helpful,[26] but only for identifying macrostructural intracranial abnormalities.[33]
- Subjectively experienced symptoms within the first 24 hours following a biomechanically plausible mechanism of injury usually represent the effects of a TBI when competing explanations for these symptoms are ruled out. For example, a new headache following an injury event might be attributable to cervical strain. Dizziness may be seen as a result of peripheral vestibular dysfunction, which can occur independent of an MTBI. Standardized symptom scales can help track recovery from MTBI, but *do not* establish the diagnosis of MTBI. Symptoms such as headache, dizziness, fatigue, difficulty concentrating, irritability, and light and noise intolerance are common following MTBI, but they are not highly specific to MTBI, acutely, subacutely, postacutely, or chronically. Orthopedically injured patients report some of these symptoms in the first week following injury. Such symptoms are sometimes endorsed by healthy people and often by people with depression, pain, and other health conditions. These factors are important to consider when a person reports symptoms weeks, months, or years following an injury.
- Neuropsychological testing can be used to examine the consequences of an MTBI, but cannot be used alone or as the primary basis for the initial diagnosis. Neuropsychological test results can be influenced by numerous demographic, situational, pre-existing, co-occurring, and injury-related factors.

■ An MTBI is diagnosed when, following a biomechanically plausible mechanism of injury, the person experiences *one or more* of the following signs that can be confidently attributed to the injury to the brain versus other confounding factors: LOC less than 30 minutes, amnesia less than 24 hours, mental status and behavioral changes, and/or neurological signs. If one or more of those signs are *not* clearly documented following a biomechanically plausible mechanism of injury (not mildly bumping one's head), a diagnosis of MTBI should be considered if a person experiences multiple acute symptoms and has at least one reliable clinical finding of cognitive impairment, balance impairment, and/or oculomotor impairment on acute clinical examination (within 72 hours).

KEY POINTS

■ There is no universally accepted definition of MTBI, but there are points of agreement among published definitions.
■ In the absence of LOC, a diagnosis of MTBI should be considered when there is an alteration in mental status immediately following head trauma or a period of amnesia that abuts the moment of impact.
■ A detailed clinical interview is often necessary to distinguish between altered mental status, amnesia, and LOC, as well as to rule out conditions other than TBI that can account for these clinical signs.
■ The ceiling threshold for MTBI is LOC for up to 30 minutes and posttraumatic confusion or amnesia lasting no more than 24 hours.

STUDY QUESTIONS

1. A patient explains that he cannot remember arriving at the hospital after a motor vehicle crash. This could be due to:
   a. Posttraumatic amnesia
   b. Opiate analgesics
   c. Psychological trauma
   d. Any of the above

2. An injury involving posttraumatic amnesia of 2 hours duration and a traumatic subdural hematoma on the day-of-injury CT scan would be:
   a. Classified as a moderate traumatic brain injury by the Department of Veterans Affairs and the Department of Defense guidelines
   b. Classified as an MTBI by World Health Organization Collaborating Centre Task Force on Mild Traumatic Brain Injury
   c. Excluded from the definition of a sport-related concussion according to the Concussion in Sport Group
   d. All of the above

3. Which of the following is most useful for grading the severity of TBI?
   a. Glasgow Coma Scale score within 30 minutes of injury
   b. Duration of posttraumatic amnesia
   c. Postconcussion symptom checklist
   d. Blood biomarkers (e.g., glial fibrillary acidic protein)

4. Which of the following provides the strongest evidence of MTBI?
   a. Irritability
   b. Repeated vomiting
   c. Difficulty following commands
   d. Glasgow Coma Scale score of 15

5. Which of the following must be present in order to diagnose an MTBI?
   a. External forces capable of impacting brain function
   b. Loss of consciousness
   c. Normal CT scan of the head
   d. Postconcussion symptoms

ADDITIONAL READING

Acute Concussion Evaluation (ACE) forms from the Centers for Disease Control and Prevention: https://www.cdc.gov/headsup/pdfs/providers/ace-a.pdf

Diagnosis/Assessment of Concussion/mTBI (Section 1) of Guideline for Concussion/Mild Traumatic Brain Injury & Prolonged Symptoms, by the Ontario Neurotrauma Foundation. https://braininjuryguidelines.org/concussion/

Crowe LM, Hearps S, Anderson V, et al. Investigating the variability in mild traumatic brain injury definitions: a prospective cohort study. *Arch Phys Med Rehabil.* 2018;99(7):1360–1369. doi:10.1016/j.apmr.2017.12.026

Silverberg ND, Iverson GL, ACRM Mild TBI Definition Expert Consensus Group and the ACRM Brain Injury Special Interest Group Mild TBI Task Force. Expert panel survey to update the American Congress of Rehabilitation Medicine definition of mild traumatic brain injury. *Arch Phys Med Rehabil.* 2020;S0003-9993(20)30970-9. Advance online publication. doi:10.1016/j.apmr.2020.08.022

Ruff RM, Iverson GL, Barth JT, et al. Recommendations for diagnosing a mild traumatic brain injury: a National Academy of Neuropsychology education paper. *Arch Clin Neuropsychol.* 2009;24(1):3–10. doi:10.1093/arclin/acp006

ANSWERS TO STUDY QUESTIONS

1. Correct Answer: d
   Memory gaps immediately following the injury are characteristic of posttraumatic amnesia. However, this finding might be explained by confounding factors, such as prescription opiates given for pain management or acute traumatic stress.

   Further Reading:
   Friedland D, Swash M. Post-traumatic amnesia and confusional state: hazards of retrospective assessment. *J Neurol Neurosurg Psychiatry.* 2016;87(10):1068–1074. doi:10.1136/jnnp-2015-312193

2. Correct Answer: d
   The definitions of MTBI referenced here differ in how they handle neuroimaging findings. A trauma-related intracranial abnormality will rule in or rule out MTBI depending on the definition used.

   Further Reading:
   Silverberg ND, Iverson GL, & ACRM Mild TBI Definition Expert Consensus Group and the ACRM Brain Injury Special Interest Group Mild TBI Task Force (2020). Expert panel

survey to update the American Congress of Rehabilitation Medicine definition of mild traumatic brain injury. *Arch Phys Med Rehabil.* 2020; S0003-9993(20)30970-9. Advance online publication. doi:10.1016/j.apmr.2020.08.022

3. Correct Answer: b
The duration of posttraumatic amnesia is widely used for grading injury severity. The Glasgow Coma Scale has been conventionally used to aid in the classification of mild, moderate, and severe TBI. However, a patient who scores less than 13 within the first 30 minutes following injury could improve such that they reach a score of 13–15 by 30 minutes post-injury, falling within the MTBI category. Patients with moderate-severe TBI do not consistently report more postconcussion symptoms than patients with MTBI. Blood biomarkers may contribute to TBI severity grading in the future, but there is currently insufficient evidence to support this application.

Further Reading:
Hawryluk GW, & Manley GT. (2015). Classification of traumatic brain injury: past, present, and future. *Handb Clin Neurol.* 2015; 127:15–21. doi:10.1016/ B978-0-444-52892-6.00002-7

4. Correct Answer: c
Postconcussion symptoms, such as irritability, are not specific to MTBI—they can be caused by other factors. Repeated vomiting has unclear diagnostic significance. A Glasgow Coma Scale score of 15 means that at the time of assessment, the patient was oriented and responsive, but it does not indicate whether there was an alteration in consciousness that resolved prior to medical evaluation. Difficulty following commands is a classic sign of brain injury.

Further Reading:
Teasdale G, Maas A, Lecky F, Manley G, Stocchetti N, & Murray G, et al. (2014). The Glasgow Coma Scale at 40 years: standing the test of time. *The Lancet. Neurology.* 2014; 13(8): 844–854. doi:10.1016/S1474-4422(14)70120-6

5. Correct Answer: a
A biologically plausible mechanism of injury involving external forces is necessary in order to diagnosis MTBI. Most MTBIs did not involve a loss of consciousness. Neuroimaging is not required to diagnose MTBI. MTBI can be diagnosed when a patient denies experiencing symptoms.

Further Reading:
Menon DK, Schwab K, Wright DW, Maas AI, & Demographics and Clinical Assessment Working Group of the International and Interagency Initiative toward Common Data Elements for Research on Traumatic Brain Injury and Psychological Health (2010). Position statement: definition of traumatic brain injury. *Arch Phys Med Rehabil.* 2010;91(11): 1637–1640. doi:10.1016/j.apmr.2010.05.017

REFERENCES

The full reference list appears in the digital product found on http://connect.springer-pub.com/content/book/978-0-8261-4768-4/part/part02/chapter/ch06

7 MILD TRAUMATIC BRAIN INJURY: INITIAL MEDICAL EVALUATION AND MANAGEMENT

MICELLE J. HAYDEL

GENERAL PRINCIPLES

Definition

Mild traumatic brain injury (MTBI) describes a forceful impact or acceleration/deceleration force to the head, associated with a transient alteration in consciousness, motor function, or cognitive ability.[1] The diagnosis of MTBI is based on the history and physical examination, which can be challenging in the setting of rapid resolution of the initial symptoms and with a normal or near-normal level of consciousness on presentation. Compared to patients with moderate or severe TBI, patients with MTBI have an extremely low likelihood of having an intracranial injury or of requiring hospitalization or neurosurgical intervention. Despite this apparent low acuity, patients do have a significant likelihood (up to 30%) of suffering from postconcussive symptoms, which makes MTBI a significant public health issue.[2]

Epidemiology

Over 2 million people in the United States seek care for MTBI each year, while it is estimated that double that amount do not seek care for sport- or recreation-related injuries.[1,3]

Classification

The Glasgow Coma Scale (GCS) is used extensively to classify TBI into levels of severity because of its inverse relationship with the incidence intracranial injury (ICI) and need for neurosurgical intervention. Patients with a normal or near-normal GCS of 14 to 15 are classified as having an MTBI. Patients with a GCS of 13, while still classified as having a MTBI, have a higher likelihood of intracranial injury on computed tomography (CT) and need for neurosurgical intervention.

Etiology

Leading causes of MTBI[4-6]:

- Falls: predominantly occurring in the very young and the very old
- Motor vehicle-related injury: primarily occurring in young adults
- Work, sports, and recreational injury

The full reference list appears in the digital product found on http://connect.springerpub.com/content/book/978-0-8261-4768-4/part/part02/chapter/ch07

- Assault
- Blast injuries: particularly in military personnel

Pathophysiology

MTBI is a complex pathophysiological process caused by direct or indirect traumatic biomechanical forces to the head. Symptoms largely reflect a functional disturbance, rather than visible structural changes on CT. The precise mechanisms responsible for the clinical features of MTBI remain unclear, with structural and functional imaging studies suggesting that TBI can be associated with varying degrees of metabolic change as well as white matter tract disruption.[7]

Mechanism of Injury

The primary injury is caused by the immediate mechanical force, whereas the secondary injury is caused by the evolving pathophysiological consequences that encompass complex neurobiological cascades, and worsened by hypoxia, ischemia, and the release of excitatory amino acids, calcium, or other neurotoxins[8] (see also Chapter 2).

DIAGNOSIS

Risk Factors

Less than 10% of patients with MTBI have ICI detectable by CT, less than 1% require a neurosurgical intervention, and 0.1% die due to their injury.[9] It is the clinician's task to screen for the small subset of patients who harbor a significant intracranial lesion, while minimizing excessive costs, radiation exposure, admissions, and unnecessary diagnostic procedures. Many of the risk factors for intracranial injury in MTBI are history- and symptom-based, which makes it imperative that the clinician secure an accurate history of presenting illness.

Clinical Presentation

Most patients with MTBI have a straightforward clinical presentation, but some have an unclear history, with little or no physical evidence of trauma. Several factors are associated with an increased risk of ICI:

- Mechanism of injury: Pedestrian struck by a motor vehicle, occupant ejected from a motor vehicle, or a fall over 3 feet or 5 stairs.[10]
- Anticoagulation: Pre-injury anticoagulant or antiplatelet use, hemophilia, or platelet disorders.[11,12]
- Past medical history: Cranial surgery, past head trauma, or immediate posttraumatic seizures.[9]
- Age: Patients over the age of 60.[9] Older age has also been shown to be an independent predictor of mortality in isolated MTBI.[13,14] Elderly patients with ICI often have fewer clinical clues and a less serious mechanism of injury than younger patients.[15]
- Reported loss of consciousness or posttraumatic amnesia: This has been shown to marginally increase the risk of ICI; conversely their absence is useful as a negative predictor if the patient has no other associated symptoms or risk factors.[9,16,17]
- Drug or alcohol use: Chronic or concurrent intoxication.[18,19]

Symptoms

- Red Flag symptoms shown to have a significantly high of a positive likelihood ratio for ICI in patients with MTBI include:
  - Persistent short-term memory deficits, seizures, deterioration in mental status, GCS <14, and focal neurological deficit.[9,20]
  - Repeated vomiting.[21]
- Headache has been associated with a small but significant increased risk of ICI in MTBI.[9] Unilateral headache can also be the presenting complaint in carotid dissection.
- Unilateral neck or face pain associated with Horner's or posterior circulation symptoms should trigger the clinician to consider a carotid or vertebral artery dissection.[22]

Physical Examination

Patients with MTBI must undergo a focused physical examination with attention to the neurological evaluation. All patients should have their cervical spine assessed promptly to determine the need for c-spine immobilization and imaging. Physical findings suggestive of a depressed or basilar skull fracture are strongly correlated with ICI, otherwise the most prognostic elements of the physical examination are the pupillary examination and the GCS.[23] The motor examination can identify subtle cranial nerve deficits,[24] as well as balance and coordination deficits that may persist long after other symptoms of MTBI have resolved.[25]

- **Pupils:** Pupillary reflexes, if abnormal, indicate both underlying pathology and severity of injury and should be monitored serially. Pupillary abnormalities in patients with a GCS over 13 are most likely due to etiologies other than TBI.[23]
- **Motor:** The cranial nerve (CN) examination should include attention to CN IV and VI, because subtle deficits may not be evident until the patient is taken through a careful extra-ocular exam.[24] Alterations in balance and gait have shown to be predictive of postconcussive symptoms.[26] Gait and balance require the complex integration of motor, visual, cerebellar, vestibular, and proprioceptive functions. Coordination can be assessed using finger-to-nose and rapid alternating hand movements.[25] Gait (straight-line and tandem) is often used in the emergency department (ED) as a marker of balance.
- **GCS:** Scoring for each component of the GCS should be documented separately in order to provide complete information for subsequent measures (e.g., GCS 10 = E3 V4 M3). Motor deficits have the strongest correlation with poor outcome in patients with TBI,[23] and a motor-only score has been shown to perform as well as the GCS.[27,28]
- **Cognitive Examination:** While it has been shown that patients with a GCS of 13 or 14 are more likely to have ICI on head CT, focused cognitive testing has revealed that the correlation between CT findings and subtle cognitive deficits (found in up to 30% of patients with MTBI) are much less clear.[29] Cognitive deficits may be identified by testing short-term memory (3-item recall, 5-number recall) and concentration (serial 7s, backward months of year or world spelling). There are also simple computer programs or apps that are being investigated as tools to help identify neurocognitive symptoms that patients with MTBI frequently encounter.[30]

Laboratory Studies

Routine laboratory and bedside studies have little value in the evaluation of patients with mild TBI, but certain groups of patients may benefit from specific studies:

- Patients with an abnormal GCS should undergo a bedside glucose, as well as electrolyte panel and toxicology screen.

- Elderly patients and those with significant co-morbid conditions or weakness should have an electrolyte panel, blood count, urinalysis, and EKG.
- Patients with known or suspected coagulation disorders, liver disease, or those taking anticoagulants would also benefit from coagulation studies.

Radiographic Assessment

Noncontrast CT is both highly sensitive and specific for the detection of fractures, contusions, epidural and subdural bleeds, and subarachnoid hemorrhage, and remains the diagnostic imaging technique of choice in patients with TBI.[31] Radiation exposure from head CT is relatively small, and purported risk of subsequent cancer is inversely related to age: a 40-year-old has a risk of approximately 1:10,000, whereas a 20-year-old has a risk of approximately 1:5,000.[32] Immediate CT is indicated in TBI patients with:

- Evidence of basilar, depressed, or open skull fracture
- Focal neurological deficits
- Altered mental status or persistent abnormal GCS

Patients without clear indications for CT can be a management challenge. To date, over 20 clinical decision rules for the use of CT in patients with MTBI have been published. Two guidelines (Table 7.1) stand out due to high sensitivity for detection of ICI (99%–100%).[10,20,33,34] Although guidelines cannot replace clinical judgment in all scenarios, in general, imaging can be avoided in patients who do not meet criteria for imaging based on well-validated clinical decision guidelines.[33,34] (See Treatment section.)

TABLE 7.1 Clinical Guidelines for CT of the Head After Mild Traumatic Brain Injury in Adults

New Orleans Criteria[20]	Canadian CT Head Rule[10]
Headache	Dangerous mechanism of injury*
Vomiting (any)	Vomiting ≥2
Age >60 years	Patient >65 years
Drug or alcohol intoxication	Glasgow Coma Score <15 at 2 hours post injury
Seizure	Any sign of basal skull fracture
Evidence of trauma above clavicles (bruise, abrasion, laceration, etc.)	Possible open or depressed skull fracture
Short-term memory deficits (anterograde amnesia)	Amnesia for events 30 minutes before injury

*Pedestrian struck by a motor vehicle, an occupant ejected from a motor vehicle, or a fall from an elevation of 3 or more feet or 5 stairs.

TREATMENT

Guiding Principles

Though patients with MTBI have a very low likelihood of harboring a clinically important ICI, they are at risk for suffering postconcussive symptoms. Therefore, the clinician has two main goals:

- To screen for the small subset of patients who have a significant intracranial lesion, while minimizing excessive costs, radiation exposure, admissions, and unnecessary diagnostic procedures.
- To provide all patients with information about the common postconcussive symptoms that occur during the first 7 to 10 days after injury as well as the resources available for follow-up should the symptoms persist.

Initial Management

Patients with MTBI should undergo a rapid and thorough assessment in order to screen for the small subset of patients who harbor a significant intracranial lesion. Unless the patient has a bleeding diathesis, evidence of basilar, depressed or open skull fracture, or focal neurological deficits, clinicians may safely follow well-established clinical guidelines (Table 7.1) to direct CT use in patients with MTBI.

Ongoing Care

Patients with ICI on CT or those with continued confusion despite a normal CT are typically admitted to the hospital for observation and/or repeat imaging. Patients who are at high risk for a delayed intracranial lesion, such as elderly patients on anticoagulants, may benefit from a period of observation and subsequent discharge only if symptom-free after 6 hours of observation. Patients with a normal CT and resolution of symptoms, or no indication for CT based on clinical guidelines may be discharged home. All patients should receive both verbal and written information about the risk of delayed ICI, as well as the possibility of immediate concussive symptoms and persistent postconcussive symptoms. Some studies suggest that over 30% of patients with a discharge diagnosis of MTBI will have symptoms at 3 months post-injury, and up to 15% will continue to be symptomatic at 1 year post injury.[35,36] See Table 7.2 for common postconcussive symptoms.

TABLE 7.2 Postconcussive Symptoms

Constitutional Symptoms	Cognitive	Mood
Headache	Difficulty concentrating	Irritability
Sleep disturbance	Memory problems	Anxiety
Dizziness/vertigo; balance problem	Difficulty thinking clearly	Depression
Nausea	Feeling cognitively slow	Emotional lability
Fatigue		
Oversensitivity to noise/light		

Treatment Controversies

Screening head CT is indicated in patients with MTBI who have a bleeding diathesis, take anticoagulants, or antiplatelet agents. Clinicians should have a low threshold for initiating factor replacement or reversal agents in patients with a bleeding disorder, on antiplatelet agents, or on anticoagulants.

- **Anticoagulants:** Patients taking anticoagulant agents have a significant increase in risk of ICI due to MTBI.[9,37] Those with an ICI on CT should undergo rapid reversal using fresh frozen plasma, prothrombin complex concentrate, or drug-specific reversal agents, and should be admitted for observation and repeat CT.[38] Delayed hemorrhage after a normal initial CT also occurs in <1% of anticoagulated patients,[39] and many experts advocate 24 hours of observation with or without a repeat CT prior to discharge for these patients.[12,37,40] Studies show that while most patients do not benefit from admission, delayed bleeds can occur up to several days after the injury.[39,41] At minimum, patients on anticoagulants must be educated about the very real risk (even days later) of delayed hemorrhage, and a shared decision-making conversation should occur when considering admission versus discharge.[12,41]

- **Antiplatelets:** Aspirin and clopidogrel have both been found to be associated with increased risk of intracranial bleed in several studies.[11,42,43] A large recent study revealed a significant increase when patients were taking both aspirin and clopidogrel.[44] Reversal of antiplatelet agents with platelet transfusions or desmopressin have not been shown to impact outcomes after TBI.[45]
- **Hemophilia:** Patients with hemophilia and MTBI have an increased risk for ICI. Clinicians should initiate factor replacement immediately in patients with hemophilia and any head injury.[46]

Additional Considerations

Most patients with MTBI will be discharged to home after their initial evaluation, and the discharge instructions play an important role in setting expectations as well as alerting the patient or family to symptoms that may signal a delayed ICI. A significant percentage of patients with MTBI will have little to no recall of verbal instructions in the days after their discharge; therefore, all patients must also be provided clear, written discharge instructions.[47]

KEY POINTS

- Clinical decision guidelines may be used to guide CT use in patients post-MTBI; these tools are well-validated for their ability to identify those at risk for detectable ICI (Table 7.1).
- Clinicians must maintain a low threshold for CT use in elderly patients with MTBI or those on anticoagulation agents.
- Written discharge instructions should address expected postconcussive symptoms (Table 7.2) as well as resources available if symptoms persist. One-third of patients with MTBI can be expected to have continued neurocognitive symptoms beyond the typical 7 to 10 day recovery period. The Centers for Disease Control and Prevention (CDC) has developed a patient discharge information sheet that provides clear information about what to expect and when to seek follow-up after discharge with MTBI.[48]
- Discharge instructions must describe the warning signs of delayed hemorrhage or occult significant ICI: repeated vomiting, worsening or unremitting headache, altered level of consciousness, confusion, agitation, seizures, visual changes, weakness, or balance difficulties.

STUDY QUESTIONS

1. A 66-year-old woman tripped and fell while standing, striking her head and sustaining a brief loss of consciousness. Her physical examination is now normal. She takes no medications other than Synthroid. Your evaluation includes:

   a. Complete blood count
   b. EKG
   c. Non-contrast CT of the head
   d. All of the above

2. Postconcussive symptoms occur in approximately 30% of patients after MTBI. These symptoms include all of the following *except*:
   a. Difficulty concentrating
   b. Anxiety
   c. Headache
   d. Seizures

3. A 45-year-old man was a restrained passenger in a motor vehicle collision. He denies loss of consciousness but reports headache, nausea, vertigo, right-sided neck and face pain. He has no past medical history and takes no medications. Your plan includes:
   a. No imaging needed. Ibuprofen and follow-up with a chiropractor or physical therapist
   b. No imaging needed. Hydrocodone and Zofran every 6 hours as needed for 3 days
   c. Plain radiographs of cervical spine
   d. Imaging study to evaluate carotid and vertebral vessels

4. A 56-year-old woman, restrained driver in moderate-speed motor vehicle collision, with a brief episode of loss of consciousness, is brought in by medics with a complaint of left wrist pain where she was struck by the airbag. The patient has soft-tissue swelling and an abrasion of the left wrist but otherwise has a normal examination. She has no past medical history, takes no medications, and her tetanus is up to date. Aside from the wrist pain, her review of systems is negative. In addition to treatment of her wrist injury, you plan to:
   a. Obtain a noncontrast CT of her head
   b. Obtain a toxicology screen to check for intoxicants
   c. Discharge with head injury precautions and concussion resources
   d. All of the above

5. An 88-year-old man on warfarin for atrial fibrillation tripped and fell while standing, striking his head, and losing consciousness for several minutes. He was confused on arrival, but his mentation is now clear, and he has a normal neurological examination. He has a small scalp abrasion and his tetanus is up to date. His head CT is normal. Which of the following is the best approach to management of this patient?
   a. After a shared decision-making discussion, the patient may be discharged home with close follow-up with his primary care provider
   b. After a shared decision-making discussion, the patient may be admitted for observation
   c. After a shared decision-making discussion, the patient may be discharged home after a repeat normal CT in 6 hours
   d. All of the above are reasonable approaches

ADDITIONAL READING

Centers for Disease Control and Prevention. *Injury Prevention & Control: Traumatic Brain Injury [Internet]*. Centers for Disease Control and Prevention. 2020. http://www.cdc.gov/TraumaticBrainInjury/index.html

Centers for Disease Control and Prevention. *Injury Prevention & Control: Traumatic Brain Injury/Resources for Health Care Providers [Internet].* Centers for Disease Control and Prevention. 2020. http://www.cdc.gov/traumaticbraininjury/providers.html

Holmes Jr, JF, Chang CH. Head injuries. In: *Harwood-Nuss' Clinical Practice of Emergency Medicine: Sixth Edition.* Wolters Kluwer Health Adis (ESP); 2014:157–164.

Silverberg ND, Duhaime AC, Iaccarino MA. Mild Traumatic Brain Injury in 2019–2020. *JAMA.* 2020;323(2):177–178. doi:10.1001/jama.2019.18134

ANSWERS TO STUDY QUESTIONS

1. Correct Answer: c

Routine laboratory and bedside studies have little value in the evaluation of patients with MTBI. Two established clinical guidelines recommend CT in patients in their 60s and above.

Further Reading:

Papa L, Stiell IG, Clement CM, et al. Performance of the Canadian CT Head Rule and the New Orleans Criteria for predicting any traumatic intracranial injury on computed tomography in a United States Level I trauma center. *Acad Emerg Med.* 2012;19(1):2–10. doi:10.1111/j.1553-2712.2011.01247.x

Smits M, Dippel DW, de Haan GG, et al. External validation of the Canadian CT Head Rule and the New Orleans Criteria for CT scanning in patients with minor head injury. *JAMA.* 2005;294(12):1519–1525. doi:10.1001/jama.294.12.1519

2. Correct Answer: d

Seizures are not a part of postconcussive symptomatology.

Further Reading:

Voormolen DC, Haagsma JA, Polinder S, et al. Post-concussion symptoms in complicated vs. uncomplicated mild traumatic brain injury patients at three and six months post-injury: results from the CENTER-TBI study. *J Clin Med.* 2019;8(11):1921. doi:10.3390/jcm8111921

Voormolen DC, Polinder S, von Steinbuechel N, et al. The association between post-concussion symptoms and health-related quality of life in patients with mild traumatic brain injury. *Injury.* 2019;50(5):1068–1074. doi:10.1016/j.injury.2018.12.002

3. Correct Answer: d

Unilateral neck or face pain with Horner's or posterior circulation symptoms should trigger the clinician to consider carotid or vertebral artery dissection.

Further Reading:

Blum CA, Yaghi S. Cervical artery dissection: a review of the epidemiology, pathophysiology, treatment, and outcome. *Arch Neurosci.* 2015;2(4). doi:10.5812/archneurosci.26670

4. Correct Answer: c

There is no indication for CT in this patient based on validated guidelines.

Further Reading:

Papa L, Stiell IG, Clement CM, et al. Performance of the Canadian CT Head Rule and the New Orleans Criteria for predicting any traumatic intracranial injury on computed tomography in a United States Level I trauma center. *Acad Emerg Med.* 2012;19(1):2–10. doi:10.1111/j.1553-2712.2011.01247.x

Smits M, Dippel DW, de Haan GG, et al. External validation of the Canadian CT Head Rule and the New Orleans Criteria for CT scanning in patients with minor head injury. *JAMA*. 2005;294(12):1519–1525. doi:10.1001/jama.294.12.1519

5. Correct Answer: d
At minimum, patients on anticoagulants must be educated about the very real risk (even days later) of delayed hemorrhage, and a shared decision-making conversation should occur when considering admit versus discharge.

Further Reading:
Menditto VG, Lucci M, Polonara S, Pomponio G, et al. Management of minor head injury in patients receiving oral anticoagulant therapy: a prospective study of a 24-hour observation protocol. *Ann Emerg Med*. 2012;59(6):451–455. doi:10.1016/j.annemergmed.2011.12.003
Cohn B, Keim SM, Sanders AB. Can anticoagulated patients be discharged home safely from the emergency department after minor head injury? *J Emerg Med*. 2014;46(3):410–417. doi:10.1016/j.jemermed.2013.08.107

REFERENCES

The full reference list appears in the digital product found on http://connect.springer-pub.com/content/book/978-0-8261-4768-4/part/part02/chapter/ch07

8 THE NATURAL HISTORY OF MILD TRAUMATIC BRAIN INJURY

GRANT L. IVERSON, DOUGLAS P. TERRY,
RAEL T. LANGE, AND NOAH D. SILVERBERG

INTRODUCTION

The natural history of mild traumatic brain injury (MTBI) is reasonably well understood. There is a body of evidence suggesting that the symptoms and problems associated with this injury are time-limited and follow a predictable course for most people.[1-7] A substantial percentage of people, however, report persistent symptoms for weeks and months following injury.[8-10] The literature on athletes with sport-related concussions and civilian trauma patients is largely distinct. Differences in patient characteristics, mechanisms of injury, study designs, and outcome measures make it difficult to integrate or even to precisely compare studies of athletes and civilian trauma patients. Moreover, little is known about people who sustain very mild injuries and experience rapid resolution of symptoms because they do not seek medical care and usually are not included in studies. It has been estimated that approximately 1 in 4 people who sustain an MTBI do not seek any healthcare.[11,12]

RECOVERY FROM SPORT-RELATED CONCUSSION

Acute Clinical Presentation

Loss of consciousness is uncommon, and posttraumatic amnesia, when present, is brief following most concussions sustained in sports.[13,14] Athletes report diverse physical, cognitive, and emotional symptoms in the acute phase. The most frequently endorsed symptoms in the initial days post-injury are headaches, pressure in head, fatigue, feeling slowed down, drowsiness, difficulty concentrating, feeling mentally foggy, and dizziness.[15-17] Impairment of balance and cognition is also common.[18]

Time Course for Recovery

Symptomatic recovery typically occurs within 2 weeks,[5,6,19] but can take considerably longer for some athletes. The effects of concussion on balance and cognition diminish rapidly between 1 and 10 days following injury[20-22] and are typically no longer detectable after 30 days following injury.[23] Physiological recovery may lag behind symptom resolution.[24]

The full reference list appears in the digital product found on http://connect.springerpub.com/content/book/978-0-8261-4768-4/part/part02/chapter/ch08

Authors' Note: The views expressed in this chapter are those of the authors and do not reflect the official policy of the Department of Defense or the U.S. Government.

Factors Associated With Slower Recovery

Systematic reviews have concluded that factors associated with slower recovery from concussion include:

- The severity of a person's acute and subacute symptoms[25]
- The development of subacute problems with headaches or depression[25]
- Personal factors such as:
  - Female gender[25]
  - A personal history of mental health problems[25]
  - Prior history of concussions[6]

There is no clear evidence at this time that a personal history of attention-deficit hyperactivity disorder (ADHD)[25,26] or migraine[25] is associated with risk for worse outcome, although studies in this area are few and methodologically limited.[25] Loss of consciousness and posttraumatic amnesia are not established predictors of worse clinical outcome, but retrograde amnesia does appear to be associated with worse outcome.[25]

Return to Sports

Most professional football players who sustain a concussion miss no more than one game before returning to play.[27] High school and college athletes take about 1 to 3 weeks, on average, to return to competition,[28,29] with more than 90% returning within 1 month.[25,28,30] Girls and women, athletes with prior concussion(s), and adolescents (versus young adults) tend to take somewhat longer to recover symptomatically and return to sports.[6,25,30–33]

RECOVERY FROM MILD TRAUMATIC BRAIN INJURY

Acute Clinical Presentation

Trauma patients report a constellation of symptoms and often perform poorly on neuropsychological tests in the initial days post injury.[34] The acute clinical presentation of MTBI in the general population can be complicated by traumatic stress and other bodily injuries.[35,36]

Time Course for Recovery

Symptoms generally improve over the first few weeks or months after MTBI.[9,37] A minority of patients continue to report symptoms at 1 year following injury.[1] Whereas headaches and dizziness are common acutely, chronic symptoms are often emotional or cognitive in nature.[37–39] It should be noted that patients with orthopedic injuries who do not experience a TBI often report similar symptoms.[1,37] Researchers have reported no or modest group differences on neuropsychological testing for those with MTBIs compared to healthy control subjects and orthopedically injured control subjects at 2 weeks[40] and 1 month[2] following injury. Multiple meta-analyses have demonstrated that by 3 months post-injury, those who have sustained MTBIs perform similarly to control participants.[3,41]

Factors Associated With Prolonged Recovery

A pre-injury history of psychiatric problems is a robust predictor of chronic symptoms.[42,43] Acute psychological distress, in the initial days following injury, is associated with persistent symptoms.[42] Developing a psychiatric condition after MTBI can also complicate recovery.[2,44] Women and older adults tend to take longer to recover,[43,45-47] although the literature is mixed on the extent to which gender and age confer this risk.

There is not a clear and consistent association between measures of TBI severity, such as loss of consciousness and posttraumatic amnesia, and long-term outcome from MTBI. Patients with complicated MTBI (e.g., MTBI with trauma-related intracranial abnormalities noted on initial brain imaging) tend to perform more poorly on neuropsychological tests than patients with uncomplicated MTBI in the first 2 months following injury, but usually on a small number of tests rather than having globally depressed scores.[48-53] When differences occur between these two groups, the effect sizes of these differences tend to be medium. At 6 months post-injury, some researchers have not reported differences in neuropsychological test performance between complicated and uncomplicated MTBI patients. Compensation-seeking is associated with prolonged recovery,[54-57] but cause and effect in this relationship is not clear.

Early Intervention

Clinicians may be able to facilitate recovery in people who have suffered an MTBI. Education and reassurance of a likely good outcome is the most researched type of early intervention. The benefits appear modest,[58-60] but given the low cost of providing information brochures, early education is probably worthwhile. Encouraging a progressive return to activity as tolerated is recommended,[61] whereas encouraging prolonged rest is discouraged.[59] There is insufficient evidence to recommend early intensive multidisciplinary intervention for the average patient with MTBI. However, targeted early intervention for patients with risk factors for prolonged recovery is prudent.[62,63]

Return to School

Although some students return to school quickly and require minimal support, other students may need accommodations because increases in activity (e.g., returning to the classroom/study and extracurricular activities) can worsen cognitive (e.g., difficulties with memory, attention, speed) and physical symptoms (e.g., headaches, fatigue, sensitivity to light/noise).[64] Several graduated return to school strategies have been recommended.[19,65] Long-term negative effects on academic performance are unlikely.[66]

Return to Work

Most studies suggest that between 60% and 90% of patients return to work within 6 months of an MTBI.[67,68] Return to work rates vary considerably across studies from different countries, due to both methodological differences in sampling, definitions across the studies, and differences in social services and healthcare systems, such as from (a) 22%[69] to 84%[70] in the first week; (b) 25%,[71] 71%,[72] and 99%[70] within the first month; and (c) 63%,[71] 76%,[73] and 83%[74] by 6 months post injury. Lower education level, occupations involving low decision-making latitude, other bodily injuries, and severe acute symptoms appear to be associated with slower return to work.[72,73,75-78]

PERSISTENT SYMPTOMS

A sizeable percentage of people who sustain an MTBI report persistent symptoms months and even years following injury.[1,8,79] Some people who sustain a mild TBI develop post-traumatic stress disorder (PTSD) in the weeks and months following the injury event,[80] and PTSD can mimic or exacerbate persistent postconcussion symptoms. Those who experience an MTBI are at increased risk for having depression months and years following their injury.[81]

When a person experiences persistent symptoms months or years following an MTBI, it is important to appreciate that those symptoms might be caused or amplified by factors unrelated to the original injury. "Postconcussion-like" symptoms are common in the general population[82–84] and they are associated with life stress,[85,86] chronic pain,[87,88] sleep problems,[89–91] anxiety,[92] traumatic stress,[93,94] and depression.[95,96] Evidence-informed treatment and rehabilitation can be useful for improving symptoms, functioning, and quality of life.[7,61,97–99]

KEY POINTS

- Individuals who sustain an MTBI may have a constellation of symptoms in the initial days following injury, and often have lower scores on neuropsychological testing. A patient's acute clinical presentation can be complicated by traumatic stress and other bodily injuries.
- Symptoms tend to improve in the initial days and weeks following an MTBI, with a small minority of patients continuing to report symptoms 1 year following injury. Patients with MTBI tend to perform as well as controls on neuropsychological tasks before 3 months post injury. Most patients (60%–90%) return to work within 6 months.
- Factors associated with prolonged recovery include pre-injury psychiatric problems, acute post-injury psychological distress, the development of a psychological disorder, and seeking compensation. Some studies show gender, age, and positive neuroimaging are associated with recovery time.
- A minority of people who have sustained an MTBI have persistent symptoms. It is important to assess for and treat potential comorbid factors that could be contributing to the patient's overall symptom presentation, given the nonspecific nature of MTBI symptoms.

STUDY QUESTIONS

1. Which is the *most common* symptom or problem experienced 1 month after an MTBI?
   a. Visual problems
   b. Nausea
   c. Headache
   d. Cognitive impairment on neuropsychological testing

2. Of these choices, which is likely the strongest predictor of a prolonged recovery from an MTBI?
   a. Gender
   b. Loss of consciousness
   c. ADHD
   d. Pre-injury psychiatric history

3. Which statement best describes the results of cognitive testing following an MTBI?
   a. Those with MTBI and controls perform similarly by or before 3 months post injury
   b. Those with MTBI and controls perform similarly by or before 1 week post injury
   c. Those with MTBI show substantial deficits at 1 to 3 months following injury
   d. Those with MTBI show substantial deficits at 3 to 6 months following injury

4. What proportion of people have returned to work by 6 months post MTBI?
   a. 10%–30%
   b. 30%–50%
   c. 60%–90%
   d. 90%–100%

5. Which is *not* considered to be a helpful intervention for MTBI?
   a. Rest until symptoms have fully subsided
   b. Pharmacological headache management
   c. Education and reassurance about the course of mild TBI recovery and how to manage symptoms
   d. Psychological treatment for those who develop mental health problems

ADDITIONAL READING

Ontario Neurotrauma Foundation. *Guidelines for Concussion/Mild Traumatic Brain Injury and Persistent Symptoms*, 3rd ed. 2018. https://braininjuryguidelines.org/concussion/fileadmin/media/Concussion_guideline_3rd_edition_final.pdf

Iverson GL, Silverberg N, Lange RT, Zasler N. Conceptualizing outcome from mild traumatic brain injury. In: Zasler ND, Katz DI, Zafonte RD, eds. *Brain Injury Medicine: Principles and Practice*, 2nd ed. Demos Medical Publishing; 2012:470–497. doi:10.1891/9781617050572.0030

Nelson LD, Furger RE, Ranson J, et al. Acute clinical predictors of symptom recovery in emergency department patients with uncomplicated mild traumatic brain injury or non-traumatic brain injuries. *J Neurotrauma*. 2018;35:249–259. doi:10.1089/neu.2017.4988

Silverberg ND, Gardner AJ, Brubacher JR, et al. Systematic review of multivariable prognostic models for mild traumatic brain injury. *J Neurotrauma*. 2015;32:517–526. doi:10.1089/neu.2014.3600

Silverberg ND, Iaccarino MA, Panenka WJ, et al. Management of concussion and mild traumatic brain injury: a synthesis of practice guidelines. *Arch Phys Med Rehabil*. 2020;101:382–393. doi:10.1016/j.apmr.2019.10.179

ANSWERS TO STUDY QUESTIONS

1. Correct Answer: c
Headache is among the most common symptoms over the first month after MTBI. Neuropsychological impairment is less common at this stage.

Further Reading:
Theadom A, Parag V, Dowell T, et al, BIONIC Research Group. Persistent problems 1 year after mild traumatic brain injury: a longitudinal population study in New Zealand. *Br J Gen Pract*. 2016;66(642):e16–e23. doi:10.3399/bjgp16X683161

2. Correct Answer: d
Although there is some mixed evidence that a loss of consciousness, gender (i.e., women), and those with ADHD may have a prolonged recovery, having a pre-injury psychiatric history is shown to be one of the most consistent and robust risk factors.

Further Reading:
Silverberg ND, Gardner AJ, Brubacher JR, et al. Systematic review of multivariable prognostic models for mild traumatic brain injury. *J Neurotrauma*. 2015;32:517–526.

3. Correct Answer: a
Meta-analyses show that there are negligible differences, if any, between MTBI patients and controls by 3 months post injury.

Further Reading:
Karr JE, Areshenkoff CN, Garcia-Barrera MA. The neuropsychological outcomes of concussion: a systematic review of meta-analyses on the cognitive sequelae of mild traumatic brain injury. *Neuropsychology*. 2014;28:321–336.

4. Correct Answer: c
Approximately 60% to 90% return to work by 6 months post injury.

Further Reading:
Bloom B, Thomas S, Ahrensberg JM, et al. A systematic review and meta-analysis of return to work after mild traumatic brain injury. *Brain Inj*. 2018;32:1623–1636.

5. Correct Answer: a
Prolonged rest is not associated with faster or better recovery from MTBI. Patients are encouraged to gradually return to activities. Prolonged rest could lead to deconditioning or other health issues.

Further Reading:
Schneider KJ, Leddy JJ, Guskiewicz KM, et al. Rest and treatment/rehabilitation following sport-related concussion: a systematic review. *Br J Sports Med*. 2017;51(12):930–934. doi:10.1136/bjsports-2016-097475

REFERENCES

The full reference list appears in the digital product found on http://connect.springer-pub.com/content/book/978-0-8261-4768-4/part/part02/chapter/ch08

SPORT-RELATED CONCUSSION I: INJURY PREVENTION AND INITIAL ASSESSMENT

PHILIP H. MONTENIGRO AND ROBERT C. CANTU

BACKGROUND AND GENERAL RECOMMENDATIONS

Concussion is among the most common injury type in amateur sports.[1-3] Sport-related concussion is defined as a traumatic brain injury (TBI) that occurs during athletic activity whether it be team sports or recreational activities. Treating and managing acute and potential long-term effects of concussion is complicated and at times controversial; therefore, prevention is an essential strategy for dealing with sport-related concussion. Prevention strategies aim to reduce the risks for concussion and improve the management of injured athletes.

There are three types of prevention: primary, secondary, and tertiary. Primary prevention aims to prevent the occurrence and diminish the effects of concussion before it occurs. Primary strategies include reducing exposure to risk factors, modifying behaviors, and increasing resistance to concussion and its effects. Secondary prevention aims to lessen the impact of concussion after it has occurred. Secondary strategies focus on earlier and more accurate detection of concussion, employing strategies to avoid a second injury or recurrence, and employing programs to restore the athlete to their baseline function in all settings, including in school, at home, and on the field. Tertiary prevention aims to ameliorate the impact of persistent and/or latent effects of concussion. Tertiary strategies include medical management and rehabilitation activities.

The past decade has seen an explosion of research studies evaluating the efficacy of prevention strategies. New legislation has been enacted to prevent and improve the management of concussion in amateur sports.[4,5] While statutes vary by state/territory, the majority have provisions that include the following: (a) limiting full-contact practice, (b) requiring education and training on concussion, (c) removing athletes suspected of having a concussion, and (d) return to play only after clearance by a qualified healthcare provider.[1,2] The following prevention recommendations are based on emerging evidence, the American Medical Society for Sports Medicine (AMSSM) Position Statement on Concussion in Sport and the 2017 Concussion in Sport Group (CISG) consensus statement.[1,2]

Primary Prevention

- Limit exposure to head impacts by restricting full-contact practice. For example, do not conduct more than one full-contact practice per week.[4,5] There is now significant evidence of potential long-term neurocognitive consequences from repetitive head impacts, with or without concussion.[6] Recent studies have also shown a significant reduction in concussion risk after implementing rule changes to limit full-contact.[7-9]
- Athletes should undergo a pre-participation history and physical to document concussion history (frequency, course, interval) and premorbid conditions that may increase susceptibility to concussion, as well as complicate the recognition, diagnosis,

---

The full reference list appears in the digital product found on http://connect.springerpub.com/content/book/978-0-8261-4768-4/part/part02/chapter/ch09

and management of concussion.[1,10] It is well-established that a history of concussion increases subsequent concussion risk.[11] Some evidence also suggests premorbid headache in the past 3 months and a diagnosis of attention deficit hyperactivity disorder may increase concussion risk.[12] Additional research is needed to confirm this observation and to evaluate prevention strategies for individuals with concussion risk modifiers.

■ Modify techniques and emphasize strategic drill training to reduce the risk of concussion.
■ Proper safety equipment should always be worn and be appropriately fitted. For example, for American football players, helmets play an important and significant role in reducing the risk for severe catastrophic injuries.
■ Proper protocols should be followed to ensure the safety of training facilities, equipment maintenance, and the availability of written emergency procedures.
■ Game officials must strictly enforce rules and coaches should support efforts to ensure safe competitions.
■ Fair play and respect should be supported as key elements of any sport, and violence should be discouraged.

Secondary Prevention

■ It is important to provide mandatory concussion education programs for all key stakeholders, including athletes, parents, coaches, referees, and athletic trainers. Though they do not reduce primary concussion risk,[9] such programs do enhance concussion recognition and management.[11]
■ Athlete education should emphasize concussion sign and symptom recognition. Common misconceptions about "mild" injuries or "dings" should be dispelled. Although concussion awareness has increased, athletes remain reluctant to report symptoms.[13]
■ Schools are encouraged to have an established concussion policy.[2] It is recommended that schools require education for all teachers and staff.
■ Some organizations endorse a one-time cognitive test at the start of the season (SCAT5, CogSport) to improve concussion diagnosis and return-to-play decision-making. That said, baseline testing is controversial and is not considered a standard of care. Baseline scores are not required for real-time post-injury score interpretation and assessment.[1]
■ Sideline assessment and observation of athletes by trained personnel, including the use of "spotters," improve early concussion recognition and initial management.[1] In addition to direct observation, video review by qualified personnel improves early recognition of subtle signs and symptoms of concussion, such as gait instability, a vacant look, or drowsiness.[1,2]
■ If a concussion is suspected, the athlete is immediately removed from play to undergo a multimodal assessment that guides clinical diagnosis.[14–16] A probable diagnosis of concussion excludes the athlete from returning to play and requires a formal follow-up evaluation.[1,2]
■ Most concussions occur without loss of consciousness and many without immediately apparent neurological signs. Therefore, athletes should continue to be monitored immediately after a suspected injury.
■ Medical clearance, usually from a physician, is required before a concussed athlete can return to play. Athletes who return to play prematurely may develop more severe symptoms, experience prolonged recovery times, and be at increased risk for a second injury.[11,17–20]
■ Additional tools to prevent and reduce the severity of concussion include incorporating neck strengthening into fitness and conditioning programs, and learning proper bracing techniques for impacts.[21,22] Both of these approaches may help to reduce head acceleration as they increase effective mass (Force = Mass × Acceleration). Effectively, if

the head is stabilized during an impact, the center of gravity shifts to include the mass of the body, thereby reducing the effect on the head. Additional research is needed to evaluate the effectiveness of these interventions.

Tertiary Prevention

- Concussion symptoms are predominantly transient, with *clinical* resolution typically resolving in days to a few weeks.[2] However, some athletes have lingering symptoms or Prolonged Postconcussion Syndrome/Symptoms (PPCS). See Chapters 15 to 17 for further discussion of this topic.
- The evidence linking a history of concussion and repetitive head impacts to long-term neurobehavioral impairment, structural and functional brain changes, neuro-degenerative biomarkers, and the disease Chronic Traumatic Encephalopathy (CTE) is growing rapidly.[6,23–37] Current or retired athletes with persistent or chronic neurobehavioral impairments should receive individualized treatment and rehabilitation aimed at improving quality-of-life and maximizing functional independence. (See also Chapter 56.)

SPORT-SPECIFIC RECOMMENDATIONS

All sports carry some risk for concussion; however, certain sports have a greater risk than others. Factors contributing to differences in risk include the types of forces experienced and the roles of different positions played. It has also been established that female athletes have a greater risk than male athletes playing the same sport, and that younger athletes have a greater risk than adults.[38]

In the paragraphs that follow, we review specific sports with a high risk of concussion. When comparing the risk of concussion among different sports, studies either report the absolute frequency of concussion or the risk of concussion in units of Athletic Exposure (AE). The absolute frequency of concussion is dependent on the number of participants in a sport, such that sports with a greater number of participants will have an inflated concussion frequency. Conversely, the number of concussions per AE defines the risk for one athlete participating in one game or practice in which they are exposed to the possibility of injury (e.g., ±3 concussions/1,000 AEs). Unlike absolute frequency, risk in terms of concussion per AE allows for comparison between different sports and is not dependent on the number of participants. Among college sports in the United States, the greatest concussion AE rates are seen in men's wrestling, men's and women's ice hockey, and men's football.[39] Men's college football and women's college soccer had the highest annual frequency of concussions, however, based on having the greatest number of participants and therefore more AEs.[39,40] Among high school sports in the United States, boys' football had the greatest concussion AE rate, followed by girls' soccer and boys' ice hockey.[40] Regardless of the sport, more than 65% of all sport-related concussions occur from direct player-to-player contact.[39]

American Football

Football is the sport associated with the greatest number of concussions in the United States, with 42.7% of high school football players reporting at least one concussion and 34.9% reporting multiple concussions.[41] Most concussions are a result of tackling, being tackled, and helmet-to-helmet impact at the top-front of the helmet during running plays, both offensive and defensive.[41,42] Recommendations for football include the following:

- Vision training intervention: A preliminary analysis of football players receiving a vision training intervention during the preseason had an 85% reduction in concussion risk.[43]
- Contact: Coaches should severely limit or remove full contact from practice.[6-8] The risk for concussion is four times higher in contact practices compared to noncontact practices.[38] In a study of high school football players, the rate of concussion was significantly lower after implementing a rule to limit the amount and duration of full-contact practice.[8]
- Position specific: Offensive linemen have the highest number of undiagnosed concussions and additional precautions should therefore be taken.[44]
- Age: Athletes younger than 14 years old (and particularly those younger than 12) should play flag football and not full-contact tackle.[45]
- Helmet-to-helmet impact, butt blocking, face tackling, and other techniques in which the helmet and facemask purposely receive the brunt of the initial impact should be discouraged in both practice and games.
- The rules prohibiting spearing should be enforced in practice and games.
- Players should avoid using their heads as battering rams when blocking, tackling, and ball carrying and keep their heads and faces out of blocking and tackling.
- Ball carriers should not lower their heads when making contact with the tackler.
- Ideally, helmets should be designed to protect the head from impact of up to 10 meters/sec, reduce linear acceleration to below 50 g, and angular acceleration to below 1,500 rads/sec^2.[46]
- All coaches, physicians, and trainers should take special care to see that the players' equipment, particularly the helmet, is properly fitted.[47]
- Neck strengthening exercises should be encouraged.[22,23]
- Any player with concussion symptoms should be examined by a member of the medical team and not be allowed to return to play until symptoms resolve.

Boxing

Boxers receive thousands of blows to the head over a typical career, and have a significantly higher risk for concussion, long-term impairment, and/or CTE. Most concussions in boxers are a result of punches directed to the side of the face or chin, such as the "hook punch" and the "upper cut," respectively.[42] Recommendations for boxing include the following:

- Changing the rules and regulations for matches, such as decreasing the number of rounds in a match or the duration of each round, as well as reducing the amount of sparring and increasing the amount of aerobic, resistive, speed, and heavy bag work.[42] Similar changes have recently been made in American-style football.
- Boxers should be examined by a member of the medical team in case of a suspected concussion.
- All boxers should be followed long term to assess for possible CTE.

Soccer

Most concussions in soccer are a result of collisions between players while attempting to head the ball, including head-to-head, elbow-to-head, fist-to-head, and foot-to-head contact.[48] Goalies have a significantly high risk of concussion.[48] Among women athletes, soccer is the sport with the highest frequency and rate of concussion.[40] Recommendations for soccer include:

- At this time, the benefit of protective headgear in soccer remains to be determined.
- Goal posts must be padded to prevent catastrophic injuries or death.

- Ball pressure should be standardized, and the ball should not be over-inflated.
- Players should be taught proper heading techniques.
- Neck strengthening exercises should be encouraged.[22,23]
- Children under 14 (and especially under 12) should be discouraged from heading the ball, and this should be considered as a new regulation in youth soccer games.
- Coaches and referees at all levels of soccer should strictly adhere to a rule change that enforces red cards for high elbows and or punches thrown during heading duels between two players for the ball.[48] There is strong evidence that enacting and enforcing this rule change significantly reduces concussion risk in soccer.[49]

Wrestling

Although the risk of concussion from wrestling is high, there exists a paucity of evidence-based recommendations for the prevention of concussion specific to wrestling. No conclusive evidence exists to support the recommendation of one type of headgear or mouthguard over another in terms of concussion prevention. Additional research is needed before specific recommendations can be made. Regardless of the lack of evidence-based guidance, protective gear should be worn in an effort to prevent more serious head and neck injuries. Coaches must be vigilant in evaluating prerequisite weight, experience, and strength before allowing an athlete to enter competition.

Baseball

In recent years, there has been a rise in the number of concussions related to baseball. Most concussions occur during a headfirst slide or when a player is struck with a thrown or batted ball. Catchers have been noted to have an increased risk for concussions, especially from foul-tipped balls, compared to other players. Recommendations for baseball include:

- Proper protection should be worn during practice and games.
- Rule changes prohibiting covering of the plate significantly reduces the risk for concussion and other injuries in baseball.[50]
- The Major League Baseball Players Association created new protocols for the league's concussion policy that established a 7-day disabled list for players with concussions. If a player has been on the list for 14 days, they will be transferred to the 15-day list to prevent further injury.
- Additionally, any player who has been diagnosed with a concussion must submit a return-to-play form to the league's medical director to be cleared to play. These guidelines should serve as examples for nonprofessional athletic associations.

Ice Hockey

Ice hockey is among the sports with the highest rate of concussion, especially among youth athletes. Body checking is associated with a significantly increased risk for concussion.[51] Recommendations for ice hockey include:

- Helmets should fit securely and be fastened tightly.
- Neck strengthening exercises should be encouraged.[22,23]
- In an effort to protect younger players, USA Hockey changed the legal age for body checking from 12 to 14 and up beginning in the 2011 to 2012 season. However, the American Academy of Pediatrics recommends delaying body checking until 15 years of age.[52] A rule change limiting body checking in youth ice hockey led to a 67% reduction in concussion risk.[8]

Cheerleading

In cheerleading, moves like tumbling runs, human pyramids, lifts, catches, and tosses have a higher risk of concussion if not performed correctly.[41] The flier position also carries an increased risk for catastrophic head and spine injuries.[41] Recommendations for cheerleading include the following:

- Pyramids over two people high should not be performed. Two-people-high pyramids should be done over mats and with proper safety precautions.
- A qualification system demonstrating the mastery of stunts is recommended.
- The coach should supervise all practices and be trained in gymnastics and cheerleading-specific safety techniques.
- The use of mini-trampolines should be prohibited.
- The safety certification by the American Association of Cheerleading Coaches and Advisors should be mandatory.

Other Sports

Some sports that lack athlete-to-athlete contact collisions, such as cycling, ice-skating, lacrosse, skiing, snowboarding, motor and equestrian sports, require protective helmets to prevent concussion and more serious head and spine injuries that occur from falling on or against a fixed surface.

LIMITATIONS AND FUTURE DIRECTIONS

- Recommendations for prevention of concussion are limited by the fact that they are generalized for all athletes, regardless of the level of play and age.
- A major issue related to enacting prevention programs, enforcing state statutes, and incorporating best practices is the associated cost. For example, effective education programs require experts in the field who can provide appropriate training to stakeholders and schools. Costs associated with sideline assessment include retaining skilled personnel who are trained to recognize subtle signs of concussion and are qualified to perform and interpret concussion screening tests.
  - Future studies would benefit from longitudinal prospective design with control groups. These studies are costly and time-consuming but are the gold standard for establishing concrete evidence.
  - Studies that compare concussion risk today with previous estimates must take into account that current improvements in sideline assessment and injury recognition likely increase current concussion risk estimates compared to decades past.

KEY POINTS

- Reducing the number and duration of full-contact practices is the most effective primary prevention intervention.
- Rapid and accurate diagnosis is an effective secondary prevention intervention.
- Football, soccer, ice hockey, and wrestling have the highest concussion rates in the United States.
- Women athletes have a higher risk for concussion than men in a given sport.
- Younger athletes have a higher risk for concussion than adults in a given sport.

STUDY QUESTIONS

1. At a follow-up visit, an athlete inquires about specific things he can do on his own to reduce his risk for a concussion in the upcoming football season. The physician highlights the limitations of concussion science but provides him with a preliminary study that reported a large risk reduction. What prevention option fits this description?
   a. Omega-3 fatty acids
   b. Custom-fitted helmet
   c. Vision training
   d. Ketogenic diet

2. The most important concussion prevention strategy is:
   a. Appropriate fitting protective equipment
   b. Increasing the age of eligibility for participation in full-contact sports
   c. Reduction of the number of contact practices
   d. Concussion education programs for teams and schools

3. In regard to soccer, what is true regarding concussion prevention?
   a. The role of protective headgear is unclear
   b. The role of gender is unclear
   c. Changing players more often during games reduces risk
   d. Covering goal posts reduces risk

4. In cheerleading, to prevent concussions, it is recommended that:
   a. Athletes properly stretch and warm up prior to practice and games
   b. Athletes properly stretch and warm up prior to two-person pyramids
   c. Programs obtain certification from the American Association of Cheerleading Coaches and Advisors
   d. Athletes obtain certification to perform complex stunts and pyramids

5. Preventing concussion is taking on greater importance because:
   a. The number of athletes that participate in contact sports has increased
   b. The treatment and management of acute and long-term effects is complicated
   c. The prevalence of Chronic Traumatic Encephalopathy is high in retired athletes
   d. The frequency of concussions has increased

ADDITIONAL READING

Teasell R, Hilditch M, Marshall S, et al. Heterotopic ossification and venous thromboembolism. In: *Evidence-Based Review of Moderate to Severe Acquired Brain Injury.* 6th ed. Module 11. https://erabi.ca/modules/module-11

Brady RD, Shultz SR, McDonald SJ, O'Brien TJ. Neurological heterotopic ossification: current understanding and future directions. *Bone.* 2018;109:35–42. doi:10.1016/j.bone.2017.05.015

Cipriano CA, Pill SG, Keenan MA. Heterotopic ossification following traumatic brain injury and spinal cord injury. *J Am Acad Orthop Surg.* 2009;17:689–697. doi:10.5435/00124635-200911000-00003

Cullen N, Bayley M, Bayona N, et al. Management of heterotopic ossification and venous thromboembolism following acquired brain injury. *Brain Inj.* 2007;21:215–230. doi:10.1080/02699050701202027

ANSWERS TO STUDY QUESTIONS

1. Correct Answer: c

   Vision training. In a study by Clark et al,[43] a preseason vision training intervention for football players was associated with an 85% concussion risk reduction. None of the other choices have been shown to reduce the risk of concussion.

   Further Reading:

   Clark JF, Graman P, Ellis JK. An exploratory study of the potential effects of vision training on concussion incidence in football. *Optometry and Visual Performance*. 2015;3(2):116–125.

2. Correct Answer: c

   New evidence from multiple studies demonstrates a clear and significant relationship between reducing the number of full-contact practices and the risk of concussion. Answer (b), increasing the age of participating in full-contact sports, is tempting but requires additional research to determine if and by how much the risk of concussion is affected. It is important that protective equipment be worn and fitted correctly (a) but evidence shows a risk reduction for catastrophic head and neck injuries more so than concussion. Education programs have not been shown to reduce the primary risk of concussion.

   Further Reading:

   Injury Prevention Legislation Database. n.d. https://www.ncsl.org/research/health/injury-prevention-legislation-database.aspx

   Kim S, Connaughton DP, Spengler J, et al. Legislative efforts to reduce concussions in youth sports: an analysis of state concussion statutes. *J Legal Aspects Sport*. 2017;27:162–168. doi:10.1123/jlas.2016-0007

   Montenigro PH, Alosco ML, Martin BM, et al. Cumulative head impact exposure predicts later-life depression, apathy, executive dysfunction, and cognitive impairment in former high school and college football players. *J Neurotrauma*. 2017;34(2):328–340. doi:10.1089/neu.2016.4413

   Montenigro PH, Bernick C, Cantu RC. Clinical features of repetitive traumatic brain injury and chronic traumatic encephalopathy. *Brain Pathol*. 2015;25(3):304–317

   Pfaller AY, Brooks MA, Hetzel S, et al. Effect of a new rule limiting full contact practice on the incidence of sport-related concussion in high school football players. *Am J Sport Med*. 2019;47(10):2294–2299. doi:10.1177/0363546519860120

   Black AM, Macpherson AK, Hagel BE, et al. Policy change eliminating body checking in non-elite ice hockey leads to a threefold reduction in injury and concussion risk in 11- and 12-year-old players. *Br J Sports Med*. 2016;50:55–61. doi:10.1136/bjsports-2015-095103

   Emery CA, Black AM, Kolstad A, et al. What strategies can be used to effectively reduce the risk of concussion in sport? A systematic review. *Br J Sports Med*. 2017;51(12), 978–984. doi:10.1136/bjsports-2016-097452

3. Correct Answer: a

   Headgear has no clear role in concussion prevention among soccer players. Answer (b) is wrong because it is known that female athletes have a greater risk than male athletes.[38] Answer (c), changing players, is hypothetical and, therefore, incorrect. Covering goalposts (d) is key to reducing catastrophic injuries and death.

Further Reading:
Clay MB, Glover KL, Lowe DT. Epidemiology of concussion in sport: a literature review. *J Chiropr Med.* 2013;12(4):230–251. doi:10.1016/j.jcm.2012.11.005

4. Correct Answer: c
   Certification by the American Association of Cheerleading Coaches and Advisors. Choices (a) and (b) are wrong because stretching has not been shown to reduce the risk of injuries. Choice (d) is wrong because no such certification for individual stunts is universal or recommended.

5. Correct Answer: b
   Treatment and management are complicated. Choice (a) is wrong because the literature reporting on changes in the number of athletes participating in different sports is conflicting. Choice (c) is wrong because the prevalence of CTE is not known. Choice (d) is wrong because the increase in frequency of concussion identified in different sports may be due to increased awareness and improved measures to diagnose concussions.

REFERENCES

The full reference list appears in the digital product found on http://connect.springer-pub.com/content/book/978-0-8261-4768-4/part/part02/chapter/ch09

SPORT-RELATED CONCUSSION II: MANAGING THE INJURED ATHLETE AND RETURN-TO-PLAY DECISION-MAKING

MARY ALEXIS IACCARINO AND ROSS ZAFONTE

BACKGROUND

As defined by the International Conference of Concussion in Sport consensus statement, a concussion is a "traumatic brain injury induced by biomechanical forces" (5th CISG).[1] It may result from a direct blow to the head or transferred force to the head from a blow to the body.[1] It results in a typical constellation of nonfocal symptoms and neurophysiological changes that are generally short lived and not associated with structural damage to the brain or abnormalities on conventional neuroimaging modalities.[1] Sport-related concussions are common. In a survey of student athletes grades 9 to 12, the Centers for Disease Control and Prevention found that 2.5 million high school students reported at least one concussion in the previous 12 months.[2] This chapter discusses assessment and management of the concussed athlete, with an emphasis on criteria and factors to consider when returning an athlete to the playing field.

Signs and Symptoms of Concussion

Observable and historical on-field or sideline signs of concussion are gait instability, a dazed or blank stare, brief confusion, slowed speech, slowed response to questions, brief anterograde amnesia, and retrograde amnesia. Traumatic loss of consciousness may occur as a part of concussion but it is not a defining clinical feature and is usually brief, only a few seconds.[3]

Symptoms reported on the sidelines include headache, feeling mentally foggy or confused, dizziness, visual symptoms, and nausea. Common symptoms reported in the first 24 hours include headache, dizziness, imbalance, nausea, fatigue, blurred vision, sensitivity to light and noise, confusion, and memory impairment. Over several days, additional symptoms of sleep disturbance, irritability, anxiety, and nervousness may occur.[4] Cognitive symptoms, such as difficulties with attention and concentration, may become apparent in the days following a concussion, particularly when the athlete returns to academic or vocational activities. It should be noted that these signs and symptoms are not unique to concussion but, when present in the context of a viable injury mechanism, concussion should be suspected, and a further assessment should be conducted to confirm the diagnosis.

The full reference list appears in the digital product found on http://connect.springerpub.com/content/book/978-0-8261-4768-4/part/part02/chapter/ch10

MANAGEMENT OF CONCUSSION

Sideline Management

Athletes suspected of concussion are removed from play for assessment and should not be allowed to return-to-play on the same day. While it was once felt that same-day return-to-play could be safe in some athletes, a more conservative approach has now been adopted. There is a subset of athletes in whom symptom recognition is delayed. The signs of concussion may not be obvious on initial sideline evaluation and may continue to evolve over time and with repeat assessment.[5] Furthermore, some athletes may underreport symptoms as they want to continue to play and may think their symptoms are mild enough that they can still play safely.

Signs that an athlete may have injuries more severe than concussion include focal neurological deficits, injury mechanism consistent with spine involvement (e.g., high velocity, fall from a height), suspected skull fracture (otorrhea, rhinorrhea, raccoon eyes, Battle's sign), bleeding from the nose or ear, and/or seizure. Initial Glasgow Coma Scale (GCS) less than 13, GCS less than 15 after 2 hours, or declining GCS is concerning for serious intracranial pathology. Athletes with these findings should undergo head and cervical spine stabilization with immediate transfer to the emergency department.[6-8]

Neuroimaging is not routinely used in concussion; when indicated, its purpose is to assess for intracranial pathology that may require neurosurgical intervention—not to make a diagnosis of concussion. Neuroimaging criteria are available that may guide decision-making for acute head injuries for children[9] and adults.[10]

Serum biomarkers are of great interest as a diagnostic tool. The combination of low serum levels of both ubiquitin carboxyl-terminal hydrolase L1 (UCHL-1) (<327 pg/mL) and glial fibrillary acidic protein (GFAP) (<22 pg/mL) within 12 hours of injury is associated with a greater than 99% probability of a negative head computed tomography (CT).[11] Within 6 hours of injury, S100B <0.10 μg/L is predictive of a negative head CT in adults. Serum biomarkers are not yet widely available for use, and they are not part of a routine concussion evaluation.[12-14]

Rest

After a concussion a period of rest is advised for athletes. The exact benefit of rest, the extent of restrictions, and duration that it should be prescribed are in question.[15] The rationale for rest after concussion is multifactorial: (a) The concussed brain is thought to be in a state of energy crisis and decreased neurometabolic demand may, theoretically, promote symptom recovery[16,17]; (b) alterations in cerebral metabolism during concussion may be amplified with overlapping injuries[18,19]; and (c) exercise after neurotrauma has suppressed markers of neuroplasticity in animal models.[20,21]

The meaning of "rest" is poorly defined, but generally includes reduced physical and cognitive activities. Cognitive rest such as staying home from school, reducing school work, limiting watching television or using electronics (computers, cell phones, games), limiting social visits, and avoiding loud noise and bright lights has unclear evidence. Thus, the prescription of rest should be directed toward limiting symptoms, while preventing social isolation and slowed progress in school. The optimal duration of rest is not known, with current recommendations based mostly on consensus. Most athletes rest for 1 to 3 days before beginning some activity.[1] There is insufficient evidence to show that prolonged periods of rest improve outcomes.[22] Furthermore, prolonged rest should be prescribed with caution as restricting athletes can lead to physiological deconditioning, depression, anxiety related to falling behind in school or work, and rumination with potential symptom amplification.[23]

Assessing Recovery

Clinical recovery is determined by (a) resolution of symptoms at rest and with physical (exercise) and cognitive (school or work) activities, (b) normalization of the physical exam, and (c) normalization of cognitive assessments. There are a variety of assessment instruments available to evaluate recovery, including the Postconcussion Symptoms Scale (PCSS), modified Balance Error Scoring System (mBESS), Standardized Assessment of Concussion (SAC), the King-Devick, ImPACT® test, Vestibular-Ocular Motor Screening (VOMS), and comprehensive neuropsychologic testing, among others. These instruments have varying degrees of reliability and validity. The mBESS, SAC, and King-Devick test have rapidly diminishing sensitivity over the first 24 to 72 hours, meaning patients may appear clinically normal on these tests but still be recovering. Due to the variability in individual tests, the most sensitive method of assessing recovery is through testing batteries that incorporate symptom scales, physical exam findings, and cognitive performance tests.[24]

Neurometabolic recovery does not necessarily correlate with clinical recovery, and diagnostic imaging studies or serological tests devised to establish a recovery trajectory are lacking. There is concern that neurometabolic recovery may lag behind clinical recovery and this is part of the rationale for a conservative approach and graded return-to-play in the asymptomatic period after concussion.[25,26]

Education and Anticipatory Guidance

A mainstay intervention in the management of concussion is athlete education. Educational interventions vary and may include one-to-one discussion with the medical provider and/or athletic trainer, handouts and brochures, referral to reliable electronic references, or a formal educational lecture. Content of educational interventions should include common symptoms, likely time course of recovery, the importance of adherence to rest and return-to-play protocols, and reassurance that the overwhelming majority of athletes make a full recovery. Careful counseling regarding potential neurological sequelae is needed to avoid elements of diagnosis threat via negative suggestion.[27,28]

Return to Learning Following Concussion

Return to the classroom is a major concern for student athletes. Normal school activities such as studying, sitting in class, looking at computers/projectors, or eating lunch in a cafeteria can be very difficult following a concussion; these activities may even exacerbate postconcussion symptoms. Teachers, parents, and other adults may not be sensitive to the discomfort of the child and may not attribute declining school performance to concussion. Although a brief absence from school may be needed for severe symptoms, return-to-school does not require the athlete to be completely symptom-free. Cognitive challenges that do not exacerbate symptoms are acceptable. Physicians should take an active role in providing a return-to-learn plan. Specific instructions should be provided to the school so that the athlete may participate as tolerated in classroom activities with accommodations and breaks when needed.[29,30] It is suggested that healthcare professionals who regularly evaluate school-age concussed patients use an accommodation form such as the one presented in Table 10.1.

All student athletes should demonstrate successful return-to-learn before returning to sports. This means that the athlete attends full days of school, completes homework and assignments without increased time, and performs at pre-concussion baseline on school exams and projects.

TABLE 10.1   **Return-to-School Accommodations Form**

Student _____ Grade ____ School _____

This student has had a concussion and may experience symptoms such as impaired concentration and memory, headache, light and noise sensitivity, dizziness, and balance problems. Please allow for the following accommodations:
___ Extra time (child may need additional time to complete assignments).
___ Please allow student to turn in assignments late.
___ Please allow student extra time to complete quizzes and tests.
___ Please allow student to take breaks if symptoms become worse.
___ Please allow student to wear sunglasses while at school.
___ Please allow student to wear ear plugs while at school.
___ Please allow student/parent to meet with guidance counselor/teachers to develop a make-up/keep-up plan for necessary assignments.
___ Student should not be required to complete standardized testing until _____.
___ This student should not be attending gym or should not be allowed to participate in physical activities during recess.
___ This student can tolerate low-level physical activities such as walking.
___ This student can participate in physical exertion but not in group physical activities.
___ This student can participate fully in gym.

Exercise and Return-to-Play Guidelines

Exercise has emerged as a potential treatment intervention for the athlete recovering from concussion. Engagement in aerobic exercise at a level that does not produce or exacerbate concussion symptoms has been found to be safe[31,32] and may hasten recovery in athletes.[33,34] Notably, the timing and intensity of exercise is not yet clear. Studies of athletes in the subacute period (about 4 weeks post-injury) show symptom reduction at a greater rate in a group that exercises using aerobics over a stretching program.[33] A recent study of acutely concussed athletes showed that when aerobic exercise was initiated in the first 7 days post-injury, time to recovery was shortened.[34] As such, it is reasonable to allow athletes to begin light aerobic exercise early in the recovery period. Early exercise should be under the supervision of a medical provider to guide and assess level of intensity of exercise and the athlete's response. Exercise protocols have been proposed to guide athletes and medical staff.[35]

Athletes must progress through a graduated return-to-play program before returning to contact sports. This begins with light aerobic exercise followed by a stepwise increase in physical exertion.[1] Each step should be separated by at least 24 hours. Any recurrence of postconcussion symptoms at a level of exertion requires the athlete to return to the previous level. For example, if an athlete is asymptomatic while riding a stationary bike (Stage 2) but develops a headache with running drills (Stage 3), then the athlete should return to biking (see Table 10.2).

For an athlete to return-to-play, they must complete the graded return-to-play protocol without symptoms and demonstrate baseline neuropsychological test performance, when such data are available. Careful attention should be paid to any medications the athlete may be taking that can ameliorate postconcussion symptoms. In general, these medications should be discontinued prior to return-to-play. However, there may be unique cases, such as an athlete with a preexisting headache disorder, in which ongoing pharmacotherapy is appropriate.

TABLE 10.2   Return-to-Play Protocol

Initial Management Following Injury

When a player shows any symptoms or signs of a concussion, the following should be applied:
The player should not be allowed to return to play the same day as the concussion.
Regular monitoring for deterioration is essential over the initial few hours after injury.
The player should be medically evaluated after the injury.
Return-to-play must follow a medically supervised stepwise process.
A player should never return to play while symptomatic.

Return-to-Play Protocol
Return-to-play after a concussion follows a stepwise process:
Stage 1: Symptom-limited activities such as daily household activities. **Goal:** Initiation of return to work and school.
Stage 2: Light aerobic exercise such as walking or stationary cycling, no resistance training. **Goal:** Increase heart rate.
Stage 3: Sport-specific exercise, for example, skating in hockey, running in soccer. **Goal:** Add movement.
Stage 4: Noncontact training drills, for example, passing drills, stick drills. Begin progressive resistance training. **Goal:** Physical and cognitive stress.
Stage 5: Full contact practice, after medical clearance. **Goal:** Restore confidence and assess skills.
Stage 6: Game play.
With this stepwise progression, the athlete should proceed to the next level if asymptomatic at the current stage. At a minimum, 1 day between stages is recommended. If postconcussion symptoms recur, the patient should drop back to the previous asymptomatic stage for 1 day and then try to progress again.

Source: Adapted from McCrory P, Meeuwisse W, Dvorak J, et al. Consensus statement on concussion in sport—the 5th International Conference on Concussion in Sport held in Berlin, October 2016. *Br J Sports Med.* 2017;51(11):838–847. doi:10.1136/bjsports-2017-097878

FACTORS THAT INFLUENCE RECOVERY

Most athletes clinically recover from concussion within 4 weeks following injury, with a minority of patients experiencing symptoms beyond 4 weeks.[1,36–38] Identifying factors that may influence recovery times can help guide concussion management. A brief review of factors that may affect recovery from concussion follows.

Age

In general, it is felt that young athletes recover more slowly than professional or adult athletes. Multiple studies show prolonged time to recovery on neuropsychological testing in high school athletes as compared to college and professional athletes.[37,39–41] Proposed theories regarding increased time to recovery in children include (a) increased sensitivity to glutamate, an excitatory neurotransmitter released during concussion; (b) increased rotational forces on the brain due to increased head-to-neck size ratio; and (c) inability to anticipate and brace for high-impact force.[26,42] Within the youth athlete population, age and recovery time may not have a linear relationship. A study of children evaluated in the emergency department after concussion found that at 4-week follow-up more children 13- to 17-years-old continued to report symptoms than those under 13 years.[43] Factors that may influence observed recovery times in children include the limited ability of young children to perceive and communicate symptoms as well as external influences on older adolescents such as psychosocial factors and academic pressures that may exacerbate symptoms.

In general, young athletes are managed more conservatively than adults, with a primary goal of returning to school, not necessarily returning to sports. There is also concern that a repeat concussion could result in potentially fatal, massive cerebral edema. This is a rare but devastating phenomenon and the overwhelming majority of cases are reported in young athletes.[44] (See also Chapter 11 for a more detailed discussion on this topic.)

Gender

Large-scale epidemiological studies have reported that females have a higher rate of concussion in sports.[45,46] The potential reasons for this gender difference are not clear. A variation in neck strength between males and females is one hypothesis that has been suggested. There may also be gender-specific differences in brain physiology that may contribute to these findings.[42,47,48] Finally, females may be more likely to report concussion, while males are more likely to underreport.[24] Symptomatology may also vary by gender. In comparison studies in high school and college athletes, females had differences in reported baseline symptoms (particularly headaches) and baseline and post-injury neuropsychological test outcomes compared to males.[49–52] Further research is needed to better understand the factors involved in these apparent gender differences.

Prior Concussion History

A history of prior concussion may impact recovery, with successive concussions being associated with increased baseline symptoms, prolonged postconcussion symptoms, and increased recovery time.[53,54] Two prospective studies, one on collegiate football players and the other on ice hockey players, found that those with three or more concussions had prolonged symptoms and delayed recovery as compared to those with fewer than three concussions.[55,56] Despite ongoing research, there is neither a consensus nor an evidence-based threshold defining the number of concussions for which athletes should be disqualified from sports. Multiple factors should be considered when determining return-to-play after multiple concussions, including symptom severity, symptom duration, time to complete recovery, and athlete's desire to continue in that sport, recognizing that those athletes who experience severe and long-standing symptoms after only mild impacts may not be well suited for contact sports.

Symptom Burden

Symptom burden has been found to be associated with prolonged recovery course in concussion. The PCSS is a self-reported, 7-point Likert scale that grades severity of 22 concussion symptoms. In a series of studies of youth through young adult athletes, higher overall score on the PCSS at initial clinical visit was an independent predictor of prolonged symptoms after concussion.[57,58] Delayed recognition of symptoms was also found to be a risk factor for prolonged symptoms, perhaps due to delayed diagnosis and continued play despite being concussed.[59]

Additional Factors

- *Migraine:* History of pre-injury migraine headache may complicate recovery although evidence for migraine as a risk factor for prolonged recovery is mixed.[59,60] The presence of posttraumatic migraine headache is associated with cognitive impairment and a protracted recovery from concussion.[61]

■ *Dizziness:* The presence of dizziness may be a predictor of prolonged symptoms after concussion. In a study of high school football players who sustained concussions, dizziness as an initial on-field symptom was the only symptom that predicted a protracted recovery (greater than 21 days).[62]

■ *Attention deficit hyperactivity disorder (ADHD):* ADHD may be a risk factor for sustaining concussion. Studies comparing student athletes with ADHD with student athletes without ADHD found athletes with ADHD reported more concussions, athletes with concussions had a higher rate of ADHD, and concussed athletes with ADHD had more concussion symptom reporting than concussed athletes without ADHD.[63,64] Evidence of ADHD as a risk factor for prolonged concussion symptoms is mixed and may be confounded by high "concussion-like" symptom reporting in those with ADHD that are not concussed.[60,65]

■ *Mood disorder:* Personal or family history of depression or other mood disorders was associated with prolonged postconcussion symptoms in athletes aged 9 to 18 years.[59] In general, personal history of pre-injury depression or psychiatric disease is associated with development of post-injury psychiatric disease after a traumatic brain injury.

■ *Genetics:* Genetic factors are postulated to play a role in recovery. In particular, the ApoE-4 allele, a marker associated with expression of Alzheimer's disease, has been of interest. The ApoE-4 allele is postulated to be a risk factor for prolonged recovery and may be associated with chronic cognitive symptoms after concussion.[53,66] However, studies on this topic have yielded mixed results and more research is needed in this area.

KEY POINTS

■ Athletes demonstrating signs or symptoms of concussion should be evaluated by medical staff and should not return to play the same day.

■ A period of rest, that is, reduced cognitive and physical activity, is recommended for athletes recovering from concussion, although the type of restrictions and exact duration of rest is not well defined in the medical literature.

■ A battery of testing focused on balance, symptom severity, and cognitive function is used to assess recovery. Anticipatory guidance and education may assist in managing expectations of recovery.

■ Athletes should follow a stage-based return-to-play exercise protocol. Student athletes should have successful return to learning before returning to play.

STUDY QUESTIONS

1. Which of the following is not thought to influence an athlete's recovery from concussion?
   a. Gender
   b. Age
   c. Past medical history of migraine
   d. Type of sport in which injury occurred

2. Which of the following statements regarding exercise and sport concussion is true?
    a. After a concussion, athletes should not begin exercise until they have completed a substantial period of rest and concussion symptoms have resolved
    b. Aerobic exercise may reduce the time to clinical recovery in athletes with concussion
    c. In the return-to-play progression, exercises, such as weightlifting and strength training, precede aerobic exercise training
    d. Exercising below the symptom threshold is an insufficient intensity to enhance concussion recovery

3. Which of the following is NOT consistent with a diagnosis of concussion?
    a. A football player suffers a blow to the body and falls to the ground. He does not strike his head but is dazed, dizzy, and mildly confused immediately after the event
    b. A soccer player sustains a head-to-head collision. She continues to play but at half time begins to have a headache and nausea. She performs poorly on balance and cognitive testing
    c. A student athlete completes a season of ice hockey. Two months later he develops a headache, nausea, and light sensitivity. He has a family history of migraine headache
    d. A snowboarder crashes after a missed landing on a half-pipe. He is unconscious for 3 minutes and upon awakening is confused, does not follow the instructions of the ski patrol, and opens his eyes only to sternal rub
    e. c and d

4. Early management of a concussed athlete includes all of the following EXCEPT:
    a. Removal from play
    b. Education of the athlete regarding symptom mitigation and natural course of recovery
    c. CT scan of the head to determine if concussion occurred
    d. A brief period of relative rest followed by gradual return to usual daily activities such as school or work

5. Which of the following injury-related factors is associated with longer recovery after concussion?
    a. Loss of consciousness
    b. Low score on the PCSS
    c. Dizziness immediately after the injury
    d. A head-to-head collision

ADDITIONAL READING

CDC's Heads Up on Brain Injury: Concussion in Sports. http://www.cdc.gov/concussion/sports/index.html
Review of Assessment Scales for Diagnosing and Monitoring Sports-Related Concussion. *https://www.ncbi.nlm.nih.gov/pmc/articles/PMC5802754/*
Collins M, Iverson G, Gaetz M, et al. Sport related concussion. In: Zasler N, Katz D, Zafonte R, eds. *Brain Injury Medicine,* 2nd ed. Demos Medical; 2013:498–516. doi:10.1891/9781617050572.0031
Ontario Neurotrauma Foundation. *Guidelines for Concussion/Mild Traumatic Brain Injury & Persistent Symptoms.* 2018; *https://braininjuryguidelines.org/concussion/*
McCrory P, Meeuwisse W, Dvorak J, et al. Consensus statement on concussion in sport-the 5th International Conference on Concussion in Sport held in Berlin, October 2016. *Br J Sports Med.* 2017;51(11):838–847. doi:10.1136/bjsports-2017-097878

ANSWERS TO STUDY QUESTIONS

1. Correct Answer: d
   There are a variety of factors that may influence concussion recovery including gender, age, and premorbid migraine headaches.

   Further Reading:
   Iverson GL, Gardner AJ, Terry DP, et al. Predictors of clinical recovery from concussion: a systematic review. *Br J Sports Med.* 2017;51(12):941–948. doi:10.1136/bjsports-2017-097729
   Kontos AP, Elbin RJ, Lau B, et al. Posttraumatic migraine as a predictor of recovery and cognitive impairment after sport-related concussion. *Am J Sports Med.* 2013;41(7):1497–1504. doi:10.1177/0363546513488751

2. Correct Answer: b
   Sub-symptom threshold aerobic exercise initiated in the first 7 days postconcussion has been shown to shorten recovery time.

   Further Reading:
   McCrory P, Meeuwisse W, Dvorak J, et al. Consensus statement on concussion in sport—the 5th International Conference on Concussion in Sport held in Berlin, October 2016. *Br J Sports Med.* 2017;51(11):838–847. doi:10.1136/bjsports-2017-097878

3. Correct Answer: e
   The skier has a GCS score of 11, compatible with a moderate traumatic brain injury, not a concussion. Loss of consciousness can occur in concussion but is not required for a diagnosis of concussion. The ice hockey player may be experiencing a migraine headache. Headaches are a symptom of concussion but should begin proximate to the time (minutes to hours) that a blow to the head or body occurs.

   Further Reading:
   McCrory P, Meeuwisse W, Dvorak J, et al. Consensus statement on concussion in sport-the 5th International Conference on Concussion in Sport held in Berlin, October 2016. *Br J Sports Med.* 2017;51(11):838–847. doi:10.1136/bjsports-2017-097878

4. Correct Answer: c
   Concussion is a clinical diagnosis. At present there is no single diagnostic test that can diagnose or exclude concussion. CT scans are used to assess for intracranial trauma that is more severe than concussion or may require neurosurgical assessment such as skull fracture or intracranial hemorrhage.

   Further Reading:
   Kuppermann N, Holmes JF, Dayan PS, et al. Identification of children at very low risk of clinically important brain injuries after head trauma: a prospective cohort study. *Lancet.* 2009;374(9696):1160–1170. doi:10.1016/S0140-6736(09)61558-0

5. Correct Answer: c
   On-field dizziness is associated with more protracted recovery after concussion. While once thought to be a measure of more severe injury, loss of consciousness does not seem to predict recovery time. Prolonged recovery is associated with more severe symptoms at time of injury (higher score on the PCSS). Head-to-head injury mechanism is not specifically associated with prolonged recovery.

Further Reading:
Lau BC, Kontos AP, Collins MW, et al. Which on-field signs/symptoms predict protracted recovery from sport-related concussion among high school football players? *Am J Sports Med.* 2011;39(11):2311–2318. doi:10.1177/0363546511410655

REFERENCES

The full reference list appears in the digital product found on http://connect.springer-pub.com/content/book/978-0-8261-4768-4/part/part02/chapter/ch10

11 SECOND IMPACT SYNDROME

GARY GOLDBERG AND WILLIAM A. ROBBINS

GENERAL PRINCIPLES

Definition

Second Impact Syndrome (SIS) refers to rapid development of cerebral hyperemia (CHE) leading to diffuse cerebral swelling (DCS) when an individual suffers a second traumatic brain injury (TBI) before symptoms related to an earlier initial TBI have fully resolved.[1,2] The second injury typically occurs within 2 weeks after the first impact, with the clinical response being well out of proportion to the severity of the second trauma, presumably related to unresolved pathophysiology from the preceding TBI. SIS occurs in the context of sport-related concussions, arising most often in contact sports.[3]

In the pediatric literature, a similar phenomenon in which CHE precipitates post-traumatic DCS has been called the "syndrome of malignant brain edema (SMBE),"[4] a condition for which a solitary TBI suffices. A typically reversible exaggerated neurological response to head trauma in children, linked to enhanced cortical spreading depression (CSD) and CHE, has been termed "juvenile head trauma syndrome (JHTS)."[5] The CHE-related neurological impairment associated with SMBE and JHTS is a rare but generally acknowledged clinical phenomenon, occurring in children and adolescents, where widespread cortical impairment ensues in the context of persisting excessive vasodilation (EVD), CHE, and increased intracranial blood volume.[4,5,6]

The presumed significant pathophysiologic overlap among these three entities, along with limited data from the few fully documented published cases of SIS, mean that the scientific underpinning of SIS prevention, the primary driver of postconcussion return-to-play guidelines and concussion legislation, is somewhat speculative.[7] Several papers have pointed to the questionable evidence of the existence of SIS as a distinct diagnostic entity.[8–12] In addressing this controversy (i.e., whether these are distinctly different phenomena), one may reconceptualize SIS as a particularly rare but especially severe and frequently lethal variant of traumatically induced CHE leading to DCS, with increased vulnerability and amplification of the pathophysiology conferred by the unresolved preceding concussion. One may consider JHTS, SMBE, and SIS as entities with a common pathophysiology on a spectrum of increasing irreversibility and severity, respectively.

The uniquely poor prognosis in SIS may be linked to persistent "second-impact dysautoregulation,"[13] wherein the frequent presence of a typically insubstantial thin subdural hemorrhage (SDH) precipitates and/or magnifies this pathophysiological process.[14–16]

Epidemiology

True SIS is exceedingly rare. While the risk of sport-related concussion is estimated to be three to six per 100 player-seasons and concussions resulting in death or major disability

The full reference list appears in the digital product found on http://connect.springerpub.com/content/book/978-0-8261-4768-4/part/part02/chapter/ch11

occur once every 20,500 player-seasons, true SIS has an estimated incidence of a single case in every 1.8 million player-seasons.[17] From 1984 to 2011, the U.S. National Center for Catastrophic Sports Injury Research in Chapel Hill, North Carolina, identified 164 cases of significant brain injury with incomplete recovery occurring in high school and college football.[18] This survey reported a single true case of SIS, in a 15-year-old who required surgery to evacuate an SDH after suffering a concussion in a head-to-head tackle while still symptomatic from a witnessed concussion that occurred 3 weeks prior.[18]

In a recent systematic review of the literature from 1996 to 2015, a total of 17 cases of reported SIS met criteria of two witnessed concussions with persistent symptoms documented across the interval between the first and second concussions.[11] All cases involved male athletes and 10 (59%) occurred in American football. All individuals who died or were left with permanent disability were younger than 20 years of age, while four of the five individuals with the best outcomes in this series were over the age of 20 years.[11] More recently, a very detailed case report from Canada of a clear-cut lethal occurrence of SIS was reported in a 17-year-old female rugby player. This account included eyewitness descriptions of the reference injury, hospital course including left hemicraniectomy and evacuation of a small SDH, and autopsy findings as well as a report from a subsequent coroner's inquest.[16] She had not reported prior symptoms to anyone in a position of authority but text messages to friends recovered from her mobile phone documented continuing symptoms including headaches from two prior undiagnosed concussions that had occurred during play within 10 days prior to the SIS-inducing injury. Concussion legislation in the province of Ontario where this case occurred was subsequently passed into law, the first such legislation in Canada.[19]

The scenario in which a young, previously healthy individual suffers rapid and dramatic neurological deterioration indicates that SIS and other injuries in which DCS develops must still be considered a very serious and potentially avoidable consequence of head trauma. While rigorously documented cases of SIS may be rare, the general notion that an individual should not be permitted to re-engage in high-risk activity until postconcussion symptoms have completely resolved remains difficult to refute.[20,21]

Pathophysiology

Initial transient responses to a significant concussion can involve brief cerebral vasodilatation and increased intracranial blood volume. To counteract the tidal wave of blood being pumped to the head by the stress-induced cardiovascular reaction, an initial autoregulatory acute "phase I" cerebrovascular response involves intense vasoconstriction and a resulting reduction in cerebrovascular capacitance with lowered intracranial blood volume.

An outright failure or insufficient persistence of this phase I reaction, however, leads to EVD, engorgement of the cerebral vasculature, massive CHE, and progressive DCS with vasogenic followed by cytotoxic edema. Elevation of intracranial pressure (ICP) then precipitates rapidly, developing inferomedial herniation of the medial temporal lobes and brainstem compression.[21,22] The interval from impact to clinical manifestations of brainstem compression in full-blown SIS can be less than 5 minutes.[21] The intracranial manifestations of DCS, including herniation and potential intracranial hemorrhage, can be demonstrated on computed tomography (CT) and magnetic resonance imaging (MRI) when imaging is obtained.[22]

Following the phase I response, a subacute phase II response involves a state of altered cerebral metabolism that may last for several days, involving decreased protein synthesis and reduced oxidative capacity.[23] Heightened vulnerability of the brain during this subacute phase of recovery is associated with relative inhibition of the acute vasoconstrictive phase I response that would normally prevent CHE, thus leading to an increased risk of CHE triggered by a second insult. At least two case series[14,15] and more recent case reports of confirmed SIS[16,24] have identified SDH as a significant factor contributing to failure of the phase I response, resulting in EVD and massive CHE. One case report suggests that early evacuation of an SDH may have a beneficial impact in SIS.[25]

Another factor which may contribute to phase I failure is migraine-linked posttraumatic dysautoregulation of cerebral blood flow[13] possibly involving the trigeminovascular (TGV) system (TGVS).[26] Persistent posttraumatic headache may be a particularly important indicator of increased second impact risk, given that vascular headache and JHTS are both thought to be related to a common pathophysiological mechanism involving anomalous TGV activation.[27,28] The TGVS is directly involved in powerfully biasing toward EVD when the trigeminoparasympathetic (TGPS) reflex is abnormally activated by head trauma, stimulating sensory afferents traversing the trigeminal ganglion.[28] This TGVS-associated EVD has been proposed as the underlying mechanism initiating CHE-related neurological impairment in JHTS.[28,29] Given that sensory collaterals of these same trigeminal ganglion cells innervate vessels in the overlying dura, even a small amount of subdural blood may irritate these autonomic afferents, provoking and potentiating the TGPS reflex response to trauma and amplifying the EVD that initiates this pathophysiological cascade.[29] This, in turn, may explain the frequent incidence of SDH in SIS. It also suggests that substances like calcitonin gene-related protein (CGRP) antagonists which block TGVS-associated EVD may prevent or slow posttraumatic CGRP-related EVD and the ominous progression to DCS.[12] While TGPS activation and related amplification of EVD as a putative pathophysiologic mechanism seems plausible, data directly supporting it remains limited at this time.

In SIS, progression from EVD to CHE to DCS to herniation can take place with dramatic neurologic deterioration occurring after an initial brief, often momentary, period of wakefulness following minor head trauma, a clinical scenario that has been labeled "talk and die."[21,30,31] With a coincident history of familial hemiplegic migraine, delayed neurologic deterioration unfolds in the presence of a specific gene mutation affecting the configuration and function of voltage-sensitive calcium channels in the cerebral cortex.[32,33] While this is a very rare genetic condition, it suggests that vascular headache, JHTS, SMBE, and SIS may share a common pathway leading to DCS precipitated by trauma-induced EVD, CHE, and augmented CSD. A recent observational case-control study of 1,342 children presenting with mild head trauma for emergency care found that the proportion of the 33 (2.5%) children diagnosed with JHTS who had first-degree relatives with migraine was significantly greater than that for children without JHTS (odds ratio 2.69; 95% confidence interval 1.16–6.22; $p = .010$).[34]

DIAGNOSIS

History

- SIS is a rare, life-threatening neurological emergency that occurs in the general context of concussion assessment and management in children and adolescents.[35]
- SIS is established through documentation of two separate sequential brain injury events with unresolved symptoms of the first brain injury persisting through to the second. Stringent diagnostic criteria for SIS require that the initial injury be witnessed and medically assessed with confirmed symptomatology persisting through to the second witnessed impact.[20]
- SIS is distinguished from repetitive head injury syndrome (RHIS) or Chronic Traumatic Encephalopathy (CTE), in which a person sustains several repeated mild traumatic brain injuries (MTBIs) spread out over time and, as a result, experiences a gradual decline in cognitive, affective, and behavioral function (see Chapter 56).

Clinical Presentation

- In the typical presentation, postconcussion symptoms occur after an initial MTBI, but before these symptoms resolve, a second relatively minor blow to the head occurs, frequently without immediate loss of consciousness.
- The individual may appear dazed or confused, but remains awake, verbal, and ambulatory. However, over the next few seconds to minutes, dramatic clinical deterioration ensues.
- There is a precipitous neurological decline with the development of a semicomatose state with rapidly dilating pupils, limited spontaneous eye movement, and respiratory failure.

Physical Examination

- In the unconscious athlete, prompt assessment and stabilization of airway, breathing, and circulation; placement of a cervical collar; and spine precautions are essential.
- Careful neurologic examination is performed including assessment of brainstem function and Glasgow Coma Scale score.
- Examination should focus on identifying evidence of elevated ICP (pupillary response, papilledema, obtundation, etc.).

Neuroimaging Assessment

- CT scan: Rules out structural damage such as intracranial hemorrhage,[36] most typically an acute SDH.
- MRI: Offers more structural detail to aid in detecting subtle structural changes associated with raised ICP and herniation but requires significantly more time to complete than CT. More advanced MR-based techniques such as perfusion MRI using arterial spin labeling and diffusion weighted imaging are promising research tools, but not relevant to routine clinical practice at this juncture.[36]
- CT angiography and perfusion scanning: Not routinely indicated after MTBI, but may be considered in situations in which this study capability is readily available, particularly if assessing cerebral blood flow patterns may alter management or if there is a concern about associated cerebrovascular anomalies.

Autopsy Findings

- Diagnosis is definitively made at autopsy: The brain shows diffuse and extensive CHE and DCS, often with evidence of transtentorial herniation.

PROGNOSIS

- SIS is linked to a common pathophysiological process shared with vascular headache, JHTS, SMBE, and "big black brain" syndrome in infants, seen most often in the context of non-accidental repetitive trauma.[37] In SIS, the susceptibility to trauma-induced EVD is significantly increased by the residual effects of the initial brain injury.
- The presence of subdural blood worsens the prognosis by further amplifying trauma-induced EVD, possibly through stimulation of autonomic sensory afferents from trigeminal ganglion cells innervating dural vessels, producing intensification of the TGPS reflex response.

■ Prognosis varies with the rapidity and degree to which this process irreversibly progresses from EVD and CHE to DCS, elevated ICP, and herniation. In JHTS, the neurological impairment is typically transient and usually fully reversible within 24 hours, while in SIS it progresses rapidly and irreversibly with devastating consequences, including 50% mortality, with most survivors left with significant permanent neurological disability.

TREATMENT

■ Treatment must be intensive and cannot be delayed.
■ The patient should be immediately stabilized with emphasis on airway management, and neurosurgery consulted.
■ Rapidly intubate and institute measures to reduce elevated ICP.
■ Treatment of impaired autoregulation of cerebral vasculature in true SIS may be difficult or impossible.
■ Emergent decompressive craniectomy and/or craniotomy with evacuation of SDH can be a lifesaving measure.[25]

PREVENTION OF SECOND IMPACT SYNDROME IN SPORTS

■ The best way to prevent SIS is to reduce the overall incidence of concussion in contact sports through protective equipment, education, and enforcement of rules designed to reduce the likelihood of significant injury (see Chapter 9).
■ **Any athlete who remains symptomatic following a concussion should not be allowed to return to play**. If symptom reporting is unreliable or the truthfulness of the patient's own report of symptoms is in question, remember: *"When in doubt, sit them out."*
■ Multiple clinical guidelines have been published advising on the timing of return-to-play and level of participation following a concussion. Such guidelines exist, at least in part, to prevent SIS.
■ Physicians with experience in concussion recognition and management should be consulted to evaluate athletes before return-to-play is authorized, in full compliance with concussion legislation that now exists in every state including the District of Columbia.
■ There is a tendency for athletes to minimize and underreport persisting postconcussion symptoms, particularly under circumstances where there are significant competitive stakes involved.[38] Education (beginning in the preseason) for the athlete[39] and family members is essential. Education for officials and coaching staff is also very important.

KEY POINTS

■ SIS is a rare but devastating and often fatal condition in which the brain swells rapidly after a person suffers a second blow to the head before symptoms from a previous brain injury have completely resolved.
■ SIS almost always occurs in children and adolescents, overlapping with JHTS, with which it may share a common pathophysiological process, although JHTS, by definition, follows a solitary head trauma.

> ▪ The underlying pathophysiology of SIS is amplified in the presence of SDH.
> ▪ Emergency measures supporting basic life functions and attempting to reduce elevated ICP are critical. Neurosurgical consultation to consider emergent decompressive craniectomy with evacuation of SDH if present can be lifesaving.
> ▪ Survivors of SIS are invariably left with irreversible neurological impairment, while those who sustain JHTS typically are not.
> ▪ The definitive and only really pragmatic approach to SIS is primary prevention. This necessitates timely and accurate concussion diagnosis, patient education, and use of structured return-to-play protocols.

STUDY QUESTIONS

1. A most often reversible exaggerated response to head trauma in children has been termed:
   a. "Big black brain"
   b. Second Impact Syndrome
   c. Syndrome of malignant brain edema
   d. Juvenile head trauma syndrome
   e. Trigeminal parasympathetic reflex response

2. The main difficulty in establishing a diagnosis of Second Impact Syndrome is:
   a. Demonstrating the presence of a subdural hemorrhage on neuroimaging
   b. Documenting the occurrence of an initial concussion with persisting symptoms
   c. Demonstrating dysregulation of cerebral blood flow
   d. Demonstrating that symptoms are disproportionate to the severity of the head trauma
   e. Demonstrating typical neuropathological findings on autopsy

3. Persistent posttraumatic headache may be an important indicator of increased risk of a subsequent exaggerated response to head trauma because it is consistent with:
   a. Anomalous function of the trigeminovascular system
   b. Significant irritation of the cerebral meninges
   c. Relative cortical ischemia and underperfusion
   d. Reduced sensitivity of the trigeminoparasympathetic reflex response to trauma
   e. Presence of a small subdural hemorrhage due to the injury

4. Vascular headache, juvenile head trauma syndrome, syndrome of malignant brain edema, and Second Impact Syndrome may all:
   a. Be entirely unrelated in terms of their underlying pathophysiology
   b. Share a common pathway
   c. Involve individuals of all ages
   d. Produce severe permanent neurological disability
   e. Be associated with cerebral vasoconstriction

5. The presence of subdural hemorrhage in suspected Second Impact Syndrome is associated with:
   a. Amplified trauma-induced excessive cerebrovascular dilatation

   b. Stimulation of autonomic sensory afferents from dural blood vessels
   c. Intensification of the trigeminal parasympathetic reflex response
   d. Worsening of prognosis
   e. All of the above

ADDITIONAL READING

Cantu RC, Gean AD. Second-impact syndrome and a small subdural hematoma: an uncommon catastrophic result of repetitive head injury with a characteristic imaging appearance. *J Neurotrauma.* 2010;27:1557–1564. doi:10.1089/neu.2010.1334

Engelhardt J, Brauge D, Loiseau H. Second impact syndrome. myth or reality? *Neurochirurgie.* 2020; S0028-3770(20)30033-3. doi:10.1016/j.neuchi.2019.12.007

May T, Foris LA, Donnally CJ. Second Impact Syndrome. *StatPearls* [Internet]. https://www.ncbi.nlm.nih.gov/books/NBK448119/

McLendon LA, Kralik SF, Grayson PA, Golomb MR. The controversial second impact syndrome. A review of the literature. *Pediatr Neurol.* 2016;62:9–17. doi:10.1016/j.pediatrneurol.2016.03.009

McCrory P, Davis G, Makdissi M. Second impact syndrome or cerebral swelling after sporting head injury. *Curr Sports Med Rep.* 2012;11:21–23. doi:10.1249/JSR.0b013e3182423bfd

ANSWERS TO STUDY QUESTIONS

1. Correct Answer: d
Answers (a), (b), and (c) are all generally associated with a nonreversible grave outcome. (e) is a postulated element of the response to head trauma in general, not specifically in children, and is not specifically linked to reversibility. Juvenile head trauma syndrome is a generally reversible exaggerated response to trauma in children that is proposed to be linked to susceptibility to migraine headache.

Further Reading:
Haas DC, Pineda GS, Lourie H. Juvenile head trauma syndromes and their relationship to migraine. *Arch Neurol.* 1975;32:727–730. doi:10.1001/archneur.1975.00490530049003
van der Veek EM, Oosterhoff M, Vos PE, Hageman G. The juvenile head trauma syndrome: a trauma triggered migraine? *Neuropediatrics.* 2015;46:116–122. doi:10.1055/s-0035-1547344

2. Correct Answer: b
Second Impact Syndrome (SIS) requires the establishment of a diagnosis of a prior concussion that continues to be symptomatic when the reference concussion occurs. The main difficulty in rigorously identifying a particular case as SIS is documentation of the prior concussion since it may not have been "officially" diagnosed but remains unreported. The other answers are evidence of possible pathophysiological components of SIS but are not necessary for the establishment of the clinical diagnosis.

Further Reading:
Saunders RL, Harbaugh RE. The second impact in catastrophic contact-sports head trauma. *JAMA.* 1984;252(4):538–539. doi:10.1001/jama.1984.03350040068030
Bey T, Ostick B. Second impact syndrome. *Western J Emerg Med.* 2009;10:6–10.
Byard RW, Vink R. The second impact syndrome. *Forensic Sci Med Pathol.* 2009;5:36–38. doi:10.1007/s12024-008-9063-7

McLendon LA, Kralik SF, Grayson PA, Golomb MR. The controversial second impact syndrome. A review of the literature. *Pediatr Neurol.* 2016;62:9–17. doi:10.1016/j.pediatrneurol.2016.03.009

Engelhardt J, Brauge D, Loiseau H. Second impact syndrome. Myth or reality? *Neurochirurgie.* 2020;S0028-3770(20)30033-3. doi:10.1016/j.neuchi.2019.12.007

3. Correct Answer: a

Anomalous function of the trigeminovascular system has been associated with migraine headache, and susceptibility to migraine headache is a presumed risk factor for exaggerated responses to trauma. Answer (d) is incorrect because it is likely that, if anything, there is increased sensitivity of the trigeminoparasympathetic reflex response to trauma with persistent posttraumatic headache. A small subdural hemorrhage may be present and produces an enhanced sensitivity of the trigeminoparasympathetic reflex but it is not necessarily present.

Further Reading:

Engelhardt J, Brauge D, Loiseau H. Second impact syndrome. Myth or reality? *Neurochirurgie.* 2020;S0028-3770(20)30033-3. doi:10.1016/j.neuchi.2019.12.007

May A, Goadsby PJ. The trigeminovascular system in humans. Pathophysiologic implications for primary headache syndromes of the neural influences on the cerebral circulation. *J Cerebral Blood Flow Metab.* 1999;19:115–127. doi:10.1097/00004647-199902000-00001

Sakas DE, Whitwell HL. Neurological episodes after minor head injury and trigeminovascular activation. *Med Hypotheses.* 1997;48:431–435. doi:10.1016/S0306-9877(97)90042-6

Sakas DE, Whittaker KW, Whitwell HL, Singounas EG. Syndromes of posttraumatic neurological deterioration in children with no focal lesions revealed by cerebral imaging: evidence for a trigeminovascular pathophysiology. *Neurosurgery.* 1997;41:661–667. doi:10.1097/00006123-199709000-00031

Squier W, Mack J, Green A, et al. The pathophysiology of brain swelling associated with subdural hemorrhage: the role of the trigeminovascular system. *Child's Nerv Syst.* 2012;28:2005–2015. doi:10.1007/s00381-012-1870-1

4. Correct Answer: b

Each of these conditions may involve some type of cerebral blood flow dysregulation that leads to altered brain hemodynamics and edema formation. Answer (b) is obviously incorrect since these conditions are presumably related. Answer (c) is incorrect since these conditions involve children and adolescents typically. Answer (d) is incorrect since juvenile head trauma syndrome typically produces a reversible neurological deficit. Answer (e) is incorrect since there may be cerebral vasodilatation leading to diffuse cerebral edema as a pathophysiological process.

Further Reading:

Saunders RL, Harbaugh RE. The second impact in catastrophic contact-sports head trauma. *JAMA.* 1984;252(4):538–539. doi:10.1001/jama.1984.03350040068030

Bey T, Ostick B. Second impact syndrome. *Western J Emerg Med.* 2009;10:6–10.

Bruce DA, Alavi A, Balanuik L, et al. Diffuse cerebral swelling following head injuries in children: the syndrome of "malignant brain edema." *J Neurosurg.* 1981;54:170–178. doi:10.3171/jns.1981.54.2.0170

Haas DC, Pineda GS, Lourie H. Juvenile head trauma syndromes and their relationship to migraine. *Arch Neurol.* 1975;32:727–730. doi:10.1001/archneur.1975.00490530049003

5. Correct Answer: e
Answers (a) through (d) can be associated with the presence of a small subdural hemorrhage linked to the presentation of second impact syndrome.

Further Reading:
Cantu RC. Dysautoregulation/second impact syndrome with recurrent athletic head injury. *World Neurosurg.* 2016;95:601–602. doi:10.1016/j.wneu.2016.04.056
Cantu RC, Gean AD. Second impact syndrome and a small subdural hematoma: an uncommon catastrophic result of repetitive head injury with a characteristic imaging appearance. *J Neurotrauma.* 2010;27:1557–1564. doi:10.1089/neu.2010.1334
Mori T, Katayama Y, Kawamata T. Acute hemispheric swelling associated with thin subdural hematomas: pathophysiology of repetitive head injury in sports. *Acta Neurochir Suppl.* 2006;96:40–43. doi:10.1007/3-211-30714-1_10
Tator C, Starkes J, Dolansky G, et al. Fatal second impact syndrome in Rowan Stringer, a 17-year-old rugby player. *Can J Neurol Sci.* 2019;46:351–354. doi:10.1017/cjn.2019.14

REFERENCES

The full reference list appears in the digital product found on http://connect.springer-pub.com/content/book/978-0-8261-4768-4/part/part02/chapter/ch11

STRUCTURAL AND FUNCTIONAL BRAIN IMAGING IN MILD TRAUMATIC BRAIN INJURY

JEFFREY DAVID LEWINE

BACKGROUND

- Almost 85% of brain injuries are classified as mild. However, such classification does not mean that the injury is insignificant. Even mild traumatic brain injury (MTBI) can have a significant effect on quality of life.
- Relevant imaging strategies include both structural and functional methods with specific recommendations varying as a patient progresses through the acute (first 24–96 hours), subacute (up to 6 months), and chronic (beyond 6 months) phases of injury.
- Computed tomography (CT) is generally appropriate for acute evaluation of head trauma as it is efficient for ruling out life-threatening injuries. However, routine clinical anatomic neuroimaging examinations using CT or even magnetic resonance imaging (MRI) are usually negative in cases of MTBI. When CT or MRI is positive for structural pathology in the acute setting of MTBI, the injury should be classified as a *complicated* MTBI.
- Advanced quantitative structural and functional brain imaging methods can sometimes provide objective evidence of brain compromise in the absence of findings on conventional imaging. Note, however, that many conditions can lead to imaging abnormalities, so advanced methods should not be considered as stand-alone diagnostic tests for MTBI. Imaging data must be considered within a multifactorial framework that includes patient history and other test results.
- This chapter is organized so as to first review types of imaging that may be encountered in managing patients with TBI, then provide a brief overview of imaging recommendation by phase of injury, and finally to touch on areas of potential future clinical application of selected advanced imaging modalities.

TYPES OF IMAGING

There are two main types of imaging methods—those that examine brain structure (CT and MRI) and those that look at brain function. Both structural and functional methods may be of utility in the evaluation of head trauma patients.[1] Structural methods like CT are appropriately employed acutely to rule out life-threating situations. Functional imaging includes methods that evaluate biochemical, metabolic, and hemodynamic features and those that directly assess brain electrophysiology. The main biochemical/metabolic/

The full reference list appears in the digital product found on http://connect.springerpub.com/content/book/978-0-8261-4768-4/part/part02/chapter/ch12

hemodynamic methods are positron emission tomography (PET), single photon emission computed tomography (SPECT), functional MRI (fMRI), and magnetic resonance spectroscopy (MRS). The main electrophysiological methods are electroencephalography (EEG) and magnetoencephalography (MEG).

During the acute phase, neither structural MRI nor functional imaging is needed for the routine clinical management of typical patients with MTBI (see Additional Reading section). Advanced structural and functional imaging methods may be of utility if there is a decline in neurological status or if symptoms persist beyond 6 weeks. These methods may also be warranted (a) in clinically complicated/atypical cases (e.g., those with seizures or those in which other diagnoses are also being considered), (b) for forensic/medicolegal purposes, and/or (c) in the context of specific *research* questions.

Structural Imaging

- **CT**—CT uses x-rays to make tomographic images of the body. CT is generally the first brain imaging method to be employed in the emergency medical management of patients with head trauma because it provides rapid identification of skull fractures and intracranial bleeds.[2,3]
  - *Findings in MTBI*: CT examination is generally within normal limits in cases of MTBI, although intracranial bleeds are sometimes seen. Nevertheless, CT is almost always recommended in cases of head trauma with loss of consciousness to rule out potentially life-threatening complications. Validated tools, such as the Canadian Head CT Rule, can serve as a valuable resource for identifying which patients with MTBI may merit CT imaging.[4]
- **MRI**—By examining how systematically applied magnetic field gradients and radiofrequency pulses alter the behavior of the hydrogen protons of water molecules, MRI provides detailed information on the soft tissues of the body. MRI is inferior to CT for identification of skull fractures and acute bleeding, but it is superior to CT for the identification of intraparenchymal abnormalities, including diffuse axonal and shear injuries.
  - *Findings in MTBI*: Most clinical MRI evaluations in MTBI are within normal limits, but sometimes clinically meaningful abnormalities are identified. Abnormal findings in MTBI may include identification of hematomas, contusions, and/or FLAIR/T2 white matter hyperintensities.[3] White matter hyperintensities are a somewhat nonspecific finding that can be seen in relationship to multiple conditions, including normal aging, small vessel ischemic disease, and TBI.[5] However, selective distribution near the gry–white matter boundary is more common in relationship to TBI than other conditions for which such findings are more common near the ventricles and in the centrum semiovale. Use of susceptibility weighted imaging (SWI) is recommended when available. SWI is highly sensitive to blood products associated with hemorrhagic lesions.[6,7] Small white matter hemorrhagic lesions near the gray–white matter boundary are a finding that is relatively specific for TBI and thought to be associated with axonal injury (see Figure 12.1).[6]
  - In the chronic post-injury period, quantitative MRI may reveal evidence of generalized and/or regional atrophy/volume reductions, even in MTBI.[8-13] Following head trauma, such analyses may reveal abnormally low or abnormally high volumes, most commonly in regions known to be especially vulnerable to traumatic forces (e.g., the hippocampi, orbital frontal cortex, temporal poles, corpus callosum).[11-13] Low volumes are believed to reflect injury-related atrophy,[8-12] whereas high volumes are most likely related to injury-induced edema, neuroinflammation, and/or compensatory mechanisms in relationship to damage in other areas.[13]

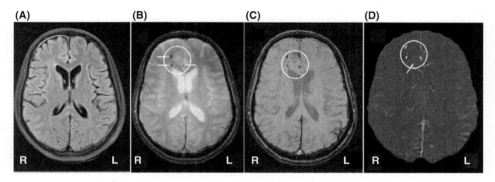

FIGURE 12.1 3T MR images of the brain of a female patient (38 years old) 2 months after a traumatic brain injury. (A) T2 flair imaging shows no abnormalities. (B) Gradient echo imaging shows three lesions in the right frontal lobe (white arrows in white circle). (C) Susceptibility-weighted imaging shows more low-intensity lesions at the same location and also in the corpus callosum (white circle). (D) Susceptibility-weighted imaging mapping shows high-intensity lesions (white circle) and deep veins (white arrow).

Source: From Liu J, Kou Z, Tian Y. Diffuse axonal injury after traumatic cerebral microbleeds: an evaluation of imaging techniques, *Neural Regen Res.* 2014;9(12):1222–1230. With permission of *Neural Regeneration Research.*

- When available, diffusion tensor imaging (DTI) may also be considered, although it requires software and hardware that are often not available at community-based hospitals. DTI can provide important information on axonal injury and the integrity of white matter pathways (as indexed by fractional anisotropy [FA] values).[1,14–17] Although the role of DTI in the clinical management of patients with MTBI remains to be fully determined, DTI is seeing increasing usage in forensic settings. In considering both clinical and forensic application, it is important to recognize that viable specification of DTI data as abnormal often cannot be done through neuroradiographic visual inspection alone. Rather, there is a need for a quantitative and statistical comparison of patient FA metrics relative to those derived from a group of gender and age range-matched neurotypical control subjects.
- For both volumetrics and DTI, it is critical to note that many neurological and psychiatric conditions other than TBI have also been associated with abnormal values.[18,19] Therefore, these quantitative methods should not be used as a stand-alone diagnostic method for trauma-related injury, although they can be important parts of a multifactorial evaluation that may support the presence of brain injury.

Functional Imaging

- **PET**—PET uses compounds labeled with positron-emitting radionucleotides to assess brain biochemistry and metabolism. Brain injury evaluations usually use fluorodeoxyglucose (FDG), and thereby measure regional metabolism, an indirect measure of neuronal activity. Clinical studies typically collect data while the brain is "at rest," whereas research and forensic studies often collect additional data during the performance of working memory or attention tasks.
  - *Findings in MTBI*: Even in cases without gross structural damage, PET images are often reported to be abnormal for days to months post MTBI. Regions of hypometabolism are most commonly identified, but both hypo- and hypermetabolic regions

may be reported. Available data indicate a variable correlation between specific PET findings and each patient's neuropsychological profile.[20-23] The role of PET in clinical management of MTBI has yet to be determined.

■ **SPECT**—SPECT is similar to PET except that relevant radionucleotides emit single photons (gamma rays) rather than positrons. As such, the spatial resolution of SPECT is slightly less than that of PET. On the other hand, the dose of radioactivity is lower for SPECT, so it is possible to perform resting and activation studies on successive days, with intrasubject comparisons. Most trauma-related studies use technetium-labeled hexamethylpropyleneamine oxime (Tc-HMPAO), with images providing information on regional blood flow, an indirect measure of regional metabolism.

 ● *Findings in MTBI*: Even in cases without gross structural damage on MRI, visual inspection of SPECT data often leads to subjective report of abnormalities following brain injury. Quantitative methods in which regional perfusion values from a patient are evaluated with respect to normative data provide more objective information (see Figure 12.2). Available data indicate that quantitative methods show moderate sensitivity to MTBI.[24-26] Frontal and temporal hypoperfusion, along with basal ganglia hypoperfusion, are most commonly reported,[24] but the scientific data are conflicted with respect to the consistency of the relationships between the location of SPECT anomalies and specific clinical profiles. SPECT is often used in forensic settings to demonstrate the presence of abnormal perfusion profiles, but observations are not diagnostically specific for MTBI, and their relevance to clinical care is presently unknown.

■ **fMRI**—The magnetic properties of oxygenated and deoxygenated blood are slightly different, so it is possible to use echo-planar, blood oxygen level-dependent (BOLD) MRI to examine regional blood flow. By comparison of data collected during rest versus active states, information can be obtained concerning how the brain activates during specific sensory, motor, or cognitive tasks. Evaluations in MTBI typically use working memory or attention tasks. There is also emerging work indicating MTBI-associated abnormalities in resting state connectivity profiles.

 ● *Findings in MTBI*: Several investigative teams have shown, in group-averaged data, atypical activation patterns during cognitive challenges related to working memory or attention. Observations include MTBI-related reductions in activity in specific network nodes or recruitment of brain regions not normally associated with completion of a particular task.[27-29] Data are also emerging to show altered patterns of functional connectivity at rest.[30-34] Generalization from group data to an individual patient is compromised by a high degree of overlap in the metrics for MTBI and control groups, so the diagnostic applicability of fMRI is generally undetermined. At the moment, fMRI is a valuable research method, but its utility in the clinical management of individual patients with MTBI remains to be demonstrated.

■ **MRS**—The local microenvironment influences the resonance frequency of protons, so it is possible to use magnetic resonance (MR) technology to measure regional concentrations of certain metabolites including N-acetyl aspartate (NAA, a neuron-specific metabolic marker), creatine (Cr, which is related to energy metabolism), and choline (Cho, a cell membrane marker).

 ● *Findings in MTBI*: Some studies have identified altered metabolite concentrations and reduced NAA/Cho and NAA/Cr ratios following mild trauma, suggesting perturbed metabolic activity in the regions measured.[35-37] At present, MRS is considered to be a research tool, with clinical and forensic applicability still under investigation.

SPECT Baseline perfusion map

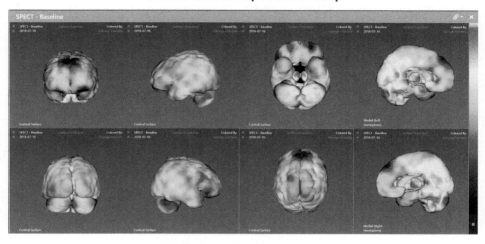

SPECT Baseline Z-score map

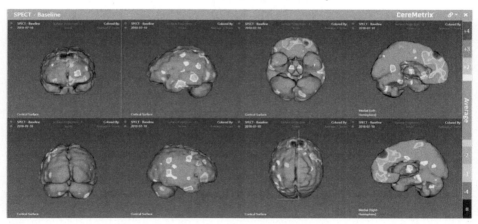

FIGURE 12.2   Use of single photon emission computed tomography (SPECT) for the evaluation of mild traumatic brain injury (MTBI). Data are shown for a 58-year-old male with uncertain loss of consciousness due to being struck on the head by a rock. Upper panels show 3D projection perfusion maps. Lower panels show quantitative maps with Z-scores calculated relative to a control database. Z-score maps in particular show focal regions of frontal hypoperfusion (dark blue zones).

Note: Although the data demonstrate clear abnormalities, SPECT findings are not diagnostically specific for TBI. However, within the context of a patient's comprehensive history, exam, and other relevant evaluations, it may be possible to specify TBI as the most likely cause of an observed objective abnormality. In this particular case it would be important to rule out a gross structural lesion or frontal lobe epilepsy as alternative explanations.

Source: Courtesy of CereScan.

■ **EEG**—EEG uses contact electrodes applied to the scalp to measure electrical potential patterns that are directly caused by changing patterns of current within brain
cells. EEG data may be visually inspected for epileptiform transients and focal or
diffuse slow waves, and it may be subjected to quantitative analyses (qEEG) with
comparison to a normative database.[38–41] While this method may be of forensic utility in the demonstration of functional compromise following head trauma, abnormal findings in isolation do not aid in determining an etiologic diagnosis. From a
clinical management perspective for MTBI, EEG is most warranted in those cases
where posttraumatic epilepsy is suspected.[42] Although not presently standard-of-
care, emerging work is demonstrating the potential utility of EEG in early "pre-iden-
tification" of focal/structural brain injury subsequently detectable on CT. This may
prove to be a useful adjunct in rapid identification and expedient management of
such injuries.[40,41]

- *Findings in MTBI*: Visual inspection of EEG following MTBI reveals abnormalities
  in less than 25% of cases, and these usually consist of nonspecific diffuse slowing of
  uncertain clinical significance. Quantitative EEG, in which patient metrics are evaluated with respect to normative values, may be abnormal in cases of MTBI,[38–45] but
  there are often concerns about the etiologic specificity of such findings with respect
  to other clinical conditions including medication effects, depression, and substance
  use disorders.[43,44] Nevertheless, while it is not a stand-alone tool for evaluation of
  MTBI, qEEG can prove useful in a forensic setting as one of several indices of brain
  dysfunction following head trauma.[45] On rare occasions, EEG reveals epileptiform
  activity following even MTBI. Depending on the clinical context, pharmacological
  management of such activity may be warranted.

■ **MEG**—MEG uses special superconducting sensors to detect the weak neuromagnetic
signals generated by the brain's electrical activity.[46] Specifically, intracellular currents
within dendrites oriented parallel to the skull are the main contributors to the MEG
signal. Simultaneous EEG data can be collected to take advantage of the complementary nature of the methods (EEG is most sensitive to currents within dendrites that are
oriented perpendicular to the skull). Both spontaneous and stimulus-evoked activity
may be gathered. Normally functioning awake brain tissue mostly generates oscillating electromagnetic signals in the theta–gamma range (6–60 Hz), with little power in
the 1 to 4 Hz delta range. Therefore, in the resting state, the presence of delta-band,
focal dipolar slow wave activity (DSWA) as a reliable sign of dysfunctional tissue can
be seen across multiple conditions, including ischemia, stroke, epilepsy, tumors, and
TBI.[46–55] In head trauma, the increase in theta and delta activity is believed to mostly
reflect compromise of thalamo-cortical projections.[52,55]

- *Findings in MTBI*: When there are clear structural lesions, sources of DSWA cluster at
  the margins of the lesions. In MTBI, where gross structural lesions are rare, sources
  of DSWA may nevertheless be seen, especially if there are persistent cognitive symptoms.[49–55] The presence of DSWA tracks with symptom severity and persistence, and
  it appears in a spatial pattern consistent with known neuroanatomical–cognitive
  relationships.[51,53] MEG slow waves resolve when symptoms resolve and they persist
  for even years after injury when symptoms persist.[49] MEG slow waves appear to
  be an objective correlate of MTBI-perturbed brain function, but in considering this,
  it must be recognized that other conditions (stroke, tumors, epilepsy, etc.) can also
  produce focal slowing.[46–48] The presence of these other conditions must therefore be
  ruled out before an observation of DSWA can be linked to a TBI (see Figure 12.3). As
  is the case with the other functional modalities discussed earlier, the role of MEG in
  the clinical management of patients with MTBI is still under investigation, but MEG
  is seeing increased usage in forensic settings, where objective correlates of brain dysfunction are sought.

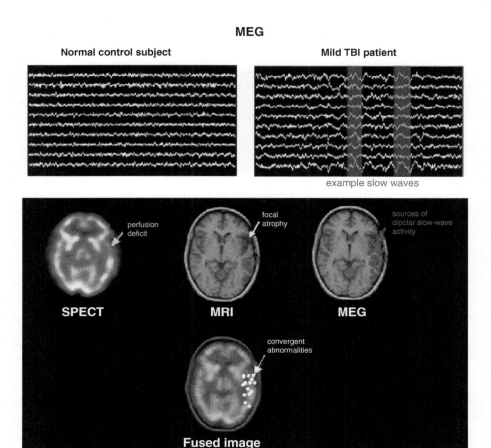

FIGURE 12.3   Multimodal imaging in mild traumatic brain injury (MTBI) with fusion of single photon emission computed tomography (SPECT), MRI, and magnetoencephalography (MEG) data. Use of MEG in the evaluation of MTBI. Upper panels show 5 seconds of representative MEG data from a normal control subject and patient with an MTBI. The patient was involved in a motor vehicle collision >1 year prior to evaluation. Large amplitude slow waves are seen in the MEG data. Lower panel shows the patient's SPECT, MRI, and MEG data. SPECT revealed hypoperfusion of the left temporal lobe. Quantitative MRI showed mild atrophy in this region (although clinically the scan was read to be without intraparenchymal abnormalities). Sources of dipolar slow wave activity in the MEG (red dots) localize to the left temporal lobe.

Note: This patient had no history of premorbid neurological or psychiatric conditions or prior head trauma, although there was note of possible ADHD. Whereas no individual finding was specific for TBI, data across modalities provided a convergent demonstration of left temporal compromise. TBI was deemed the most likely cause of the observed multimodal abnormalities.

TYPE/TIMING OF IMAGING

Acute Phase of Injury

In the acute care setting, well-established clinical criteria exist (New Orleans Head CT Criteria, Canadian Head CT Rule) to aid in determining which patients may require CT imaging.[2-4] (Specific clinical guidelines delineating indications for imaging in MTBI are addressed further in Chapter 7. See also Additional Reading section.) According to most published guidelines, acute MRI is generally warranted only if there is a significant deterioration in clinical status.[2-4] The one exception comes from the Defense and Veterans Brain Injury Center (DVBIC), which recommends MRI if there is a memory loss of greater than 15 minutes and persistent symptoms for more than 72 hours, or a history of multiple prior concussions during the past 12 months (see Additional Reading).

Subacute Phase of Injury

At present, there are no specific published guidelines with respect to recommendations for imaging in the subacute phase. MRI (or repeat CT if MRI is not available) may be warranted if there is any type of neurological deterioration during the subacute phase or if there are ongoing neurological concerns that persist beyond the period of anticipated symptom resolution and that are not well explained by clinical context and/or initial imaging.

Chronic Phase of Injury

The evaluation and treatment of MTBI patients who have symptoms that persist into the chronic period (>6 months) is especially challenging. There is often a disconnect between the self-reported severity of symptoms on subjective questionnaires versus what can be documented using objective and formal neurological and/or neuropsychological evaluation.

Standard CT and MR structural imaging are typically within normal limits in the chronic period, even for patients diagnosed as having had a complicated MTBI. On the other hand, advanced structural methods show some sensitivity to injury during the chronic period.

Hemosiderin (iron) deposits associated with microbleeds into the brain parenchyma are not readily reabsorbed, so old bleeds can be identified using SWI, even decades after the initial bleed. However, this means that caution must be used in trying to link SWI findings to a specific remote traumatic event. The data must be carefully considered within a framework of the patient's entire medical history.

ADVANCED IMAGING: POTENTIAL APPLICATIONS/ ONGOING INVESTIGATION

In a research context, volumetric and DTI strategies demonstrate utility at the group level for demonstrating differences in gray and white matter brain integrity for subjects with chronic sequelae of TBI versus normal controls. Individual subjects may also demonstrate values that are clearly outside of normal limits. Both abnormally low and abnormally high regional brain volumes[9-13] and FA values[1,14-17] have been reported following TBI, but such findings are not diagnostically specific for TBI. In all settings (research, clinical, and forensic), individual patient-specific data must be cautiously interpreted within a comprehensive historical and diagnostic framework. Use of quantitative statistical methods with comparison of individual subject data relative to a large gender and age range-matched normative sample is required. Approaches to individual subjects, while viable, must be applied with care and are presently of limited clinical utility.

Functional imaging methods including PET, SPECT, EEG, and MEG can be useful for the objective identification of persistent brain dysfunction during the chronic phase post-injury, but these are not diagnostic tests for TBI. Abnormal findings may provide objective evidence of brain dysfunction, but linkage to a specific traumatic event in both clinical and forensic settings requires a comprehensive evaluation to identify other underlying or unrecognized conditions which can present with similar imaging findings. Because of these limitations, use of these modalities for evaluation of MTBI remains limited, with no broadly recognized guidelines recommending their routine clinical use for MTBI at this time.

KEY POINTS

Structural Imaging

- Even mild trauma can infrequently lead to life-threatening injury. Validated parameters exist for identifying patients most at risk for significant intracranial injury requiring expedient CT imaging.
- MRI can be useful as a complement to CT in selected circumstances, such as the presence of prolonged, progressing, or unexplained symptoms, particularly when advanced imaging sequences (diffusion-weighted imaging [DWI]/SWI) and quantification methods are available.

Functional Imaging

- Functional modalities may provide objective evidence of brain dysfunction in the absence of gross lesions on structural imaging.
- Although functional imaging methods are sensitive for detecting abnormalities even in the setting of mild trauma, there is a general lack of specificity of findings. Also, functional findings only rarely provide clinically actionable information. Their role in the routine clinical evaluation of MTBI patients is therefore generally limited.

STUDY QUESTIONS

1. Why is CT often recommended within the acute setting of TBI?
   a. It is highly sensitive to soft tissue damage
   b. It is highly sensitivity to skull fractures and intracranial bleeds
   c. It is highly sensitive to axonal damage
   d. It provides information on brain metabolism

2. When is structural MRI most appropriate?
   a. During the acute phase of injury
   b. Whenever there has been a loss of consciousness
   c. During the subacute recovery phase
   d. When there is an unexpected decline in clinical status

3. Which is generally true with respect to diffusion tensor imaging (DTI)?
   a. DTI provides stand-alone diagnostic information on TBI
   b. Visual inspection of DTI data often provides strong evidence of injury
   c. Quantitative DTI analyses can provide objective evidence of a compromise of white matter integrity
   d. DTI is the preferred method for examining gray matter volume loss

4. Which is generally true with respect to SPECT?
   a. SPECT selectively evaluates brain electrophysiology
   b. Quantitative SPECT is often used to guide clinical management in the acute phase of injury
   c. In isolation, quantitative SPECT observations are NOT diagnostically specific for MTBI
   d. SPECT observations are diagnostically specific for MTBI

5. Which is true with respect to EEG?
   a. qEEG can be used as a stand-alone diagnostic test for MTBI in the clinical setting
   b. EEG may be useful clinically when posttraumatic epilepsy is suspected
   c. EEG provides a direct measure of brain biochemistry
   d. EEG is only useful as a research tool

ADDITIONAL READING

DCoE Clinical Recommendations. Neuroimaging following mild traumatic brain injury in the non-deployed setting. https://dvbic.dcoe.mil/system/files/resources/588.1.2.2_NeuroimagingCR_508.pdf

American College of Emergency Room Physicians Guideline for neuroimaging in mTBI. www.nimbot.com/Med/Head%20Trauma-%20Guidelines%20for%20Imaging/ACEP%20Clinical%20Policy%20-%20Neuroimaging%20and%20Decisionmaking%20in%20Acute%20Adult%20Mild%20TBI.pdf

Ricker JH, Arenth P. Functional neuroimaging of TBI. In: Zasler ND, Katz DI, Zafonte RD, eds. *Brain Injury Medicine: Principles and Practice.* Demos Medical Publishing; 2006:149–156.

Belanger HG, Vanderploeg RD, Curtiss G, Warden DJ. Recent neuroimaging techniques in mild traumatic brain injury. *J Neuropsychiatry Clin Neurosci.* 2007;19:5–20. doi:10.1176/jnp.2007.19.1.5

Wilde E, Bouix S, Tate DF, et al. Advanced neuroimaging applied to veterans and service personnel with traumatic brain injury: state of the art and potential benefits. *Brain Imaging Behav.* 2015;9:367–402. doi:10.1007/s11682-015-9444-y

ANSWERS TO STUDY QUESTIONS

1. Correct Answer: b
CT is used acutely because of its high sensitivity to skull fractures and intracranial bleeds—potentially life-threatening situations.

Further Reading:
Jagoda AS, Bazarian JJ, Bruns JJ Jr, et al. Clinical policy: neuroimaging and decision-making in adult mild traumatic brain injury in the acute setting. *Ann Emerg Med.* 2008;52:714–748. doi:10.1016/j.annemergmed.2008.08.021
Orrison WW, Lewine JD. Neuroimaging in closed head injury. In: Rizzo M, Tranel D, eds. *Head Injury and Post-concussive Syndrome.* Churchill Livingstone; 1995:71–88.
Stiell IF, Wells GA, Vandemheen K, et al. The Canadian CT Head Rule for patients with minor head injury. *Lancet.* 2001:357:1391–1396. doi:10.1016/S0140-6736(00)04561-X

2. Correct Answer: d
MRI is not generally recommended for routine use following MTBI. However, it is appropriate in the clinical setting whenever there is an unexpected change in neurological status or unexplained persistence of symptoms into the chronic period. MRI may also be of utility in forensic settings.

Further Reading:
Jagoda AS, Bazarian JJ, Bruns JJ Jr, et al. Clinical policy: neuroimaging and decision-making in adult mild traumatic brain injury in the acute setting. *Ann Emerg Med*. 2008;52:714–748. doi:10.1016/j.annemergmed.2008.08.021
Orrison WW, Lewine JD. Neuroimaging in closed head injury. In: Rizzo M, Tranel D, eds. *Head Injury and Post-concussive Syndrome*. Churchill Livingstone; 1995:71–88.

3. Correct Answer: c
Quantitative DTI is not a stand-alone diagnostic test for TBI and visual inspection lacks sensitivity and objectivity with respect to subtle white matter damage. Quantitative methods involving evaluation of client FA values with respect to gender and age range-matched control subjects can provide objective evidence of brain compromise, this being most useful in a research or forensic setting.

Further Reading:
Wilde E, Bouix S, Tate DF, et al. Advanced neuroimaging applied to veterans and service personnel with traumatic brain injury: state of the art and potential benefits, *Brain Imaging Behav*. 2015;9:367–402. doi:10.1007/s11682-015-9444-y
Liu J, Kou Z, Tian Y. Diffuse axonal injury after traumatic cerebral microbleeds: an evaluation of imaging techniques. *Neural Regen Res*. 2014;9(12):1222–1230. doi:10.4103/1673-5374.135330
Hulkower M, Poliak DB, Rosenbaum SB, et al. A decade of DTI in traumatic brain injury: 10 years and 100 articles later. *AJNR Am J Neuroradiol*. 2013;34:2064–2074. doi:10.3174/ajnr.A3395
Lipton ML, Kim N, Park YK, et al. Robust detection of traumatic axonal injury in individual mild traumatic brain injury patients: intersubject variation, change over time and bidirectional changes in anisotropy. *Brain Imaging Behav*. 2012;6(2):329–342. doi:10.1007/s11682-012-9175-2
Croall ID, Lohner V, Moynihan B, et al. White matter correlates of cognitive dysfunction after mild traumatic brain injury. *Neurology*, 2014;83:494–501. doi:10.1212/WNL.0000000000000666
Dennis EL, Wilde EA, Newsome MR, et al. Military brain injury: a coordinated meta-analysis of diffusion MRI from multiple cohorts. *Poc IEEE Int Symp Biomed Imaging*. 2018;1386–1389.
Zahr NM. Structural and microstructural imaging of the brain in alcohol use disorders. *Handbk Clin Neurol*. 2013;125:275–290. doi:10.1016/B978-0-444-62619-6.00017-3

4. Correct Answer: c
SPECT measures brain perfusion. Both hypo- and hyperperfusion can be seen in multiple conditions, so observations are not diagnostically specific in insolation. The role of SPECT in the clinical management of MTBI patients is not clear at present.

5. Correct Answer: b
EEG is the gold-standard for evaluating epileptic activity.

REFERENCES

The full reference list appears in the digital product found on http://connect.springer-pub.com/content/book/978-0-8261-4768-4/part/part02/chapter/ch12

13 SELECTED SOMATIC DISORDERS ASSOCIATED WITH MILD TRAUMATIC BRAIN INJURY: FATIGUE, DIZZINESS AND BALANCE IMPAIRMENT, AND WHIPLASH INJURY

ELIE P. ELOVIC AND MICHAEL HENRIE

INTRODUCTION

Common somatic aliments seen in association with mild traumatic brain injury (MTBI) include balance deficits, dizziness, fatigue, headache, nausea, visual disturbances, tinnitus (particularly with blast injury or MTBI associated with damage to the internal auditory canal), slurred speech, dysesthesias, generalized nonspecific weakness, and musculoskeletal complaints such as cervical spine injury and whiplash-associated disorders (WADs). In general, the initial symptoms directly attributable to traumatic brain injury (TBI) occur as a result of neurometabolic processes.[1] One must also consider that some symptoms may result from the associated cranial and soft tissue injury that often accompanies MTBI. The most important of these manifestations not discussed elsewhere in this text are discussed in the following sections.

FATIGUE

Definition

Fatigue can be defined as reduced capacity for mental and/or physical activity and is common after acquired brain injury.[2] It has also been defined as: (a) that state following a period of mental or bodily activity, characterized by a lessened capacity for work and reduced efficiency of accomplishment, usually accompanied by a feeling of weariness, sleepiness, or irritability; and (b) a sensation of boredom and lassitude due to absence of stimulation, monotony, or lack of interest in one's surroundings.[3]

Classification

Fatigue can be classified as: (a) central fatigue, resulting from supratentorial structures; or (b) peripheral fatigue, which has a physical, metabolic, or muscular origin. It can be further subdivided as either physical or mental/cognitive. There is substantial overlap between central and peripheral processes governing fatigue.[4] In addition, excessive daytime sleepiness (i.e., the inability to maintain wakefulness and alertness) is common following TBI[5]

The full reference list appears in the digital product found on http://connect.springerpub.com/content/book/978-0-8261-4768-4/part/part02/chapter/ch13

and should be viewed as a separate but related construct; it should be differentiated from fatigue, although they often coexist.

Post-TBI fatigue is not merely a subjective complaint; those with fatigue even after successful rehabilitation demonstrate impaired performance over time on cognitive tasks when compared to controls.[6] Furthermore, long-standing fatigue after TBI has a negative effect on employment status.[7]

Epidemiology

A recent review of the literature showed an incidence of fatigue after TBI varying from 32.4% to 73%.[2] It is one of the most common postconcussion symptoms and may persist even after other symptoms have resolved.[8]

Pathophysiology

Centrally mediated fatigue results from direct injury to central structures such as the reticular activating system and basal ganglia. A number of other factors that may contribute to fatigue include depression, decreased levels of the amino acids tryptophan and tyrosine, and alterations in cholinergic, serotonergic, and histaminergic pathways.[4] Endocrine disease, including deficiencies in growth hormone, cortisol, testosterone, and thyroid hormones, can also produce fatigue.[9] In addition, there is evidence to suggest that the injured brain is subject to fatigue because it needs to "work harder" in order to compensate for cognitive impairments such as decreased processing speed and attention.[10] A more recent publication opines that cellular injury, inflammation, and the acute stress response could lead to neural network dysfunction via a mechanism which is thus far poorly understood.[11] Finally, in Gulf War Illness, which affects 25% of returning Gulf War veterans and has cognitive fatigue as one of its major symptoms, the fronto-striatal-thalamic circuit and the caudate nucleus were implicated in fatigue. Those suffering from this condition demonstrated greater activation in the frontal and parietal regions than healthy controls.[12]

Diagnosis

Clinical Presentation

Fatigue can affect an individual's cognitive function, ability to successfully perform activities of daily living, quality of life, and employment. When obtaining a history, the line of questioning should help differentiate between fatigue and sleepiness and should include identification of possible psychological, neurological, or endocrine abnormalities.

Examination and Laboratory Assessment

Several subjective scales have been used to measure fatigue in brain-injured patients—Fatigue Severity Scale, Visual Analog Scale for Fatigue, Fatigue Impact Scale, Barrow Neurological Institute (BNI) Fatigue Scale, and Cause of Fatigue (COF) Questionnaire. The BNI and COF Questionnaires were designed specifically for brain-injured patients.[4,13] Systematic screening for endocrine dysfunction is also recommended in all patients with TBI and persistent fatigue.[9]

Treatment

Nonpharmacological management of fatigue includes the following:

- Establish a routine home exercise program with the goal of optimizing cardiovascular health and improving physical well-being.
- Follow good dietary habits with the goal of weight reduction to improve energy efficiency.

■ Educate patients on appropriate sleep hygiene and address any treatable sleep disorders.
■ Address depression if present.
■ Introduce compensatory activities and activity modification to conserve energy.[4]

Pharmacological management should be initiated if conservative measures fail. Management includes discontinuation or appropriate substitution of any medications with the potential to cause fatigue. One common problem (particularly in the setting of moderate to severe TBI) is the inappropriately prolonged use of anticonvulsants. If post-traumatic epilepsy is present, the least sedating medication should be used. Other medications that are commonly prescribed in this population will include muscle relaxants, pain medications, and hypnotics. While sometimes necessary, the risk/benefit ratio of using these medications must be evaluated.

Endocrine deficiencies requiring immediate treatment include diabetes insipidus, adrenal insufficiency, and secondary thyroid insufficiency. Treatment of gonadal and growth hormone deficiencies, on the other hand, should be postponed until the need for such therapy is confirmed by appropriate retesting, typically at least 1 year after injury.[9]

Use of neurostimulants for post-TBI fatigue has met with mixed results. Studies have shown efficacy of stimulants for treatment of cognitive impairment, but generally not for fatigue, post TBI.[14] That said, in other populations these agents have demonstrated a positive effect on fatigue. For example, the dopaminergic agents methylphenidate and dextroamphetamine have demonstrated benefit in treating HIV-related fatigue.[15] Modafinil has been reported to be of benefit in stroke, multiple sclerosis, and depression.[16,17] A recent publication suggests that modafinil may also be helpful with fatigue post TBI.[18] Regarding methylphenidate, a recent meta-analysis concluded that the published data to date do not demonstrate a beneficial effect for post-TBI fatigue.[19] Finally, a recent small study (28 subjects) looked at a novel agent currently referred to as OSU-6162, a partial agonist at D2 and 5HT2, and found that activity level and mental fatigue improved with use of this agent.[20]

In summary, based on current published medical evidence, the use of neurostimulants for post-TBI fatigue remains under investigation, and no specific medication can be recommended for use at this juncture.

BALANCE AND DIZZINESS

Definition

The term "dizzy" is nonspecific and can refer to lightheadedness, a sense of an impending fainting, vertigo, a sense of imbalance, or dizziness due to pathology affecting sensory organ input.[21]

Classification

Dizziness following brain injury can be broadly categorized by etiology as vestibular and nonvestibular.

Epidemiology

Dizziness may affect up to 20% to 50% of individuals with mild to moderate TBI. It is one of the five most common complaints that distinguish postconcussive patients from healthy controls.[22] In the military population, 80% of service members identified as having sustained a TBI reported balance dysfunction.[23]

Pathophysiology

The balance system is complex and consists of multiple sensory inputs including the visual, somatosensory, and proprioceptive systems in addition to the vestibular end organs. Injury to any of the components can lead to complaints of dizziness and imbalance.[24] In addition, injury to the head, which does not necessarily result in TBI, may account for the symptoms. Vestibular causes include benign positional vertigo that may result from displacement of calcium crystals from the otoliths into the semicircular canal, and labyrinthine concussion caused by violent head movements. Labyrinthine concussion can occur in the absence of a temporal bone fracture and is often used to describe the spectrum of inner ear symptoms that occur following brain injury. Less common causes include ischemia, hemorrhage, or direct trauma to one or more components of the vestibular system, as well as perilymphatic fistula and posttraumatic Meniere's syndrome. Decreased processing speed, migraine headache, and concomitant injuries to the visual system or musculoskeletal system should also be considered as potentially affecting the vestibular system's output.[21]

There is little information available in the literature regarding nonvestibular causes of dizziness following TBI. Causes likely include positional orthostasis, cervical spine injury, medications such as antihypertensives and anticonvulsants, hyponatremia, and rarely vestibular epilepsy.[21] A recent imaging study looked at pathological connectivity post-TBI and showed that those with balance disorder after TBI demonstrated different modulation of their cognitive function, with increased activation of the lateral occipital cortex to pre-supplementary motor cortex pathway.[25] This may also potentially represent a pathophysiological mechanism for the presence of complaints of imbalance and dizziness post TBI.

In the military population, development of these symptoms probably occurs via the effect of the blast pressure wave on inner ear structures.[23] Others have suggested that it may also be a manifestation of posttraumatic stress, vestibular migraines, microstructural injury to the brain, or anxiety.[26]

Diagnosis

Clinical Presentation

Symptoms are often poorly or vaguely described. Common complaints include lightheadedness, feeling drunk, a spinning or rotating sensation, or trouble with balance. Dizziness may contribute to balance difficulty, falls, problems with transfers and activities of daily living, as well as psychological distress.[21] A detailed neurotological history is the most important factor in determining diagnosis and treatment course, and therefore must be accurately obtained.[24]

Examination

Metrics used to assess dizziness include both objective and self-reported measures, with the *Dynamic Gait Index* and *Measures of Gait Velocity* being examples of the former and the Dizziness Handicap Inventory, Vertigo Handicap Questionnaire, and Vertigo Symptom Scale being examples of the latter.[21] Balance can also be measured with metrics such as the Balance Error Scoring System (BESS).[27] If benign positional vertigo is suspected, the Dix–Hallpike test should be performed.[24]

Laboratory and Radiologic Assessment

Formal audiometric testing should be strongly considered given the anatomic relationship between the peripheral vestibular and auditory systems. Radiographic evaluation and laboratory vestibular/balance testing can confirm a lesion site, but are less likely to drive treatment decisions.[24]

Treatment

Balance rehabilitation therapy (BRT), also known as vestibular rehabilitation, is the most frequently used form of treatment for dizziness and vestibular disorders.[21,24] Vestibular rehabilitation employs balance exercises that enhance central nervous system compensation for vestibular dysfunction. Although a few studies have looked at BRT in TBI, some with encouraging results, it is still unclear if this intervention is effective.[21]

The most common use of medications is the short-term use of vestibular suppressants. Vestibular suppressants include anticholinergics (scopolamine), antihistamines (meclizine and promethazine), benzodiazepines, and phenothiazine. Vestibular suppressants have an effect that can significantly slow the body's natural compensation process and can exacerbate cognitive complaints; they should therefore only be used on a short-term "as needed" basis, if at all. An alternative approach involves use of N-acetyl-cysteine, which was shown to be effective in ameliorating dizziness, vertigo, memory issues, headaches, and sleep issues in a military population 7 days after a blast injury.[28] Though no long-term follow-up studies have been performed which clearly demonstrate sustained efficacy, its use may be worth considering because of its favorable safety profile and potential symptomatic benefit.[29]

Chronic medication use has little benefit, unless directed at treatment of secondary causes of dizziness/poor balance, such as migraine headaches or psychologic disorders. Surgery is generally reserved for cases involving temporal bone fracture or perilymphatic fistula.

WHIPLASH-ASSOCIATED DISORDERS

Definition

The Quebec Task Force on WAD defines whiplash as "an acceleration–deceleration mechanism of energy transfer to the neck. It may result from rear-end or side-impact motor vehicle collisions, but can also occur during diving or other mishaps. The impact may result in a variety of clinical manifestations."[30,31]

Classification

The Quebec Task Force developed the classification taxonomy listed in Table 13.1.[31]

Epidemiology

The literature regarding whiplash disorders associated with MTBI is limited. A recent study found all hockey players sustaining concussion complained of symptoms of WAD.[32] The incidence of claims for whiplash in the general population is 1 to 6 per 1,000 people per year. Most patients recover quickly with only 15% to 20% of patients remaining symptomatic after 12 months.[30]

TABLE 13.1   Quebec Task Force Classification of Whiplash-Associated Disorders

Grade 0	No complaint or physical sign
Grade 1	Neck complaint (pain, stiffness, or tenderness) without physical signs
Grade 2	Neck complaint with musculoskeletal signs (range of motion [ROM] loss or tenderness)
Grade 3	Neck complaint and neurological signs
Grade 4	Neck complaint and fracture or dislocation

Source: Reproduced with permission from Liebenson C, Skaggs C. The role of chiropractic treatment in whiplash injury. In: Malanga GA, Nadler SF, eds. *Whiplash*. Hanley & Belfus; 2002.

Pathophysiology

Whiplash is a result of injury to soft tissues of the neck resulting from an acceleration–deceleration event. Common associated injuries include articular pillar fracture and subchondral plate fracture, annulus fibrosus tear and endplate avulsion/fracture, hemarthrosis of the facet joint, contusion of the intra-articular meniscus of the facet joint, rupture of the joint capsule, and anterior longitudinal ligament injury.[33]

Whiplash is considered to be a result of neck injury as opposed to brain injury. The impact on balance can be additive, however. A study which used the BESS in an MTBI population found that those with whiplash in addition to MTBI had a statistically higher score on the BESS than those with MTBI alone. From a neuroanatomic perspective, another study found that corticoreticulospinal tract volume is decreased in those with whiplash and MTBI when compared to those with MTBI alone.[27]

Diagnosis

Clinical Presentation
Head, neck, and upper thoracic pain typically dominate the clinical picture. Initial symptoms are often delayed for several hours after the injury. Balance complaints may also be reported; the combination of MTBI and whiplash is associated with a higher incidence of balance problems than for MTBI alone.[34]

Examination
A comprehensive biomechanical and neurological examination should be performed. The area of tissue injury and pain generator should be identified. Examination should include cervical range of motion in all planes, palpation for focal tenderness over spinous processes as well as the cervical paraspinal muscles, and observation of any postural irregularities. Look for areas of kinetic chain dysfunction and biomechanical overload and any adaptive mechanisms.

Radiologic Assessment
The American College of Radiology's Appropriateness Criteria for Imaging and Treatment Decisions states that in acutely symptomatic patients with neck pain, with or without neurological deficit, initial cervical spine imaging is indicated. If there is radiographic evidence of instability or focal neurological deficits, more advanced imaging should be obtained.[35]

Treatment

Acute care consists of reassurance, activity modification, and pain control. Recommendations of the Quebec Task Force include the following:

- No medications for grade 1 injury and short-term use of nonsteroidal anti-inflammatory drugs (NSAIDs) and nonnarcotic analgesics for grades 2 and 3 injury.
- Narcotics should not be prescribed for grades 1 and 2, but can be used for a limited time in grade 3 injury.
- Muscle relaxants should not be used in the acute phase of treatment.

An individualized behavioral treatment plan can also be effective, administered either via a face-to-face format or through the Internet.[36]

   Although the literature regarding medical management of whiplash injury is sparse,[37] low back pain treatment, which has been more extensively studied, may offer additional treatment options. Muscle relaxants have been shown to be effective in treating muscle spasm associated with acute low back pain, but are cognitively sedating, and therefore should be avoided, as discussed previously. Gabapentin and tricyclic antidepressants have been used effectively to treat radicular pain and may have a role in treating refractory/persistent pain.[37] Rehabilitation should focus on identifying and correcting biomechanical deficits and adaptive patterns in the kinetic chain.[38]

KEY POINTS

- Fatigue is a common problem after TBI and is multifactorial in nature.
- Treatment of posttraumatic fatigue can be challenging and includes identification and treatment of related conditions, nonpharmacological and pharmacological approaches.
- Dizziness and balance disorders can be found in up to 50% of civilian survivors of mild to moderate TBI and up to 80% of those from the military, with blast injury a likely source for the increased rate.
- Whiplash, an acceleration–deceleration mechanism of energy transfer to the neck, can account for symptoms after TBI and should be considered as a potential cause of persistent somatic symptoms.

STUDY QUESTIONS

1. Fatigue after MTBI
   a. Can result in reduced capacity for mental and/or physical activity
   b. Can have a negative impact on employment status
   c. Should initially be managed by nonpharmacological means
   d. All of the above

2. Treatments for fatigue after MTBI include:
   a. Activity modification and good dietary habits to promote conservation of energy
   b. Home exercise program

    c. Use of medications such as methylphenidate or modafinil
    d. Both a and b

3. Dizziness/balance disorder:
    a. Is rarely seen after MTBI
    b. May be a result of a head injury or a brain injury
    c. Is generally not seen in the absence of post-TBI cognitive issues
    d. Is measured via the Quebec Task Force classification schema

4. With respect to whiplash:
    a. It results from an acceleration–deceleration mechanism of energy transfer to the neck
    b. The majority of patients are still symptomatic at 1 year
    c. Symptoms develop immediately after injury
    d. Imaging is recommended only for patients with neurological findings

ADDITIONAL READING

https://msktc.org/lib/docs/Factsheets/TBI_Balance_Problems_and_TBI.pdf
Cantor JB, Ashman T, Bushnik T, et al. Systematic review of interventions for fatigue after traumatic brain injury: a NIDRR traumatic brain injury model systems study. *J Head Trauma Rehabil.* 2014;29(6):490–497. doi:10.1097/HTR.0000000000000102
Hoffer ME, Balaban C, Nicholas R, et al. Neurosensory sequelae of mild traumatic brain injury. *Psychiatric Annals.* 2013;43(7):318–323. doi:10.3928/00485713-20130703-06
Spitzer WO, Skovron M, Salmi L, et al. Scientific monograph of the Quebec Task Force on Whiplash-Associated Disorders: redefining "whiplash" and its management. *Spine.* 1995;20(8 suppl):1S–73S.

ANSWERS TO STUDY QUESTIONS

1. Correct Answer: d
All of these statements are correct.

Further Reading:
Henrie M, Elovic EP. Fatigue assessment and treatment. In: Zasler ND, Katz DI, Zafonte RD, eds. *Brain Injury Medicine: Principles and Practice*, 2nd ed. Demos; 2013. doi:10.1891/9781617050572.0042
Palm S, Ronnback L, Johansson B. Long-term mental fatigue after traumatic brain injury and impact on employment status. *J Rehabil Med.* 2017;49:228–233. doi:10.2340/16501977-2190

2. Correct Answer: d
Multiple modalities for treatment have been suggested to be potentially efficacious. While some data suggest benefit, there remains a relative paucity of evidence regarding use of medications such as methylphenidate and modafinil for treatment of TBI-related fatigue.

Further Reading:
Henrie M, Elovic EP. Fatigue assessment and treatment. In: Zasler ND, Katz DI, Zafonte RD, eds. *Brain Injury Medicine: Principles and Practice*, 2nd ed. Demos; 2013. doi:10.1891/9781617050572.0042

3. Correct Answer: b
This issue can result from an injury to the brain or cranial peripheral structures.

Further Reading:
Maskell F, Chiarelli P, Isles R. Dizziness after traumatic brain injury: overview and measurement in the clinical setting. *Brain Inj*. 2006;20:293–305. doi:10.1080/02699050500488041
Fife TD, Kalra D. Persistent vertigo and dizziness after mild traumatic brain injury. *Ann N Y Acad Sci*. 2015;1343:97–105. doi:10.1111/nyas.12678
Shepard NT, Handelsman JA, Clendaniel RA. Balance and Dizziness. In: Zasler ND, Katz DI, Zafonte RD, eds. *Brain Injury Medicine: Principles and Practice*, 2nd ed. Demos; 2013. doi:10.1891/9781617050572.0047

4. Correct Answer: a
Whiplash occurs as "a result of injury to soft tissues of the neck resulting from an acceleration–deceleration event." Symptoms often don't appear until hours to several hours after the injury occurs.

Further Reading:
Teasell R, Shapiro A. The clinical picture of whiplash injuries. In: Malanga GA, Nadler SF, eds. *Whiplash. Hanley and Belfus*; 2002. doi:10.1016/B978-1-56053-438-9.50011-4

REFERENCES

The full reference list appears in the digital product found on http://connect.springer-pub.com/content/book/978-0-8261-4768-4/part/part02/chapter/ch13

14 COGNITION IN MILD TRAUMATIC BRAIN INJURY: NEUROPSYCHOLOGICAL ASSESSMENT

ERIC B. LARSON AND HEATHER G. BELANGER

GENERAL PRINCIPLES

Definition

Neuropsychological assessment (NPA) is the quantitative and qualitative evaluation of clinical history and neurobehavioral status that typically includes assessment of cognitive performance and psychological/behavioral functioning. Mild traumatic brain injury (MTBI), also commonly referred to as concussion, occurs when an external force is transmitted to the brain and alters its functioning. The Department of Veterans Affairs (VA) and Department of Defense (DoD) define a concussion as an injury that results in normal structural neuroimaging and up to 24 hours alteration of consciousness (AOC), up to a day of posttraumatic amnesia (PTA), or up to 30 minutes of loss of consciousness (LOC).[1] It is important to distinguish concussions from moderate, severe, and penetrating TBIs, which generally have longer duration of LOC/PTA/AOC, may have abnormal structural neuroimaging, and typically result in worse outcomes. NPA may or may not be utilized in the management of MTBI, as the vast majority of people experience complete cognitive recovery within 3 months.[2]

Purpose

The purposes of an NPA following MTBI are to:

- Assist in determining whether an MTBI occurred through assessment of the historical event and any subsequent alteration of cerebral function, often using a structured interview such as the Ohio State TBI Identification Interview (OSU TBI-ID).[3]
- Identify/describe the nature and extent of any cognitive deficits and psychological changes as well as provide prognosis.
- Determine the need for treatment and inform the development of an individualized treatment plan to address any cognitive, emotional, or behavioral needs.
- Evaluate the effectiveness of interventions in terms of their immediate and long-term impacts on proximal (e.g., specific cognitive or psychological problems) or distal outcomes (e.g., return to work, social integration).

The full reference list appears in the digital product found on http://connect.springerpub.com/content/book/978-0-8261-4768-4/part/part02/chapter/ch14

COMPREHENSIVE NEUROPSYCHOLOGICAL ASSESSMENT

A comprehensive NPA consists of a thorough clinical interview and testing that may include verbal and nonverbal tests, paper-and-pencil tests, motor and constructional tasks, and self-report questionnaires. Though the vast majority of individuals who sustain an MTBI will recover completely, comprehensive NPA may be indicated if an individual continues to experience cognitive deficits several months after MTBI. The following are essential components to comprehensive NPA.

Clinical Interview

A thorough clinical history provides context for understanding the neuropsychological test data. Important issues to address during a clinical interview following MTBI include:

- Description of the injury—Determine how the injury occurred, duration of any alteration in mental status (e.g., confusion, PTA), or LOC. It is best to ask about the injury and any subsequent sequelae in an open-ended fashion.
- Description of current functioning—Ask the individual about what they do during a typical day and get a sense of their activity level and overall functioning.
- Comprehensive history—In addition to information about the current injury, it is important to determine if a person has sustained multiple MTBIs, as well as find out about their overall health/medical history, including any past psychiatric diagnoses or treatment. Assessment of substance abuse is particularly important to obtain details that individuals may otherwise omit or minimize.
- Review of imaging studies—Inquire about what tests were done in the emergency department or immediate post-injury period and whether the results are available. Those with abnormalities on initial computed tomography (CT) scans may have worse outcomes.[4,5]
- Comorbid conditions—These could account for the person's symptoms/cognitive performance/functional status.
- Social, educational/academic, and employment history—Be sure to determine if there is a history of attention deficit hyperactivity disorder (ADHD) and/or learning disability. Similarly, be sure to obtain a family history of neurological disorder or psychiatric illness to assess risk for conditions with a strong hereditary component.

Neuropsychological Testing

The data gathered in an NPA comes from standardized tests designed to quantify cognitive, psychological, and behavioral functioning.

- Domains—The cognitive performance domains to be assessed following MTBI include attention/concentration, speed of information processing, learning/encoding of new information, fine motor speed, memory, verbal and nonverbal fluency, and executive functions (problem-solving, planning, organization, strategizing, etc.). Assessment of dysexecutive behaviors such as impulsivity, apathy, risk taking, and irritability should also be included. Finally, an estimate of the person's premorbid abilities is essential to understanding the context of current cognitive performance level. Estimates of premorbid function are based on educational and vocational history and on tests designed to assess premorbid cognitive ability (e.g., Wechsler Test of Adult Reading, Test of Premorbid Functioning, National Adult Reading Test).
- Instrument selection—Select tests that are sensitive to the subtle cognitive changes that are characteristic of MTBI. Tests with a low ceiling or intended for use as screening tools

(e.g., mini mental status examinations) are not useful in assessing potential changes related to MTBI. Instrument selection should be tailored to the client; this is not a one-size-fits-all determination. That said, some commonly used instruments include the Wechsler Memory Scale (WMS), the Repeatable Battery for Neuropsychological Status (RBANS), the Trailmaking Test, and the Wisconsin Card Sorting Test (WCST), to name but a few.

- Assessment of mood—Psychological distress may exacerbate the person's perceptions of the extent of their cognitive deficits and compound their functional impairments. Individuals with a history of MTBI commonly experience depression, anxiety, and emotional dysregulation. These changes in mood may be related to the injury event itself, may represent an exacerbation of preexisting conditions, or may be secondary to physical injuries, pain, and fatigue. Posttraumatic stress disorder (PTSD) can co-occur with MTBI, particularly when the circumstances leading to the injury were traumatic or combat related.[6]

- Symptoms—Assess what, if any, symptoms the person is experiencing, their attributions as to the cause, and any resulting functional impairment. Standardized symptom checklists may be helpful, especially when combined with follow-up questions assessing the patient's beliefs regarding pre-injury severity, time of post-injury onset, and subsequent course.[7]

- Validity—Given our litigious society, and the fact that financial and other incentives can have a substantial effect on cognitive performance in those with MTBI,[8] it is important to assess both performance validity and symptom validity. This should be accomplished using both stand-alone and embedded measures when possible.

Feedback and Recommendations Following the Assessment

- Feedback—It is appropriate to provide feedback to the client and their family about the findings of NPA. Feedback should be provided in language that is understandable to the client/family members. Allow the client and family the opportunity to ask questions. Address both weaknesses and strengths. Focus on how assessment findings compare to what the patient and family expected to hear. Discuss the role of expectations in the etiology and maintenance of certain symptoms.

- Recommendations
  - Treatment planning—Use the results of the NPA to identify appropriate interventions. This will often include psychological interventions to address any psychiatric disorders, physical/behavioral interventions to address deconditioning/lack of activity, and education to address common misperceptions about MTBI (e.g., that Chronic Traumatic Encephalopathy [CTE] is common following MTBI or that MTBI invariably leads to poor long-term outcomes). Evidence suggests that psychological interventions are effective in those with a history of MTBI.
  - Referrals for further evaluation or diagnostic testing—Determine whether the observed sequelae of MTBI require additional diagnostic evaluations by another specialist and make appropriate referrals.

OTHER TYPES OF ASSESSMENT FOLLOWING MILD TRAUMATIC BRAIN INJURY

Brief Cognitive Assessments

Brief cognitive assessments are routinely performed by a variety of health professionals (physicians, nurses, physical therapists, occupational therapists, speech pathologists, etc.) to assess the presence of cognitive deficits. Several brief screening instruments exist (e.g., Mini Mental Status Examination, Montreal Cognitive Assessment, Clock Drawing Test, Standardized Assessment of Concussion). Although these instruments may be useful in detecting gross impairments, they are unlikely to detect subtle changes in cognitive functioning. Indeed, some individuals with MTBI will perform on these assessments without any difficulty despite having demonstrable impairments when given more extensive NPAs. Therefore, clinicians should not solely rely on brief assessments to identify post-MTBI cognitive deficits or changes in cognitive function when a person continues to report challenges several months after injury.

Computerized Assessments

Several computerized cognitive tests (CCTs) have been developed to assess changes in cognition. CCTs are used widely for assessing sport-related injuries. Examples of popular CCTs include the Cambridge Neuropsychological Test Automated Battery (CANTAB), the Automated Neuropsychological Assessment Metrics (ANAM), the Immediate Postconcussion Assessment and Cognitive Testing (ImPACT), the Cognistat Cognitive Assessment (Cognistat), and CNS Vital Signs.

■ Advantages—Availability of alternate forms, automated output that provides performance and variability-in-performance indices, shorter administration time, accessibility, and automation of administration, scoring, and data storage.
■ Disadvantages—Little normative data exist for some CCTs and the reliability and validity of some of these assessments have not been adequately demonstrated. CCTs can be administered without professional supervision and/or in group settings (e.g., sports teams undergoing preseason baseline assessments), leading to unknown adverse effects on validity/accuracy. Test results still require interpretation by a trained clinician.

Post-injury use of CCTs should only be employed as one component of a thorough clinical evaluation by a qualified provider.

ISSUES RELATED TO NEUROPSYCHOLOGICAL ASSESSMENT FOLLOWING MILD TRAUMATIC BRAIN INJURY

Controversies Surrounding Neuropsychological Assessment Following Mild Traumatic Brain Injury

Although an NPA is a recommended part of repeat assessment following MTBI in athletes and military servicemembers and is part of well-established guidelines thereof, there is some controversy surrounding the utility of baseline and repeat neuropsychological testing following MTBI given the lack of sensitivity to change and lack of incremental utility beyond symptom resolution.[9-11] There is also a concern that baseline assessments may have unacceptably high rates of invalid data, especially in pediatric populations, possibly due to group administration protocols.[12]

Examiner Qualifications

Formal graduate school training in neuropsychology, clinical psychology, and structured postdoctoral training in NPA is required to properly interpret the results of NPA.[13] Board certification in clinical neuropsychology (e.g., from the American Academy of Clinical Neuropsychology) is the gold standard for demonstrating one's competence in clinical neuropsychology.

Repeated Testing

Practice effects secondary to frequent testing with similar measures can threaten the validity of subsequent NPAs. Physicians and rehabilitation clinicians should avoid using common neuropsychological measures to conduct frequent "check-up" cognitive evaluations during office visits, because this may threaten measurement validity in subsequent NPAs due to practice effects. If more frequent assessment is required (e.g., to measure changes in performance associated with interventions in a research context), alternate forms of cognitive tests or measures not included in the baseline NPA assessment should be used. In clinical settings, reassessment is indicated at least 12 months following initial assessment when changes in performance (decline or improvement) are reported by the patient.

KEY POINTS

- NPA, though not routinely indicated following an MTBI, may be used for diagnostic purposes, treatment planning, treatment evaluation, and/or in forensic cases.
- NPA consists of (a) a thorough clinical interview, including a description of the injury, TBI history, current symptomatology, and a review of medical, psychiatric, academic, vocational, and social history and (b) neuropsychological testing.
- NPA should be supervised and interpreted by qualified professionals with specialized training.

STUDY QUESTIONS

1. MTBI is typically defined by:
   a. Abnormal structural neuroimaging
   b. Loss of consciousness for at least 1 day
   c. A day or less of posttraumatic amnesia
   d. No alteration of consciousness

2. Following MTBI, cognitive recovery
   a. Is determined by the amount of brain tissue bleeding
   b. Is commensurate with neuroimaging abnormalities
   c. Is never complete
   d. Is typically complete within 3 months

3. A commonly used structured interview to determine if an MTBI occurred is
   a. Ohio State TBI Identification Interview (OSU TBI-ID)
   b. The Structured Concussion Tool
   c. The ACME Interview of TBI
   d. The Beck Depression Inventory

4. Why is it important to consider performance and symptom validity in neuropsychological evaluations?
   a. Because subsequent referrals may be needed
   b. Because financial and other incentives can have a substantial effect on performance during the evaluation

   c. Because attorneys may bias the patient
   d. Because many tests are produced by publishing companies with profit motives

5. A common comorbidity in those with combat-related MTBI might be
   a. Obsessive-compulsive disorder
   b. Fractures
   c. Visual problems
   d. PTSD

ADDITIONAL READING

https://www.psych.on.ca/getattachment/Resources/OPA-Guidelines/Guidelines-for-Best-Practices-in-the-Assessment-of/OPAConcussionGuidelinesFINAL2018.pdf.aspx?ext=.pdf

Belanger HG, Tate D, Vanderploeg RD. Concussion and mild traumatic brain injury. In: *Textbook of Clinical Neuropsychology.*, 2nd ed. Taylor and Francis; 2017:411–448. doi:10.4324/9781315271743-18

Lezak M, Howieson DB, Loring DW. *Neuropsychological Assessment.* Oxford University Press; 2004.

Strauss E, Sherman EMS, Spreen O. *A Compendium of Neuropsychological Tests.*: Oxford University Press; 2006.

Tate RL. *A Compendium of Tests, Scales and Questionnaires.* Psychology Press; 2010.

ANSWERS TO STUDY QUESTIONS

1. Correct Answer: c
The Department of Veterans Affairs (VA) and Department of Defense (DoD) define a concussion as an injury that results in normal structural neuroimaging and up to 24 hours alteration of consciousness (AOC), up to a day of posttraumatic amnesia (PTA), or up to 30 minutes of loss of consciousness (LOC).

Further Reading:
Department of Veterans Affairs/Department of Defense. *VA/DoD clinical practice guideline for the management of concussion-mild traumatic brain injury.* Edited by Group TMoC-mTBIW2016.

2. Correct Answer: d
The vast majority of people who sustain MTBI experience complete cognitive recovery within 3 months.

Further Reading:
Belanger HG, Curtiss G, Demery JA, et al. Factors moderating neuropsychological outcome following mild traumatic brain injury: a meta-analysis. *J Int Neuropsychol Soc.* 2005;11:215–227. doi:10.1017/S1355617705050277

3. Correct Answer: a
The OSU TBI-ID is a structured interview that is used to help determine whether an MTBI occurred through assessment of the historical event and any subsequent alteration or loss of consciousness.

Further Reading:
Corrigan JD, Bogner J. Initial reliability and validity of the Ohio State University TBI Identification Method. *J Head Trauma Rehabil.* 2007;22:318–329. doi:10.1097/01.HTR.0000300227.67748.77

4. Correct Answer: b
Because financial and other incentives can have a substantial effect on performance during the evaluation.

Further Reading:
Binder LM, Rohling ML. Money matters: a meta-analytic review of the effects of financial incentives on recovery after closed-head injury. *Am J Psychiatry*. 1996;153:7–10. doi:10.1176/ajp.153.1.7

5. Correct Answer: d
PTSD is a common comorbidity among those whose circumstances leading to the injury were particularly traumatic or combat related.

Further Reading:
Stein MB, McAllister TW. Exploring the convergence of posttraumatic stress disorder and mild traumatic brain injury. *Am J Psychiatry*. 2009;166:768–776. doi:10.1176/appi .ajp.2009.08101604

REFERENCES

The full reference list appears in the digital product found on http://connect.springer-pub.com/content/book/978-0-8261-4768-4/part/part02/chapter/ch14

15 POSTCONCUSSION SYNDROME: DIAGNOSTIC CHARACTERISTICS AND CLINICAL MANIFESTATIONS

ERICA BELLAMKONDA AND FELISE S. ZOLLMAN

GENERAL PRINCIPLES

Definition

Individuals sustaining a traumatic brain injury (TBI) often report a constellation of physical, cognitive, and emotional/behavioral symptoms. These symptoms typically resolve in days to weeks after the initial injury, but in some individuals symptoms can persist beyond 3 months and may be referred to as postconcussion syndrome (PCS).[1-3] The term "postconcussion syndrome" is still commonly used, but since the symptom clusters are nonspecific and not a distinct syndrome associated with a disease or disorder, the term is falling out of favor and being replaced by the symptom-focused term "persistent postconcussive symptoms" (PPCS).[4]

(Note that throughout this text you will see the terms PCS, PPCS, and postconcussion disorder [PCD] used interchangeably.)

There is debate in the literature on a universally accepted definition of PCS; however, the *International Classification of Diseases*, 10th revision (*ICD-10*), and *Diagnostic and Statistical Manual of Mental Disorders*, 5th edition (*DSM-5*), provide diagnostic guidelines as well as research criteria for diagnosis of PCS.[1,2]

- *ICD-10* clinical description and diagnostic guideline for F07.2: Postconcussional syndrome:[1]
  - History of head trauma, usually sufficiently severe to result in loss of consciousness
  - At least three of the following present:
    - Headache
    - Dizziness, usually without features of true vertigo
    - Fatigue
    - Irritability
    - Memory impairment
    - Difficulty concentrating and performing mental tasks
    - Insomnia
    - Reduced tolerance of alcohol, stress, or emotional excitement
  - Symptoms may be accompanied by depression or anxiety due to loss of self-esteem and fear of permanent brain damage.
  - Preoccupation with symptoms may lead to a search for diagnosis and cure; the patient may adopt a persistent sick role or identity.

The full reference list appears in the digital product found on http://connect.springerpub.com/content/book/978-0-8261-4768-4/part/part02/chapter/ch15

- *ICD-10* diagnostic criteria for research for F07.2: Postconcussional syndrome[2]
  - A history of head trauma with loss of consciousness, preceding onset of symptoms by up to 4 weeks
  - Symptoms from at least three of the following categories are present:
    - Headache, dizziness, malaise, fatigue, or noise intolerance
    - Irritability or emotional lability that is easily provoked; may be accompanied by depression and/or anxiety
    - Subjective complaints of difficulty with concentration, memory, or performing mental tasks without clear objective evidence of impairment
    - Insomnia
    - Reduced tolerance of alcohol
    - Preoccupation with symptoms, fear of permanent brain damage, and/or adoption of sick role
- *DSM-5* criteria:
  - The *DSM-5* defines TBI as an injury resulting from impact to the head or other mechanism causing the brain to shift within the skull, with at least one of the following: loss of consciousness, posttraumatic amnesia, disorientation/confusion, or neurologic signs such as evidence of injury on neuroimaging, seizures, loss of smell, or hemiparesis.[5]
  - Unlike the preceding edition, the *DSM-5* does not contain the diagnosis postconcussion disorder. In the *DSM-5*, persistent concussive symptoms are captured in the neurocognitive disorder (NCD) category, which describes disorders with acquired cognitive dysfunction as the core feature.[5] Unlike previous *DSM* editions, the *DSM-5* offers criteria for diagnosing a TBI event and its severity and considers the potential neurocognitive/neuropsychiatric sequelae attributed to it.
  - The *DSM-5* diagnostic criteria for Mild and Major NCD due to TBI include evidence of cognitive decline from a previous level of performance not occurring exclusively in the context of a delirium and not better explained by another mental disorder (e.g., major depressive disorder, schizophrenia), with onset immediately following the occurrence of a TBI.[5]

The essential distinction between Mild NCD due to TBI and Major NCD due to TBI is that, in the latter instance, cognitive deficits interfere with ability to perform everyday activities, necessitating the assistance of another.

In every circumstance, one must first ascertain that a precipitating TBI did in fact occur. If occurrence of a TBI cannot be assertained, then PCS and/or NCD due to TBI cannot be diagnosed.

EPIDEMIOLOGY

- The literature widely cites the estimation that 1 year after injury, approximately 10%–20% of persons will have persistent posttraumatic symptoms.[4] However, the accurate incidence and prevalence of PCS have not been established despite decades of research, largely because of limitations in subject recruitment (i.e., not all persons who suffer a mild TBI [MTBI] come to medical attention), varied criteria used for diagnosis, general lack of diagnostic specificity (diagnosis based on subjective report of nonspecific symptoms), and symptom fluctuations over time.[6-8]

- Individuals with positive early neuroimaging findings after MTBI have outcomes similar to those with moderate TBI,[8] that is, protracted symptoms are more common in this subset of MTBI patients.
- Recurrent MTBI may be associated with long-term neurocognitive impairment.[5]

PATHOPHYSIOLOGY

The initial symptom constellation reflects the neurometabolic cascade that occurs immediately following a TBI (described in Chapter 2). Symptom persistence has been attributed to both physiological and psychological causes; however, it is significantly influenced by a variety of factors that ultimately affect how persons perceive their symptoms after MTBI. Such confounding factors include personality traits, affective disorders, pain disorders, and medication side effects, among others[9–11] (see Figure 15.1).

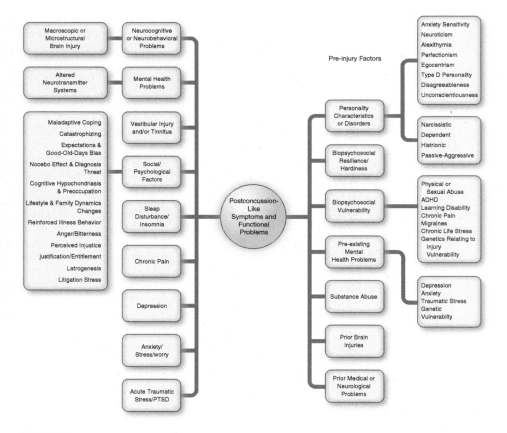

FIGURE 15.1 Factors that may influence symptom persistence after mild traumatic brain injury.

Source: From Iverson GL, Silverberg N, Lange RT, Zasler ND. Conceptualizing outcome from mild traumatic brain injury. In: Zasler ND, Katz DI, Zafonte RD, eds. *Brain Injury Medicine: Principles and Practice*. Demos Medical Publishing; 2013:470–497.

Selected factors worth further mention include the following:

- Personality
  - Certain personality traits or disorders are considered vulnerable to poor outcome: the overachieving, the dependent, the insecure, the grandiose, and those with borderline personality characteristics.[12,13] Alexithymia, characterized by difficulty identifying and describing feelings, externally oriented thinking, and limited imaginary thinking ability, and type D personality, characterized by negative affectivity and social inhibition, are also associated with an increased likelihood of experiencing PPCS.[14]
- Social-psychological
  - Nocebo effect—Symptoms are caused by expectation of experiencing certain symptoms and problems after injury.
  - Diagnosis threat—Adverse effect on task performance as a result of expectation-setting based on perception that symptoms experienced reflect persistent sequelae of TBI.[14,15]
  - Stereotype threat—Negative stereotype associated with having an injury adversely affects task performance.
  - Good-old-days bias—Overestimation in difference between pre- and post-injury symptoms/functioning.[4,16]
- Expectation as etiology—Anticipation or expectation of certain symptoms causes misattribution of future normal, everyday symptoms to the remote injury, or failure to appreciate the relationship between more proximate factors (life stress, poor sleep, mild depression, medication side effects) and symptoms.[4,14]
- Symptom exaggeration—Amplification of a symptom or sign that has a true physiological or psychological basis; most commonly seen in cases involving personal injury litigations, worker's compensation claims, and disability evaluations.[17]
- Malingering—Intentional exaggeration of symptoms or feigning symptoms for an external reward; less common than symptom exaggeration.

DIAGNOSIS

Clinical Presentation

- Common symptoms include fatigue, headache, and dizziness/lightheadedness. Other frequently reported symptoms include blurry/double vision, irritability, poor concentration, impairment in memory and attention, sensitivity to light/noise, and sleep disturbance.[18]
- Diagnosis is largely based on symptom presentation in the setting of a verified precipitating TBI; no symptom or sign is pathognomonic for PCS. Healthy persons as well as persons with a variety of conditions (e.g., depression, fibromyalgia, chronic pain, orthopedic injuries, whiplash, stress disorders, sleep disorders) frequently report symptom constellations that can meet criteria for PCS in the absence of any head injury[19,20] (see Table 15.1).

EVALUATION

- PCS should be considered a diagnosis of exclusion, as the symptoms are not specific to one condition.

TABLE 15.1   Percentages of Subjects Endorsing Symptoms at a Mild or Moderate to Severe Level (British Columbia Postconcussion Symptom Inventory)

Items	Healthy Community Volunteers		Patients With Depression		Patients With Fibromyalgia	
	Mild	Moderate to Severe	Mild	Moderate to Severe	Mild	Moderate to Severe
Headaches	19.6	3.2	59.4	28.1	72.2	37.0
Dizziness/ lightheaded	11.4	1.3	31.2	10.9	37.0	7.4
Nausea/feeling sick	133	0.0	40.6	10.9	35.2	18.5
Fatigue	27.8	5.1	85.6	57.8	96.3	79.6
Extra sensitive to noises	11.4	1.3	50.0	18.8	68.5	44.4
Irritability	21.5	5.1	76.6	35.9	53.7	25.9
Sadness	18.4	1.3	76.6	56.3	55.6	33.3
Nervous or tense	16.5	1.3	65.6	35.9	59.3	33.3
Temper problems	15.8	5.1	37.5	15.6	27.8	7.4
Poor concentration	16.5	3.2	78.1	46.9	75.9	44.4
Memory problems	13.3	3.8	70.3	42.2	74.1	44.4
Difficulty reading	8.2	1.9	40.6	23.4	48.1	24.1
Poor sleep	22.8	5.1	78.1	53.1	87.0	59.3

Healthy adults ($N = 158$), patients with depression ($N = 64$), and patients with fibromyalgia ($N = 54$).

Source: Adapted from Iverson GL, Zasler ND, Lange RG. In: Zasler ND, Katz DI, Zafonte RD, eds. *Brain Injury Medicine: Principles and Practice. Post-Concussive Disorder*. Demos Medical Publishing; 2007:377–379.

- Obtain a detailed history of the injury, ascertaining whether an inciting TBI did in fact occur, and elicit a description of the onset and progression of symptoms.
- Neuropsychological testing (NPT) is generally not required in the setting of PPCS but may aid in more thoroughly characterizing the nature/extent of cognitive/behavioral/ affective deficits when unexplained symptoms persist. NPT may also be useful as an educational tool, providing a framework for discussion of areas of relative strength or weakness. Caution must be exercised in interpreting results, however, because many of the aforementioned confounding factors (e.g., mood disorder, medication use, and malingering) can result in significant abnormal test results even in the absence of TBI (see Table 15.1).
- Differential diagnosis includes, but is not limited to, head and/or neck pain due to cervical injury whiplash-associated disorder or precipitation/aggravation of migraine, exacerbation of other chronic pain conditions, mood disorder (depression, anxiety), stress disorder (including PTSD), sleep disorder, and iatrogenesis/medication side

effects. Before concluding that the patient's symptoms are due to PCS, the provider must evaluate and treat confounding problems that may account for the clinical presentation (e.g., pain, insomnia, mood disorder, and medication side effects). It is important to note that concussion can exacerbate premorbid conditions, which can, in turn, be responsible for ongoing symptoms.

■ Posttraumatic symptoms that do not follow a typical course of resolution or are characterized by delayed clinical deterioration should trigger an evaluation for other conditions.

TREATMENT

Management of PCS is discussed in detail in Chapter 16. Basic principles include (a) identifying and addressing confounding factors, (b) education/reassurance, (c) introduction of behavioral modifications/lifestyle changes if indicated, (d) engagement in progressive aerobic exercise, (e) judicious, modest use of medication where appropriate, and (f) counseling the patient in safety practices to avoid repeat injury.[21]

KEY POINTS

■ There is no universally accepted definition of PCS. The syndrome-focused term PCS is still commonly used but the symptom-focused term PPCS is also gaining favor.

■ In the *DSM-5*, PCD is no longer described and has been subsumed under NCDs.

■ After a TBI, posttraumatic symptoms typically resolve over the course of a few weeks but symptoms can persist. Look for confounding factors such as mood disorder, medication side effects, or pain, which may account for these symptoms.

■ Diagnosis of PCS is largely based on subjective nonspecific symptom reporting and should be considered a diagnosis of exclusion.

STUDY QUESTIONS

1. Which of the following statements about PCS is true?
   a. Depending upon the symptoms experienced, PCS may be diagnosed immediately following a documented MTBI
   b. The presence of headache is required to assert a diagnosis of PCS
   c. PCS refers to a nonspecific constellation of symptoms which persist for an extended period post MTBI
   d. PCS is common; the majority of those who experience an MTBI will have PCS for at least some period of time post injury

2. Which of the following scenarios most likely represents PCS?
   a. A 35-year-old male status post-cycling injury with persistent neck pain and irritability 6 weeks post injury
   b. A 50-year-old male with a pre-injury history of migraine and depression who complains of persistent headaches and fatigue 3 months post MTBI

   c. A 17-year-old soccer player status post on-field collision resulting in confusion, removed from play for concussion, with migraines and insomnia x 2 weeks, now resolved.

   d. A 25-year-old female with no past medical history, 4 months post-MTBI, with persistent fatigue, mental fogginess, and irritability

3. Social-psychological factors which may contribute to symptom persistence post-TBI include all of the following except:

   a. Diagnosis threat

   b. Good-old-days bias

   c. Nocebo effect

   d. Malingering

4. Approximately what percent of persons experience persistent symptomatology 1 year or more after injury?

   a. 1%–2%

   b. 10%–20%

   c. 40%–50%

   d. 70%–80%

5. A core principle in management of persistent postconcussive symptomatology is

   a. Limit activity/stimuli as much as possible

   b. Address and treat confounding/comorbid conditions

   c. Utilize prescription medications to treat each symptom as it arises

   d. Consider pre-injury biopsychosocial factors unlikely to play a significant role in PCS

ADDITIONAL READING

Guidelines for Concussion/Mild Traumatic Brain Injury & Prolonged Symptoms, Third Ed for Adults Over 18 Years of Age, 2019: https://braininjuryguidelines.org/concussion/

Alexander MP. Mild traumatic brain injury: pathophysiology, natural history, and clinical management. *Neurology.* 1995;45(7):1253–1260. doi:10.1212/WNL.45.7.1253

Marshall S, Bayley M, McCullagh S, et al. Updated clinical practice guidelines for concussion/mild traumatic brain injury and persistent symptoms. *Brain Inj.* 2015;29(6):688–700. doi:10.3109/02699052.2015.1004755

Rickards TA, Cranston CC, McWhorter J. Persistent postconcussive symptoms: A model of predisposing, precipitating, and perpetuating factors. *Appl Neuropsychol Adult.* 2020;1–11 (Online ahead of print). doi:10.1080/23279095.2020.1748032

Silverbert ND, Iverson GL. Etiology of the postconcussion syndrome: physiogenesis and psychogenesis revisited. *NeuroRehabilitation.* 2011;29:317–329. doi:10.3233/NRE-2011-0708

ANSWERS TO STUDY QUESTIONS

1. Correct Answer: c

The term PCS is used to describe persistent symptoms experienced by a minority of patients after TBI, not immediate post-injury symptoms. It is typically considered when symptoms persist for 3 months or more. There is no single complaint or combination of symptoms which is pathognomonic for PCS.

Further Reading:

World Health Organization. *The ICD-10 Classification of Mental and Behavioral Disorders: Clinical Descriptions and Diagnostic Guidelines (aka the "Blue Book")*. Author; 2010:63–64.

World Health Organization. *The ICD-10 Classification of Mental and Behavioral Disorders: Diagnostic Criteria for Research* (aka the "Green Book"). Author; 1993: 60–61.

Rickards TA, Cranston CC, McWhorter J. Persistent postconcussive symptoms: a model of predisposing, precipitating, and perpetuating factors. *Appl. Neuropsychol. Adult.* 2020:1–11 (Online ahead of print). doi:10.1080/23279095.2020.1748032

2. Correct Answer: d

   Whether using *ICD-10* or *DSM-5* criteria, the term PCS is used to apply to someone who experiences persistent symptoms post-TBI not otherwise explained by other comorbid conditions. Answer (a) is wrong because it describes a scenario consistent with likely whiplash injury, (b) describes exacerbation of premorbid migraines and depression, and (c) symptom resolution without any symptom persistence.

   Further Reading:

   World Health Organization. *The ICD-10 Classification of Mental and Behavioral Disorders: Clinical Descriptions and Diagnostic Guidelines (aka the "Blue Book")*. Author; 2010:63–64.

   World Health Organization. The ICD-10 Classification of Mental and Behavioral Disorders: Diagnostic Criteria for Research (aka the "Green Book"). Author; 1993: 60–61.

   Rickards TA, Cranston CC, McWhorter J. Persistent postconcussive symptoms: a model of predisposing, precipitating, and perpetuating factors. Appl. *Neuropsychol Adult.* 2020:1–11.

   American Psychiatric Association. *Diagnostic and Statistical Manual of Mental Disorders,* (DSM 5). 5th ed. 2013. doi:10.1176/appi.books.9780890425596

3. Correct Answer: d

   Items (a) to (c) are social-psychological factors which may contribute to symptom persistence post TBI. Malingering is a term used to describe intentional symptom exaggeration for secondary gain or benefit.

   Further Reading:

   Silverbert ND, Iverson GL. Etiology of the postconcussion syndrome: physiogenesis and psychogenesis revisited. *Neuro Rehabilitation.* 2011;29:317–329. doi:10.3233/NRE-2011-0708

4. Correct Answer: b

   While a true/accurate figure is not attainable (an unknown number of MTBI cases are mild and medical care is not sought; there is significant variability in diagnosing PCS), it is estimated that 10% to 20% of those who experience a TBI will continue to experience some symptoms 1 year out.

   Further Reading:

   Guidelines for Concussion/Mild Traumatic Brain Injury & Prolonged Symptoms, Third Ed. for Adults Over 18 Years of Age. http://braininjuryguidelines.org/concussion/ (accessed 5/3/21).

5. Correct Answer: b
When symptom persistence is prolonged after MTBI, all potential contributing factors (e.g., exacerbation of premorbid headache disorder, medication side effects, mood disorder) should be considered and management strategies employed accordingly.

Further Reading:
Marshall S, Bayley M, McCullagh S, et al. Updated clinical practice guidelines for concussion/mild traumatic brain injury and persistent symptoms. *Brain Inj*. 2015:29(6):688–700. doi:10.3109/02699052.2015.1004755

REFERENCES

The full reference list appears in the digital product found on http://connect.springer-pub.com/content/book/978-0-8261-4768-4/part/part02/chapter/ch15

POSTCONCUSSION SYNDROME: SYMPTOM MANAGEMENT

WILLIAM C. WALKER AND RICHARD D. KUNZ

TREATMENT OF POSTCONCUSSION SYNDROME

Introduction

A minority of patients who sustain mild traumatic brain injury (MTBI; concussion) have persistent symptoms. Postconcussion syndrome (PCS) is the persistence of postconcussion symptoms and related difficulties for at least several months after MTBI, and is further defined in Chapter 15. The focus of this chapter is the treatment of PCS; for the treatment of MTBI itself, refer to Chapter 7. Evidence to guide treatment of PCS in the form of randomized controlled trials is limited, but review of the literature reveals a relative expert consensus concerning appropriate treatment principles. This chapter reviews these principles along with author recommendations on specific interventions.

Guiding Principles of Postconcussion Syndrome Management

- Management of persistent postconcussion symptoms (PPCS) should focus on promoting recovery and avoiding harm.
- Patients with entrenched PPCS are often suffering and distressed. Education, support, understanding and guidance are crucial components of treatment.
- A patient-centered approach[1] should be used to provide the needed reassurance and motivation.
- Treatment of somatic complaints (e.g., insomnia, dizziness/incoordination, nausea, alterations of smell/taste, appetite problems, vision/hearing changes, numbness, headache, fatigue) should be based on individual factors and symptom presentation.
- Any medications added for symptom control must be carefully prescribed after consideration of sedating properties or other side effects.
- In patients with PPCS that have been refractory to treatment, consideration should be given to other factors including psychiatric, psychosocial support, and issues of compensation/litigation. A comprehensive multidisciplinary treatment approach for such patients should also be considered, but scientific proof of its efficacy beyond the non-specific effects of extra attention is scant.
- Potential comorbidities contributing to PPCS such as depression, sleep apnea, and endocrine disorders should be sought and treated regardless of possible relation to the MTBI.[2,3]
- One effective semiquantitative way to monitor the course of PCS and success of applied treatments is by quantifying the number and intensity of individual symptoms using one of the available standardized inventories such as the PCS Checklist,[4] Rivermead Postconcussion Symptoms Questionnaire,[5] Concussion Symptom Checklist,[6] or Neurobehavioral Symptom Inventory (NSI).[7]

The full reference list appears in the digital product found on http://connect.springerpub.com/content/book/978-0-8261-4768-4/part/part02/chapter/ch16

Education

Education is the mainstay of PCS treatment. A randomized controlled trial in which patients with concussion received telephone counseling focused on education and symptom management showed significantly less PCS symptoms at 6 months post-injury compared to patients who received standard hospital discharge materials.[8]

- Assure the patient that symptoms are part of the normal recovery process, and not a sign of permanent brain dysfunction.
- Noncontact, aerobic, and recreational activities should be encouraged within the limits of the patient's symptoms; increased headache or irritability suggests that this level has been exceeded. (See Physical Rehabilitation for further details.)
- Encourage resumption of occupational, educational, and social responsibilities in a graded fashion to minimize stress and avoid fatigue.
- Ascertain current sleep–wake cycle and provide counseling regarding appropriate sleep hygiene as needed (see Table 16.1).[9]
- Education, counseling, and joint goal-setting should cover all aspects of lifestyle that may impact brain health including stress management, nutrition, and substance use.
- Provide printed and verbal education.

TABLE 16.1   Education for Sleep Hygiene

- Avoid going to bed too early in the evening
- Avoid stimulants, caffeinated beverages, power drinks, and nicotine during the evening
- Avoid stimulating activities before bedtime (e.g., exercise, video games, TV)
- Avoid alcohol
- Restrict the nighttime sleep period to about 8 hours
- Wake up and arise from bed at a consistent time in the morning (e.g., 7 a.m.)
- Reduce (to less than 30 minutes) or abolish daytime naps
- Engage in daytime physical and mental activities (within the limits of the individual's functional capacity)

Source: Reproduced with permission from Irish LA, Kline CE, Gunn HE, Buysse DJ, Hall MH. The role of sleep hygiene in promoting public health: a review of empirical evidence. *Sleep Med Rev.* 2015;22:23–36. doi:10.1016/j.smrv.2014.10.001

Physical Rehabilitation

- There is mounting evidence for the safety and benefit of graded aerobic exercise in PCS.[10,11] A caveat is that physical (or cognitive) exertion can temporarily increase postconcussion symptoms at any point in recovery. Although long-term ill effects from this are not demonstrated, to be safe keep exercise intensity and duration below symptom threshold.
- Gradually increase duration and intensity to accommodate the activity intolerance and fatigue that is commonly associated with PCS.
- A general exercise program that includes strength training, core stability, aerobic activities, and range of motion is ideal.
- Targeted and customized vestibular, visual, and proprioceptive therapeutic exercises are recommended for persistent dizziness, disequilibrium, and spatial disorientation impairments.[12,13]
- Targeted therapeutic exercise is also recommended for any persisting focal musculoskeletal impairments.
- If a person's normal activity involves significant physical activity, exertional testing (i.e., stressing the body) should be conducted before permitting full resumption.

Psychological Treatment

- Psychotherapy for PCS is commonly recommended, although evidence of efficacy is limited. A recent meta-analysis found the best evidence exists for counseling and to a lesser degree cognitive behavioral therapy (CBT).[14]
- Some research also suggests that psychological treatment early after sustaining MTBI may protect against developing PCS, but the benefit may be limited to those at high risk for PPCS (e.g., history of chronic depression).[14]
- Counseling typically includes education, reassurance, and teaching of anxiety reduction techniques, while CBT seeks to target and modify cognitive biases and misattribution. Psychotherapy can also be useful in identifying psychosocial factors contributing to symptom presentation and teaching specific coping skills for dealing with psychosocial pressure.[15]
- In these authors' opinion, referral to a neuropsychologist or psychologist with expertise in PCS is indicated when there is failure to respond to initial treatments, worsening stress, deterioration in function, or significant impairment in vocational or social function.

Cognitive Rehabilitation

Patients who have cognitive symptoms that do not resolve or have been refractory to treatment should be considered for referral for neuropsychological assessment. Individuals with memory, attention, and/or executive function deficits that do not respond to initial treatment (e.g., reassurance, management of sleep dysfunction, mood disorders, and somatic complaints) may benefit from cognitive therapy (e.g., speech and language pathology, neuropsychology, or occupational therapy) for development of compensatory strategies (e.g., use of external memory aids such as a smartphone or notebook).

PHARMACOLOGICAL MANAGEMENT OVERVIEW

Postconcussion symptoms are frequently treated with medications despite the paucity of randomized controlled trials. A survey of treatments prescribed by a representative sample of physicians showed that nonsteroidal anti-inflammatory analgesics were most often recommended. Antidepressant medications were the second most commonly prescribed overall, and the treatment preferred by neurologists.[16] Where evidence-based data exist to direct pharmacotherapeutic decision-making, it will be presented; where such data are not presented, the recommendations made represent the opinions of the author.

Thorough medication reconciliation is crucial. The existing medication list should be reviewed for agents that can cause neurological abnormalities (centrally acting medications, pain medications, sleep aids, anticholinergics, etc.). If a medication with neurological side effects is identified, consider discontinuing or decreasing dose and re-evaluate after 1 week.

Headache

Headache is the most common PCS symptom. Management should be tailored to the subtype of headache (see Chapter 56 for a detailed discussion of this subject).

Mood Disorders

■ Anxiety and depression symptoms can be treated with a variety of medications. The choice is usually dictated by comorbid symptoms and the side effect profile of the various agents. In general, selective serotonin reuptake inhibitors (SSRIs; e.g., sertraline, citalopram, fluoxetine, paroxetine) are preferred first-line agents. Serotonin–norepinephrine reuptake inhibitors (SNRIs; e.g., duloxetine, venlafaxine) and "atypical" antidepressants (e.g., mirtazapine, bupropion) may also be considered.

■ Irritability and anger are common complaints. If depression or anxiety are ruled out or are well controlled, then antiepileptic mood stabilizers (e.g., valproic acid and carbamazepine) are reasonable options. A randomized control trial showed amantadine improved irritability and aggression in chronic TBI of mixed severity with the caveats that PCS post-MTBI was not specifically studied, and observer ratings did not improve relative to placebo.[17,18]

Fatigue and Inattention

■ Fatigue symptoms may be secondary to comorbid conditions. After conditions such as depression, insomnia, and sleep apnea have been ruled out or treated, stimulant medications may be appropriate.

■ An activating antidepressant (e.g., fluoxetine) is a reasonable agent to try initially. If the patient is already on an antidepressant medication, consider switching to one with a less sedating profile.

■ Modafinil, a medication approved by the Food and Drug Administration (FDA) for narcolepsy and shift work sleep syndrome, has been advocated by some, but there is no evidence of benefit in TBI populations.[19,20]

■ Similarly, amphetamine-type simulants (e.g., methylphenidate) are used for mental fatigue or inattention, but only low-quality studies have shown any benefit in TBI populations.[9,19] Thus, they are best suited for patients with a preinjury history of attention deficit disorder.

■ Amantadine has mixed evidence of efficacy for fatigue symptoms in multiple sclerosis and is considered by some to be an option for PCS-related fatigue.

Sleep Dysfunction

■ Primary sleep disorders should be considered and ruled out with a sleep study as indicated.

■ Behavioral interventions, including meditation, relaxation training, and white noise devices, are preferred over pharmacotherapy (see Table 16.1).

■ Benzodiazepines should be avoided.

■ Additional management recommendations can be found in Chapter 53.

Dizziness and Disequilibrium

■ Medication review and reconciliation are crucial because numerous medications have dizziness as a potential side effect.

■ Vestibular suppressants (e.g., meclizine) have not been shown to be effective in chronic dizziness after concussion.[21]

■ The mainstays of treatment for persisting symptoms are the aforementioned vestibular exercises in combination with habituation and coping strategies.

■ Specific treatments may be indicated for some subtypes (e.g., Semont and modified Epley maneuvers for benign paroxysmal positional vertigo).

> **KEY POINTS**
>
> ▪ Symptom persistence after MTBI occurs in a minority of patients and, if present for an extended period and unexplained by other co-occurring conditions, is termed PCS.
> ▪ Why most individuals have complete recovery after MTBI and some have persisting symptoms is unclear; convincing objective data are lacking and misattribution is suspected in many cases.
> ▪ State-of-the-art treatment is a practical holistic symptom-based approach that addresses psychosocial and lifestyle factors as well as specific somatic or cognitive complaints.
> ▪ Comprehensive education and counseling are cornerstones of treatment.

STUDY QUESTIONS

1. What strategy is least helpful for patients with persistent PPCS?
   a. Physical exercise
   b. Stimulant medication
   c. Sleep hygiene
   d. Stress management
   e. Cognitive compensatory strategies

2. Which PCS symptom is most amenable to physical therapy?
   a. Fatigue
   b. Tinnitus
   c. Depression
   d. Dizziness
   e. Headache

3. Which intervention has the most basic science and clinical research evidence of benefit and safety in patients with PPCS?
   a. Aerobic (cardio) exercise at sub-symptom threshold levels
   b. Aerobic (cardio) exercise at symptom-provoking levels
   c. Resistance (strengthening) exercise at sub-symptom threshold levels
   d. Resistance (strengthening) exercise at symptom-provoking levels
   e. None of the above; all exercise should be avoided

4. Which of the following is NOT among the recommendations for proper sleep hygiene in the setting of PPCS?
   a. Avoid caffeine and other stimulants in the evening hours before bed
   b. Take a long nap during the day if tired
   c. Avoid alcohol
   d. Wake at a scheduled time (e.g., 7 a.m.)
   e. Don't watch television or electronic screens in bed

5. Which statement about the use of psychotherapy for patients with PCS is most accurate?
   a. Psychotherapy should always include cognitive behavioral therapy
   b. Cognitive behavioral therapy has no role in treatment of PPCS

   c. Psychotherapy is indicated for all PCS patients
   d. Psychotherapy is primarily appropriate for PCS patients with comorbid PTSD
   e. Psychotherapy is most appropriate when PCS patients have not responded well to symptom-based medical treatments and their stress levels are high

ADDITIONAL READING

Va/DoD Clinical Practice Guideline for Management of Concussion/Mild Traumatic Brain Injury (MTBI). Version 2. 2016. https://www.healthquality.va.gov/guidelines/Rehab/mtbi/mTBICPGFull-CPG50821816.pdf

Silver JM. Persistent symptoms after mild traumatic brain injury. In: Silver JM, McAllister TW, Arciniegas DB, eds. *Textbook of Traumatic Brain Injury*, 3rd ed. American Psychiatric Pub; 2018:699–714. doi:10.1176/appi.books.9781615372645

Walker WC, Lacey R. Post concussive syndrome (PCS). In: Eapen B, Cifu DX, eds. *Eapen: Concussion Assessment, Management and Rehabilitation*. 2019. doi:10.1016/B978-0-323-65384-8.00004-3

Mittenberg W, Canyock EM, Condit D, Patton C. Treatment of post-concussion syndrome following mild head injury. *J Clin Exp Neuropsychol*. 2001;23(6):829–836. doi:10.1076/jcen.23.6.829.1022

ANSWERS TO STUDY QUESTIONS

1. Correct Answer: b
Optimizing lifestyle factors is the pillar of treatment for PPCS. There are significant inherent risks in using stimulant medications and there is no good evidence of meaningful benefit in the TBI population. Methylphenidate trials in the TBI population have shown improved neuropsychological test scores but neither functional benefit nor improved engagement in rehabilitation therapies.

Further Reading:
Dougall D, Poole N, Agrawal N. Pharmacotherapy for chronic cognitive impairment in traumatic brain injury. *Cochrane Database Syst Rev*. 2015;(12):CD009221. doi:10.1002/14651858.CD009221.pub2
Chien YJ, Chien YC, Liu CT, et al. Effects of methylphenidate on cognitive function in adults with traumatic brain injury: a meta-analysis. *Brain Sci*. 2019 24;9(11): pii: E291. doi:10.3390/brainsci9110291
Walker WC, Lacey R. Post concussive syndrome (PCS). In: Eapen B, Cifu DX, eds. *Eapen: Concussion Assessment, Management and Rehabilitation*. 2019. doi:10.1016/B978-0-323-65384-8.00004-3

2. Correct Answer: d
Dizziness is the best answer. There is some decent research evidence and ample experiential evidence that vestibular type physical therapy is the treatment of choice for dizziness or imbalance after mild TBI. Headache will only potentially respond to physical therapy if there is a cervicogenic component. Fatigue and depression may respond to a home exercise program with formal physical therapy reserved for those that can't safely perform or tolerate home exercise.

Further Reading:
Murray DA, Meldrum D, Lennon O. Can vestibular rehabilitation exercises help patients with concussion? A systematic review of efficacy, prescription and progression patterns. *Br J Sports Med*. 2017;51(5):442-451. doi:10.1136/bjsports-2016-096081

Gurley JM, Hujsak BD, Kelly JL. Vestibular rehabilitation following mild traumatic brain injury. *Neuro Rehabilitation*. 2013;32(3):519–528. doi:10.3233/NRE-130874

Walker WC, Lacey R. Post concussive syndrome (PCS). In: Eapen B, Cifu DX, eds. *Eapen: Concussion Assessment, Management and Rehabilitation*; 2019. doi:10.1016/B978-0-323-65384-8.00004-3

3. Correct Answer: a

There is abundant scientific evidence that aerobic exercise, more than any other type of exercise, has benefit not only for patients with PPCS, but also in TBI recovery, dementia prevention, and healthy and diseased brain function in general. Because the long-term potentially negative effects of provoking symptoms are unknown, the safest practice is to keep intensity and duration below the level of triggering or significantly worsening any symptoms during exercise. In general, duration and intensity can be gradually titrated up over time as tolerated.

Further Reading:

Leddy JJ, Haider MN, Ellis M, Willer BS. Exercise is medicine for concussion. *Curr Sports Med Rep*. 2018;17(8):262–270. doi:10.1249/JSR.0000000000000505

Ritter KG, Hussey MJ, Valovich McLeod TC. Subsymptomatic aerobic exercise for patients with postconcussion syndrome: a critically appraised topic. *J Sport Rehabil*. 2018:1–6.

4. Correct Answer: b

Napping during the day for longer than 1 hour or later than 3 p.m. is discouraged in the setting of insomnia as it can exacerbate sleeplessness at night. The other recommendations in the list are common and appropriate sleep hygiene practices for treatment of insomnia.

Further Reading:

Irish LA, Kline CE, Gunn HE, et al. The role of sleep hygiene in promoting public health: a review of empirical evidence. *Sleep Med Rev*. 2015;22:23–36. doi:10.1016/j.smrv.2014.10.001

5. Correct Answer: e

Psychotherapy can be a helpful intervention for patients with PCS as an adjunct to the primary provider's education, reassurance, and informal counseling. It is most appropriate for patients with high stress levels who have not responded well to initial education and symptom-based medical treatments. The specific method of psychotherapy varies. Currently, the method with most evidence for efficacy in PCS is formal counseling. Cognitive behavioral therapy is a promising method and may be appropriate, but has less evidence for efficacy.

Further Reading:

Sullivan KA, Kaye SA, Blaine H, et al. Psychological approaches for the management of persistent postconcussion symptoms after mild traumatic brain injury: a systematic review. *Disabil Rehabil*. 2019:1–9.

REFERENCES

The full reference list appears in the digital product found on http://connect.springer-pub.com/content/book/978-0-8261-4768-4/part/part02/chapter/ch16

CONFOUNDING FACTORS IN POSTCONCUSSIVE DISORDERS

NATHAN D. ZASLER

INTRODUCTION

The diagnosis of postconcussive disorders may be complicated by a number of confounding factors that practitioners should keep in mind when assessing this group of patients. The purpose of this chapter is to identify some of the key issues that complicate assessment of claimed concussion and provide guidelines for addressing them. Even if a concussion or mild traumatic brain injury (MTBI) is diagnosed based on diagnostic criteria at the time of an accident, one cannot necessarily conclude that symptoms occurring after the event are in fact causally related to the concussion. Additionally, abnormal physical exam findings cannot be causally related to the injury in question without being able to confirm those findings were not in fact present prior to the concussion and/or caused by other etiologies than traumatic brain injury (TBI). (The challenges of opining on causality and apportionment are beyond the scope of this chapter; see Chapter 62 for information on this topic.) A patient's pre-injury history, temporal onset of signs and symptoms post-injury, as well as symptom quality, severity, frequency, evolution and response to treatment must be considered in the context of differential diagnosis after claimed concussion. Clinicians need to consider potential confounding issues that make assessing and managing this group of patients so challenging.[1-3]

NOMENCLATURE

Cerebral concussion (Latin: *commotion cerebri*) is a phraseology that has been around since the time of Hippocrates. There remains some debate as to whether concussion and MTBI are analogous, although most clinicians and researchers do not make a clinical distinction. Some have advocated for avoiding the MTBI terminology altogether and instead classifying such injuries as "concussive brain injury" (CBI), avoiding the adjectival descriptor of "mild."[4] Others have advocated for dispensing with the nomenclature of "concussion," as well as "postconcussion syndrome" (PCS) due to their perceived unhelpfulness in terms of expressing the spectrum of impairment severity and/or duration of same that may occur.[5] The Centers for Disease Control and Prevention (CDC) defines a timeframe of 3 months for endorsing PCS; in the ICD-10, PCS is defined as occurring when there is an injury "usually sufficiently severe to result in loss of consciousness" followed by an onset of at least three of eight symptoms within 4 weeks of the injury.[6,7] A syndrome is a consistent set of findings associated with a condition with symptom linkage and coupling of symptom resolution. There is neither consistency to the signs or symptoms of concussion nor is there any symptom/set of symptoms or signs that are in and of themselves a priori diagnostic of CBI.[8]

The full reference list appears in the digital product found on http://connect.springerpub.com/content/book/978-0-8261-4768-4/part/part02/chapter/ch17

Therefore, the use of the phrase "postconcussive syndrome" is in reality a misnomer and leads to "lumping" symptoms and potentially over-diagnosing concussive injury and/or persistent impairment from same. Instead, developing a unified classification of the severity of TBI coupled with a careful attempt to identify the underlying cause for any persistent posttraumatic symptoms appears to be the current trend of thinking in the field.[4,5,9]

The phrases "brain injury" and "head injury" are often used interchangeably, although these are two distinct terms. The former describes insult/trauma to the cerebrum and the latter connotes traumatic injury to the cranium or its surrounding structures. Both injuries can produce a number of parallel symptoms including headache, dizziness, hearing loss, smell loss, among other complaints and should therefore be distinguished appropriately and not analogized.[10]

When postconcussive symptoms (to be referred to as PCS in this chapter) become persistent is unclear and varies across definitional criteria and between sport-related concussion and civilian concussion literature. The phrase "persistent postconcussion symptoms" (PPCS) is an unclear terminology as well, as persistence has been defined variably from weeks in some definitions to months in others.[11] There is additionally no specific symptom burden defined for diagnosis of PPCS.[8] Recent writings have suggested an early phase of symptoms with a more organic basis and a late-phase symptom complex which is highly influenced by a number of psychosocial factors and has little specificity for brain injury per se.[12] A history of multiple concussions seems to increase the risk of more severe and protracted symptoms.[3,12] The bottom line is that the longer symptoms persist after concussion, the more likely it is that confounding factors are playing a contributory role above and beyond the original neurological injury,[1,3,12] although that does not negate the possibility of persistent neurogenic impairment due to the original concussion.

DIFFERENTIAL DIAGNOSTIC ISSUES

The aim of evaluation following a claimed concussion should be to appropriately understand the pre-injury, injury, and post-injury history to facilitate accurate diagnosis. Thorough and appropriate differential diagnosis requires pursuing the potential etiologies for the presenting symptoms and/or signs while avoiding generic diagnoses for subjective complaints (somatic and otherwise) such as posttraumatic headache, dizziness, smell or hearing loss, or tinnitus, as these provide no specific etiology or direction for appropriate treatment.[8,10,12] Understanding the myriad posttraumatic impairments that might produce symptoms attributed to concussion but that in fact have noncerebral origins is particularly important.[5,8,10,12] Conditions such as posttraumatic stress disorder (PTSD) and other anxiety disorders, depression, chronic pain, and insomnia, among others, can be misdiagnosed as PCS given the overlap of symptomatology.[10] When present, these aforementioned conditions can complicate the clinical assessment and treatment of such patients as well as protract postconcussive symptomatology. Good differential diagnosis is only possible with an eye to garnering sufficient historical information and performing an appropriately focused physical examination that should include both neurological and musculoskeletal assessments based on complaints and injury history. Ideally, clinicians should also seek corroboratory information from injury witnesses and/or individuals familiar with the injured persons both pre-injury and post injury.

History

Obtaining a detailed history regarding pre-injury, injury, and post-injury symptoms and signs can be very helpful in elucidating the nature of the patient's current complaints and their apportionment.[1,2,8,12] Evaluation of postconcussive symptoms poses a number of confounds in part due to the subjective nature and non-specificity of said symptoms. The common symptoms of concussion are fairly prevalent in the general population.[1] In some cases, persistent symptoms appear to be an extension of acute symptoms that are taking longer than usual to resolve.[12] In other cases, pre-existing conditions or a prior history of problems that parallel postconcussive symptoms (e.g., dyssomnias, migraine-related disorders, vertigo, tinnitus) may confound diagnosis and protract recovery.[10] It should be noted that the method of assessment influences PCS base rates, such that symptom elicitation decreases relative to the reduction in prompting associated with each assessment methodology. Clinicians need to consider how their chosen assessment method may be influencing the symptoms reported by their patients regardless of the presence of potential secondary gain influences.[13] Certain factors have been shown to assist in prediction of risk of protracted postconcussional symptoms. These include prior brain injury, acute and sub-acute symptom burden, pre-injury mental health issues, poor coping/resilience, substance abuse, post-insult depression, headache disorders such as migraine, pre-injury or post injury.[1,10,12] Interestingly, recent research suggests that attention deficit hyperactivity disorder (ADHD) and/or learning disabilities do not appear to be significantly related to greater risk of slower recovery.[10]

Pre-injury medical, military, and scholastic records including standardized testing should be requested for review when possible to provide better objective baselines for both medical and cognitive-behavioral status. There are certainly some patients who come to treatment with premorbid and undiagnosed conditions such as hypertension, diabetes mellitus, sleep apnea, as well as psychiatric disorders that can potentially complicate assessment as well as treatment.

Injury-related historical issues that should be explored by the examining clinician include[1,2,13]:

- The specifics of the incident responsible for the claimed MTBI (e.g., vehicular accident, fall, assault, sports injury) and details of same
- Memory for preconcussive as well as postconcussive events
- Any gap in memory and, if present, its duration
- Any loss of consciousness and, if present, its duration (as well as corroboration)
- Any history of direct cranial/facial impact injury including facial trauma
- History of neck injury and/or cervicalgia

Post-injury history should seek to clarify symptom onset and progression/resolution, specific complaints experienced by the patient, evaluations and treatments to date including prior medications, dosing and duration of medication treatment, type of therapeutic interventions administered and response to same, as well as injury-related functional consequences and their evolution over time. An adequate history should be taken to explore for symptoms that may be consistent with physiological, visuo-vestibular, and/or cervicogenic patterns of postconcussive findings and/or associated injuries.[14] Use of age appropriate rating scales should be encouraged, whereas use of baseline computerized cognitive assessments is not generally recommended.[15]

PHYSICAL EXAMINATION

Subtle neurological findings may be seen in persons after concussion, including smell or hearing loss, vestibular dysfunction, visual impairments such as convergence insufficiency, higher level balance impairment, kinetic tremor, slowed reaction time, and/or frontal motor impairments, among other potential findings.[2,4,8,12,14] Areas of clinical function that should be assessed based on a systematic review following sport-related concussion include neurological, vestibular, ocular motor, visual, neurocognitive, psychological, and cervical domains.[16] The clinician should do a careful exam focusing on the patient's known injury history and current somatic complaints. Examination should include a thorough cervical assessment given the role of the neck in many symptoms that are also seen in concussion.[8,17] Cervical assessment should be done even in the absence of complaints of neck pain. Elemental neurological examination that includes careful assessment of smell, higher level balance, visuo-vestibular, and cognitive behavioral function should be conducted.[8,12] The ability to recognize non-organic and functional symptoms and signs is essential.[18-21] Clinicians should also conduct an appropriate musculoskeletal examination of the face, head, neck, and shoulder girdles as clinically indicated.[8,12,22] Exercise tolerance testing should also be considered when warranted based on clinical presentation.[8]

Screening cognitive assessments should be considered when symptoms persist for more than a month and certainly when they have not cleared by 3 months to serve as a baseline for future comparison.[2,8,12] When there are concerns about secondary behavioral impairments, standardized and normed psychoemotional batteries such as the Minnesota Multiphasic Personality Inventory-2-RF, Personality Assessment Inventory, and Millon Clinical Multiaxial Inventory-IV as well as focused assessment for conditions such as PTSD (e.g., Trauma Symptom Inventory-2 or Detailed Assessment of Posttraumatic Stress) or poor pain coping (Pain Catastrophizing Scale) should be considered. In the context of such assessments, performing validity checks are important, particularly in certain at-risk populations, such as athletes incentivized to perform poorly on preseason screening or persons with secondary gain incentives, such as a legal case, who may be incentivized to magnify their complaints (consciously or unconsciously).[18-22]

Further elaboration on assessment strategies and differential diagnosis of postconcussive/posttrauma symptoms can be found in the Additional Reading section. If symptoms persist beyond 2 weeks in adults or 4 weeks in adolescents, then referral to a multidisciplinary center that focuses on CBI is recommended.

DIAGNOSTIC ASSESSMENT

A few of the more commonly used and more sensitive testing approaches include early neuroimaging (traditionally computed tomography [CT] or magnetic resonance imaging [MRI]), electrophysiological (i.e., electroencephalogram [EEG]), neuro-otological, neuro-ophthalmological, chemosensory, and/or neuropsychological testing. It is critical for clinicians to also understand the appropriate applications and limitations of such tests, including their validity (i.e., internal, external, ecological) and reliability (i.e., test–retest), as well as their sensitivity and specificity for detecting changes that are causally related to the history of concussion with a degree of medical probability.[23-26] There is often over-reliance on diagnostics, in particular imaging studies, as a means of legitimizing claimed symptoms as concussion-related, when in fact literature has demonstrated a lack of significant association between many such findings and postconcussive symptom report.[27] Newer technologies such as MRI diffusion tensor imaging (DTI), functional MRI (fMRI), and volumetric analysis may hold promise in verifying brain dysfunction/injury due to concussion but remain of unresolved utility mainly due to the fact that other conditions can affect findings of these imaging technologies.

Use of symptom-limited aerobic exercise and mental activity, focused physical therapy, primary symptom modulation (including sleep, mood, and pain), appropriately focused patient and family education, and a multidisciplinary medical as well as interdisciplinary rehabilitation approach generally have been found to produce the best results and assist in clarifying confounds.[8,15,28]

Pathologies That May Produce Signs and Symptoms Parallel to Those of Concussion

Cranial Trauma

Trauma to the cranium can produce an array of symptoms that parallel postconcussive ones without having any concurrent brain injury.[1,8,29] Some of the problems that may be seen after these types of injuries include headache, tinnitus, hearing loss, hyperacusis, vestibulopathies, olfactory impairments, and visual dysfunction. Appropriate practitioner understanding of the differential diagnosis of each of the aforementioned conditions is therefore critical in optimizing both assessment accuracy and treatment outcomes.

Cervical Injuries

Injuries to the neck, such as through acceleration/deceleration or direct trauma, may produce an array of problems that may be mistaken for PCS, including referred cervicogenic headache, tinnitus, cervical vertigo, visual problems including blurry vision, autonomic dysfunction symptoms (including orthostatic hypotension) and photosensitivity, as well as retro-orbital pain.[29–31] Clinicians should be aware of the role of the trigeminocervical network in terms of its ability to promulgate a variety of PCS-type symptoms through cervical afferent nociceptive input.[17,29,30] Practitioners should also be familiar with the literature on how neck trauma can masquerade as PCS and methods to fully assess for neck injury and related impairment.[17,30,31]

Chronic Pain

Posttraumatic pain disorders are an often-overlooked concomitant of cranial and cervical trauma as well as concussion itself. When pain becomes chronic (i.e., more than 6 months duration), it typically becomes more challenging to identify the primary pain generators due to central sensitization phenomena, as well as secondary psychoemotional responses to chronic pain. Pain may also have adverse consequences on sleep and cognition, which further complicates both assessment and treatment of postconcussive symptoms.[32–34]

Affective Issues

Patients may develop secondary psychological reactions either to the trauma itself or to the consequences thereof. Clinicians working with such patients should be familiar with anxiety spectrum disorders including PTSD, depression, and adjustment disorders. Occasionally, patients may present with organic affective lability with a propensity to become easily tearful. Some have speculated that psychoemotional issues are predominantly responsible for persistent postconcussive symptom complaints beyond the 6- to 12-month mark, which would be another reason to intervene early to minimize, and ideally negate, secondary adverse responses to injury and losses, as well as bolster coping and resilience.[1,10,12,24,35]

Somatic Symptoms and Related Disorders

In the fifth edition of the *Diagnostic and Statistical Manual of Mental Disorders* (DSM–5), there has been a restructuring of terminology and diagnostic categories. This restructuring has attempted to get away from the mind–body dualism promulgated in prior versions which overemphasized the centrality of medically unexplained symptoms. The current categories under somatic symptom and related disorders include somatic symptom disorder, illness anxiety disorder, functional neurological symptoms disorder (FNSD; what used to called conversion disorder), psychological factors affecting other medical conditions, factitious disorder, other specified somatic symptom and related disorder as well as unspecified somatic symptom and related disorder. It is essential to differentiate FNSD pseudo-neurological presentations from presentations which are directly due to sequelae of TBI as the treatments are highly divergent. In that regard, it is also important to understand that the diagnoses are not mutually exclusive. All clinicians treating individuals following concussion must understand how these conditions may create vulnerabilities for protracted symptomatology following concussion and/or develop subsequent to concussion.[36-40] There is a dearth of literature on this topic aside from a number of studies that have looked at the correlation of somatization symptoms and TBI, both in terms of pre-injury vulnerability issues and post-injury development of same.

Symptom Magnification and Malingering

Factitious disorder is a challenging diagnosis to make and implies that a patient is consciously feigning symptoms/impairment for purposes of so-called primary gain.[41,42] Both malingering and factitious disorder involve feigning (consciously mediated efforts to mislead the assessor); however, the former is associated with secondary gain as opposed to primary gain incentives. Florid malingering is an extremely rare event. Symptom magnification, however, is extremely common and may not necessarily be consciously mediated. It is of utmost importance that practitioners understand validity assessment in the context of the clinical workup of such patients to be able to more accurately opine on the relevant clinical diagnoses.[18,20,21,43-45] Making these clinical distinctions can sometimes be quite challenging; the same patient may present with a combination of the aforementioned clinical conditions.[46,47]

IATROGENESIS

The phenomenon of iatrogenesis can work in two directions, neither of which, ultimately, is in the best interest of the patient. Doctors who dismiss symptoms that are truly neurological following concussion do the patient a disservice by not treating what truly "ails" them. Furthermore, such practice risks promulgating adverse adaptive responses, including anxiety, depression, insomnia, stress, and potential worsening of pain, which will likely result in protraction of impairment and any related functional disability.[3,12,32,48,49] On the other hand, clinicians who over-diagnose concussion-related impairments may actually be producing a nocebo effect; that is, they are instilling negative expectancies in the patient, which may ultimately manifest as maladaptive behaviors, reinforce disability/illness behavior (whether true impairment is present or not), and perpetuate inappropriate diagnostic labels, as well as lead to ineffective and clinically unnecessary, as well as often costly, treatments.[50-53]

OTHER FACTORS TO CONSIDER

Clinicians should be aware of the literature examining the impact of pre-injury personality (including resilience, coping skills, and stress tolerance), psychosocial factors, and litigation on symptom reporting, clinical presentation, prognosis, and treatment response.[3,12,27,28,54-56] An important but often ignored area of clinical and neuropsychological assessment is that of validity assessment including effort and response bias testing. Effort testing is important to ensure that both symptom and performance validity are acceptable.[20,21,57-59] In the context of postconcussion assessment, response bias testing allows the practitioner to determine the response style of the patient relative to whether they are providing unbiased responses or coloring them in a particular direction (i.e., symptom minimizing versus symptom magnifying). In this latter context, practitioners need to be aware of how factors such as psychosocial and pre-injury psychiatric problems, post-injury psychological reactions, expectancy and nocebo effects, poor coping, anger, post-injury stress, litigation, good-old-days bias, stereotype and/or diagnosis threat may affect both response style and effort in order to fully evaluate the validity of interview data and diagnostic testing results.[60–62]

Some patients may fear that they will have permanent brain damage which may worsen the original symptoms secondary to the potential for aforementioned nocebo effects of the diagnosis. Preoccupation with the injury may be accompanied by the assumption of a "sick role" and hypochondriasis. Legal proceedings, including social security disability cases, worker's compensation claims, and personal injury litigation can promulgate this focus and maintain illness behavior.[21,50,51,63]

The concept of diagnosis threat as related to negative expectations on cognitive performance after concussion, as first posited by Suhr and Gunstad, involves the hypothesis that focusing on the fact that someone had a concussion and/or on the consequences of same, may in and of itself lead to worse performance on testing compared to the patient for whom the consequences of the injury are not a focus[64]; however, some studies have called this into question.[65]

CONCLUSION

Practitioners must take an array of confounding variables into consideration when assessing and treating persons following concussion. Comprehensive assessment of pre-injury, injury, and post-injury history, and a well-informed knowledge of concussion guidelines and current concussion science, as well as an eye to differential diagnosis (with the inclusion of effort, performance and symptom validity, and response bias assessments) will result in optimizing diagnostic accuracy and treatment outcomes.

KEY POINTS

- Know the patient you are treating; that is, explore pre-injury, injury, and post-injury history to better understand factors potentially confounding the clinical presentation.
- Think about the contributions of cranial/cranial adnexal and cervical injury to the symptom presentation and do not assume that postconcussive symptoms are necessarily due to the concussion; there are many conditions that may be potentially responsible and some patients may have a combination of concussion-related impairment with other comorbid trauma-related consequences both psychological and physical.
- Ameliorate/modulate complicating factors that can confound through promulgation and/or aggravation/exacerbation post-injury symptoms including dyssomnias, chronic pain, PTSD, and other affective issues such as depression or other anxiety disorders and/or sensory impairment (hearing loss, tinnitus, dizziness, lightheadedness, etc.).
- Understand the contributions of pre-injury personality, including coping skills/resilience in symptom reporting and concussion recovery.
- Examine for sign/performance and symptom validity including gauging response bias and effort to better define post-injury impairments and confounds.

STUDY QUESTIONS

1. What are the symptoms of concussion that make it apropos to label persistent symptoms as a postconcussion syndrome?
   a. Dizziness
   b. Headache
   c. Imbalance
   d. Memory problems
   e. None of the above

2. Which of the following might be inappropriately mistaken for postconcussive symptomatology?
   a. Chronic pain
   b. PTSD
   c. Dyssomnias
   d. Depression
   e. All of the above

3. Which of the following factors has been correlated with a higher risk of protracted recovery course after concussion?
   a. Acute symptom burden
   b. ADHD
   c. Poor coping resources
   d. a and c
   e. b and c

4. Cervical examination is important following concussion:
   a. Due to the fact that cervical pathology can manifest as postconcussive symptoms
   b. Due to the fact that forces associated with concussion commonly also produce cervical whiplash injuries
   c. Due to the fact that cervical trauma following concussion often leads to the need for surgery
   d. a and b
   e. a and c

5. Incorrectly diagnosing someone with a concussion who does not have one, or no longer has the original concussion as the explanation for ongoing symptoms, creates the following risk(s):
   a. Creating or reinforcing illness behavior
   b. Causing a nocebo effect
   c. Inducing depression and anxiety
   d. Worsening pain
   e. All the above

ADDITIONAL READING

www.concussionsontario.org/wp-content/uploads/2017/06/ONF-Standards-for-Post-Concussion-Care-June-8-2017.pdf

Carone DA, Bush SS (eds.). *Mild Traumatic Brain Injury: Symptom Validity Assessment and Malingering*. Springer Publishing Company; 2013.

Dwyer B, Katz DI. Post-concussion syndrome. *Handb Clin Neurol*. 2018;158:163–178. doi:10.1016/B978-0-444-63954-7.00017-3

Waljas M, Iverson GL, Lange RT, et al. A prospective biopsychosocial study of the persistent post-concussion symptoms following mild traumatic brain injury. *J Neurotrauma*. 2015;32(8):534–547. doi:10.1089/neu.2014.3339

Zasler N, Haider MN, Grzibowski NR, et al. Physician medical assessment in a multidisciplinary concussion clinic. *JHTR*. 2019:34(6):409–418: doi:10.1097/HTR.0000000000000524

ANSWERS TO STUDY QUESTIONS

1. Correct Answer: e

None of these symptoms are pathognomonic for concussion and no clearly characterized syndromal condition exists following this type of injury as noted in the text.

Further Reading:

Sharp DJ, Jenkins PO. Concussion is confusing us all. *Pract Neurol*. 2015;15:172–186. doi:10.1136/practneurol-2015-001087

Zasler N, Haider MN, Grzibowski NR, et al. Physician medical assessment in a multidisciplinary concussion clinic. *JHTR*. 2019:34(6):409–418. doi:10.1097/HTR.0000000000000524

2. Correct Answer: e

All these conditions can present with symptoms that parallel symptoms of concussion and could therefore be confused with same when there is a history suggestive of such injury.

Further Reading:

Iverson GL, Lange RT, Gaetz M, Zasler N. Mild traumatic brain injury. In: Zasler ND, Katz DI, Zafonte R, eds. *Brain Injury Medicine: Principles and Practice*, 2nd ed. Demos; 2013:434–469. doi:10.1891/9781617050572.0029

Zasler N, Haider MN, Grzibowski NR, et al. Physician medical assessment in a multidisciplinary concussion clinic. *JHTR*. 2019:34(6):409–418. doi:10.1097/HTR.0000000000000524

3. Correct Answer: d

Systematic reviews have selectively found that acute symptom burden is one of the most predictive indicators of protracted symptomatology following concussion among numerous other factors both pre-injury and post injury. Additional factors include coping resources and resilience.

Further Reading:

Dwyer B, Katz DI. Post-concussion syndrome. *Handb Clin Neurol*. 2018;158:163–178. doi:10.1016/B978-0-444-63954-7.00017-3

Iverson GI, Gardner A, Terry D, et al. Predictors of clinical recovery from concussion: a systematic review. *BJSM*. 2017;51(12):941–948. doi:10.1136/bjsports-2017-097729

Iverson GL, Lange RT, Gaetz M, Zasler N. Mild traumatic brain injury. In: Zasler ND, Katz DI, Zafonte R, eds. *Brain Injury Medicine: Principles and Practice*, 2nd ed. Demos; 2013:434–469. doi:10.1891/9781617050572.0029

4. Correct Answer: d

Cervical injury associated with concussion can produce many of the symptoms of concussion, and continue to perpetuate symptoms even after post-whiplash pain has resolved. The forces necessary to produce brain injury are such that they would also have a predilection for causing associated forces across the neck, potentially inducing injury there as well.

Further Reading:
Ellis MJ, McDonald PJ, Olson A, et al. Cervical spine dysfunction following pediatric sports-related head trauma. *JHTR*. 2019;34(2):103–110. doi:10.1097/HTR.0000000000000411
Zasler N, Haider MN, Grzibowski NR, et al. Physician medical assessment in a multidisciplinary concussion clinic. *JHTR*. 2019:34(6):409–418. doi:10.1097/HTR.0000000000000524

5. Correct Answer: e
Observed reactions to being told that one is brain injured include anxiety, negative expectancies, and other potentially adverse emotional consequences. These experiences may generate further symptom persistence based on a nocebo effect.

Further Reading:
Bender SD, Matusewicz M. PCS, iatrogenic symptoms, and malingering following concussion. *Psychol Inj Law*. 2013;6(2):113–121. doi:10.1007/s12207-013-9156-9
Polich G, Iaccarino MA, Kaptchuk TJ, et al. Nocebo effects in concussion: is all that is told beneficial? *Am J Phys Med Rehabil*. 2020;99(1):71–80. doi:10.1097/PHM.0000000000001290
Vanderploeg RD, Belanger HG, Kaufman PM. Nocebo effects and mild traumatic brain injury: legal implications. *Psychol Inj Law*. 2014;7:245–254. doi:10.1007/s12207-014-9201-3
Mittenberg W, DiGiulio DV, Perrin S, Bass AE. Symptoms following mild head injury: expectation as aetiology. *J Neurol Neurosurg Psychiatry*. 1992;55:200–204. doi:10.1136/jnnp.55.3.200

REFERENCES

The full reference list appears in the digital product found on http://connect.springer-pub.com/content/book/978-0-8261-4768-4/part/part02/chapter/ch17

RECOGNIZING MANIFESTATIONS OF POSTTRAUMATIC STRESS DISORDER IN PATIENTS WITH TRAUMATIC BRAIN INJURY

ERIC B. LARSON AND HEATHER G. BELANGER

BACKGROUND

Definition

Psychological trauma and traumatic brain injury (TBI) are both historical events that must be distinguished from their consequences. Not all psychological trauma results in persistent distress and not all injuries result in persistent disability or psychiatric complications. One syndrome that may persist after exposure to a traumatic event is posttraumatic stress disorder"(PTSD), a constellation of emotional, behavioral, and cognitive symptoms that may follow exposure to significant threat to life, serious physical injury, or sexual violence. Following moderate to severe TBI, persistent sequelae are common and PTSD is sometimes confused with other psychiatric disorders associated with injury such as adjustment disorder or personality change due to TBI. Following mild TBI, a full recovery is typical but in those with persistent psychiatric complications, differential diagnosis can be particularly complicated.[1] This chapter offers a brief summary of issues related to assessment and management of PTSD in these populations.

Diagnostic Criteria

Problems from each of the following five categories must be observed for a diagnosis of PTSD[2]:

- History of exposure to trauma
- Intrusion of trauma-related symptoms after the event
- Avoidant behavior
- Dysfunctional changes in cognition and mood associated with trauma
- Increased autonomic arousal

Diagnosis further requires that duration of symptoms is more than 1 month, and that these symptoms result in significant distress or functional impairment.

Epidemiology

In the general population, lifetime prevalence of PTSD is 7.8%. In patients with mild TBI (MTBI), estimates of prevalence range from 10% to 27%. Prevalence of PTSD has been shown to be the same among MTBI patients as it is among patients with other traumatic injuries.[3] In patients with severe TBI, the best estimate of prevalence is 3%, although self-report of symptoms is much higher.[4]

The full reference list appears in the digital product found on http://connect.springerpub.com/content/book/978-0-8261-4768-4/part/part02/chapter/ch18

Etiology

A Behavioral Account

Most forms of anxiety are a result of appraisal of an impending (future) threat. PTSD involves processing a *past* trauma as a current threat, possibly because of activation of implicit memories of the traumatic events. Discrimination between current experience and past implicit memories may be more difficult because the latter are more vaguely defined than are explicit memories.[5]

A Neurobiological Account

The implicit learning involved in PTSD may be mediated by neural circuits that are characterized by:

- Inadequate frontal inhibition (associated with inability to suppress attention to stimuli related to trauma)
- Excessive amygdala response (associated with conditioned fear and reactivity to potential threats)
- Compromised hippocampus function (associated with deficient ability to distinguish safe and unsafe environments)[6]

Pathophysiology

Inconsistent evidence of atrophy in the hippocampus and in the anterior cingulate cortex has been reported in structural imaging studies of PTSD patients. Some have proposed these are stress-induced changes, but twin studies suggest that reduced volume in these structures is a pretrauma vulnerability factor.[7] Similarly, comparisons of structural, perfusion, and diffusion magnetic resonance imaging (MRI) data in 17 veterans with PTSD and in 15 age-matched veterans without PTSD showed increased regional cerebral blood flow in the right parietal and superior temporal cortices, and reduced functional anisotropy in white matter regions near the anterior cingulate, prefrontal lobe, and the posterior angular gyrus. As in previous imaging studies, it was concluded that these abnormalities may be the result of PTSD or may be risk factors that cause individuals to be predisposed to the disorder.[8]

DIAGNOSIS

Risk Factors

Knowledge of characteristics that leave patients vulnerable to PTSD can help determine if that disorder is present in a TBI survivor with an ambiguous clinical presentation.

- **Pretrauma risk factors:** Sex and marital status are the strongest demographic predictors of PTSD. Women and previously married (e.g., divorced or widowed) individuals have the highest risk for PTSD.[9]
- **Trauma-related risk factors:** For men, the highest risk for PTSD is for those who have been in combat and for those who have witnessed someone being killed or severely injured. For women, the highest risk is associated with rape or sexual molestation.
- **Posttrauma risk factors:** A lack of subsequent social support and experience of additional life stressors are both stronger predictors of PTSD than pre-trauma risk factors.[10]
- **Poor cognitive function:**[11] A pretrauma cognitive deficit may leave an individual less able to cope with stressors, which may make them more vulnerable to PTSD.

■ TBI patients are at increased risk for PTSD at 6 months after injuries if they experienced acute stress disorder after their injuries, if they exhibited symptoms of depression and anxiety within 1 week of injuries, if they have previous histories of psychiatric disorders, or if they had memories of the traumatic events.[12]

Clinical Presentation

Both people with PTSD and those with a history of TBI may complain of noise sensitivity, fatigue, anxiety, insomnia, poor concentration, poor memory, and irritability. The presence of these symptoms alone is not diagnostic of either disorder because all have high base rates in the general population as well.

Symptoms

■ Intrusion symptoms
  ● Recurrent involuntary, intrusive distressing recollections of the traumatic event. Such memories are sudden, unwanted, and disruptive to one's activities
  ● Recurrent distressing dreams of the event (nightmares)
  ● Dissociative behavior in which one acts or feels like the event is recurring (e.g., flashbacks). This involves perception that the trauma is happening in the present and differs from remembering the traumatic event as a past occurrence. Contact with present reality is diminished and in extreme cases may be entirely lost.
  ● Intense psychological distress at exposure to trauma-related cues
  ● Physiological reactivity on exposure to trauma-related cues
■ Persistent avoidance
  ● Efforts to avoid thoughts or feelings associated with the trauma
  ● Efforts to avoid activities or situations that arouse recollections of trauma (e.g., appointment cancellations, failed appointments, and tardiness to treatment sessions)
■ Maladaptive changes in mood and cognition
  ● Inability to recall an important aspect of the trauma, only if determined not to be because of posttraumatic amnesia
  ● Persistent and overgeneralized dysfunctional beliefs about oneself, other individuals, or the world
  ● Persistent and distorted thoughts of blame
  ● Markedly diminished interest in significant activities that are still available despite physical disability
  ● Feeling of detachment or estrangement from others
  ● Persistent inability to experience positive emotions
  ● Reckless or self-destructive behavior
■ Maladaptive changes in arousal and reactivity
  ● Difficulty falling or staying asleep
  ● Irritability or outbursts of anger
  ● Difficulty concentrating
  ● Hypervigilance—which does not necessarily exclude situations in which an individual's perception of threat is justified by actual danger in their environment
  ● Exaggerated startle response

Evaluation

■ **Symptom checklists:** Questionnaires that rely on self-report like the PTSD Checklist for *DSM–5* (PCL-5)[13] require little time to complete (5 minutes or less) and may be used as screening measures but should not be used for diagnosis given their poor specificity.

That is, instruments designed to assess symptom type and severity are not helpful in identifying the specific mechanism responsible out of the many disorders in the differential. Further, in TBI patients, self-report is notoriously inaccurate.

■ **Structured interviews:** The "gold standard" for PTSD diagnosis, clinician interviews require extended time to complete (30–120 minutes). They also require formal training to ensure inter-rater reliability. Measures include the Clinician-Administered PTSD Scale for *DSM-5* (CAPS-5)[14] and the Structured Clinical Interview for *DSM-5* Disorders—Clinician Version (SCID-5-CV).[15]

■ **Neuropsychological evaluation:** Standardized psychological assessment provides a detailed description of the nature of cognitive impairment and emotional distress. However, in cases where it is unclear whether a patient has sustained an MTBI, identifying cognitive impairment does not assist with differential diagnosis, because such impairment can be seen in individuals with PTSD alone.[16]

Controversies

It has been suggested that TBI does not produce PTSD because the disturbance of consciousness that must occur in the former interferes with formation of memories of trauma, which is presumably the cause of symptoms in the latter.[17] Although some evidence supports this conclusion, other studies show that PTSD exists in individuals who lost consciousness at the time of their injuries.[12,18] The formation of implicit memories (that may not require clear consciousness at the time of trauma and that may exist in the absence of explicit recall) has been offered as an explanation for this counterintuitive finding.

TREATMENT

Guiding Principles

Exposure and Avoidance

Treatment that increases exposure to trauma-related stimuli in a supportive, controlled environment is effective at reducing symptoms. Avoidance of stimuli that provoke distress results in increased anxiety when those triggers can no longer be escaped.

Medication and Cognition

Some pharmacological interventions are effective at short-term management of anxiety but can result in iatrogenic cognitive impairment, which makes them bad choices for TBI survivors.

Psychopharmacology

■ Sertraline, paroxetine, fluoxetine, or venlafaxine are effective and are strongly recommended for people with PTSD who choose not to engage in or are unable to access trauma-focused psychotherapy. Divalproex, tiagabine, guanfacine, risperidone, benzodiazepines, ketamine, hydrocortisone, or D-cycloserine are all ineffective, harmful, or both for people with PTSD. Practice guidelines strongly recommend that practitioners avoid prescribing these agents.[19]

Psychotherapy

■ For patients capable of participation, there is high strength of evidence of a medium to large magnitude benefit for the critical outcome of PTSD symptom reduction for

Prolonged Exposure therapy. Similarly, there is moderate strength of evidence of a medium to large magnitude benefit for Cognitive Processing Therapy, Cognitive Therapy and Mixed Cognitive-Behavioral Therapy.[20]

■ Therapy can be introduced early for patients with MTBI and later in the course of recovery for moderate to severe TBI patients. Memory deficits are a substantial obstacle to efficacy; in fact, such impairment may never resolve to the point that psychotherapy is possible.

■ Referral to cognitive-behavioral specialists can be particularly helpful. Centralized referral databases are now offered (listed in the Additional Reading section).

Treatment Controversies

Eye Movement Desensitization and Reprocessing

An ongoing debate continues about the efficacy of eye movement desensitization and reprocessing (EMDR). Although several outcome studies support the use of this technique, many clinicians argue that it is effective because it includes elements of exposure therapy, and that there are no advantages to EMDR over traditional exposure therapy.[21]

Additional Considerations

Disability Evaluations

In veterans, a diagnosis of PTSD may be used to support claims of disability. Disabled veterans can receive disability income if they can substantiate these claims. Secondary monetary gains may result in many false disability claims.

Personal Injury Cases

Individuals who file personal injury lawsuits may argue that their injuries resulted in PTSD. Again, secondary gains may influence symptom reporting. Consider referral for evaluation by a PTSD specialist and/or neuropsychologist who can determine the extent to which this influence may result in symptom magnification or malingering.

KEY POINTS

■ People with PTSD and those with a history of TBI may both complain of noise sensitivity, fatigue, anxiety, insomnia, poor concentration, poor memory, and irritability. The presence of these symptoms alone is not diagnostic of either disorder because all have high base rates in the general population as well.

■ Structured interviews are the gold standard for PTSD diagnosis. Due to poor specificity, self-report measures should not be used for this purpose.

■ Prolonged Exposure, Cognitive Processing Therapy, Cognitive Therapy and Mixed Cognitive-Behavioral Therapy have all been shown to have significant benefit in PTSD. Psychopharmacology can also have value, especially in individuals with memory impairment complicating response to psychotherapy.

STUDY QUESTIONS

1. PTSD is a psychiatric syndrome that may follow exposure to all of the following except:
   a. significant threat to life
   b. financial exploitation

   c. serious physical injury
   d. sexual violence

2. Which of the following treatments has high strength of evidence of a medium to large magnitude benefit for PTSD symptom reduction?
   a. Prolonged Exposure therapy
   b. Avoidant behavior
   c. Sedative hypnotics (e.g., benzodiazepines)
   d. Cognitive processing therapy

3. Which of the following is an example of an intrusion symptom?
   a. Efforts to avoid thoughts or feelings associated with the trauma
   b. Persistent and distorted thoughts of blame
   c. Recurrent distressing dreams of the event (nightmares)
   d. Irritability or outbursts of anger

4. The gold standard for PTSD diagnosis is
   a. Neuropsychological evaluation
   b. Structured clinical interview
   c. The PTSD Checklist for *DSM-5* (PCL-5)
   d. Polygraphy

5. Which of the following is the strongest risk factor for PTSD?
   a. Female sex
   b. Pretrauma divorced marital status
   c. Pretrauma widowed marital status
   d. Posttrauma lack of social support and experience of additional life stressors

ADDITIONAL READING

Practice Guideline (Pocket Guide): http://www.healthquality.va.gov/ptsd/ptsd_poc2.pdf

Forbes D, Bisson JI, Monson CM, Berliner L. *Effective treatments for PTSD: Practice guidelines from the international society for traumatic stress studies.* 3rd ed. Guilford Press; 2020.

Gill IL, Mullin S, Simpson J. Psychosocial and psychological factors associated with post-traumatic stress disorder following traumatic brain injury in adult civilian populations: a systematic review. *Brain Inj.* 2014;28(1):1–14. doi:10.3109/02699052.2013.851416

McAllister TW. Psychopharmacological issues in the treatment of TBI and PTSD. *Clin Neuropsychol.* 2009;23(8):1338–1367. doi:10.1080/13854040903277289

To find a cognitive behavioral therapist: https://www.findcbt.org/FAT

Vanderploeg RD, Belanger HG, Curtiss G. Mild traumatic brain injury and posttraumatic stress disorder and their associations with health symptoms. *Arch Phys Med Rehabil.* 2009;90(7):1084–1093. doi:10.1016/j.apmr.2009.01.023

ANSWERS TO STUDY QUESTIONS

1. Correct answer: b
   Posttraumatic stress disorder (PTSD), a constellation of emotional, behavioral, and cognitive symptoms that may follow exposure to significant threat to life, serious physical injury, or sexual violence. Although financial exploitation may accompany other forms of abuse, when it occurs in isolation it is not a recognized trigger of PTSD as defined in the *DSM-5*.

Further Reading:
American Psychiatric Association. *Diagnostic and Statistical Manual of Mental Disorders.* 5th ed. American Psychiatric Association; 2013.

2. Correct answer: a
   Avoidant behavior is a symptom of PTSD and not a treatment. Sedative hypnotics are specifically contraindicated due to harmful effects. A systematic review of outcome research showed that prolonged exposure therapy has a high strength of evidence of a medium to large magnitude benefit for PTSD symptom reduction, while cognitive processing therapy has moderate strength of evidence.

Further Reading:
American Psychological Association. *Clinical practice guideline for the treatment of posttraumatic stress disorder (PTSD) in adults.* Author; 2017.
Department of Veterans Affairs, Department of Defense. *VA/DoD clinical practice guideline for the management of posttraumatic stress disorder and acute stress disorder.* 2017. www.healthquality.va.gov/guidelines/MH/ptsd/VADoDPTSDCPGFinal.pdf

3. Correct answer: c
   In the *DSM-5,* efforts to avoid thoughts or feelings are considered a form of avoidance, persistent and distorted thoughts of blame are classified as maladaptive changes in mood and cognition, and irritability is listed as a form of maladaptive change in arousal. Nightmares are considered an intrusion symptom.

Further Reading:
American Psychiatric Association. *Diagnostic and Statistical Manual of Mental Disorders.* 5th ed. Author; 2013.

4. Correct answer: b
   Structured clinical diagnostic interviews are the gold standard against which other approaches (e.g., self-report questionnaires like the PCL-5) are evaluated.

Further Reading:
Spoont M, Arbisi P, Fu S, et al. *Screening for Post-Traumatic Stress Disorder (PTSD) in Primary Care: A Systematic Review [Internet].* Department of Veterans Affairs (US); 2013.

5. Correct answer: d
   A lack of subsequent social support and experience of additional life stressors are both stronger predictors of PTSD than pre-trauma risk factors.

Further Reading:
Brewin CR, Andrews B, Valentine JD. Meta-analysis of risk factors for posttraumatic stress disorder in trauma-exposed adults. *J Consult Clin Psychol.* 2000;68(5):748–766.

REFERENCES

The full reference list appears in the digital product found on http://connect.springer-pub.com/content/book/978-0-8261-4768-4/part/part02/chapter/ch18

III MODERATE TO SEVERE TRAUMATIC BRAIN INJURY

FIELD MANAGEMENT: PREHOSPITAL CARE

JOSHUA B. GAITHER

GENERAL PRINCIPLES

The goal of prehospital management of moderate to severe traumatic brain injury (TBI) is to prevent secondary brain insult (e.g., due to hypoxia, hypotension, hypoglycemia, or inadvertent hyperventilation following intubation), and, by reducing secondary brain injury, improve patient outcome.[1]

Aims of Prehospital (Field) Care

Goal-directed patient care includes rapid patient assessment, intervention to prevent secondary brain injury, early transport (scene time less than 10–15 minutes), and direct transport to an appropriate trauma receiving facility.

ASSESSMENT

Scene Assessment

Ensuring scene safety and donning appropriate personal protective equipment is the first step in management of TBI.

- Initial assessment and management of the patient may have to wait until the scene is safe.
- If the patient is trapped, work with other rescue personnel to formulate an extrication plan and ensure responder safety.

Patient Assessment

Initial assessment should focus on identification and management of life-threatening injuries using a structured assessment:

- *Airway*—Evaluate the ability to maintain an open airway while limiting cervical spine motion.
- *Breathing*—Evaluate the respiratory rate and pattern, and evaluate for external chest injury.
- *Circulation*—Identify significant external hemorrhage and access perfusion. Measure blood pressure (BP) and heart rate (HR). Evaluation of peripheral pulses or capillary refill time may also be used if BP cannot be obtained.

The full reference list appears in the digital product found on http://connect.springerpub.com/content/book/978-0-8261-4768-4/part/part03/chapter/ch19

- *Disability*—Document blood glucose, Glasgow Coma Score (GCS), pupil size and reactivity, and evidence of seizure or focal motor deficits.
- *Exposure*—Remove clothing to evaluate for life-threatening injury. Avoid hypothermia or hyperthermia.

Common problems identified during patient assessment include airway obstruction, hypoventilation, hypoxemia, hypo- or hypertension, and reduced level of consciousness. Extracranial injuries such as life-threatening external hemorrhage, tension pneumothorax, and spinal cord injury are common. Initial management should ensure hemorrhage is controlled. Spinal injury should be assumed in all patients with head injury.

MANAGEMENT

Goals of patient management—The management strategy outlined in the following is based on the treatment recommendations released by the Brain Injury Foundation (BIF) and focuses on the rapid identification and correction of hypoxia, hypotension, hypoglycemia, and prevention of hyperventilation.[2] Large population studies have shown that implementation of these guidelines dramatically improves patient outcomes.[3]

Airway Management

- *Goal*: Prevent hypoxia
- *Indications*:
  - Evidence of upper airway obstruction.
  - Advanced airway management should be considered when insertion of an oropharyngeal airway (OPA)/nasopharyngeal airway (NPA) and ventilation with a bag-valve mask (BVM) with high-flow oxygen does not maintain oxygen saturation >90%.
- *Management*:
  - *Basic airway management:* Insertion of an OPA or NPA and application of a nonrebreather (NRB) mask with high-flow oxygen.
  - *Advanced airway management*: Insertion of a supraglottic airway or endotracheal intubation (ETI).
- *Complications*: Prehospital ETI can lead to inadvertent hypoxia, and unrecognized esophageal intubation is fatal. Increased intracranial pressure (ICP), aspiration of gastric contents, and hypo- or hypertension can also occur.

Discussion
In patients with airway obstruction, insertion of an OPA/NPA can be sufficient to open the airway and allow effective oxygenation and ventilation. Successful prehospital ETI requires both provider expertise and involved medical oversight. Evidence for the benefit of advanced airway management is conflicting; some studies have shown improved morbidity and mortality with prehospital ETI,[4,5] while other others have not.[6,7] Supraglottic airways are an alternative to ETI and are easy to insert and achieve faster time to ventilation than ETI.[8] Advanced airway management requires use of end-tidal CO_2 ($EtCO_2$) to ensure tube placement and prevent hyperventilation.

Breathing/Ventilation

- *Goal:* Ensure adequate oxygenation (O_2 saturation >90%) and ventilation ($EtCO_2$ = 35–45)

- *Indications:* O_2 saturation less than 90% despite use of high-flow oxygen indicates the need for assisted ventilation.
- *Management:*
  - Administer high-flow oxygen by NRB mask, if inadequate oxygenation, assist ventilation with a BVM.
  - Optimal ventilation is best achieved when continuous O_2 saturation and $EtCO_2$ monitoring is utilized.
- *Complication:* Hyperventilation ($EtCO_2$ <35) is associated with significant increase in morbidity and mortality.

Discussion

Hypoxia and hyperventilation (low CO_2) increase mortality following TBI.[9] Inadvertent hyperventilation is common in intubated patients and if available, $EtCO_2$ monitoring should be utilized. Adjust the ventilation rate and tidal volume to reach a goal $EtCO_2$ of 35 to 45. If $EtCO_2$ is not available, the goal respiratory rate for patients with TBI is as follows: adults: 10 breaths/min; children (2–14 years): 15 breaths/min; and neonates (0–1 years): 25 breaths/min. Use of a pressure-controlled bag for ventilation can reduce the risk of hyperventilation and lung injury.

Circulatory Management Goal

- *Goal:* Maintain systolic blood pressure (SBP) >90.
- *Indications:* SBP <90 or if a significant drop in SBP occurs.
- *Management:* Administer isotonic 500 mL crystalloid fluid boluses, or if available, blood products to maintain SBP >90.
- *Complications:* Hypothermia, coagulopathy, volume overload, pulmonary edema, and respiratory failure.

Discussion

A single episode of hypotension doubles the risk of mortality in severe TBI.[10] The BIF recommends that SBP be maintained above 90 mmHg. However, in the prehospital setting across large populations with TBI, mortality is the lowest when SBP is near 140.[11] Therefore, when an initial BP is obtained that is less than 140 and subsequent BP values decrease, field providers should consider starting fluid resuscitation. Both administration of isotonic fluids and blood products have been shown to improve outcomes in patients with TBI. Use of vasopressors and administration of hypertonic fluids in the field have thus far been impractical or not associated with a clear mortality benefit.[12–15]

Disability

- *Goal:* Identify and treat hypoglycemia. Identify neurological injury and increased ICP.
- *Indication:*
  - Blood glucose <70 in adults or <50 in children.
  - Evidence of increased ICP including unilateral pupillary dilatation with decreased GCS
- *Management:*
  - Administer dextrose to maintain a normal blood glucose level.
  - Routine hyperventilation is no longer recommended to decrease ICP; however, it may be beneficial in patients who demonstrate signs of herniation.
- *Complications:* Hyperventilation will reduce ICP but does so at the expense of reduced cerebral blood flow, and therefore should only be administered when clinically indicated, and should be monitored via capnography.[9]

Discussion

Historically, the prehospital treatment of increased ICP by therapeutic hyperventilation has been the mainstay of TBI management. However, the BIF has significantly reduced the emphasis on treatment of increased ICP in favor of treating or preventing other causes of secondary injury. Assess periodically for signs of raised ICP (i.e., declining GCS, pupil dilatation and/or reduced reactivity, increasing systemic hypertension with reflex bradycardia). Providers could consider a 30° head-up tilt of spinal board if evidence of increased ICP is present. Current data do not support prehospital administration of mannitol or hypertonic saline.[13,14]

Spinal Immobilization

Most head-injured patients require application of spinal motion restriction techniques. Common tools used to prevent spinal motion include the application of a cervical collar and immobilization of the patient on the transport stretcher. Historically, long spinal boards have been used to prevent spinal motion; however, use of long spinal boards for more than a short period of time (patient extraction) has fallen out of favor and is no longer generally recommended.

Patient Destination

Trauma patients have improved outcomes when treated in a facility with an experienced trauma team, ready access to neuroimaging, and ideally neurosurgery on site.[15] Direct and rapid transport to facilities with these resources, possibly utilizing air-transport when conditions make prolonged ground transport likely, can improve outcomes.

KEY POINTS

- In the prehospital setting, prevention of secondary brain injury is critical to improving patient outcomes.
- Particular attention should be paid to monitoring for the development of hypoxia, hypotension, hypoglycemia, and/or iatrogenic hyperventilation, which are known to cause secondary injury.
- Prehospital treatment of moderate to severe TBI should focus on maintaining oxygen saturation above 90%, maintaining SBP above 90 mmHg, and preventing hyperventilation.

STUDY QUESTIONS

1. Prehospital treatment of moderate to severe TBI should focus on:
   a. Prevention and treatment of hypoxia
   b. Prevention and treatment of spinal injury
   c. Prevention and treatment of increased intracranial pressure
   d. Prevention and treatment of hyperglycemia

2. The goal of treating hypoxia is to maintain an oxygen saturation above:
   a. 80%
   b. 85%

   c. 90%
   d. 95%

3. The goal of treating hypotension is to maintain a systolic blood pressure above:
   a. 90 mmHg
   b. 100 mmHg
   c. 110 mmHg
   d. 120 mmHg

4. Hyperventilation is defined as an $EtCO_2$ less than:
   a. 35
   b. 40
   c. 45
   d. 50

5. Which of the following has been shown to improve outcomes in patients with hypotension in the prehospital or field setting?
   a. Administration of hypertonic saline
   b. Administration of vasopressors
   c. Administration of isotonic fluids
   d. Administration of glucose

ADDITIONAL READING

Brain Trauma Foundation website. https://braintrauma.org

Gaither JB, Spaite DW, Bobrow BJ, et al. Balancing the potential risks and benefits of out-of-hospital intubation in traumatic brain injury: the intubation/hyperventilation effect. *Ann Emerg Med.* 2012;60(6):732–736. doi:10.1016/j.annemergmed.2012.06.017

Hammell CL, Henning JD. Prehospital management of severe traumatic brain injury: a clinical review. *BMJ.* 2009;338:b1683. doi:10.1136/bmj.b1683

Parr M. Prehospital airway management for severe brain injury. *Resuscitation.* 2008;76(3):321–322. doi:10.1016/j.resuscitation.2008.01.001

Stahil PF, Smith WR, Moore EE. Hypoxia and hypotension, the "'ethal duo'"in traumatic brain injury: implications for prehospital care. *Intensive Care Med.* 2008;34(3):402–404. doi:10.1007/s00134-007-0889-3

ANSWERS TO STUDY QUESTIONS

1. Correct Answer: a
Prevention and treatment of hypoxia. Hypoxia during the prehospital interval is independently associated with increased mortality. Similarly, prehospital treatment of hypoxia is thought to be a key component to improved survival.

Further Reading:
Badjatia N, Carney TJ, Crocco, et al. Guidelines for prehospital management of traumatic brain injury, 2nd edition. *Prehosp Emerg Care.* 2008;12(suppl 1):S1–S52. doi:10.1080/10903120701732052

2. Correct Answer: c
Maintaining an oxygen level above 90% has been associated with improved outcomes following TBI. Although high oxygen levels may be beneficial, there is currently no strong evidence to suggest that higher oxygen saturations are helpful.

Further Reading:
Badjatia N, Carney TJ, Crocco, et al. Guidelines for prehospital management of traumatic brain injury 2nd edition. *Prehosp Emerg Care.* 2008;12(suppl 1):S1–S52. doi:10.1080/10903120701732052

3. Correct Answer: a
90 mmHg. Hypotension is independently associated with increased mortality and treatment of hypotension through administration of isotonic fluids is thought to be critical in improving outcomes in patients with TBI.

Further Reading:
Badjatia N, Carney TJ, Crocco, et al. Guidelines for prehospital management of traumatic brain injury 2nd edition. *Prehosp Emerg Care.* 2008;12(suppl 1):S1–S52. doi:10.1080/10903120701732052

4. Correct Answer: a
Hyperventilation following advanced airway management has been associated with increased mortality. Maintaining $EtCO_2$ levels above 35 is thought to be a critical component of improving survival after TBI

Further Reading:
Gaither JB, Spaite DW, Bobrow BJ, et al. Balancing the potential risks and benefits of out-of-hospital intubation in traumatic brain injury: the intubation/hyperventilation effect. *Ann Emerg Med.* 2012;60(6):732–736. doi:10.1016/j.annemergmed.2012.06.017

5. Correct Answer: c
Administration of isotonic fluids in patients with hypotension (systolic blood pressure <90 mmHg) is thought to be critical in improving outcomes in patients with severe head injury treated in the field.

Further Reading:
Spaite DW, Bobrow BJ, Keim SM, et. al, Association of statewide implementation of the prehospital traumatic brain injury treatment guidelines with patient survival following traumatic brain injury: the Excellence in Prehospital Injury Care (EPIC) study. *JAMA Surg.* 2019;154(7). doi:10.1001/jamasurg.2019.1152

REFERENCES

The full reference list appears in the digital product found on http://connect.springer-pub.com/content/book/978-0-8261-4768-4/part/part03/chapter/ch19

EMERGENCY DEPARTMENT MANAGEMENT AND INITIAL TRAUMA CARE CONSIDERATIONS

MATTHEW KOCHUBA AND MARIE CRANDALL

GENERAL PRINCIPLES

Introduction

Traumatic brain injury (TBI) is one of the leading causes of disability in the United States.[1] TBI is a heterogeneous disease in terms of injury severity, mechanism of injury (blunt, penetrating), and pathophysiology. Clinical severity is classified using the Glasgow Coma Score (GCS). A GCS of 13 to 15 is considered mild, 9 to 12 moderate, and 3 to 8 severe.[2-4] This chapter focuses on initial management of moderate to severe TBI.

Pathophysiology

The pathophysiology of TBI is divided into primary and secondary injury. (See Chapter 2 for additional information on this topic.) The primary insult results in tissue damage, impaired cerebral blood flow (CBF) regulation, and alterations in brain metabolism with upregulation of inflammatory mediators, oxidative stress, and vasospasm. This process ultimately leads to cell death.[5] Surgical treatment of primary brain lesions is central to the initial management of severe brain injuries.

The pathophysiology of secondary injury due to cerebral edema or the presence of a space-occupying lesion is based on the understanding of the Monro–Kellie hypothesis. The total intracranial volume is made up of brain tissue, cerebral spinal fluid (CSF), venous blood, and arterial blood. CBF is usually tightly autoregulated to maintain constant CBF over a range of blood pressures. If one compartment is increased (cerebral edema), then there is a compensatory decrease in another compartment to prevent intracranial hypertension. If intracranial hypertension develops, then there is subsequently a detrimental decrease in cerebral perfusion pressure (CPP). A decrease in CPP implies a decrease in CBF, and ultimately leads to ischemia and hypoxia and worsening of the initial TBI insult by secondary injury.[5-7] The prevention of such a secondary brain injury is the principal focus of the neuro-intensive care unit. (See Chapter 23 for further information on this topic.)

DIAGNOSIS

Clinical Presentation

The mechanism of the patient's injury should be obtained from the patient (if possible), as well as from bystanders or prehospital care providers. In patients with blunt trauma,

---

a cervical spine injury must be assumed until disproved. Any trauma patient presenting with an altered or decreased level of consciousness should be assumed to have a TBI unless/until it has been ruled out.

Symptoms

Any change in mental status, including the duration of any loss of consciousness, should be identified. Complaints of headache, vertigo, nausea, vomiting, weakness, ataxia, or other neurological symptoms should be sought. History of recent drug or alcohol use should be obtained in addition to past medical history and current medications (with special attention to any anticoagulant medications).

Physical Examination

Initial management of a patient with suspected TBI is executed according to the Advanced Trauma Life Support (ATLS) protocol.[8] Upon arrival to the emergency department (ED), a detailed medical and surgical history should be obtained, including an accurate description of the patient's baseline. Attention must also be paid to any prehospital medications used for sedation, pain control, or intubation that may interfere with an accurate neurological exam.[9]

An accurate neurological exam on admission to the ED is essential to determine diagnosis, treatment strategies, and prognosis. A GCS score ≤8 is considered an indication for intubation and serves as a marker for severe TBI. Decorticate (flexor) or decerebrate (extensor) posturing, if observed, is of particular concern as they may be indicative of cerebral herniation. Decorticate posturing presents with flexion of the upper extremities and may indicate damage to the cerebral hemisphere or midbrain. Decerebrate posturing, characterized by extension of the upper extremities, is a more ominous physical exam finding and may indicate compression of the midbrain.[10]

As the secondary survey continues, attention to the pupillary exam can give some clue to the presence of a potential space-occupying lesion. A nonreactive and dilated pupil may indicate compression of the oculomotor nerve (cranial nerve III) due to uncal herniation and should alert the treating physician to proceed with emergency interventions aimed to decrease intracranial pressure (ICP). Another sign of impending herniation is the Cushing response (hypertension and bradycardia). This is a compensatory mechanism aimed to increase CBF; thus, the bradycardia and hypertension should not be treated with pharmacological agents targeting hemodynamics but with adjuncts aimed at decreasing ICP.[10]

The remainder of the secondary survey should focus on a thorough head and neck exam as well as careful inspection for any evidence of trauma, with special attention to the ears (hemotympanum or otorrhea), the nose (rhinorrhoea), Battle's sign (retroauricular hematoma), or raccoon's eyes (periorbital ecchymoses), all indicators of a potential basilar skull fracture.[8]

Diagnostic Evaluation/Laboratory Studies

The gold standard for initial diagnostic evaluation of the moderate to severely head-injured patient is a rapid noncontrast computed tomography (CT) scan of the head. The findings being sought on CT scan include skull fracture, epidural hematoma, subdural hematoma, subarachnoid hemorrhage, cerebral contusion, intraventricular hemorrhage, blurring of the gray–white margins, and diffuse edema. Significant head trauma is often associated with cervical spine fractures, so a C-collar should be applied, and cervical spine imaging should be considered in conjunction with brain imaging whenever possible.

There are validated clinical decision-making tools available to the ED team that aid in determining who warrants a head CT scan. The Canadian Head CT Rule has the highest sensitivity (100%) and specificity (60%). See Table 20.1.[11] Negative predictive value for the clinical decision rule was 100% with a positive predictive value of 5%.[12]

Patients ≥65 years of age should undergo a screening CT of the head regardless of GCS or prehospital use of anticoagulation. Patients <65 years of age can be selectively screened based on presenting complaints, mechanism of injury, and/or use of anticoagulation, as detailed earlier.[13]

Routine lab work should be obtained on any patient presenting with a suspected TBI. An ethanol level, toxicology screen, complete blood count, basic metabolic panel (electrolytes, GLUCOSE), prothrombin time (PT), and thromboelastography (TEG) should be performed.[14,15]

TABLE 20.1   Canadian Head CT Rule, Consider CT of the Head if:

1. GCS <15 at 2 hours after injury
2. Suspected open or depressed skull fracture
3. Any sign of basal skull fracture
4. Vomiting ≥2 episodes
5. Age ≥65 years
6. Amnesia for events ≥30 min before impact
7. Dangerous mechanism (pedestrian struck by vehicle, occupant ejected, fall from elevation)

Source: Reproduced with permission from Stiell IG, Wells GA, Vandemheen K, et al. The Canadian CT Head Rule for patients with minor head injury. *Lancet*. 2001;357(9266):1391–1396. doi:10.1016/S0140-6736(00)04561-X.

TREATMENT

Guiding Principles

A major component of TBI treatment is prevention of secondary injury. Prevention of hypoxemia, hypercarbia, and hypotension is essential to preventing secondary brain injury; all are associated with an increased morbidity and mortality.[16]

Initial Management

Early treatment of TBI ideally starts prehospital. Early administration of oxygen therapy or endotracheal intubation with oxygen saturation monitoring is recommended if injury severity/respiratory status merit it, because prehospital hypoxia has been shown to be an independent predictor of increased mortality in TBI.[17] Crystalloid and/or blood products should be administered, if appropriate, in an effort to maintain ideal CPP. Hypotension is associated with increased mortality in patients with GCS ≤12.[18]

In the ED setting, initial management of TBI patients must follow the ATLS algorithm. Initial airway management is crucial upon arrival to the trauma bay. Endotracheal intubation should be done for a trauma patient who is unable to protect their airway, with a GCS ≤8, has inability to maintain SpO_2 >90% despite supplemental oxygen, or has signs of clinical herniation.[8] Endotracheal intubation is a definitive management technique, but if unable to be done due to facial trauma, then a surgical airway is needed. Ketamine has been shown to be a good drug for induction of rapid sequence intubation due to its favorable hemodynamic profile. Despite its theoretical risk of increasing ICP, a systematic review of the use of ketamine in TBI did not show an increase in ICP.[19]

Next, oxygenation and CO_2 levels must be assessed. The current recommendation for $PaCO_2$ levels for patients with a TBI is 35 to 45 mmHg $PaCO_2$. Extremes have been shown to be detrimental to cerebral perfusion in brain-injured patients and have been shown to be predictors of increased morbidity and mortality.[20]

Circulation is assessed in an attempt to recognize and avoid hypotension. TBI patients should have large bore IV access placed immediately, in keeping with ATLS protocol.[8] TBI is known to have the potential to induce a coagulopathy, likely related to the release of tissue factors coupled with hypoperfusion. This may also be exacerbated with crystalloid resuscitation, due to a dilution effect. A balanced volume resuscitation with equal parts blood, fresh-frozen plasma, and platelets has been shown in multiple studies to be beneficial in trauma patients requiring transfusion and likely for inpatients with TBI as well.[21–23]

A neurological exam should be completed as soon as possible to determine clinical severity of the TBI. This consists of a GCS and pupillary exam, with a repeat exam performed at regular, frequent intervals. This evaluation should focus on pupillary exam, assessing for lateralizing signs suggestive of a mass lesion with increased ICP, and GCS to stratify TBI severity. Clinical deterioration may occur in the initial hours after injury. When indicated, pauses in sedation to accurately assess GCS score and/or use of invasive monitoring to follow ICP status should be considered.

Evaluation and management of increased ICP must begin immediately in the trauma bay. Lifesaving measures must be initiated immediately in patients with clinical signs of impending or ongoing herniation. In the most severely injured TBI patients, or in those who are deteriorating, treatment with an osmotic diuretic, usually mannitol 0.25 to 1 g/kg IV, or hypertonic saline may improve the patient's condition through the reduction of cerebral edema.[24] Note that per the Fourth Edition of the *Brain Trauma Foundation* (BTF) guidelines, current evidence is insufficient on effects and clinical outcome to support specific recommendations with regard to use of any particular hyperosmolar agent.[25] A subsequent systematic review by Li et al., however, concluded that hypertonic saline was more effective than mannitol at reducing ICP in TBI patients.[26]

Hyperventilation, while available as an option for ICP management, should only be used as a temporary stabilizing technique to prevent impending herniation. Decreasing the patient's $PaCO_2$ to 30 mmHg will cause a temporary decrease in the (elevated) ICP through cerebral vasoconstriction with subsequent decrease in CBF. This should be done only for a brief period of time, and serum CO_2 levels should be monitored by arterial blood gas (ABG) measurement or end-tidal CO_2 values (after being correlated with $PaCO_2$ from an ABG measurement), because an undesirable side effect of this action is further cerebral ischemia with increased secondary brain injury.[27]

Ongoing Care

Ongoing treatment is aimed at ICP management, maintaining an adequate CPP; optimizing oxygenation/CO_2 levels, blood pressure management, temperature management, glucose control, seizure prevention, addressing coagulopathy, if present; and preventing other potential secondary brain insults. Neurosurgery should be consulted early for any potential anticipated need for surgical intervention, if merited based on initial imaging. (See Chapter 22 for more information on neurosurgical intervention in TBI.)

Invasive ICP monitoring is recommended for patients with a severe TBI (GCS 3–8 after resuscitation) and an abnormal CT scan. It is also recommended in the setting of severe TBI with a normal CT scan if two or more of the following features are noted at admission: age over 40 years, unilateral or bilateral motor posturing, or systolic blood pressure (BP) <90 mmHg.[25]

Fluid management should be used to maintain euvolemia with isotonic solutions, with saline preferred over albumin due to the increased mortality with albumin (42% vs. 22%, p <.001).[28] BP must be monitored continuously to avoid hypotension. Guidelines recommend maintaining a systolic blood pressure ≥100 for patients 50-69 and ≥110 for patients 15-49 or >70 years of age.[29]

CPP autoregulation, which maintains normal cerebral vascular flow across wide maps (50–150 mmHg), is disrupted in approximately one-third of patients with severe TBI.[30,31] (Management of CPP is further addressed in Chapter 22.)

Hypoxia should be avoided, with a goal PaO_2 of >60.[29] Acute hypercarbia can cause elevated ICP, and hypocarbia can cause cerebral ischemia.[25] (See Chapter 22 for further discussion of this topic.)

Temperature management is also key for patients with severe TBI. Fever should be avoided; it is likely related to worse outcome with TBI and also worsens ICP control through an increase in metabolic demand, blood flow, and blood volume.[32]

A recent randomized clinical trial compared neurological outcomes among patients with severe TBI with early prophylactic hypothermia versus normothermia. Normothermia had similar outcomes to prophylactic hypothermia based on comparison of 6-month neurological outcomes.[33] Shivering must be monitored for and treated aggressively due to the fact it may complicate treatment and increase metabolic demand worsening brain injury.[34]

Glucose should be maintained to avoid extremes; current ranges target 140 to 180 mg/dL.[25] Both hyperglycemia and hypoglycemia are associated with worse outcomes in severe TBI.[35]

Treatment Controversies

■ The current Fourth Edition of the BTF guidelines still recommends invasive ICP monitoring. There is a paucity of data showing a decrease in morbidly and mortality due to limited comparative studies. One trial looking at ICP monitoring for patients with severe TBI versus care based on imaging and clinical examination for monitoring and treatment of intracranial hypertension, has been published.[36] More studies are needed to determine whether invasive ICP monitoring meaningfully improves outcomes.

■ Patients with TBI are at significant risk for developing venous thromboembolism (VTE).[37,38] TBI has been associated with up to 54% incidence of deep vein thrombosis without prophylactic treatment, and even with use of sequential compression devices, a 25% incidence of VTE has been reported.[39,40] The optimal timing of VTE prophylaxis is still unknown. More studies are needed to better understand when the beneficial effects of VTE prophylaxis outweigh the potential negative consequences.

KEY POINTS

■ The primary principle guiding ED and initial trauma care in TBI is prevention of secondary brain injury due to systemic hypotension, hypoxia, hypercarbia, increased ICP, fever, seizures, and/or hypo-/hyperglycemia.

■ Elevated ICP must be aggressively managed immediately in the trauma bay. Treatment consists of either mannitol (0.25–1 g/kg IV) or—particularly if hemorrhagic shock or osmotic edema is a concern—hypertonic saline.

■ Hyperventilation should only be used as a temporary stabilizing technique to prevent impending herniation.

STUDY QUESTIONS

1. A 30-year-old man is admitted to the neurological ICU for management of a severe TBI resulting from an unhelmeted motorcycle collision. On admission, vital signs are

blood pressure 148/75 mmHg, heart rate 128 beats/min, respiratory rate 23 breaths/min (overbreathing the ventilator), temperature 37.8°C, and GCS of 6T.* An external ventricular drain (EVD) is placed for ICP monitoring. ICP is 28 mmHg and remains elevated for 30 minutes. The head is elevated, and he receives sedation consisting of fentanyl and propofol. Which of the following is the most appropriate next step in management?

a. Pentobarbital coma
b. Implement hypothermia to 33°C
c. Neurosurgery evaluation for decompressive craniectomy
d. Drainage of cerebrospinal fluid by EVD

---

* "T" designates an intubated patient who is unable to verbally communicate. These patients are only evaluated with respect to motor and eye opening responses, and get the lowest verbal score of "1."

2. A 35-year-old man is evaluated in the emergency department after a motorcycle collision. He is obtunded. He does not open his eyes to voice or painful stimuli. He makes mumbling sounds and withdrawals to painful stimuli. Vital signs are blood pressure 80/48 mmHg, heart rate 150 beats/min, respiratory rate 23 breaths/min, and oxygen saturation 92% on nonrebreather face mask. He is intubated and remains hypotensive after 2 units of blood. Focused assessment with sonography for trauma (FAST) exam reveals free fluid in the right upper quadrant. He undergoes a damage control laparotomy with splenectomy and pelvic packing. A CT scan of the head postoperatively reveals a frontal intraparenchymal hemorrhage and scattered subarachnoid hemorrhage, but no midline shift or mass effect. His neurological exam remains unchanged, and he is transferred to the ICU intubated. Which is the most appropriate recommendation for neuromonitoring?

a. Hourly clinical assessment inclusive of serial neurological exams
b. Continuous sedation with continuous electroencephalogram (EEG) monitoring
c. Hourly clinical assessment inclusive of serial neurological exams, repeat head CT scan in 12 to 24 hours, and ICP monitoring
d. Hourly clinical assessment inclusive of serial neurological exams, repeat head CT scan in 12 to 24 hours, and continuous EEG monitoring

3. A 55-year-old woman presents after being found down on the side of a highway. She has abrasions to her left temporal area with a deep laceration exposing the skull. Her GCS is 8. Vital signs are blood pressure 77/48 mmHg, heart rate 99 beats/min, respiratory rate 23 breaths/min, and oxygen saturation 88% on pulse oximetry. An ABG reveals a PaCO2 55 mmHg and PaO2 58 mmHg. A CT scan of the head is done and shows no abnormalities. Which of the following would be an indication for an ICP monitor?

a. PaO_2 of less than 65 mmHg
b. Le Fort fractures seen on CT maxillofacial scan
c. Systolic blood pressure of 77 mmHg
d. $PaCO_2$ of more than 50 mmHg

4. A 70-year-old woman presents after falling on her floor at home and striking her head. Family states that she was confused immediately after, but now her GCS is 15. She denies any medical history or use of anticoagulants. She has small abrasions to her left temporal area. Vital signs are blood pressure 145/80 mmHg, heart rate 70 beats/min, respiratory rate 18 breaths/min, and oxygen saturation 98% on room air. Which of the following would be the appropriate next step?

a. Discharge home with family
b. Admission for observation
c. Neurosurgery consult
d. CT scan of head

5. A 72-year-old man presents after being found down at home with obvious head trauma. Family states that they heard a bang and then found him in a pool of blood. They are unsure of any medical history or anticoagulation use. GCS is 6T on arrival (E1V1M5). Vital signs are blood pressure 90/40 mmHg, heart rate 110 beats/min, respiratory rate 20 breaths/min (on mechanical ventilation), and oxygen saturation 98%. Which of the following characteristics is the strongest predictor of outcome?
a. Hypotension
b. GCS eye exam
c. GCS motor exam
d. Age

ADDITIONAL READING

Brain Trauma Foundation guidelines: https://braintrauma.org/uploads/03/12/Guidelines_for_Management_of_Severe_TBI_4th_Edition.pdf

Moore, E. E., Feliciano, et al. *Trauma*. McGraw-Hill Education; 2017.

Saadeh Y, Gohil K, Bill C, et al. Chemical venous thromboembolic prophylaxis is safe and effective for patients with traumatic brain injury when started 24 hours after the absence of hemorrhage progression on head CT. *J Trauma Acute Care Surg*. 2012;73(2):426–430. doi:10.1097/TA.0b013e31825a758b

Jeremitsky E, Omert LA, Dunham CM, et al. The impact of hyperglycemia on patients with severe brain injury. *J Trauma*. 2005;58(1):47–50. doi:10.1097/01.TA.0000135158.42242.B1

Badr A, Esposito D, Rock W, et al. Thromboelastogram as a screening tool for hypercoagulability in traumatic brain injury. *Crit Care*. 2004;8:104. doi:10.1186/cc2571

ANSWERS TO STUDY QUESTIONS

1. Correct Answer: d
   The BTF guidelines encourage ICP monitoring by EVD, which allows cerebrospinal fluid drainage for ICP control. The current Fourth Edition would recommend ICP monitoring due to an abnormal CT scan and evidence of severe TBI based on the patient's presenting GCS. If ICP remains elevated despite this intervention, then neurosurgical evaluation may be needed for possible craniectomy.

   Further Reading:
   Brain Trauma Foundation, American Association of Neurological Surgeons, Congress of Neurological Surgeons, Joint Section on Neurotrauma and Critical Care, AANS/CNS, et al. Guidelines for the management of severe traumatic brain injury. VIII. Intracranial pressure thresholds. *J Neurotrauma*. 2007;24(Suppl 1):S155–S58.
   Chesnut RM, Temkin N, Carney N, et al. A trial of intracranial-pressure monitoring in traumatic brain injury. *N Engl J Med*. 2012;367(26):2471–2781. doi:10.1056/NEJMoa1207363

2. Correct Answer: c
   ICP monitoring would be warranted for this patient based on the current Fourth Edition of the BTF guidelines, in the setting of severe TBI based on GCS after resuscitation, and

an abnormal CT scan. Continuous EEG monitoring is currently not recommended for routine TBI management.

Further Reading:
Brain Trauma Foundation, American Association of Neurological Surgeons, Congress of Neurological Surgeons, Joint Section on Neurotrauma and Critical Care, AANS/CNS, et al. Guidelines for the management of severe traumatic brain injury. VIII. Intracranial pressure thresholds. *J Neurotrauma.* 2007;24 Suppl 1:S155–S58. doi:10.1089/neu.2007.9988

3. Correct Answer: c
According to the BTF Fourth Edition, one indication for invasive ICP monitoring would be severe TBI with a normal CT scan if two or more of the following features are noted at admission: age over 40 years, unilateral or bilateral motor posturing, or systolic blood pressure BP < 90 mmHg.

Further Reading:
Brain Trauma Foundation, American Association of Neurological Surgeons, Congress of Neurological Surgeons, Joint Section on Neurotrauma and Critical Care, AANS/CNS, et al. Guidelines for the management of severe traumatic brain injury. VIII. Intracranial pressure thresholds. *J Neurotrauma.* 2007;24 Suppl 1:S155-S58. doi:10.1089/neu.2007.9988

4. Correct Answer: d
The Canadian Head CT Rule is a widely used screening tool which aids in determining which trauma patients require a CT scan of the head. Inclusion criteria are loss of consciousness, amnesia, disorientation, GCS 13 to 15, age ≥16 years, no coagulopathy or anticoagulation, and no seizures. If none of the following are present a head CT is not warranted: age ≥65, >2 episodes vomiting, suspected open skull fracture, signs of basilar skull fracture (hemotympanum, racoon eyes, CSF otorrhea or rhinorrhea, or battle's sign), GCS <15 at 2 hours post-injury, retrograde amnesia >30 minutes, or dangerous mechanism (pedestrian struck by, or ejection from, a motor vehicle; or fall >3 feet or 5 stairs).

Further Reading:
Stiell IG, Wells GA, Vandemheen K, et al. The Canadian CT Head Rule for patients with minor head injury. *Lancet.* 2001;357(9266):1391–1396. doi:10.1016/s0140-6736(00)04561-x
Moore MM, Pasquale MD, Badellino M. Impact of age and anticoagulation: need for neurosurgical intervention in trauma patients with mild traumatic brain injury. *J Trauma Acute Care Surg.* 2012;73:126–130. doi:10.1097/TA.0b013e31824b01af

5. Correct Answer: d
Both the International Mission for Prognosis and Analysis of Clinical Trials in TBI (IMPACT) and the Corticosteroid Randomization After Significant Head injury (CRASH) data sets have been shown to be useful as predictors of outcomes in patients with moderate to severe TBI. Both models show worsening prognosis with advanced age, followed by the presenting motor score. Pupillary reactivity, hypoxia, and hypotension also had strong prognostic values. Both models do not account for anticoagulation use, which has also been shown to worsen outcome.

REFERENCES

The full reference list appears in the digital product found on http://connect.springer-pub.com/content/book/978-0-8261-4768-4/part/part03/chapter/ch20

21   IMAGING IN MODERATE TO SEVERE TRAUMATIC BRAIN INJURY

DAVID N. ALEXANDER AND ELLEN C. WONG

BACKGROUND: IMAGING TECHNIQUES

The two most commonly used imaging procedures in traumatic brain injury (TBI) are computed tomography (CT) of the brain and magnetic resonance imaging (MRI) or MR of the brain. Less commonly used imaging procedures that are helpful in selected patients with brain injury for specific purposes include lateral and AP (anteroposterior) skull x-rays (SXRs), cerebral angiography, CT angiography (CTA), magnetic resonance angiography (MRA), magnetic resonance venography (MRV), single-photon emission computerized tomography (SPECT), positron emission tomography (PET), diffusion tensor imaging (DTI), and functional MRI (fMRI). Each of these techniques has its own principles, benefits, and limitations. They have been employed in some settings and will be briefly described; however, the primary focus of this chapter is CT and MR.

Computed Tomography

CT measures the density of structures in the brain displayed in two-dimensional slices that vary in thickness from 2 mm to 1 cm. CT is the initial imaging procedure of choice in acute moderate to severe TBI. CT is readily available, with rapid scanning time, and has excellent imaging of acute blood, fractures, foreign bodies, and hemorrhagic contusion.

High-density structures, such as bone and acute blood, appear white on CT, whereas low-density structures, such as air or cerebrospinal fluid (CSF), appear dark. The white matter of the brain is slightly less dense than gray matter, so white matter is darker than gray matter on CT imaging. Edema reduces the density of the brain, making it appear darker. So density, and therefore whiteness on the scan, is as follows: bone > acute blood > gray matter > white matter > CSF > air. One can choose to view a specific range or a subset of the data obtained, referred to as "windowing." Generally, the CT scan is windowed to visualize brain matter best; a second set of images are windowed to highlight bone densities ("bone windows") to allow better visualization of fractures.

Magnetic Resonance Imaging

MRI is the best single test for assessing injury to the brain in moderate and severe TBI in the subacute or chronic phase after TBI. Its advantages over CT in the subacute phase include excellent imaging of the posterior fossa, assessment of axonal injury, and visualization of cortical and subcortical nonhemorrhagic contusions and edema. The signal characteristics of hematomas on MRI are highly variable. The appearance is greatly influenced by the state of hemoglobin (ferrous vs. ferric), the field strength of the magnet, the pulse

---

The full reference list appears in the digital product found on http://connect.springerpub.com/content/book/978-0-8261-4768-4/part/part03/chapter/ch21

sequence used, the status of the RBCs (intact vs. lysed), the age of the clot, the hematocrit, state of oxygenation, and size of the clot.

MRI is an imaging procedure without ionizing radiation. The basic principle of MRI is the imaging of proton magnetism. Protons, a component of water, are ubiquitous in the body and brain. The magnetic field lines up the charged protons like little magnets, then the magnetic field is removed or perturbed. Sequences of perturbation and data acquisition determine imaging characteristics:

- T1-weighted images show the general structure of the brain. White matter is hyperintense on T1 and gray matter is hypointense.
- T2-weighted and T2-fluid attenuated inversion recovery (T2-FLAIR) images show white matter changes, and generally are most sensitive to intracerebral pathology. On T2, white matter is hypointense, gray matter is hyperintense, and CSF is hyperintense. T2-FLAIR appears similar to T2-weighted imaging, except the CSF signal is suppressed and appears dark.
- Diffusion weighted imaging (DWI) and derived apparent diffusion coefficient (ADC) maps are sensitive to early swelling of cells in ischemic infarction and disruption of white matter tracts, thus may show injured neurons and glia in TBI.
- Gradient recalled echo (GRE) and susceptibility weighted imaging (SWI) sequences are used to visualize blood on MRI. They are very sensitive to paramagnetic compounds (including deoxyhemoglobin, ferritin, and hemosiderin) seen in blood products, which show up as hypointense lesions.

MR requires a longer scan time than CT and is therefore less useful for agitated patients or patients who cannot remain still during the test. MR is not useful for bone imaging or for fractures. MR cannot be used in patients with pacemakers, or a variety of other metallic implants. MR is more sensitive than CT in visualizing reversible signal changes that are the result of seizure activity, which can include focal cortical lesions, focal swelling, and sulcal enhancement, and these findings need to be differentiated from structural injury due to TBI

Skull X-Rays

Historically, SXR was the initial neuroradiological procedure for imaging head trauma. Conventional radiographs were used as early as the Spanish–American War to evaluate the cranial vault for depressed fractures and for localizing radiopaque materials. SXRs have been supplanted by CT scan, although a modified lateral SXR is generally obtained as a "scout film" in preparation for the CT.

Angiography, Including CT Angiography and MR Angiography/Venography

Angiography defines the intra- and extracranial circulation to the brain. Improvements in CT angiography make this noninvasive study the imaging procedure of choice for visualizing the anatomy of the cerebral vasculature, resulting in less need for conventional angiography. CTA is less invasive and intravenous contrast media is used in doses similar to that of a CT brain with contrast. Catheter cerebral angiogram is used uncommonly in TBI, and then generally for treatment of an identified vascular malformation, such as an incidental aneurysm or arteriovenous malformation (AVM). Both CTA and catheter angiography may be contraindicated for patients with allergy to contrast media, or if kidney injury is present. Time of flight MR angiography (TOF-MRA) is an alternative imaging procedure to study cerebral vasculature, requiring no contrast agent, but it does have less spatial resolution and less sensitivity than CTA or catheter angiography. If cerebral venous thrombosis is suspected, MRV is a useful and sensitive test.

Single-Photon Emission CT

SPECT is a nuclear medicine tomographic imaging technique using γ rays and a γ camera. A common γ-emitting isotope used in SPECT, technetium 99m-hexamethylpropylene amine oxime (99mTc-HMPAO), is useful in the detection of regional cerebral blood flow. SPECT is uncommonly used in TBI and its clinical value is limited.

Positron Emission Tomography

PET utilizes positron-emitting radiopharmaceuticals to map the physiology, biochemistry, and hemodynamics of the brain. 2-Deoxy-2-[18F]fluoro-D-Glucose (FDG) is the most common radiopharmaceutical used in PET to measure regional glucose metabolism in the brain. A variety of other substrates and radiolabeled compounds can be injected and a cross-sectional map of the brain shows the quantitative distribution, utilization, or binding of these substrates in the brain. The radiation exposure from a PET scan is about the same as a CT. The clinical value of PET in TBI is under investigation.

Diffusion Tensor Imaging

DTI measures the diffusion of water molecules and their vectors/direction along white matter tracts, using MR techniques. The most commonly studied result is the fractional anisotropy (FA) value, which reflects the degree to which molecular diffusion is linear. It is measured on a unit-less scale from 0 to 1. CSF, with no directional diffusion, is zero, and extreme unidirectional diffusion (e.g., along an axon) is maximal at 1, representing infinite anisotropic diffusion. The FA maps are typically color coded such that fibers traveling left to right or vice versa are red, fibers traveling in AP direction are green, and fiber tracts traveling vertically (superior ↔ inferior) are blue. Disruption of white matter tracts, as is typically seen in the context of diffuse axonal injury (DAI), is more dramatically visualized with DTI. Further research is needed to establish the clinical utility of this test.[1]

Functional MR Imaging

fMRI measures changes in blood oxygenation levels in specific volumes (voxels) of the brain. The brain rapidly changes its blood flow/oxygen delivery to parts of the brain as they become metabolically more or less active. Both resting state and connectivity patterns can be examined. A small minority of patients with severe brain injury and in a minimally conscious state or vegetative state have shown metabolic patterns that indicate consciousness using fMRI to measure response to questions/commands.[2]

PATHOLOGY: IMAGING APPEARANCE OF ACUTE TO SUBACUTE TBI

The pathological changes typically associated with moderate to severe closed head injury include traumatic diffuse axonal injury, intra- and extra-axial hemorrhages, focal cortical contusions (FCCs), and hypoxic-ischemic injury (HII). Open or penetrating head injury leads to direct disruption of brain parenchyma. Other phenomena include skull fractures and diffuse brain swelling. The main mechanical phenomena causing brain damage are that of contact and acceleration (Table 21.1).

TABLE 21.1 **Summary of Traumatic Brain Injury Pathology**

Extracerebral hemorrhagic lesions: SDH, EDH, SAH, IVH
Intracerebral hemorrhagic lesions: FCC, IPH, DAI-TTH
Intracerebral nonhemorrhagic lesions: FCC, edema, HII, DAI

DAI, diffuse axonal injury; EDH, epidural hematoma; FCC, focal cortical contusion; HII, hypoxic–ischemic injury; IPH, intra-parenchymal hematoma; IVH, intraventricular hemorrhage; SAH, subarachnoid hemorrhage; SDH, subdural hematoma; TTH, tissue-tear hemorrhage.

Extracerebral Hemorrhagic Lesions

Subdural Hematoma

Subdural hematomas (SDHs) are common in severe head injury, occurring in 12% to 29% of patients admitted with severe TBI.[3] SDHs are caused by tears of bridging veins that connect the superficial cerebral veins with the dural venous sinuses, and are generally seen unilaterally over the frontal and parietal convexities. They appear as crescent-shaped, high-density extra-axial fluid collections. They can be isodense during the subacute phase, generally between 10 days and 3 weeks. At that time, they are seen on CT as a displacement of the gray and white matter interface or displacement of surface veins during contrast administration.

MRI easily identifies the isodense subacute phase of SDHs: they are bright on T1, particularly on coronal images. MRI also improves visualization of SDHs that are bilateral, small, interhemispheric, subtemporal, subfrontal, or tentorial (Figure 21.1).

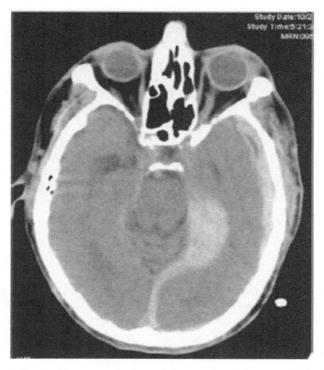

FIGURE 21.1 Patient with traumatic brain injury and a left temporal and left tentorial subdural hematoma as seen on computed tomography head.

Epidural Hematoma

Epidural hematoma (EDH) refers to bleeding that occurs between the skull and the dura mater. The vascular origins of EDH are (a) middle meningeal artery (50%); (b) meningeal vein (30%); or (c) laceration of dural venous sinuses, diploic veins, or internal carotid artery (20%). The arterial bleeding strips away the dura, which is normally tightly adherent to the inner table of the skull. EDHs are generally small, biconvex (or lens-shaped), high-density extra-axial masses with sharp anterior and posterior margins because of their firm dural attachments (Figure 21.2). Two thirds of the time they occur over the temporal or parietal region. Any extra-axial high-density mass lesion crossing the midline and depressing the superior sagittal sinus is an EDH. SDHs do not cross the midline but instead track along the falx or tentorium.

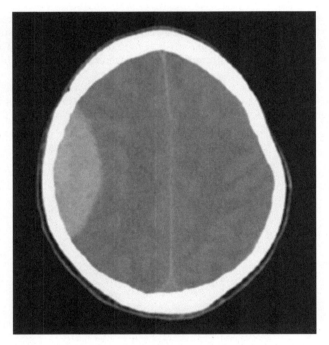

FIGURE 21.2   CT head showing epidural hematoma. Note the midconvexity, high-density biconvex lens–shaped appearance.

Subarachnoid / Intraventricular Hemorrhage

Traumatic subarachnoid hemorrhage (SAH) is a common finding in TBI, occurring in approximately 35% of patients.[4] Traumatic SAH can be seen as subtle increased density along the falx, a feathery appearance due to blood in the sulci over the convexity, or in the interpeduncular fossa, particularly with the patient lying supine during scanning procedures. Intraventricular hemorrhage (IVH) can also occur (the subarachnoid and intraventricular space are contiguous) and may be seen as an accumulation of blood in the occipital horns of the lateral ventricles.

Intracerebral Nonhemorrhagic Lesions

Parenchymal Contusions (See Also Intracerebral Hemorrhagic Lesions)

Parenchymal contusion is focal bruising that occurs most commonly along the inferior, lateral, and anterior aspects of the frontal and temporal lobes (Figure 21.3). The irregular bony contours of the floor of the anterior and middle cranial fossae predispose to this focal injury. MRI is superior to CT in visualizing nonhemorrhagic contusion. On CT, nonhemorrhagic contusion may appear as subtle hypodensity reflective of cerebral edema, while on MRI, the cerebral edema present in a nonhemorrhagic contusion will be obviously hyperintense on T2/FLAIR sequence.

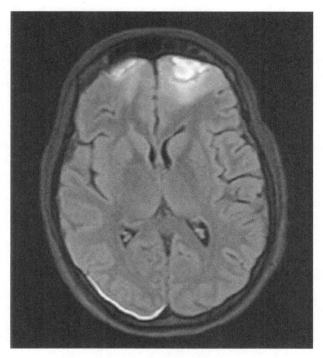

FIGURE 21.3   FLAIR MRI of bifrontal contusions, likely hemorrhagic based on appearance of circumscribed hyperintense frontal lesions with surrounding hyperintense cerebral edema, and a right posterior thin subdural hematoma in a 31-year-old woman who fell off a skateboard 4 months prior to this scan, now presenting with seizures.

Edema

Brain edema is most commonly divided into vasogenic edema and cytotoxic edema; both mechanisms are seen in TBI. Vasogenic edema is best visualized on MR, with fingers of edema following white matter tracts. Cytotoxic edema, typically caused by dying neurons and glia because of hypoxic or ischemic injury, can result in generalized brain edema and herniation (Figure 21.4). Osmotic edema occurs when there is a difference in the solute concentrations between the brain parenchyma and the blood plasma, such as in hyponatremia (common with syndrome of inappropriate antidiuretic hormone [SIADH] and cerebral salt wasting which can occur with TBI, discussed in Chapter 48) and can have both vasogenic and cytotoxic components.[5]

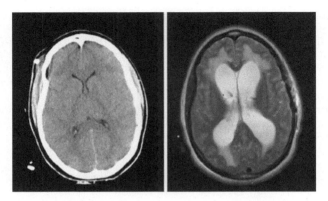

FIGURE 21.4   **Traumatic brain injury in a teenager due to motor vehicle collision, initially presenting with mild cerebral edema and small ventricles, seen on CT head (left). Three months post-injury, this same patient has hydrocephalus due to shunt failure, combined with encephalomalacia or atrophy from neuronal and glial loss, seen on T2-weighted MRI (right).**

Hypoxic–Ischemic Injury

TBI is often associated with hypoperfusion of the brain. Areas of the brain particularly sensitive to hypoxic injury include the hippocampus CA1 pyramidal cells (crucial for memory acquisition), layers 3, 5, and 6 of the cerebral cortex, and Purkinje cells in the cerebellum and striatal neurons. Hypoperfusion may affect watershed areas in the cortex. HII recovers less well than DAI because of the necrosis of large numbers of cortical neurons. CT is insensitive to hypoxic injury, but may show watershed infarctions. MR is relatively insensitive to HII but may show subtle changes including bright cortical signal on T1 (indicating cortical laminar necrosis)[6] or on DWI (indicating infarction due to edema).

Intracerebral Hemorrhagic Lesions

Parenchymal Contusions

Hemorrhagic FCC is seen on CT scan as a mottled area of high density, reflecting the petechial bleeding associated with capillary rupture. Contusions appear as inhomogeneous areas of high and low density because of the mixture of blood and edema, varying from minimal focal edema to scattered high-density foci with massive edema. Hemorrhagic contusion is seen on MRI as hypointense lesions on GRE/SWI. Cerebral edema surrounding hemorrhagic foci will appear hypodense on CT and hyperintense on T2/FLAIR sequences of MRI. FCC without hemorrhage are low density on CT, and therefore darker than normal brain tissue.

■ **Coup-Contrecoup Injury**

Coup-contrecoup injury refers to a common pattern of parenchymal contusion seen in non-penetrating head trauma. Contusions are seen at both the site of the impact (coup injury) and at the area of the brain opposite to the site of the original injury (contrecoup injury). The most frequently affected areas are the inferior surface of the frontal lobes and temporal poles.

Intraparenchymal Hematomas

Traumatic intraparenchymal hematomas can occur in any region of the brain, most commonly in the basal ganglia and the internal capsule.

Cerebral Microhemorrhages

Cerebral microhemorrhages, also known as "tissue tear hemorrhages," are frequently associated with DAI. These tend to occur at the boundary of gray and white matter, in the periventricular white matter, and the corpus callosum. They can be seen most sensitively on higher field strength magnets using GRE (T2-weighted) or SWI, and appear as tiny ovoid hypointensities.[7]

Diffuse Axonal Injury

DAI is a frequent underlying pathology in TBI. The initial pathology of DAI consists of retraction balls with severed, broken, and swollen axons. The axonal or white matter shearing injuries are better evaluated on MRI than CT. Nevertheless, the shearing may cause microhemorrhages, which can be seen on CT scan. DAI can occur from the level of the gray–white matter junction down to the deep white matter and brainstem structures (Figure 21.5). With more severe injuries, the force tends to be transmitted to the deep middle portion of the brain, with particular involvement of the corpus callosum, dorsal lateral midbrain, white matter at the gray–white junction, and cerebellar white matter near the dentate nucleus.

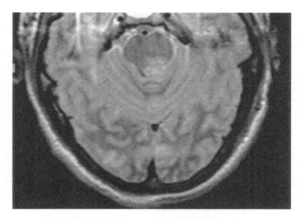

FIGURE 21.5   T2-weighted MRI showing dorsolateral pontomesencephalic axonal injury in a traumatic brain injury patient with diffuse axonal injury and right frontal contusion.

Extracerebral Lesions

Skull Fractures

CT scanning with bone windowing is needed for an evaluation of suspected fracture. Skull fractures vary from small linear fractures to displaced and complex fractures. Fractures will appear as linear discontinuities in the bone which may or may not be displaced, and must be distinguished from normal suture lines, which will appear more uniform in nature. Basilar skull fractures are not well visualized unless the CT is viewed with bone windows. If the clinical situation suggests a basilar skull fracture, with hemotympanum (blood behind the ear drum), Battle's sign (purplish bruising and ecchymosis in the mastoid region), or leakage from the ear, then a CT scan with bone windows is needed, even if a SXR was done and was negative. MRI is insensitive to cortical bone and therefore does not visualize fractures well.

Pneumocephalus

Pneumocephalus is intracranial air or gas, which can be seen in the setting of a penetrating injury or as post-operative sequelae (often after craniotomy/craniectomy, or external ventricular drain placement). Air on CT has very low density, appearing completely black.

On MRI, air appears completely black in all sequences, so depending on the sequence care must be taken not to mistake it for blood product or flow voids.

Cervical Spine Injury

Cervical spine films at the onset of head injury are important because of the 6% co-occurrence of cervical spine injury in TBI patients. The digital lateral skull radiograph obtained during CT scan of the head as a scout film should be reviewed, because it may include a portion of the cervical spine to look for cervical spine pathology.

PATHOLOGY: IMAGING APPEARANCE OF SUBACUTE TO CHRONIC TRAUMATIC BRAIN INJURY

Subacute to chronic imaging in TBI reveals sequelae of brain tissue damage. Some pathology is common to all forms of chronic parenchymal injury, including encephalomalacia and Wallerian degeneration. Others may be sequelae of surgical intervention for TBI, including syndrome of the trephined. Hydrocephalus can be seen in multiple circumstances as described in the following.

Encephalomalacia

TBI can lead to encephalomalacia, or the atrophy of brain tissue. Encephalomalacia is often the sequelae of severe intracerebral damage. On CT, it is seen as a region of hypoattenuation and volume loss in a previously damaged area. On MRI, the signal of encephalomalacia depends on the sequence, but follows CSF signal (see Figure 21.4).

Wallerian Degeneration

Wallerian degeneration is common after severe TBI, occurring as a result of neuronal injury. On MRI the different phases of Wallerian degeneration can be distinguished, with the early subacute phase appearing as hyperintensity on T1 and hypointensity on T2, and vice versa in the late subacute phase (Figure 21.6).

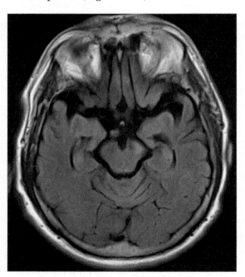

FIGURE 21.6   T2-FLAIR imaging shows hyperintensity in the left cerebral peduncle, consistent with Wallerian degeneration.

Sinking Skin Flap Syndrome

Sinking skin flap syndrome, also known as "syndrome of the trephined" or paradoxical brain herniation, is a rare complication after craniectomy, which can be life-threatening. Imaging will show a craniectomy with marked concavity of the overlying skin flap, with underlying mass effect including sulcal effacement and midline shift (Figure 21.7). Clinically, manifestations are widely variable, including altered mental status, headache, seizures, focal deficits, or dysautonomia. Treatment includes replacing the bone flap as soon as possible.[8]

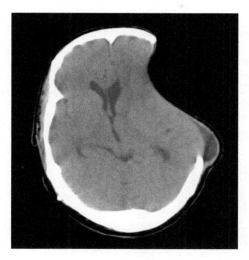

FIGURE 21.7   CT head showing sinking skin flap syndrome. Note the large left craniectomy, concavity, and 9-mm midline shift.

Hydrocephalus

Hydrocephalus refers to the buildup of CSF and resultant enlargement of the ventricles of the brain. This topic is covered in detail in Chapter 45.

KEY POINTS

- CT and MR are the mainstays of imaging in TBI, and readily show the key pathologic changes of TBI:
  - Extracerebral hemorrhagic lesions: Subdural and EDHs, and sub-arachnoid hemorrhage.
  - Intracerebral hemorrhagic lesions: FCCs, intra-parenchymal hemorrhages, and DAI with TTHs.
  - Intracerebral nonhemorrhagic lesions: FCCs, edema, HII, and DAI.
  - Subacute to chronic lesions include encephalomalacia, Wallerian degeneration, sinking skin flap syndrome, ventricular enlargement, and hydrocephalus
- Emerging procedures, particularly DTI and fMRI, show changes in metabolism and white matter tract dysfunction in TBI, in addition to identifying anatomic lesions, although they are not in routine clinical use and require further study.

STUDY QUESTIONS

1. Which of the following is the accurate ordering of density on CT, from most to least dense?
   a. Bone > acute blood > gray matter > white matter > CSF > air
   b. CSF > acute blood > gray matter > bone > white matter > air
   c. Air > bone > acute blood > white matter > gray matter > CSF
   d. Bone > acute blood > white matter > gray matter > air > CSF

2. Which MR imaging sequence is best for visualizing blood?
   a. T1
   b. T2/FLAIR (fluid attenuated inversion recovery)
   c. Diffusion weighted imaging (DWI)
   d. Gradient recalled echo (GRE) / susceptibility weighted imaging (SWI)

3. Which of the following shows an epidural hematoma?
   a.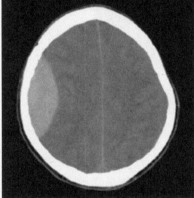

   b.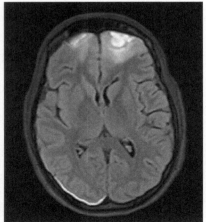

c.

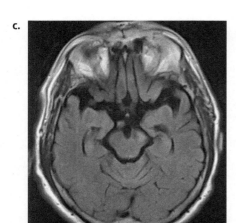

d.

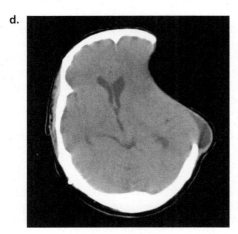

4. What is the most common vascular origin of epidural hemorrhage?
   a. Bridging veins
   b. Middle meningeal artery
   c. Vertebral artery
   d. Middle cerebral artery

5. Which statement is true regarding MRI sequences?
   a. T1-weighted imaging shows white matter as hypointense and gray matter as hyperintense
   b. GRE sequence is the best for assessing white matter lesions and general pathology
   c. T2-weighted imaging is ideal for imaging blood products, which appear hypointense
   d. DWI and ADC are sensitive for ischemic changes

ADDITIONAL READING

https://radiopaedia.org/articles/traumatic-brain-injury

Griffin AD, Turtzo LC, Parikh GY, et al. Traumatic microbleeds suggest vascular injury and predict disability in traumatic brain injury. *Brain*. 2019;142(11):3550–3564. doi:10.1093/brain/awz290

Haghbayan H, Boutin A, Laflamme M, et al. The prognostic value of MRI in moderate and severe traumatic brain injury: a systematic review and meta-analysis. *Crit Care Med*. 2017;45(12):e1280–e1288. doi:10.1097/CCM.0000000000002731

Mutch CA, Talbott JF, Gean A. Imaging evaluation of acute traumatic brain injury. *Neurosurg Clin N Am*. 2016;27(4):409–439. doi:10.1016/j.nec.2016.05.011

Smith LGF, Milliron E, Ho M-L, et al. Advanced neuroimaging in traumatic brain injury: an overview. *Neurosurg Focus*. 2019;47(6): E17. doi:10.3171/2019.9.FOCUS19652

ANSWERS TO STUDY QUESTIONS

1. Correct Answer: a
   High-density structures, such as bone and acute blood, appear white on CT, whereas low-density structures, such as air or cerebrospinal fluid (CSF), appear dark. The white matter of the brain is slightly less dense than gray matter; so white matter is darker than gray matter on CT imaging. Edema reduces the density of the brain, making it appear darker. So density, and therefore whiteness on the scan, is as follows: bone > acute blood > gray matter > white matter > CSF > air.

   Further Reading:
   Robert D. CT and MRI. In: Lewis PR, Pedley TA, eds. *Merritt's Neurology*. 12th ed. Lippincott Williams & Wilkins; 2010:62–73.

2. Correct Answer: d
   Gradient recalled echo (GRE) and susceptibility weighted imaging (SWI) sequences are preferred for visualization of blood on MRI. They are very sensitive to paramagnetic compounds (including deoxyhemoglobin, ferritin, and hemosiderin) seen in blood products. They show up as hypointense lesions.

   Further Reading:
   Robert D. CT and MRI. In: Lewis PR, Pedley TA, eds. *Merritt's Neurology*. 12th ed. Lippincott Williams & Wilkins; 2010:62–73.

3. Correct Answer: a   Answer (a) shows epidural hematoma. Both (b) and (c) show subdural hematomas, with (c) also showing bifrontal contusions. (d) shows sinking skin flap syndrome.

   Further Reading:
   Le TH, Gean AD. Neuroimaging of traumatic brain injury. *Mt Sinai J Med*. 2009;76(2):145–162. doi:10.1002/msj.20102

4. Correct Answer: b
   Epidural hematoma (EDH) refers to bleeding that occurs between the skull and the dura mater. The vascular origin of EDH is middle meningeal artery (50%); meningeal vein (30%); and laceration of dural venous sinuses, diploic veins, and internal carotid artery (20%).

Further Reading:

Le TH, Gean AD. Neuroimaging of traumatic brain injury. *Mt Sinai J Med*. 2009;76(2):145–162. doi:10.1002/msj.20102

5. Correct Answer: d

Diffusion weighted imaging (DWI) and derived apparent diffusion coefficient (ADC) maps are sensitive to early swelling of cells in ischemic infarction and disruption of white matter tracts, thus may show injured neurons and glia in TBI.

Further Reading:

Robert D. CT and MRI. In: Lewis PR, Pedley TA, eds. *Merritt's Neurology*. 12th ed. Lippincott Williams & Wilkins; 2010:62–73.

REFERENCES

The full reference list appears in the digital product found on http://connect.springer-pub.com/content/book/978-0-8261-4768-4/part/part03/chapter/ch21

NEUROSURGICAL MANAGEMENT OF SKULL FRACTURES AND INTRACRANIAL HEMORRHAGE

JOSHUA M. ROSENOW

SKULL FRACTURES

General Principles

Epidemiology

There are more than 2.5 million brain injuries in the United States annually, with approximately one third sustaining a skull fracture from the injury.[1]

Classification

Pattern

- Linear—A simple, straight single fracture line.
- Complex or comminuted—Multiple intersecting or radiating fracture lines.
- Nondisplaced—The fractured sections of skull are separated by the fracture line but still aligned.
- Displaced (A.K.A. depressed)—The fractured sections of skull are misaligned by a variable distance. The thickness of the skull is often the defining distance for denoting the displacement as clinically significant.
- Diastatic—The fracture traverses and separates one of the cranial sutures.

Scalp Integrity

- Closed—There is no connection between the fracture and the atmosphere.
- Open—The scalp overlying the fracture has been lacerated to such an extent as to expose the fracture to the atmosphere.
- Skull base fracture—Involves the bones of the skull base, rather than the cranial vault. These bones include the sphenoid, temporal, and occipital bones, as well as the clivus and orbital roof.
- Open depressed fractures expose the patient to an increased risk of intracranial infection and cerebrospinal fluid (CSF) leak due to the chance of a dural tear caused by the depressed fragment. This results in a communication between the intradural space and the atmosphere.

Etiology

Blunt trauma is the most common etiology. The topography of the fracture is dependent on the force of the injury and the surface against which the skull strikes. Striking the skull against a smaller surface increases the force per unit area, thus increasing the chance of a complex and/or depressed skull fracture. Skull fractures may also be caused by penetrating injuries such as projectiles (bullets, commonly), and other sharp objects driven through the skull.

The full reference list appears in the digital product found on http://connect.springerpub.com/content/book/978-0-8261-4768-4/part/part03/chapter/ch22

Diagnosis

Clinical Presentation/Symptoms/Physical Examination

- Asymptomatic—This is the most common presentation of a skull fracture, especially closed, linear, nondisplaced fractures.
- Arterial epidural hemorrhage—Fracture lines may cross the paths of major dural arteries such as the middle meningeal artery (MMA). This causes epidural arterial hemorrhage that may rapidly expand and cause significant neurologic deficit, including cerebral herniation. Evacuation of the hemorrhage and coagulation of the bleeding point is often indicated.
- Venous epidural hemorrhage—Fracture lines may cross the paths of major venous sinuses, such as the transverse sinus or superior sagittal sinus. These are high-flow spaces between dural leaves; sinus lacerations can result in substantial hemorrhage. Occipital fractures that cross the transverse sinus can result in epidural hemorrhage in the posterior fossa.
- Carotid injury—The traumatic force sustained by the skull can not only cause bony fractures but can also lead to injury of intracranial vessels due to transmission of this force to the vessels. For example, fractures of the temporal bone that extend across the carotid canal or clival fractures involving the cavernous sinus may lead to carotid dissection and pseudoaneurysm formation.[2] Carotid-cavernous fistulas (CCFs) may also be formed. These may present with pulsatile exophthalmos.
- Cranial nerve (CN) deficits—Basal skull fractures crossing the course of CNs may lead to specific deficits as follows:
  - Olfactory nerve (CN I) injury—Although the olfactory nerve may be injured simply by shear injury without a concomitant skull fracture, disruption of the cribriform plate will also result in loss of olfaction because of shearing off of the olfactory processes that extend through the anterior skull base into the upper nasal cavity.
  - Optic nerve (CN II) injury—Anterior skull base and orbital fractures. Clival fractures may result in midline optic chiasm injury causing bitemporal hemianopia.
  - Oculomotor nerve (CN III) injury—Skull base fractures across the cavernous sinus.
  - Abducens nerve (CN VI) injury—Clival fractures.
  - Facial nerve (CN VII), auditory nerve (CN VIII)—Peripheral-pattern facial weakness, dry eye, and hearing loss—temporal bone fractures.
  - Glossopharyngeal nerve (CN IX), vagus nerve (CN X), spinal accessory nerve (CN XI)—Dysphagia, hoarseness, weakness of trapezius—posterior fossa fractures through the jugular foramen.
  - Hypoglossal nerve (CN XII)—Weakness of tongue protrusion—fractures through the occipital condyle and foramen magnum.
- CSF leak
  - CSF rhinorrhea—Anterior skull base pathology such as fractures of the cribriform plate or frontal sinus with associated dural tear. Fractures of the temporal bone with an associated dural tear may also lead to CSF flow down the nasopharynx via the Eustachian tube.
  - CSF otorrhea—Temporal bone fracture and overlying dural tear leading to CSF egress via ear if the tympanic membrane is violated.
  - CSF leakage may lead to the development of meningitis.[3]
- Open fractures may present with obvious signs of displaced/protruding skull pieces with or without CSF leakage.
- Encephalocele—If the fracture defect is large enough and there is an adjacent associated dural tear, a portion of the brain may herniate through the defects. This may be associated with CSF leakage but this is not always present.

- Anterior skull base—Encephaloceles may involve the orbit or ethmoid sinuses.
- Temporal bone—Brain may protrude into the mastoid air cells.
- External signs of hemorrhage
  - Battle's sign (ecchymosis in the mastoid region) or hemotympanum because of temporal bone fracture.
  - Raccoon eyes—Periorbital ecchymosis due to anterior skull base fracture.

Radiographic Evaluation

- X-rays—These identify fractures very well, but have been largely replaced by computed tomography (CT) scan.
- Ultrasound—In the pediatric population, ultrasound is increasingly used because of its lack of associated radiation.[4]
- CT scan—Allows for definition of the morphology of a skull fracture, its relationship to the underlying brain and venous sinuses, and for evaluation for associated hemorrhage.

Specific Circumstances Requiring Special Evaluation

- Fractures across venous sinuses—CT venography may be considered if concern for sinus occlusion is present.
- Fractures through the carotid canal or midline sphenoid bone (cavernous carotid)—CT angiography is useful for identifying vascular dissection.
- If there is suspicion of CCF—CT angiography may help diagnose this but ultimately catheter angiography will be needed to definitively identify the site of arterial injury.
- "Growing skull fractures" in children[5-6]—Otherwise known as posttraumatic leptomeningeal cysts. These are seen in fewer than 1% of pediatric skull fractures and present as an enlarging scalp mass. They result from a dural tear that allows the arachnoid to progressively herniate through the fracture defect. Secure dural closure is required.

Treatment

Guiding Principles

The assessment of the patient with a skull fracture should be directed toward assessing any neurological injury from the originating trauma, as well as assessing the extent of the fracture and then devising a management plan.

- Simple linear fractures—These are managed conservatively.
- Indications for surgery—Open and depressed fractures[7]:
  - Depression greater than the thickness of the skull
  - Open depressed fracture
  - Obvious CSF leakage
  - Neurological deficit due to cerebral compression from fractured segment
  - Frontal sinus fractures with displacement of the inner table and/or fractures of both the inner and outer tables may be considered for cranialization of the sinus with exenteration of sinus contents and packing of the frontonasal ducts. This is done to prevent the development of a mucocele with epidural extension and resulting abscess

Additional Considerations

- Fractures across venous sinuses—Bleeding from venous sinus lacerations can be especially significant and difficult to control. Unless there is a critical reason to intervene, such as open fracture with CSF leakage, neurological deficit from sinus obstruction[8] or brain compression, or active sinus hemorrhage, consideration may be given to deferring elevation of the fracture segment.

- Tension pneumocephalus—Increasing pneumocephalus due to progressive air trapping (often from anterior skull base fractures extending into the nasal sinuses) may cause increased intracranial pressure (ICP) requiring operative intervention.
- Anterior skull base fractures—Avoid passing nasogastric tubes in these patients because of the risk that the tube will pass intracranially through a fractured skull base.

INTRACRANIAL HEMORRHAGE

General Principles

Definition

- Bleeding within the cranial cavity may be of several different types and many etiologies. Types of hemorrhage include epidural, subdural, intracerebral, intraventricular, and subarachnoid.

Epidemiology

- In a survey of 90,250 hospitalized patients with brain injury,[9] 30.6% had traumatic intracranial hemorrhage (ICH).
- Types of hemorrhage included: subarachnoid—47.9%, subdural—40.6%, epidural—17.5%, intracerebral—14.0%, and intraventricular—4.3%.

Classification

ICH is generally classified by location. The following may be considered a general schema:

- Extra-axial hemorrhage
  - Subdural (acute, subacute, chronic)
  - Subarachnoid
  - Epidural
- Intracerebral (A.K.A. traumatic cerebral contusion)
  - Lobar
  - Basal ganglia (most commonly thalamic or putaminal)
  - Brainstem (midbrain, pons)
  - Coup contusions—Occur on the same side of the impact
  - Contrecoup contusions—Occur contralateral to the side of impact
- Intraventricular

Etiology

- Traumatic ICH is most commonly caused by either direct impact of the brain on the inner skull surface or by shearing or tearing of vascular structures.
- Epidural hematomas are classically caused by rupture of a dural vessel (more commonly arterial) associated with a skull fracture crossing its path. Subdural hematomas are caused by tearing of draining veins that bridge the subdural space on their way from the cerebral surface to the venous sinuses.
- Contusions in the frontal, occipital, and temporal poles are due to direct impact of the brain while basal temporal and basal frontal/gyrus rectus contusions are more likely to be due to scraping of the brain on the middle and anterior fossa floors, respectively. Contusions may initially be caused by impact resulting in hemorrhage, but may expand over time because of necrosis, infarction, further hemorrhage, and cerebral edema.
- Deep traumatic hemorrhages in the basal ganglia or brainstem are likely caused by shearing of perforating vessels.

■ Intraventricular hemorrhage (IVH) may be caused by tearing of the deep venous system that lines the walls of the lateral and third ventricle, as well as by damage to the vascularized choroid plexus.

Diagnosis

Risk Factors

■ Any significant trauma places the patient at risk for ICH.
■ Minor head injury may also cause ICH on occasion.
■ Use of anticoagulants/antiplatelet agents increases the risk both for ICH in general as well as for ICH expansion.
■ Patients with a known bleeding diathesis or reason for impaired hemostasis (i.e., chronic liver disease) are at risk both for ICH in general as well as for ICH expansion.

Clinical Presentation

■ Epidural hematoma (EDH)—Classically described brief loss of consciousness followed by a lucid interval before neurological decline; this occurs in fewer than 30% of patients.[10]
■ Intracerebral hemorrhage/contusion—The clinical presentation is dependent on size and location; contusions may cause focal deficits if they are located in the eloquent cortex.
■ Subdural hematoma—Patients with substantial acute SDHs are often severely neurologically ill owing to the significant impact forces involved in these injuries. These patients often have poor neurological outcomes, even with the most aggressive and rapid treatment. Subacute/chronic SDH may present with progressive neurological decline over anywhere from hours to weeks.
■ Substantial IVH often obstructs the flow of CSF through the ventricles and cerebral aqueduct, leading to obstructive hydrocephalus and increased ICP.
■ Traumatic subarachnoid hemorrhage often does not initially produce symptoms, but focal cerebral vasospasm may occur several days after the acute event, leading to focal deficits due to cerebral ischemia.

Physical Examination

■ The examination of the patient with traumatic ICH should first concentrate on ensuring that the patient has a patent airway and is hemodynamically stable. Following this, a thorough trauma survey and a focused neurological exam should be performed.
■ The neurological exam should include determination of the patient's Glasgow Coma Scale (GCS) score as well as elucidation of any focal CN, motor, or sensory deficits.

Radiographic Assessment

■ CT scan is the best study for diagnosis and monitoring of traumatic intracerebral hemorrhage.
■ Acute blood is typically hyperdense to the brain parenchyma, but in certain circumstances, such as rapid hemorrhage or low hematocrit, it may be iso- or hypodense.
■ The typical appearance of EDH is a biconvex, lenticular lesion caused by the stripping of the dura away from the skull by the hematoma. Lateral spread stops at the sutures where the dura is most tightly adherent, leading to an increase in hematoma thickness.
  ● Hemorrhage causing significant mass effect or neurological deficit requires emergent evacuation.
  ● Very thin EDH (less than 5 mm) may not require evacuation. However, if the decision is made to observe, these lesions require very close clinical and imaging monitoring as patients (especially children) may deteriorate rapidly. In general, there should be a low threshold for surgical intervention.

- Because there are few barriers to the spread of hemorrhage along the hemispheric surface, SDH are often crescentic, holohemispheric lesions.
- Cerebral contusions are often hyperdense on initial CT scan and will often develop a surrounding area of hypodense edema over the first several hours to days. These typically occur in areas where the polar aspects of the lobes (frontal, temporal, occipital) strike the skull, or where the surface of the brain rubs on the irregular surface of the skull base (inferior frontal, temporal lobes). Shearing of white matter tracts may cause small deep contusions.
  - Coup contusions—Occur on the same side of the impact.
  - Contrecoup contusions—Occur contralateral to the side of impact.
- Substantial IVH often obstructs the flow of CSF through the ventricles and cerebral aqueduct, leading to obstructive hydrocephalus and increased ICP.

Treatment

Guiding Principles

- Traumatic ICH must be treated aggressively to prevent neurological decline due to increased ICP or cerebral herniation due to mass effect.
- If it is decided to clinically follow ICH, close radiographic and clinical monitoring needs to be considered.

Initial Management

- TBI may be associated with coagulopathy due to systemic fibrinolysis.[11,12] For this reason, coagulation parameters should be monitored closely and corrected as needed to prevent expansion of contusions.
- For EDH, surgical treatment involves evacuation of the hemorrhage, coagulation of the bleeding point, and tacking up the dura to eliminate the epidural space and prevent reaccumulation. The craniotomy should be large enough to encompass the hematoma.
- Contusions are at high risk for expansion in the first several days following injury due to both expansion of the hemorrhage and increasing surrounding edema. This may lead to an increase in ICP, causing neurological decline and the need for further treatment. Because of this, CT scans should be intermittently repeated.
- Contusions in the temporal lobe may be especially dangerous because of their location adjacent to the brainstem. Expansion may lead to precipitous neurological decline and uncal herniation. Substantial temporal lobe contusions need to be monitored especially closely and surgeons should have a lower threshold for evacuation.
- Surgical evacuation of contusions may be indicated in the setting of neurological deterioration or significant ICP increase.[13]
- Patients with substantial acute SDHs are often severely neurologically ill owing to the significant impact forces involved in these injuries. These patients often have poor neurological outcomes, even with the most aggressive and rapid treatment.
- Hemorrhage causing significant mass effect or neurological deficit requires emergent evacuation. Small SDHs in patients with good neurological examinations may sometimes be observed. However, if the decision is made to observe, these lesions require very close clinical and imaging monitoring.
- Surgical treatment involves craniotomy for evacuation of the hemorrhage with coagulation of the bleeding point. Burr holes are not adequate for treatment of acute SDH because the clot is often too solid and extensive to be sufficiently treated through such a small exposure. The craniotomy should be large enough to allow sufficient access to the thickest part of the hematoma and to allow visualization of the majority of the subdural space.

■ If the brain is significantly swollen at the time of surgery, a decompressive craniectomy may be of use in alleviating the increased ICP. Many of these patients may also require ICP monitoring. A decompressive craniectomy must be generous enough to allow the brain to herniate through the defect without strangulating the herniated portion, thus leading to ischemia and further cerebral edema. The dura must be patched open to allow for this expansion. Despite the fact that this technique has been called into question by some, it continues to be used routinely; published studies to date have either been retrospective case series, small series (both prospective and retrospective), or randomized trials with significant methodological flaws.[14,15]

■ Obstructive hydrocephalus caused by significant IVH should be treated with external ventricular drainage. In cases of massive IVH, it may be difficult to keep the drain from becoming repeatedly clogged.

KEY POINTS

■ Most skull fractures do not require surgical treatment.

■ Significantly depressed or open skull fractures may require elevation and/or debridement along with exploration and repair of the dura to prevent infection and CSF leak.

■ Patients with skull base fractures or those that cross venous sinuses may require additional imaging to exclude associated vascular injury.

■ Traumatic ICH may require emergent evacuation due to mass effect and increased ICP.

■ Close clinical and radiographic follow-up needs to be considered for any patient with traumatic ICH.

■ Traumatic ICH is at high risk for expansion in the near term after initial injury.

STUDY QUESTIONS

1. Skull fractures often require surgery when which of the following conditions are met?
   a. The fracture line crosses a cranial suture
   b. The fracture involves the carotid canal
   c. The fracture is depressed more than the thickness of the skull
   d. The fracture involves the temporal bone

2. Traumatic brain contusions:
   a. Are not hemorrhagic
   b. Tend to expand a week after the initial trauma
   c. May expand in the hours after trauma
   d. Do not require surgery

3. Skull fractures that cross venous sinuses can cause issues due to:
   a. Traumatic rupture of the venous sinus
   b. Traumatic occlusion of the venous sinus
   c. CSF leak due to dural tear
   d. a and b

4. The spread of an epidural hematoma:
   a. Is often more extensive than that of subdural hematomas
   b. Is often bounded by cranial suture lines
   c. Is more rapid than that of acute subdural hematomas
   d. Rarely causes clinical symptoms

5. The initial management of a patient with TBI and an anterior skull base fracture DOES NOT include which of the following measures:
   a. Placing a nasograstric tube
   b. Securing the airway
   c. Maintaining adequate ventilation
   d. Fluid resuscitation to maintain adequate blood pressure

ADDITIONAL READING

AANS/CNS Joint Section on Neurotrauma and Critical Care. http://www.neurotraumasection.org

Chesnut RM, Temkin N, Carney N, et al. A trial of intracranial-pressure monitoring in traumatic brain injury. *N Engl J Med*. 2012 27;367(26):2471–2481. doi:10.1056/NEJMoa1207363

Edwards P, Arango M, Balica L, et al. CRASH trial collaborators. Final results of MRC CRASH, a randomised placebo-controlled trial of intravenous corticosteroid in adults with head injury—outcomes at 6 months. *Lancet*. 2005;365(9475):1957–1959. doi:10.1016/S0140-6736(05)66552-X

Gregson BA, Rowan EN, Francis R, et al. Surgical Trial In Traumatic intraCerebral Haemorrhage (STITCH): a randomised controlled trial of early surgery compared with initial conservative treatment. *Health Technol Assess*. 2015;19(70):1–138. doi:10.3310/hta19700

Hawryluk GWJ, Rubiano AM, Totten AM, et al. Guidelines for the management of severe traumatic brain injury: 2020 update of the decompressive craniectomy recommendations. *Neurosurgery*. 2020;87(3):427–443. doi:10.1093/neuros/nyaa278

ANSWERS TO STUDY QUESTIONS

1. Correct Answer: c
Fractures that are displaced more than the thickness of the skull can cause injury to the underlying dura and brain and should be elevated.

Further Reading:
Ullman J, Raksin P. *Atlas of Emergency Neurosurgery*. Thieme; 2015.

2. Correct Answer: c
Brain contusions are traumatic hemorrhages that may expand in the hours after trauma and require evacuation if they result in increased intracranial pressure.

Further Reading:
Loftus CM. *Neurosurgical Emergencies*, 3rd ed. Thieme; 2017.

3. Correct Answer: d
Skull fractures that cross venous sinus lines can tear the dural covering of a venous sinus, resulting in epidural or subdural hemorrhage, or may depress the sinus, resulting in thrombosis and occlusion of the sinus.

Further Reading:
Bokhari R, You E, Bakhaidar M, et al. Dural venous sinus thrombosis in patients presenting with blunt traumatic brain injuries and skull fractures: a systematic review and meta-analysis. *World Neurosurg*. 2020;142:495–505.e3. doi:10.1016/j.wneu.2020.06.117

4. Correct Answer: b
Traumatic epidural hematomas may rapidly enlarge due to the causative arterial hemorrhage and require surgical evacuation. Their spread is often bounded by the firm attachment of the dura to the skull at suture lines.

Further Reading:
Ullman J, Raksin P. *Atlas of Emergency Neurosurgery*. Thieme; 2015.

5. Correct Answer: a
Nasogastric tube placement is contraindicated in patients with anterior skull base fractures due to the risk that the tube could travel through the fracture into the skull.

Further Reading:
Greenberg MS. *Handbook of Neurosurgery*, 9th ed. Thieme; 2019

REFERENCES

The full reference list appears in the digital product found on http://connect.springer-pub.com/content/book/978-0-8261-4768-4/part/part03/chapter/ch22

THE NEUROINTENSIVE CARE UNIT: INTRACRANIAL PRESSURE AND CEREBRAL OXYGENATION

BRANDON A. FRANCIS AND MATTHEW B. MAAS

GENERAL PRINCIPLES

Once a traumatic brain injury (TBI) occurs, little can be done to reverse the initial injury. The main aim of TBI management therefore focuses on minimizing secondary injury.

Secondary Brain Injury

Cerebral Vasospasm

While aneurysmal subarachnoid hemorrhage (aSAH) is the prototypic disease associated with vasospasm, the same process can occur in TBI if there is sufficient blood coating the vessels in the circle of Willis. TBI causes endothelial damage and extravasation of blood which, through a variety of mechanisms, irritates the blood vessels themselves leading to vasospasm.[1] Vasospasm can lead to downstream ischemia.

Secondary Brain Ischemia

Cerebral ischemia can occur whenever cerebral oxygen demand exceeds oxygen supply. This metabolic mismatch can occur following a TBI due to a cascade of events, including release of inflammatory cytokines, vascular abnormalities, changes in neuronal metabolism, and susceptibility to infection. These mechanisms may be related to systemic changes, intracranial changes, or both. No pharmacological agent has proven effective at reducing secondary ischemic injury in this population.[2]

Brain Compression

Intracranial pressure (ICP) values are often conceptualized as a whole brain measurement, but in reality there are regional variations and gradients of ICP. One common area for these regional variations would be the posterior fossa, where large changes in ICP locally may not be accurately captured by frontally placed bolts or external ventricular drains (EVDs). This is most apparent when one considers that herniation syndromes can occur in the setting of apparently normal ICP values. When ICP is high and compensatory mechanisms have been exhausted, herniation can occur. Recent research suggests ICP values greater than 19 mmHg are associated with mortality and poor functional outcomes.[3] Emergently, herniation syndromes may be managed by providing an alternative path for the excess pressure (such as EVDs or surgical decompression), by decreasing the available fluid in the intracellular space (hyperosmolar therapy), or by decreasing cerebral blood flow (hyperventilation and hemodynamic parameter manipulation). If left untreated, acute herniation syndromes can be fatal.[4]

The full reference list appears in the digital product found on http://connect.springerpub.com/content/book/978-0-8261-4768-4/part/part03/chapter/ch23

Mechanisms of Traumatic Brain Injury Morbidity

Nosocomial Infection

Patients with TBI are considered to be at increased risk of nosocomial infections compared to general surgical patients and other types of neurosurgical patients, most commonly ventilator associated pneumonia (8.4%), surgical site infections (4.25%), and meningitis (2%).[5]

Cardiac Instability

Stress induced cardiomyopathy, or Takotsubo cardiomyopathy, is common in TBI patients.[6] The mechanism is not fully understood but appears to be related to catecholamine elaboration following brain injury. Cardiac instability may manifest as arrhythmias, diastolic or systolic heart failure, autonomic dysfunction, or pulmonary hypertension.

Seizures

Seizures are common in patients with TBI. In one cohort of 94 patients, 22% of TBI patients had seizures, 52% of which had nonconvulsive seizures that were only appreciated on electroencephalography (EEG).[7]

Pathophysiology of Cerebral Perfusion (How Are Cerebral Vasospasm, Secondary Brain Ischemia, and Brain Compression Linked?)

The intracranial compartment is composed of the following components: blood, cerebrospinal fluid (CSF), and brain parenchyma. The Monro–Kellie hypothesis states that the volume inside the skull is fixed, so that if there is an increase in the volume of any of the components, there must be a decrease in volume of another component.[8] For example, CSF may be shunted into the spinal canal in the setting of a brain mass. Once the compensatory abilities are overwhelmed, pressure in the intracranial cavity will rise rapidly. The relationship between the change in pressure (ICP) and the change in volume can be conceptualized by the cerebral compliance curve[9] (Figure 23.1).

Cerebral perfusion pressure (CPP; CPP = Mean arterial pressure [MAP] − ICP) is the pressure gradient driving blood into the brain.[1] If CPP is too low, the brain can become ischemic. When cerebral autoregulation is intact, blood vessels will constrict or dilate in order to keep cerebral blood flow constant. After TBI, cerebral autoregulation is often dysfunctional, so ICP measurement is often utilized to accurately determine CPP and prevent cerebral ischemia. Hypercapnia strongly stimulates cerebral vasodilation and an increase in cerebral blood flow. Conversely, hypocapnia (hyperventilation) leads to cerebral vasoconstriction. If the hyperventilation is prolonged or severe, it can lead to cerebral ischemia, which ultimately can worsen neurological outcomes.[10]

Frequent causes of elevated ICP in TBI are impaired autoregulation, diffuse cerebral edema, focal brain contusion, intracerebral hemorrhage, epidural hematoma or subdural hematoma, hydrocephalus, and venous sinus thrombosis. Additionally, if there is associated intraventricular hemorrhage (IVH), obstructive hydrocephalus may develop and may present another cause of elevated ICP.

DIAGNOSIS AND MONITORING

Clinical Presentation of Elevated Intracranial Pressure

Initial presentation is variable but can include agitation, somnolence, confusion, vomiting, unilaterally or bilaterally dilated pupils, sluggish or absent reaction of pupil to light, and motor posturing.

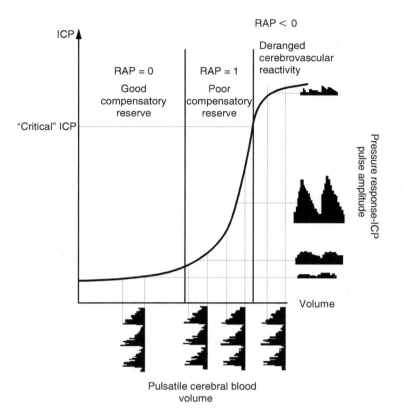

FIGURE 23.1 **Cerebral compliance curve. In a simple model, pulse amplitude of intracranial pressure (ICP) (expressed along the y-axis on the right side of the panel) results from pulsatile changes in cerebral blood volume (expressed along the x-axis) transformed by the pressure–volume curve. This curve has three zones: a flat zone, expressing good compensatory reserve; an exponential zone, depicting poor compensatory reserve; and a flat zone again, seen at very high ICP (above the "critical" ICP) depicting derangement of normal cerebrovascular responses. The pulse amplitude of ICP is low and does not depend on mean ICP in the first zone. The pulse amplitude increases linearly with mean ICP in the zone of poor compensatory reserve. In the third zone, the pulse amplitude starts to decrease with rising ICP.**

RAP, index of compensatory reserve.

Source: From Czosnyka M, Pickard JD. Monitoring and interpretation of intracranial pressure. *J Neurol Neurosurg Psychiatry.* 2004;75:813–821. doi:10.1136/jnnp.2003.033126. Used with permission from BMJ Publishing Group Ltd.

 Blood pressure may be elevated as a reflex to maintain CPP. The Cushing reflex may be observed—the triad of hypertension, bradycardia, and irregular breathing.[11]

 Papilledema or absent venous pulsations may be observed on fundoscopic exam. Additionally, there has been some data to support optic nerve sheath ultrasound measurements as a method for evaluation for elevated ICP, although the stretch in the optic nerve sheath may remain even after the ICP crisis has resolved.[12] The utility of serial optic nerve sheath diameter measurement needs further study. Papilledema, absence of venous pulsations, and increased optic nerve sheath diameter may all occur at different points in time and may not all be apparent in the hyperacute setting.

Radiographic Assessments

Computed tomography (CT) scan is indicated to evaluate for:

- Intra- and extra-axial hemorrhage
- Cerebral edema
- Hydrocephalus or compression of ventricles
- Midline shift
- Effacement of the suprasellar or quadrigeminal plate cisterns
- Effacement of sulci and gyri
- Infarction, such as a large ischemic middle cerebral artery (MCA) syndrome or an infarction in the posterior fossa (where even a small increase in pressure can result in dramatic neurological consequences given the limited space).

Neuromonitoring Approaches

Rationale for Neuromonitoring

Invasive and noninvasive neuromonitoring for the critically ill patient, in addition to frequent and active clinical assessment, is often necessary to optimize evaluation and treatment (see Table 23.1).[13] Advanced or multimodality monitoring can assist the clinicians' decision-making process by tracking biomarkers associated with complicated physiologic derangements.

TABLE 23.1   Reasons Why We Monitor Patients With Neurological Disorders Who Require Critical Care

Detect early neurological worsening before irreversible brain damage occurs

Individualize patient care decisions

Guide patient management

Monitor the physiological response to treatment and to avoid any adverse effects

Allow clinicians to better understand the pathophysiology of complex disorders

Design and implement management protocols

Improve neurological outcomes and quality of life in survivors of severe brain injuries

Through understanding disease pathophysiology, begin to develop new mechanistically oriented therapies where treatments currently are lacking or are empiric in nature

Source: From Le Roux P, Memon DK, Citerio G, et al. Consensus summary statement of the International Multidisciplinary Conference on multimodality monitoring in neurocritical care: a list of recommendations and additional conclusions: a statement for healthcare professionals from the Neurocritical Care Society and the European Society of Intensive Care Medicine. *Intensive Care Med*. 2014;40(9):1189–1209. doi:10.1136/jnnp.2003.033126. Used with permission.

Surveillance Neurological Exams and Neuroimaging

Patients with severe neurological injury are often best managed in an intensive care unit setting, where appropriate hemodynamic and neurological monitoring can be performed. Surveillance neurological assessment ("neurochecks") consists of consistent, regular, reproducible evaluations by trained staff to monitor and in some cases quantify neurological clinical parameters. They have been shown to reliably detect neurological changes in patients with neurological injury and can be considered a clinically meaningful biomarker.[14] When combined with appropriate neuroimaging, neurochecks have been shown to detect clinically meaningful neurological changes.[15] Similarly, neuroimaging repeated at regular intervals can be used to monitor changes in cerebral edema, brain compression, and focal hematomas.

Invasive and Noninvasive ICP Monitoring

The Brain Trauma Foundation (BTF) guideline recommends ICP monitors be placed in patients with Glasgow Coma Scale (GCS) of ≤8 with an abnormal head CT scan, as well as patients with GCS ≤8 with normal head CT but age greater than 40 years, systolic blood pressure (SBP) less than 90 mmHg, or motor posturing.[16]

The Trial of Intracranial Pressure Monitoring in Traumatic Brain Injury was designed to detect whether or not protocol-guided management using ICP monitors impacted the primary outcome of survival time, impaired consciousness, and functional status versus neurochecks and surveillance neuroimaging alone.[17] They found that ICP-guided care with a goal ICP of ≤20 mmHg did not improve outcomes (functional status $p = .49$; 6-month mortality $p = .6$; length of stay $p = .25$).

A variety of techniques are under development to approximate ICP by noninvasive measurements, including optic nerve sheath diameter, transcranial Doppler indices, and automated pupillometry measurements. Many of these measurements have been shown to correlate to ICP, but only moderately, such that no noninvasive method has supplanted invasive ICP monitoring in usual care.[18]

Cerebral Oxygenation Monitoring

There are multiple known methods to measure cerebral perfusion. Some measure cerebral blood flow directly, but the more commonly used technologies measure delivery of oxygen to the brain. Low cerebral oxygen tension has been associated with poor outcomes, but therapy guided by brain oxygenation measurements has not been shown to improve outcomes. This may be in part due to regional differences in oxygen tension between the sampling site and other injured regions. To date, there are no prospective, randomized trials to offer guidance in this regard.[19]

EEG Monitoring

Seizures can occur in approximately 8% of the general intensive care unit (ICU) population while seizures can occur in upward of 30% in the neuro-ICU.[20] EEG monitoring can be used to identify seizure activity and monitor response to treatment. If a seizure is detected, a diagnostic workup should be performed to evaluate for causes other than the primary brain injury such as toxins, medications or, in the right clinical scenario, infections. There are also a host of other metabolic and physiological derangements that can occur in the setting of seizures including acid–base disturbances, respiratory compromise, and cardiac arrhythmias—all of which require close monitoring. As discussed earlier, seizures in TBI patients are common, especially in the acute setting. The European Society of Intensive Care Medicine (ESICM) strongly recommends continuous EEG monitoring in TBI patients with persistent and unexplained altered consciousness.[21] Nonconvulsive status epilepticus (NCSE) is difficult to diagnose clinically, and given that up to 48% of comatose patients in an ICU have been found to be in NCSE, it is important to consider as an etiology for persistent altered consciousness. In a study of 110 ICU patients, continuous EEG (cEEG) found that 95% of conscious patients had their first seizures within 24 hours; however, only 80% of comatose patients had their first seizures by that same time. By the 48-hour mark, 98% of comatose patients had their first seizures. It therefore may require longer than 24 hours to diagnose NCSE in the comatose patient.[22] Epileptiform abnormalities detected during the acute period also indicate higher risk for posttraumatic epilepsy developing within the first year, though expectant prophylaxis in the absence of ictal activity has not been shown to be of benefit in this population, and is not recommended beyond the first 7 days post injury.[23]

Neuromonitoring Controversies and Uncertainties
A. *Does invasive ICP monitoring have a role?*

Currently, there are no definitive prospective, randomized-controlled trials that demonstrate improvement in mortality by managing TBI patients with invasive ICP monitors. Recently, TBI experts met to discuss the BEST TRIP ICP Trial (Benchmark Evidence from South American Trials: Treatment of Intracranial Pressure) and offer their interpretations of the evidence on the utility of ICP monitors in TBI patients.[24] The group issued seven statements that highlighted the concept that, while elevated ICP has been associated with worse outcomes, the benefit of basing intervention on ICP in TBI patients remains unclear.

B. *What is the ideal protocol for clinical-radiological monitoring?*

Currently, there is no evidence-based optimal protocol for clinical-radiological monitoring. Most experts would agree that neurochecks and surveillance neuroimaging at regular intervals are reasonable during the acute period following the injury. Beyond the acute phase, it is reasonable to pursue additional imaging based on clinical exam changes.

TREATMENT

Initial Management of Elevated Intracranial Pressure

Position
Optimal head position improves cerebral venous drainage and consequently prevents venous congestion, which increases ICP. Raise the head of bed to at least 30°, keep the head midline, and make sure the cervical collar (if present) is not too tight. Proper head positioning may reduce aspiration risk as well.

Access
All patients undergoing ICP management should have a central venous catheter placed for the administration of medications and monitoring of central venous pressure. Arterial catheters are helpful in closely monitoring MAP and calculating CPP.

Respiration
Patients with inability to protect the airway for a variety of reasons such as altered sensorium, or head or neck trauma, should be intubated and mechanically ventilated.

Hyperventilation (target $PaCO_2$ 30–35 mmHg) decreases ICP by causing cerebral vasoconstriction, thereby decreasing cerebral blood volume. Hyperventilation is associated with diminished cerebral perfusion and should be used cautiously. Hyperventilation is an acute treatment and will only work for a short time. Acute elevations in $PaCO_2$ should be prevented.

The exact arterial partial pressure of oxygen (PaO_2) goal is unknown for this patient population, but oxyhemoglobin saturation less than 90% correlates with worse outcome. Some data suggest that a minimum PaO_2 of 100 mmHg should be maintained to prevent cerebral hypoxia.[25]

CSF transits hydrostatically into the cerebral venous system. Therefore, increases in venous pressure may elevate ICP by impeding CSF resorption. Patients with a small gradient between ICP and central venous pressures are more likely to experience significant ICP elevations with application of positive end-expiratory pressure, presumably due to increased intrathoracic pressure increasing central venous pressure.[26] Sustained episodes of intracranial hypertension can be induced by positioning changes and suctioning as well.[27]

Blood Pressure

A SBP less than 90 mmHg should be avoided. Even a single episode of SBP less than 90 mmHg doubles mortality.[28]

MAP goal is greater than 80 mmHg until CPP can be measured.

CPP goal is 50 to 70 mmHg. CPP of greater than 70 mmHg has been associated with an increased risk of acute respiratory distress syndrome, and is not routinely indicated.[29,30] If fluid resuscitation does not meet MAP or CPP goals, vasopressors should be started.

Cerebrospinal Fluid Drainage

If an EVD is in place, CSF can be drained to reduce ICP. EVD placement may be considered in severely impaired patients, especially in the context of high ICP.

Osmotherapy

Either mannitol or hypertonic saline are equally efficacious as osmotic diuretics in TBI.[31] It should be noted that the reflection coefficient (the marker of a substance's ability to cross the blood–brain barrier [BBB]) suggests hypertonic saline would be superior, however, and it may be the preferred agent in certain clinical situations such as in the setting of renal failure.[32]

Mannitol

Initially, 1 to 2 g/kg initial bolus, then 0.25 to 1 g/kg ever 4 to 6 hours. Serum osmolality and the osmolar gap should be assessed prior to initiating therapy to determine therapeutic need and assess for incomplete clearance (elevated osmolar gap), which increases the risk for acute tubular necrosis and resulting renal failure. Mannitol is a diuretic and may cause hypovolemia.

Hypertonic Saline

30 mL of 23.4% NaCl over 10 minutes or 250 mL of 3% NaCl over 30 minutes every 4 to 6 hours for bolus dosing, or a continuous infusion of 3% NaCl. Serum sodium should be assessed regularly to determine therapeutic efficacy targeting a clinical marker such as ICP or neurological exam. Serum sodium levels must be monitored carefully in the context of renal replacement. Iso-osmolar dialysate used with hemodialysis and continuous venovenous hemofiltration will work to normalize the sodium concentration, and the resulting decrease in serum osmolality may exacerbate cerebral edema.

Sedation and Analgesia

Adequate sedation and analgesia can decrease cerebral metabolism and therefore oxygen demand. One should consider the concept of context-sensitive half-time, which describes the elimination of an infused drug based on the duration of time it has been administered. For example, fentanyl may have a relatively short half-life; however, if that infusion is continuous for over an hour, the context (the hour it was infusing) dramatically increases the half-time from 10 minutes to over 100 minutes.[33] First-line sedatives include lorazepam, midazolam, morphine, fentanyl, and propofol. Because of their adverse properties (long half-life, hypotension, myocardial depression), barbiturates are often reserved for management of elevated ICP refractory to other medical treatment. Barbiturates (often pentobarbital) are often used with continuous EEG and titrated to burst suppression.

Chemical Paralysis

Chemical paralysis is used for refractory ICP elevations, especially in patients with significant shivering or ventilator dyssynchrony. Neuromuscular blockade may decrease metabolic rate and lower intrathoracic pressure, thereby reducing intracranial blood volume. Daily holidays from sedation are advised as it improves outcomes,[34] but adequate sedation is recommended in patients who are chemically paralyzed. Train-of-four peripheral nerve stimulation monitoring should be employed for a goal of 1 to 2 of four twitches during the use of neuromuscular blocking agents as the fewer the twitches the greater the neuromuscular blockade. The greater the blockade, the longer it will take to reverse.[35]

Intra-Abdominal Hypertension

Intra-abdominal hypertension should be avoided. This may require medications to promote adequate bowel motility. There are case series indicating efficacy of decompressive laparotomy in reducing refractory ICP.[36]

Craniectomy

Surgical removal of part of the skull can reduce ICP and allow the brain to expand. In one major clinical trial for patients with diffuse, severe TBI who have refractory ICP elevation, bifrontal decompressive craniectomy was shown to decrease ICP and hospital length of stay but was associated with worse outcomes and no improvement in mortality.[37] A more recent trial in a similar patient population also showed effective ICP control that resulted in lower mortality, but a greater number of patients surviving with severe disability or in a vegetative state.[38] There is some controversy with respect to how to interpret these studies' findings, but the consensus remains that surgical decompression is appropriate in certain specific contexts.[39] (See also Chapter 22 for more on this topic.)

Temperature Management

Fever control helps lower ICP. Normothermia should be the therapeutic goal. Cooling measures include acetaminophen 650 mg every 6 hours, intravenous cooled saline, and surface cooling devices. For every 1°C cooler the core gets, the brain decreases metabolism by 3% to 7%.[40] This is hypothesized to decrease risk of supply-demand mismatch, which can lead to apoptosis.[41,42]

Seizure Prophylaxis and Treatment

Seizures worsen outcomes in patients with TBI. The American Academy of Neurology recommends providing seizure prophylaxis for 7 days to prevent early posttraumatic seizures.[43] Prophylaxis beyond the first 7 days is not recommended due to decreased risk of seizures. Phenytoin has been associated with fevers and worse outcomes after brain hemorrhage, and is generally avoided in TBI for similar concerns,[44] and because it may adversely impact neural plasticity. (See also Chapter 46 for a more detailed discussion of posttraumatic seizures.)

Cerebral Oxygenation Management

Brain tissue oxygen monitors are intraparenchymal probes inserted via a burr hole into the white matter of the brain. A treatment threshold of less than 15 mmHg is affirmed by the latest BTF guidelines,[16] although as previously discussed there is no direct evidence that management by intraparenchymal oxygen monitors improves outcomes. Treatment options for low brain oxygen include lowering ICP, increasing CPP (some patients do require CPP values above 70 mmHg for adequate perfusion), decreasing $PaCO_2$, increasing PaO_2, and increasing hemoglobin. Maintaining PaO_2 greater than 90 mmHg is recommended, as lower levels are associated with higher mortality. Jugular vein oxygen saturation less than 50% is likewise associated with worse outcomes, although placement requires a fiberoptic catheter and the incremental benefit of jugular oxygen monitoring is not established.[45]

KEY POINTS

- Most of the management principles in TBI center around minimizing secondary injury.
- The brain is vulnerable to secondary injury after TBI, in part because the volume inside the skull is fixed such that an increase in one component results in a decrease in at least one of the other components (Monro–Kellie hypothesis).
- Cerebral autoregulation may be disrupted.
- Measurement (or calculation) of cerebral perfusion pressure is central to determining appropriate intervention in the ICU.

STUDY QUESTIONS

1. You are caring for a 29-year-old man who suffered a severe traumatic brain injury one day prior. Initial imaging showed 1.5 mm of subarachnoid blood along the lateral left temporal and inferior frontal lobes. You are discussing the risk of secondary cerebral vasospasm, and whether a specific treatment is indicated. Which of the following has been shown to improve secondary ischemia in patients with severe traumatic brain injury?
   a. Nimodipine
   b. Phenytoin
   c. Acetazolamide
   d. None
   e. Acetaminophen

2. A patient with traumatic brain injury develops pneumonia with septic shock, likely attributable to aspiration of gastric contents shortly after injury. Intracranial pressure (ICP) is being monitored and is intermittently elevated. Norepinephrine is being infused to maintain a target mean arterial pressure (MAP). What is the relationship between cerebral perfusion pressure (CPP), systemic MAP and ICP?
   a. MAP = CPP/ICP
   b. CPP = 2 x ICP – MAP
   c. CPP = MAP – ICP
   d. ICP = MAP x MAP/CPP
   e. CPP x MAP = ICP/MAP

3. A 48-year-old male pedestrian presents after being hit by a motor vehicle. He is unconscious, vital signs are within normal limits, and no cranial nerve abnormalities are identified on exam. He does not respond to noxious stimulation. The treating team proceeds with intubation and mechanical ventilation for airway protection. CT scan of the head reveals moderate, diffuse subarachnoid hemorrhage and a small right-sided subdural hematoma. The consulting neurosurgeon determines that no immediate intervention is indicated at this time. Which of the following is the next best step?

    a. Obtain continuous (>24 hours) electroencephalography (cEEG)
    b. Repeat a CT scan of the head
    c. Obtain somatosensory evoked potentials
    d. Measure the serum concentration of neuron specific enolase
    e. Obtain a routine (20–40 min) electroencephalogram

4. A 65-year-old woman presents after a fall down a flight of stairs. The systolic blood pressure is 180 mmHg. Serum chemistries are within the normal reference range. On initial examination, the patient demonstrates asymmetric pupils that are minimally reactive. The patient is intubated and mechanically ventilated. The CT scan shows a loss of gray-white differentiation, decreased prominence of the sulci, and effacement of the cisterns. What is the next best step in management?
    a. Intravenous furosemide 40 mg bolus
    b. Mannitol 1 g/kg bolus
    c. Lactated Ringer's 30 cc/hr continuous infusion
    d. 23.4% saline 1 L bolus
    e. Obtain an emergent magnetic resonance imaging (MRI) scan of the brain

5. What is the role of craniectomy in TBI?
    a. There is no role for craniectomy in TBI
    b. Craniectomy improves functional outcomes in all patients with TBI
    c. Only patients with mild traumatic brain injury (MTBI) are candidates for craniectomy
    d. Only small frontal craniectomy is indicated in TBI
    e. Craniectomy can improve mortality in certain patients with severe TBI

ADDITIONAL READING

http://www.braintrauma.org
Lee K, ed. *The Neuro ICU Book: Neurocritical Care Monitoring.* McGraw Hill; 2012.

ANSWERS TO STUDY QUESTIONS

1. Correct Answer: d
No pharmacological agents have been proven to improve outcomes related to delayed ischemia in patients with severe TBI.

Further Reading:
Dearden NM. Mechanisms and prevention of secondary brain damage during intensive care. *Clin Neuropathol.* 1998;17(4):221–228.

2. Correct Answer: c
CPP = MAP – ICP. This relationship demonstrates the importance of hemodynamic monitoring and, at times, hemodynamic augmentation in the setting of elevated ICP.

Further Reading:
Kirkman MA, Smith M. Intracranial pressure monitoring, cerebral perfusion pressure estimation and ICP/CPP-guided therapy: a standard of care or optional extra after brain injury. *Br J Anaesth.* 2014;112(1):35–46. doi:10.1093/bja/aet418

3. Correct Answer: a
   Obtain continuous (>24 hours) electroencephalography. Seizures are one of the primary concerns in comatose patients, especially in the setting of brain injury. Seizures are common in patients with traumatic brain injury. In some cases, it can take up to 48 hours to identify seizures in comatose patients, supporting the idea that brief EEGs are not sufficient. Repeating the CT scan of the head would most likely show continued evidence of the brain injury but would not exclude a contributing clinical scenario such as seizures. Neuron specific enolase can be a helpful marker of neuronal damage but this test can take significant time to obtain a result, it is non-specific for the etiology of the neurological injury, and does not exclude seizures as a component of the clinical picture.

   Further Reading:
   Friedman D, Claassen J, Hirsch LJ. Continuous electroencephalogram monitoring in the intensive care unit. *Anesth Analg*. 2009;109(2):506–523. doi:10.1213/ane.0b013e3181a9d8b5

4. Correct Answer: b
   This patient has both clinical and radiographic signs concerning for cerebral edema. Mannitol 1 g/kg is a reasonable next step to address life-threatening cerebral edema. Furosemide, a diuretic, is unlikely to increase the osmotic gradient by a large enough magnitude to reduce cerebral edema of this magnitude. Lactated Ringer's is effectively iso-osmolar and would not alter cerebral edema. 23.4% saline is an appropriate intervention, however, the usual dose is 30 mL over 10 minutes. A 1-L bolus of 23.4% saline is dangerously excessive. An emergent MRI of the brain might help define the extent of brain injury but would not be indicated at this time due to untreated, uncontrolled cerebral edema.

   Further Reading:
   Cook AM, Jones GM, Hawryluk GWJ, et al. Guidelines for the acute treatment of cerebral edema in neurocritical care patients. *Neurocrit Care*.2020;32:647–666. doi:10.1007/s12028-020-00959-7

5. Correct Answer: e
   Craniectomy can improve mortality in certain patients with TBI. There is controversy regarding how to interpet the various studies that evaluate the effect of neurosurgical craniectomy in TBI. Craniectomy remains an important treatment modality in severe TBI that can improve mortality in certain patients.

   Further Reading:
   https://braintrauma.org/guidelines/guidelines-for-the-management-of-severe-tbi-4th-ed#/:guideline/decompressive-craniectomy

REFERENCES

The full reference list appears in the digital product found on http://connect.springer-pub.com/content/book/978-0-8261-4768-4/part/part03/chapter/ch23

ANOXIA COMPLICATING TRAUMATIC BRAIN INJURY

CAROLINE SIZER AND GARY GOLDBERG

INTRODUCTION

This chapter addresses clinical concerns when hypoxic/ischemic brain injury (HIBI) and traumatic brain injury (TBI) overlap. Simultaneous HIBI and TBI are known to occur,[1-3] although research on the incidence and prevalence of coinciding HIBI and TBI remains limited. To date, there are only a few published studies that specifically investigate overlapping HIBI and TBI (O/HIBI+TBI). Recent animal models of O/HIBI+TBI provide some insight into the unique pathophysiology and functional recovery of O/HIBI+TBI, and argue for more aggressive identification and treatment of post-TBI hypoxemia.[4,5] Establishment of the diagnosis of both HIBI and TBI concurrently remains challenging, limiting detailed clinical study. Nevertheless, it is expected that early recognition and diagnosis of O/HIBI+TBI may increase with more sophisticated neurointensive care techniques.[6] This chapter describes the epidemiology, diagnosis, selected medical complications, treatment, and prognostication in patients suspected to have O/HIBI+TBI.

DEFINITIONS

■ **Hypoxic brain injury:** Hypoxic brain injury (HBI) is defined as a global disturbance in brain function due to a decrease or loss of oxygen supply to the brain. Since tissue oxygenation is related to the product of deliverable blood oxygen content and blood flow, tissue hypoxia can result from a significant reduction in either or both of these factors (i.e., hypoxemia and ischemia, respectively). The resultant effect of brain hypoxia depends on the degree to which the tissue oxygen supply is reduced, and the duration of the reduction. Hypoxia thus leads to a continuum of injury severity. Mild hypoxia produces generally reversible tissue dysfunction. However, prolonged hypoxia induces neuronal cell death resulting in irreversible brain injury. The term "anoxia" is intended to refer to a complete loss of tissue oxygenation. This condition can result from hypoxemia (i.e., a severe reduction in deliverable blood oxygen content) but more often is due to ischemia (i.e., a severe disruption in perfusing blood flow, e.g., as a result of cardiac arrest or hypovolemic shock). Brain tissue hypoxia can also result from hypoxemia alone in the presence of normal brain perfusion, as in the case of carbon monoxide poisoning or suffocation.

Pure HBI with major compromise of brain perfusion is rarely associated with TBI unless there has also been a cardiac event leading to pump failure, or hypovolemic shock due to blood loss. Compromise of respiratory function due to thoracic injury or reduced ventilatory drive related to the TBI can also reduce brain oxygenation due to hypoxemia.

The full reference list appears in the digital product found on http://connect.springerpub.com/content/book/978-0-8261-4768-4/part/part03/chapter/ch24

▪ **Ischemic brain injury:** Ischemic brain injury (IBI) occurs when there is decreased brain oxygenation due to reduced oxygen delivery resulting from reduced brain perfusion. Brain ischemia can be either focal (i.e., due to blockade of flow through a particular cerebral artery, as occurs most commonly in thrombo-embolic cerebrovascular pathology or traumatic vascular injury) or global (i.e., due to pump failure, e.g., in cardiac arrest).

▪ **Hypoxic/ischemic brain injury:** In their purest forms, hypoxemic and ischemic brain injuries can have very different presentations: In hypoxemic injury, the normally more active oxygen-sensitive areas of the brain are especially susceptible, whereas with ischemic injury, brain territories supplied through specific vascular structures are more vulnerable. Most often, these disorders clinically overlap. This overlapping hypoxic/ischemic injury, which is the most typical presentation associated with TBI, is the primary focus of this chapter.

EPIDEMIOLOGY

▪ HIBI can complicate TBI, and has been reported to occur in 35% to 44% of individuals who sustain moderate to severe TBI based on demonstration of hypoxia on initial emergency medical services (EMS) pulse oximetry measurements.[3,6,7]

▪ This prevalence of O/HIBI+TBI is anticipated to rise with advancements in critical care medicine, which improve survival rates after HIBI,[8] as well as with improved diagnosis and management.

▪ Frequently, O/HIBI+TBI is seen in the setting of polytrauma, which is often complicated by hypotension associated with hypovolemic shock, airway obstruction, and respiratory failure due to chest injury (such as hemopneumothorax and lung contusion). Furthermore, the TBI itself can potentially exacerbate the HIBI by reducing respiratory drive due to brainstem injury, thereby causing a concurrent HIBI.[6,9]

▪ Recognition and diagnosis of O/HIBI+TBI is important in guiding treatment decisions, projecting expected outcome, and predicting the course of recovery.

▪ A handful of studies have directly assessed outcome from HIBI and TBI in case-controlled designs, offering a glimpse into differences in outcomes from pure HIBI referenced to expected outcome from TBI under otherwise equivalent conditions. The results of those studies will be discussed further in the Prognosis section.[8,10–12]

MAKING THE DIAGNOSIS

Comparisons can be drawn readily between TBI and HIBI in the rehabilitation setting, due to the current pragmatic practice of admitting individuals with either traumatic or hypoxic-ischemic encephalopathy to the same brain injury rehabilitation unit, utilizing the same treatment team and approach.[8,10–15] A number of key clinical factors can distinguish HIBI from TBI, or suggest concomitant HIBI and TBI with the production of additional superimposed impairment.

History

Risk factors for concomitant HIBI and TBI include documented hypoxic pulse oximetry in the field and/or at initial presentation, seizures, cardiac or respiratory arrest, chest trauma, near drowning, attempted hanging, anesthetic accidents, vehicular trauma with prolonged extrication and/or delayed resuscitation, carbon monoxide poisoning, and various metabolic encephalopathies.[8,10,11] Available medical records should be carefully reviewed for evidence of impaired oxygenation, respiratory insufficiency, and/or reduced cerebral perfusion as well as the timing, severity, and duration of such impairment. Circumstantial evidence such as initial vital signs in the field, delays in initiation of resuscitation, cyanosis, and evidence of systemic hypoperfusion (e.g., hypovolemic shock due to hemorrhage) can also suggest superimposed HIBI-related impairment.

Physical Examination

Abnormal or ataxic gait, movement disorders,[10] significantly poorer performance on the mental status exam in the realms of visuospatial cognition, attention, calculation, and memory (particularly short-term memory and visual memory),[16] spastic quadriparesis in the absence of spinal trauma, profound and fluctuating anosognosia, and prolonged disorders of consciousness, all suggest possible concomitant HIBI.[12]

Neuropsychological Testing

Moderate to severe memory impairment, psychomotor slowing, profound and fluctuating memory deficits, decreased psychomotor speed, impaired insight, and abnormal visuospatial processing are all more characteristic of O/HIBI+TBI than TBI alone. Executive function and attention appear to be less severely affected by HIBI.[10,12,16]

Neuroimaging

HIBI is associated with characteristic patterns of disproportionate damage to more highly metabolic areas of the brain and areas more vulnerable to globally reduced perfusion, namely, specific gray matter structures (cerebral cortex, basal ganglia, pyramidal cell loss in the hippocampi, and Purkinje cell loss in the cerebellum).[8,10,17,18] In IBI in particular, one may expect to see damage to vascular watershed areas.

Magnetic resonance imaging (MRI) findings demonstrate distinct characteristics that delineate four discrete phases of HIBI.[19] Broadly, early MRI findings are characterized by diffuse edema (hours to weeks), evolving to chronic diffuse atrophy (3 or more weeks out). These findings are summarized in Table 24.1.

SELECTED UNIQUE SYNDROMES SEEN IN HYPOXIC/ISCHEMIC BRAIN INJURY

- **Movement disorders:** These are more prevalent in HIBI due to involvement of subcortical brain structures involved in the organization of voluntary movement.[12]
  - **Subtle generalized convulsive state (also referred to as "myoclonic status epilepticus"):** Typically occurs in the first 12 hours after injury in 30% to 40% patients who sustain a severe HIBI and are in the comatose state.[20] This condition is defined as at least 30 minutes of sustained generalized myoclonic twitches of the facial and/or axial muscles. This does not respond well to antiepileptic drugs and is frequently noted to precede death due to the severity of the underlying HIBI and the associated poor prognosis.[21]
- **Post-hypoxic action myoclonus:** Also known as "Lance–Adams syndrome." This condition typically appears days to weeks after severe HIBI, most often in survivors of cardiac arrest, and is thought to be secondary to hypoxic damage to Purkinje cells in the cerebellar cortex.[22] It is a relatively rare movement disorder, with less than 200

TABLE 24.1 **Distinctive MRI Findings by Phase in Hypoxic/Ischemic Brain Injury**

MRI Protocol	Acute Phase (<24 hr)	Early Subacute (24 hr–13 days)	Late Subacute (14–20 days)	Chronic Phase (≥21 days)
T1	Normal	Normal	(+): subcortical WM, BG, pons	Normal
T2	(+): cortex >BG and thalamus	(+): BG, thalamus (–): subcortical WM	(+): cortex, thalamus, BG, and pons	Normal
DWI	Earlier findings, and more sensitive to mild hypoxic BI than T2 (+): cortex >BG and thalamus	(+): cortex, BG and thalamus	(+): *decreased* compared to early subacute of the cortex, BG and thalamus	Normal
T1 + gadolinium	Normal	Subcortical enhancement with cortical laminar necrosis	Subcortical enhancement	Normal

BG, basal ganglia; BI, brain injury; WM, white matter.

Notes: + indicates hypersignal; – indicates hyposignal.

Source: Adapted with permission from Weiss N, Galanaud D, Carpentier A, et al. Clinical review: prognostic value of magnetic resonance imaging in acute brain injury and coma. *Crit Care.* 2007;11(5):1–12. doi:10.1186/cc6107

reported cases in the literature.[23] Regardless of medication used to attempt to reduce the frequency of the myoclonic jerks, the response is characteristically incomplete. Despite this incomplete treatment response, and in contrast to the acute post-hypoxic myoclonus associated with subtle generalized convulsive state, post-hypoxic action myoclonus is not uniformly associated with a poor prognosis.[20]

TREATMENT

Acute Setting

A great deal of neurocritical care focus addresses the mitigation of cerebral hypoxia. Therapy targeted at maintaining adequate brain tissue oxygenation (BtO_2) can improve outcome after TBI. Prolonged brain hypoxia after severe TBI has been shown to be an independent factor linked to less favorable short-term outcomes. Unfortunately, BtO_2-targeted therapy can be technically challenging to execute, thus limiting its wider implementation.[24] For more specific information, please see the dedicated Chapters 19, 20, 22, 23, respectively on Field, Emergency, Neurosurgical, and Neurocritical care of individuals with TBI regarding monitoring for and prevention of HIBI in the context of acute TBI.

Rehabilitation Setting

■ **Acute inpatient rehabilitation:** The handful of studies that compare pure TBI with HIBI patients describe the practice that exists across many rehabilitation centers: HIBI and TBI patients are frequently treated by the same rehabilitation team on the same rehabilitation unit. This allows for direct comparison of the relative progress of both groups of patients using a case-control design. The majority of the case-control studies comparing HIBI and TBI demonstrate a slower rate of recovery and poorer overall outcome in the HIBI groups compared to those with pure TBI. Despite this finding, patients with HIBI have been shown to benefit significantly from acute inpatient rehabilitation.[8,10–12] In contrast to these reports, two studies by the same group of investigators have demonstrated similar functional outcomes between HIBI and TBI in the acute inpatient rehabilitation setting.[11,15] It is important to note that all of the studies comparing HIBI and TBI suffer from significant methodological challenges, not the least of which include very small sample sizes. Selected specific results of these studies are presented in Table 24.2 in the Prognosis" section.

■ **Pharmacotherapy:** The evidence for use of pharmacotherapeutics for the treatment of the cognitive sequelae in HIBI is limited, and is comprised primarily of retrospective studies, case series, and case reports:

  ● **Methylphenidate and amantadine:** A retrospective study of 588 patients who sustained HBI and disorders of consciousness following cardiac arrest compared the group to 16 patients who were treated with either amantadine ($n = 8$), methylphenidate ($n = 6$), or both ($n = 2$), and demonstrated improved rates of emergence of consciousness with treatment with either amantadine, methylphenidate, or both.[25]

  ● **Levodopa +/– bromocriptine:** One case series describes the beneficial effects of levodopa and/or bromocriptine for the treatment of the cognitive impairments seen in five individuals who sustained HBI, noting significant improvements in agitation, apathy, and involuntary movements, and mild improvements in memory.[26]

  ● **Zolpidem:** A single case report describes a patient with HBI and decreased arousal refractory to amantadine and methylphenidate, who demonstrated improved arousal with the administration of twice-daily zolpidem, and worsening with withdrawal of the medication.[27]

PROGNOSIS

Of great importance to the patient, their family, and the rehabilitation physician, is prognostication. It is prudent to note that HIBI generally carries a poorer prognosis than TBI. A patient who sustains O/HIBI+TBI is expected to progress more slowly and to ultimately achieve a lower level of functional independence than an otherwise matched individual who sustained a pure TBI.[12]

For the purposes of this chapter, we will focus on prognosis after HIBI, and direct comparisons that have been described between TBI and HIBI outcomes. For more information about prognosis after TBI, please see Chapter 40.

Outcomes in HIBI and Comparison of Outcomes in Hypoxic/Ischemic Brain Injury Versus Traumatic Brain Injury

Acute care predictors of long-term outcome after acquired brain injury of any kind remain an area of continued interest, particularly in individuals with disorders of consciousness (DOC). Patients who sustain O/HIBI+TBI are more likely to present with DOC. A particularly interesting and exciting recent study suggests that in patients with intact olfaction, a "sniff test"[28] may prove a means to detect a minimally conscious state. This is an intriguing notion which will require further validation before clinical applicability can be ascertained.

Although HIBI patients tend to have lower admission and discharge Functional Independence Measure (FIM) scores, and lower FIM efficiency than TBI patients, they do demonstrate meaningful improvements in function with acute inpatient rehabilitation.[14,29] Table 24.2 describes outcomes in HIBI, and where indicated, comparison of specific outcomes in HIBI to those of TBI, based on the available literature to date.

TABLE 24.2   Outcomes in Hypoxic/Ischemic Brain Injury

Parameter	Outcome
Mortality	85% die within the 1st month, or remain in a persistent VS.[29]
Emergence from VS	VS at 2 weeks: Chance of emergence is 13%.[30] VS >3 months: 5% to 11% recover consciousness.[31] *Unlikely* to emerge (NPV of 100%): • If at 6 months post-injury *any* of the following are noted: • CRS-R <6 • SEP bilaterally absent • Absent pupillary light reflex • Absent facial or motor response to noxious stimuli • Absence of PSH[32]
FIM efficiency	When matched for admission FIM scores to TBI patients, HIBI patients demonstrated lower discharge FIM scores despite longer lengths of stay (lower FIM efficiency).[8] Functional measures of ADLs and cognitive function appear to account for the majority of this inferior functional outcome among individuals with HIBI compared to those with TBI.[10,12]
Rehabilitation LOS	One study found *longer* rehabilitation LOS for HIBI compared to TBI (3 months vs. 2 months).[8] Another study found *shorter* LOS, as the HIBI patients frequently reached their mobility potential faster than their fellow TBI patients, but lagged in their ADL and cognitive performance, and this finding was associated with increased discharge to institutional settings rather than home.[33]
Complete independence	HIBI: 10% TBI: 60% (small study, *n* = 20)[27]
Discharge destination	Home: HIBI: 45% to 57% TBI: 80% to 85%[12,14] Long-term institutional care: HIBI: 33%; TBI: 11%[12]
Return to work	In a study of 31 individuals who underwent acute inpatient rehabilitation for HIBI, 14% returned to work in some capacity, and only one individual returned to their previous level of employment.[13]

ADLs, activities of daily living; CRS-R, JFK Coma Recovery Scale-Revised; HIBI, hypoxic/ischemic brain injury; LOS, length of stay; NPV, negative predictive value; PSH, paroxysmal sympathetic hyperactivity; SEP, somatosensory evoked potentials; TBI, traumatic brain injury; VS, vegetative state.

SUMMARY

Few studies have been published that address effects of concurrent diagnoses of HIBI and TBI and their interaction. Most currently available studies compare performance and outcome of purely TBI or HIBI injured individuals, which can help with general, but not specific, discussions of expected prognosis for individuals with O/HIBI+TBI. Unfortunately, there are no specific statistics that address the incidence, rehabilitation, or outcome in patients with O/HIBI+TBI pathology as of this date, nor are there clinically applicable metrics to determine which of the two pathologies might be driving the majority of an individual's impairment and disability. One could speculate that a patient who sustains both HIBI and TBI by history, and who demonstrates relatively rapid improvements in mobility with atypical lagging progress in ADL performance, memory tasks, orientation, social pragmatics, and executive function, may be manifesting evidence of a suspected HIBI-related influence on recovery from the TBI. With advances in diagnostic technologies and clinical metrics, and further research specifically evaluating relative recovery patterns in this particular population, this assertion may become more clearly supported with observational data.

KEY POINTS

- HIBI is known to complicate TBI, with estimates of O/HIBI+TBI in up to 44% of patients who sustain moderate to severe TBI.
- Diagnosis of O/HIBI+TBI is difficult, as a TBI is almost always readily apparent, and validated diagnostic criteria for O/HIBI do not currently exist.
- O/HIBI+TBI must be considered when counseling patients and their loved ones regarding progress and specific impairments, as an O/HIBI would be expected to be associated with a more prolonged recovery and poorer overall prognosis.

STUDY QUESTIONS

1. A patient with TBI complicated by a prolonged post-TBI cardiac arrest struggles with progress in physical therapy 2 weeks post injury. His therapists describe new onset of involuntary rapid limb movements every time he tries to initiate a transfer, bathing, or dressing tasks. He has no alteration of consciousness during these episodes. This presentation is most consistent with which of the following complications of his associated anoxic brain injury?
   a. Myoclonic status epilepticus
   b. Delayed post-hypoxic leuko-encephalopathy
   c. Post-hypoxic action myoclonus
   d. Simple focal motor seizures

2. In studies comparing individuals to their traumatically brain injured counterparts, individuals who sustain anoxic brain injury differ in which of the following ways with regard to functional outcome?

a. About 80% fewer patients with anoxic brain injury go home on discharge from an inpatient level of care, compared to those with TBI only
b. Individuals with an anoxic brain injury are six times less likely than those with TBI to achieve complete functional independence
c. Individuals with anoxic brain injury have higher FIM efficiency in acute inpatient rehabilitation compared to their TBI counterparts
d. Individuals with TBI are more likely than those with anoxic brain injury to discharge to long-term institutional care

3. Which of the following is FALSE with regard to brain tissue oxygen (BtO_2) targeted therapy in acute management of traumatic brain injury?
   a. Detection of hypoxia (via BtO_2 measurement) is an independent predictor of outcome in TBI.
   b. ICP+BtO_2-targeted therapy reduces mortality and is associated with better long-term functional outcome when compared to standard ICP targeted therapy
   c. BtO_2-targeted therapy has been shown to be of uncertain benefit with respect to clinical outcomes post TBI
   d. A major barrier to implementation of BtO_2-targeted therapy is protocol complexity

4. The susceptibility of different regions of the brain to hypoxemia is primarily dependent upon:
   a. The particular cerebral arterial supply territory that has been affected
   b. The basal rate of metabolism of particular cell populations in specific cerebral tissues
   c. The relative sparing of regions with overlap of arterial supply in so-called "watershed" regions
   d. The posture of the patient at the time of onset of the hypoxemia
   e. The duration of the period of hypoxemia

5. The suspicion of a significant hypoxic–ischemic contributing component in a patient recovering from severe TBI would be raised by the observation of all of the following EXCEPT:
   a. Impaired executive function
   b. Profound fluctuating memory impairment
   c. Persistently slowed psychomotor processing speed
   d. Persistent severe short-term memory impairment
   e. Persisting lack of insight

ADDITIONAL READING

Hypoxic brain injury review: https://www.ncbi.nlm.nih.gov/books/NBK537310

https://radiopaedia.org/articles/hypoxic-ischaemic-encephalopathy-adults-and-children?lang=us

Anderson CA, Arciniegas DB. Cognitive sequelae of hypoxic-ischemic brain injury: a review. *NeuroRehabilitation*. 2010;26(1):47–63. doi:10.3233/NRE-2010-0535

Busl KM, Greer DM. Hypoxic-ischemic brain injury: pathophysiology, neuropathology and mechanisms. *NeuroRehabilitation*. 2010;26(1):5–13. doi: 10.3233/NRE-2010-0531

Harbinson M, Zarshenas S, Cullen NK. Long-term functional and psychosocial outcomes after hypoxic-ischemic brain injury: a case-controlled comparison to traumatic brain injury. *PM R.* 2017;9(12):1200–1207. doi:10.1016/j.pmrj.2017.04.015

ANSWERS TO STUDY QUESTIONS

1. Correct Answer: c
   The correct answer is "post-hypoxic action myoclonus" or Lance–Adams syndrome, most often seen clinically as a delayed onset of action-associated myoclonic jerks after cardiac arrest. Focal motor seizures would tend to produce tonic-clonic rather than myoclonic movements and this is not myoclonic status since the movements are isolated and episodic rather than continuous.

   Further Reading:
   Malhotra S, Mohinder K. Lance-Adams syndrome: difficulties surrounding diagnosis, prognostication, and treatment after cardiac arrest. *Anesth Essays Res.* 2012;6(2):218–222. doi:10.4103/0259-1162.108339

2. Correct Answer: b
   Individuals with only a TBI are far more likely to achieve functional independence than those with a combination of TBI and significant anoxic injury. Answers (c) and (d) are clearly incorrect since they both suggest better outcomes for anoxic brain injury compared to TBI. Answer (a) overestimates the negative impact of anoxic brain injury on discharge home compared to TBI.

   Further Reading:
   Fitzgerald A, Aditya H, Prior A, et al. Anoxic brain injury: clinical patterns and functional outcomes. A study of 93 cases. *Brain Inj.* 2010;24:1311–1323. doi:10.3109/02699052.2010.506864
   Cohen SI, Duong TT. Increased arousal in a patient with anoxic brain injury after administration of zolpidem. *Am J Phys Med Rehabil.* 2008;87:229–231. doi:10.1097/PHM.0b013e318161971b

3. Correct Answer: c
   BiO_2-targeted therapy does have a definite favorable impact on post-TBI outcomes. All the other statements are true with regard to this study.

   Further Reading:
   Oddo M, Levine JM, Mackenzie L, et al. Brain hypoxia is associated with short-term outcome after severe traumatic brain injury independently of intracranial hypertension and low cerebral perfusion pressure. *Neurosurgery.* 2011;69(5):1037–1045. doi:10.1227/NEU.0b013e3182287ca7

4. Correct Answer: b
   The neural cell populations in regions of gray matter in the brain that have the highest basal metabolic rate such as pyramidal neurons of the hippocampus (CA1 region), pyramidal neurons of the cerebral cortex (layers 3, 5, and 6) which leads to "laminar necrosis," the death of neurons in the basal ganglia (caudate nucleus and putamen), and the Purkinje cell layer of the cerebellum are most susceptible to hypoxemia. Answers (a) and (c) refer to ischemia rather than hypoxemia. The posture of the patient affects the distribution of intracranial pressures and venous drainage. Posture may be influential in precipitating symptoms such as headache in the presence of intracranial hypotension. The duration and the severity of hypoxemia may affect the degree of reversibility of the injury but not the region of the brain that would be most likely to be affected.

Further Reading:
Lacerte M, Shapshak AH, Mesfin FB. Hypoxic brain injury. *StatPearls*. https://www.ncbi.nlm.nih.gov/books/NBK537310/

5. Correct Answer: a

All of the answer choices would raise suspicion of significant hypoxic–ischemic brain injury except for impaired executive function which is typically seen in frontal lobe injury due to head trauma.

Further Reading:
Cullen NK, Weisz K. Cognitive correlates with functional outcomes after anoxic brain injury: a case-controlled comparison with traumatic brain injury. *Brain Inj*. 2011;25:35–43. doi:10.3109/02699052.2010.531691

REFERENCES

The full reference list appears in the digital product found on http://connect.springerpub.com/content/book/978-0-8261-4768-4/part/part03/chapter/ch24

THE ROLE OF NEUROPROTECTIVE INTERVENTIONS IN TRAUMATIC BRAIN INJURY

JACOB R. JOSEPH AND DAVID O. OKONKWO

BACKGROUND

Definitions

- *Primary injury:* neuronal death or dysfunction as a consequence of initial impact.
- *Secondary injury:* progressive ischemic, inflammatory, and cytotoxic processes initiated or potentiated by systemic and/or intracranial insults.
  - Systemic insults: hypoxia, hypotension, hyperthermia, hyperglycemia
  - Intracranial insults: intracranial hypertension, cerebral edema, mass lesion, cerebral vasospasm
- *Neuroprotective intervention:* treatment initiated prior to and/or at the onset of secondary injury with the aim of minimizing its intensity or immediate effects.

General Principles

- Prophylaxis and early treatment of secondary insults may mitigate secondary injury and improve outcome following traumatic brain injury (TBI). Secondary insults such as hypoxemia, hypotension, hypercarbia, hyperthermia, electrolyte disturbances, increased intracranial pressure, and seizures potentiate secondary injury through ongoing ischemic, inflammatory, and cytotoxic cascades. In turn, these potentiate a vicious circle of further metabolic compromise, oxidative stress, inflammation, vascular dysfunction, apoptosis, and neuroregeneration.
- Vast research has been conducted delineating the cascade of factors responsible for secondary injury following TBI, with a subsequent focus on a host of potential agents directed at ameliorating these insults. Putative therapeutic targets to counteract secondary insults in TBI can be categorized by the core pathophysiological processes from which they are derived:
  - Neuronal, axonal, and astroglial damage
    - N-methyl-D-aspartic acid (NMDA) and α-amino-3-hydroxy-methyl-4-isoxazolyl-propionic acid (AMPA) receptor antagonists—Suppression of the excitotoxic response that follows TBI
    - Cyclosporin A analogues and caspase inhibitors—Target mitochondrial dysfunction and its interplay with apoptosis
    - Prostacyclin—Produces vasodilation, also inhibits leukocyte adhesion and platelet aggregation theoretically decreasing secondary ischemia
    - Stem cell–based therapies—Cell replacement for neurons or supporting cells that are damaged during primary or secondary injury. These therapies may also

The full reference list appears in the digital product found on http://connect.springerpub.com/content/book/978-0-8261-4768-4/part/part03/chapter/ch25

separately work to modulate the inflammatory response in secondary injury. Preclinical work has been promising, and multiple human clinical trials are ongoing, though none have reached phase III to date.[1,2]

- Astrogliosis and neuroinflammation
  - Progesterone—Down-regulates synthesis of proinflammatory cytokines, while decreasing immune cell migration and proliferation
  - Recombinant human IL-1 receptor antagonist—Reduces the secretion of pro-inflammatory cytokines while increasing the release of anti-inflammatory mediators
- Disrupted integrity of the blood–brain barrier
  - Mesenchymal stem cells—mediate the repair of the blood–brain barrier in addition to providing immunomodulation
- Despite promising experimental results all phase III randomized clinical trials evaluating neuroprotection via pharmacological interventions have failed to show an improvement in outcome following TBI.[3]
- Various reasons have been postulated for the lack of successful translation of preclinical studies into human clinical trials:
  - Complexity and poor understanding of the pathophysiological mechanisms at play in TBI
  - Heterogeneity of the condition and patient population
  - Flaws in trial design and outcome assessment
- Given the plurality of mechanisms responsible for cellular injury, it remains unlikely that any single-agent treatment can address all aspects of TBI pathophysiology.
- The only widely accepted neuroprotective strategies at present target systemic and intracranial insults readily amenable to common therapeutic interventions (e.g., hypoxemia, hypotension, hyperthermia, and hyperglycemia).

HYPOXEMIA

Guiding Principles

- The brain accounts for 20% of the body's oxygen consumption. Blood oxygen content exceeds the brain's utilization by only a factor of 2 or 3, leaving the brain vulnerable to small changes in oxygen supply.
- Primary injury stresses the tenuous balance between supply and demand, making the brain more susceptible to secondary ischemic insults.
- The detrimental effect of secondary ischemic damage is well documented; both depth and duration of hypoxemia are significantly associated with increased morbidity and mortality.
- Cerebral oxygen delivery is a function of cerebral blood flow (CBF) and arterial oxygen content.

Diagnosis and Treatment

- Although no treatment threshold exists per se, studies have found severe morbidity and mortality to be associated with PaO_2 less than 60 mmHg and O_2 saturation less than 90%.[4] Hyperventilation, except as a brief temporizing maneuver in the setting of elevated intracranial pressure (ICP), should be avoided.[5]
- Multiple therapies directed at increasing oxygen delivery and utilization have been investigated (e.g., normo- and hyperbaric hyperoxia, brain oxygen tension [$PbtO_2$]

directed therapy), but have produced only equivocal results.[6] However, new trials are forthcoming.

- Direct measures of the cerebral metabolic rate of oxygen consumption ($CMRO_2$) have shown no increase in brain O_2 utilization with normobaric hyperoxia. Hyperbaric treatment has been shown to increase $CMRO_2$; however, a clear clinical benefit has yet to be demonstrated. A phase III trial is currently underway as of the publication of this edition.[7]
- Studies have shown poor outcome with hypoxic brain oxygen tension ($PbtO_2$ <15 mmHg).[8] A recent phase II study investigating a treatment protocol utilizing ICP monitoring coupled with $PbtO_2$ monitoring showed a trend toward lower mortality and improved outcomes.[9] The treatment threshold for this study was $PbtO_2$ ≤20. A phase III trial is currently underway.[10]

■ Potential toxicity of hyperoxia:
- Prolonged high fraction of inspired oxygen (FiO_2) has been associated with injury to the lens of the eye, lungs, heart, brain, and gastrointestinal tract, and may also lead to cerebral vasoconstriction.
- High positive end expiratory pressure (PEEP >15–20 mmHg) should be avoided; PEEP is transmitted through lungs to thoracic vessels leading to cerebral venous congestion and increased ICP.[11]

■ The potential risks in combination with no clear benefit should preclude the use of empiric hyperoxia until RCTs demonstrate a clear advantage.

■ Goals of ventilator management should be sufficient oxygen delivery to avoid hypoxemia or brain hypoxia, while also avoiding ventilation-induced lung injury and acute respiratory distress syndrome. Specifically, this employs protective ventilation using low tidal volumes (Vt, 6–8 mL/kg), plateau pressure less than 30 cm H_2O, and adequate PEEP levels.[11] A goal of eucapneic ventilation ($PaCO_2$ 35–40 mmHg) is especially important in those suffering intracranial hypertension.[12]

HYPOTENSION

Guiding Principles

■ Hypotension is one of the most powerful predictors of outcome—a relationship that is independent of Glasgow Coma Scale (GCS) score, age, or intracranial lesion. Cerebral ischemia may occur in the acute post-injury phase in as many as 35% of patients independent of systemic hypotension.[4]

■ The critical threshold for CBF, below which irreversible tissue damage occurs, can shift following TBI to 15 mL/100 g/min, versus 5 to 8.5 mL/100 g/min in healthy brain tissue.[13]

■ Major influences on CBF include adequate blood pressure, flow-metabolism coupling, $PaCO_2$, and cerebral autoregulation; dysfunction in any or all post-TBI puts patients at risk for hyperemia and/or ischemia.
- The relationship of CBF to blood pressure and vascular resistance is demonstrated by the equation CBF = CPP/CVR; where cerebral perfusion pressure (CPP) is the difference between mean arterial pressure (MAP) and ICP is divided by cerebrovascular resistance (CVR).

■ Changes in CBF following TBI generally occur in three phases:
- Hypoperfusion and ischemia: 6–12 hours post injury
- Hyperemia and concomitant ICP increases: 24–48 hours
- Vasospasm with decreased perfusion: >72 hours

- Posttraumatic cerebral vasospasm is pathological narrowing of intracranial blood vessels with or without resultant ischemia that is precipitated by blood in the subarachnoid space and direct vascular injury by impact or stretch.[14]
  - Occurs in 10% to 30% of severe TBI patients, with 4% to 16% experiencing resultant neurological deficits.
  - Begins 1 to 3 days post-injury and follows a more abbreviated course than vasospasm secondary to aneurysmal subarachnoid hemorrhage (SAH).
  - The risk of developing vasospasm is associated with greater volumes of subarachnoid blood as well as blast-induced neurotrauma.

Diagnosis and Treatment

- Systolic blood pressure (SBP) or CPP can be used as surrogates for estimating CBF with goal thresholds being an SBP greater than 110 (or SBP greater than 100 in patients ages 50–69) and CPP values of 60 to 70 mmHg. Indiscriminate maintenance of CPP greater than 70 mmHg has been associated with increased ICP, acute respiratory distress syndrome (ARDS), and mortality.
- Computed tomography (CT) perfusion studies provide quantitative information regarding CBF, mean transit time (MTT) or time to peak (TTP), and cerebral blood volume (CBV).
- Therapies to treat symptomatic posttraumatic vasospasm include intra-arterial calcium channel blockers and balloon angioplasty.[14] Oral nimodipine, which has been demonstrated to improve outcomes in aneurysmal sub-arachnoid hemorrhage, has also been trialed in posttraumatic vasospasm. However, the preponderance of evidence suggests that nimodipine does not improve outcomes in TBI, likely due to its hypotensive effect.[15]

HYPERTHERMIA

Guiding Principles

- Hyperthermia in the acute post-injury phase is associated with longer intensive care unit (ICU) stay and worsened neurological outcome.[16]
- Temperature surges occur in up to 67% of TBI patients within the first 72 hours after admission, and may result from multiple causes (hypothalamic disruption, inflammation, medications, surgery, etc.).

Diagnosis and Treatment

- Core temperature should be monitored (preferably by brain temperature probe or rectal thermometer) and temperature spikes ≥38°C should be avoided and aggressively treated.[17]
- In addition to the common methods of identifying causative factors accompanying fever (e.g., infection), one should also consider central causes of temperature dysregulation.
- Published literature indicates prophylactic hypothermia does not provide primary neuroprotection after severe TBI, and study results show consistent risk of harm with primary prophylactic hypothermia in TBI.[18]
- Antipyretics, extra-corporeal cooling, gastric lavage, and intravascular cooling catheters have all been investigated as means to prophylactically control temperature

in TBI patients. Intravascular cooling catheters have shown the most consistency in induced normothermia, without increases in rates of infection, antibiotic, or sedation usage.[17,19]

HYPOCAPNIA

Guiding Principles

- Hypocapnia ($PaCO_2$ ~30–35 mmHg) is generally caused by intended or accidental hyperventilation (e.g., with therapeutic hyperventilation in managing increased ICP).[4]
- The ability of hyperventilation (and hypocapnia) to reduce CBV is achieved at a disproportionate cost to CBF, which may be especially harmful in the first 24 hours post injury.[12]
- The effects of hypocapnia on vascular smooth muscle are pH-mediated; cerebral and renal buffering returns pH to normal within 4 to 6 hours, eliminating this effect and precluding the use of sustained hypocapnia. Additionally, this buffering leads to pH-overshoot and subsequent rebound hyperemia/increased ICP.

Diagnosis and Treatment

- Prophylactic hyperventilation should not be used, as it has been associated with worsened ICP control and poor neurological outcome.[4,19]
- Brief (e.g., 20 minutes) moderate hyperventilation for ICP reduction should be undertaken cautiously and only until a pathology-specific intervention can be instituted.

HYPERGLYCEMIA

Guiding Principles

- The massive stress response following TBI results in elevated circulating catecholamine levels with subsequent increases in serum glucose.
- Hyperglycemia, which leads to intracellular acidosis, is associated with the development of reactive oxygen species, especially during the acute ischemic phase of TBI, exacerbating secondary brain injury.
- Admission and early post-operative hyperglycemia (serum glucose ≥200 mg/dL) have been associated with worse neurological and mortality outcomes.[20]

Diagnosis and Treatment

- A target serum glucose no greater than 180 to 200 mg/dL decreases episodes of hyperglycemia and has been associated with decreased mortality.[20]
- Note that intensive insulin therapy (target glucose 80–110 mg/dL) results in an increased risk of hypoglycemic episodes without conferring mortality benefits. Conservative treatment of glucose levels greater than 180 mg/dL is generally accepted as striking the best balance.

POSTTRAUMATIC SEIZURES

Guiding Principles

- Posttraumatic seizures (PTS) may occur in 20% to 25% of all patients suffering moderate to severe TBI (see also Chapter 46).[21] PTS can be classified by time of onset: immediate (first few hours), early (occurring during the first week), and late (greater than 1-week post injury).
- Late posttraumatic epilepsy is associated with severity and type of injury (subdural and intracerebral hemorrhage, skull fractures, neurological dysfunction)[22]; biochemical and structural alterations have been the main pathophysiological mechanisms proposed.

Diagnosis and Treatment

Studies to date have not addressed effects of PTS on secondary injury. However, early short-term prophylactic treatment with antiepileptic drugs antiepileptic drugs (AEDs) (i.e., for the first week post-injury) has been shown to decrease the relative risk of early PTS; although this is without a concordant decrease in development of late seizures (i.e., posttraumatic epilepsy), morbidity, or mortality.[23] Most studies have not shown marked differences in rates of PTS when using levetiracetam versus phenytoin.[18] (See Chapter 46 for further recommendations regarding management of PTS.)

KEY POINTS

- Current neuroprotective strategies target prophylaxis against and early treatment of secondary systemic and intracranial insults to mitigate secondary injury.
- Hypoxemia and/or hypocapnia significantly increases the risk of post-TBI ischemic brain injury. Therapeutic goals should target PaO_2 >60 mmHg, O_2 saturation> 90%, eucapneic ventilation ($PaCO_2$ 35–40 mmHg), and brain oxygen tension >15 mmHg.
- Hypotension and its corollary, diminished cerebral blood flow, remains one of the most powerful predictors of outcome. Thresholds for adequate cerebral blood flow include maintaining SBP >110 (or >100 in patients ages 50–69) and CPP value of 60–70 mmHg.
- Hyperthermia in the acute post-injury phase negatively impacts outcome and should be avoided and aggressively treated through induced normothermia.
- Early post-TBI hyperglycemia leads to intracellular acidosis, reactive oxygen species, and worse overall outcome. A target serum glucose <180–200 mg/dL decreases hyperglycemic episodes and is associated with improved outcome.

STUDY QUESTIONS

1. What is the minimum target systolic blood pressure after severe TBI in a 60-year-old patient?
   a. 80 mmHg
   b. 90 mmHg
   c. 100 mmHg

    d. 110 mmHg
    e. 120 mmHg

2. Which of the following is the preferred agent for prevention of early posttraumatic seizures?
    a. Valproic acid
    b. Levetiracetam
    c. Phenytoin
    d. Lacosamide
    e. None of the above

3. For how long do the effects of sustained hypocapnia on intracranial pressure last?
    a. 20 minutes
    b. 1 hour
    c. 6 hours
    d. 12 hours
    e. 24 hours

4. What is the target temperature for patients after severe TBI?
    a. 30–32°
    b. 32–34°
    c. 34–36°
    d. 36–37.5°

5. What pharmacological agents have shown efficacy in improving patient outcomes in severe TBI?
    a. Dexamethasone
    b. Cyclosporin A
    c. Erythropoietin
    d. Progesterone
    e. None of the above

ADDITIONAL READING

Progesterone and neuroprotection: https://www.ncbi.nlm.nih.gov/pmc/articles/PMC6463867/

Bahr M. *Neuroprotection: Models, Mechanisms, and Therapies.* Wiley-VCH; 2004:95–115:chap 6. doi:10.1002/3527603867

Guidelines for the management of severe traumatic brain injury. *Neurosurgery.* 2017;80(1):6–15.

Kabadi SV, Faden AI. Neuroprotective strategies for traumatic brain injury: improving clinical translation. *Int J Mol Sci.* 2014;15(1):1216–1236. doi:10.3390/ijms15011216

Kochanek PM, Jackson TC, Ferguson NM, et al. Emerging therapies in traumatic brain injury. *Semin Neurol.* 2015;35(1):83–100. doi:10.1055/s-0035-1544237

ANSWERS TO STUDY QUESTIONS

1. Correct Answer: c
   SBP should be maintained greater than 110 mmHg for patients less than 50 years old or greater than 70 years old. For patients aged 50 to 69, SBP should be greater than 100 mmHg.

Further Reading:
Carney N, Totten AM, O'Reilly C, et al. Guidelines for the management of severe traumatic brain injury. *Neurosurgery*. 2017;80(1):6–15. doi:10.1227/NEU.0000000000001432

2. Correct Answer: e
While phenytoin is the most widely studied agent, there have not been any demonstrated benefits for specific anti-epileptic drugs when compared against each other.

Further Reading:
Carney N, Totten AM, O'Reilly C, et al. Guidelines for the management of severe traumatic brain injury. *Neurosurgery*. 2017;80(1):6–15. doi:10.1227/NEU.0000000000001432

3. Correct Answer: c
The effects of sustained hypocapnia last for approximately 4–6 hours, and then can result in rebound hyperemia and increased ICP. Sustained hypocapnia is not recommended for patients with severe TBI.

Further Reading:
Carney N, Totten AM, O'Reilly C, et al. Guidelines for the management of severe traumatic brain injury. *Neurosurgery*. 2017;80(1):6–15. doi:10.1227/NEU.0000000000001432

4. Correct Answer: d
36–37.5°C Hyperthermia has shown to be harmful in severe TBI, while prophylactic hypothermia has had largely poor outcomes.

Further Reading:
Carney N, Totten AM, O'Reilly C, et al. Guidelines for the management of severe traumatic brain injury. *Neurosurgery*. 2017;80(1):6–15. doi:10.1227/NEU.0000000000001432

5. Correct Answer: d
There have not been any medications which have demonstrated improved patient outcomes in severe TBI.

REFERENCES

The full reference list appears in the digital product found on http://connect.springerpub.com/content/book/978-0-8261-4768-4/part/part03/chapter/ch25

NUTRITIONAL CONSIDERATIONS

MELISSA A. NESTOR AND BARBARA MAGNUSON-WOODWARD

GENERAL PRINCIPLES

■ Moderate to severe traumatic brain injury (TBI) patients often require nutrition support with either enteral nutrition (EN) or parenteral nutrition (PN) due to intubation, dysphagia, or low Glasgow Coma Scale (GCS) score.
■ Controversy exists regarding optimal feeding route with respect to gastric versus small bowel delivery:
  ● Intolerance to gastric feeding with high gastric residuals may lead to subsequent aspiration pneumonia.
  ● Preference for duodenal or jejunal feedings often avoids gastric intolerance and optimizes EN delivery, avoiding malnutrition, and resulting immunocompromise.[1–5]
  ● The Brain Trauma Foundation Guidelines recommend that moderate to severe TBI patients receive full caloric replacement by day 7 after injury (with no specification of route), and suggest initiating feeding within 72 hours after injury and targeting 100% to 140% of estimated resting metabolism expenditure (18%–25% of those calories being protein).[6]
■ The American Society of Parenteral and Enteral Nutrition (ASPEN) Critical Care and the Society of Critical Care Medicine (SCCM) Guidelines both recommend early EN as the initial route, and that it be initiated within 24 to 72 hours for critically ill patients.[7]

DIAGNOSIS

Clinical Presentation

■ TBI patients presenting with malnutrition, wounds, and other chronic disease states require an immediate nutrition assessment to optimize nutrition and minimize further malnutrition-associated complications.
■ Frequently reassess the ability to swallow, the need for a temporary nasoduodenal (ND) or nasojejunal (NJ) feeding tube (placed at bedside), or the need for more secure feeding access (gastrostomy tube [G-tube]).
■ G-tubes are indicated when a patient presents with dysphagia for a prolonged period of time (i.e., >2–3 weeks). TBI patients are more likely to tolerate gastric feedings as the acute phase of illness subsides. Typically by week 2 or 3 after TBI, gastric administration of feedings, medications, and maintenance fluids are well tolerated. That said, some data suggest that, in patients for which a G-tube will be required, earlier placement (within 7 to 14 days after injury) may be beneficial.[8]

The full reference list appears in the digital product found on http://connect.springerpub.com/content/book/978-0-8261-4768-4/part/part03/chapter/ch26

- PN should only be considered in patients with early feeding difficulty and inability to establish access (i.e., due to severe facial fractures or severe intestinal injury), or who do not tolerate EN within the 4 days after injury. The benefits of early nutrition must be balanced with the high dextrose load, large fluid volume, and infectious risks of PN.[9]

TREATMENT

Guiding Principles

- Prompt nutrition assessment is needed to establish goals for optimal calories, protein, and fluids.
- Caution should be exercised with application of various equations utilized to predict energy expenditure that incorporate age, weight, and height.
  - None are specific to TBI and all have a degree of inaccuracy.[7]
  - A weight-based equation (25–35 kcal/kg) is often utilized, but again caution with obese or underweight patients should be exercised, as this lends to further the inaccuracy.
- Indirect calorimetry (IC) is the current gold standard for accuracy of energy expenditure, but is more costly.[10]
- Recognize changing nutritional needs: repeating IC readings is warranted as clinical status changes, for example, immediately after TBI, as sedation and/or neuromuscular blockade is decreased, and during the convalescent phase.
- Aggressively address electrolyte abnormalities:
  - Hypophosphatemia, hypokalemia, and hypomagnesemia develop due to intercellular shifts when carbohydrates are initiated with nutrition support.
  - Avoid hyponatremia and hyperglycemia.
- Avoid overfeeding by accounting for the lipid caloric provision: propofol and clevidipine are in a lipid emulsion solvent. Propofol provides 1.1 kcal/mL and clevidipine provides 2 kcal/mL.[11,12]
  - Lipids in PN regimens are often discontinued while the patient is receiving propofol.
- Despite comatose appearance, TBI patients have increased metabolic needs (~120%–140% of resting metabolic expenditure) because of hypercatabolic response. The Harris Benedict, Ireton-Jones 1992, Penn State 2003, and Swinamer equations are frequently utilized to determine calorie needs. Estimates may be as high as 160% in pediatric patients and adults with multitrauma.[13]
- Conversely, needs may be as low as 80% in pharmacologically induced coma.[14]
- Protein requirements range from 1.2 to 2 g/kg depending on degree of hypercatabolism, wounds present, and if continuous renal replacement therapy is utilized.[15]
  - 1.5 g/kg is a typical starting protein dose.
- Large volumes of salt-free water and other hypotonic fluids should be avoided to prevent exacerbation of cerebral edema or hyponatremia.

Initial Management

- Establish postpyloric feeding access as soon as possible.[8,9]
- Administer a calorically dense EN product as early as possible (preferably within 48 hours after injury).[7]
- Provide at least 18% to 25% of calories as protein to account for protein catabolism.

- Some studies suggest success in starting EN near goal rate; common practice tends to focus on slowly increasing EN rate to goal over 12 to 48 hours, depending on patient tolerance.[16,17]
- Re-evaluate metabolic needs as the patient convalesces and clinically improves.

Glycemic Control

- The optimal range of glucose values is an often debated topic in critically ill individuals.
- Hyperglycemia (>200–225 mg/dL) may be associated with increased morbidity and mortality in TBI patients.[18,19]
- The rate of infectious complications, immune dysfunction, and other noninfectious complications such as polyneuropathy are closely associated with elevated glucose levels.[20]
- Hypoglycemia has been associated with increased mortality in critically ill individuals.[21]
- TBI patients exhibit some differences in brain glucose metabolism and likely require slightly higher glucose values to ensure appropriate brain metabolism.
  - Maintenance of serum glucose values between 80 and 110 mg/dL ("intensive insulin") may result in cerebrospinal fluid (CSF) glucose values below the normal threshold.[22,23]
  - Serum glucose values of 140 to 180 mg/dL should result in improved CSF glucose values and reduce the risk of hypoglycemia.

Treatment Controversies

- Timing—If early enteral nutrition is not feasible, PN should not be initiated in the first week except in the setting of severe malnutrition on admission.[24]
  - If PN is used, clinicians should be vigilant to avoid permissive delays in EN initiation while providing early PN (i.e., clinicians should still be aggressive in attempting to start EN as soon as possible). Note that no benefits were realized with supplemental early PN compared to late PN (i.e. initiated after 7 days).[7]
  - Caution should be used in patients with intracranial hypertension or cerebral edema due to the large volume of dextrose and fluids required in PN to meet nutritional needs.
- Management of hyperglycemia
  - The American Diabetes Association (ADA) and ASPEN recommend a target glucose range of 140 to 180 mg/dL for critically ill patients.[7,25]
  - *The Brain Trauma Foundation Guidelines* do not comment on a recommendation for glucose control specific to TBI.
- Immunonutrition—Role of immunonutrients such as glutamine, arginine, and omega-3 fatty acids in the inflammatory response of TBI patients is ill-defined.[26]
  - Theoretical suppositions can be made based on the pathophysiology of TBI and the mechanism of action of these immunonutrients, but clinical data are lacking.
  - Very few studies have evaluated combinations of pharmaconutrients in TBI patients to recommend its net benefit or harm.
  - Based on the current understanding of the mechanism of action of each individual nutrient, caution should be exercised when evaluating the use of immunonutrients.
  - Glutamine could possibly be deleterious due to the potential conversion to glutamate, an excitatory neurotransmitter known to be a major factor in the pathology of secondary brain injury, but a 2014 study showed this theory may not be a significant clinical concern.[27]
  - Controversy exists as to whether arginine confers a potential net clinical benefit or harm in patients with TBI:

- While arginine is likely beneficial for multi-trauma and burn patients due to the nitric oxide–mediated perfusion and enhanced immune function, the data in TBI patients are sparse. Increasing nitric oxide in cerebral circulation may theoretically increase cerebral blood volume and intracranial pressure. Other studies, however, have shown improved cerebral blood perfusion with arginine administration early after injury.[28,29]
- Preclinical literature suggests that omega-3 fatty acids, specifically docosahexaenoic acid (DHA), may be able to mitigate the central inflammatory response and propagation of lipid peroxidation, due to the ischemia and metabolic dysfunction seen after severe TBI, by shunting prostaglandin production away from arachidonic acid and associated metabolites. However, further clinical studies are still required to validate these findings.
  - ASPEN guidelines continue to suggest the use of either arginine-containing immune-modulating formulations of EPA/DHA supplement with standard enteral formulation in patients with TBI.[7]
- Optimal timing of reductions in calories and protein as the TBI patient improves clinically is not well defined. Clinicians should continue to monitor caloric needs, nutrition tolerance, and caloric intake, even after the acute illness subsides.

KEY POINTS

- Initiate nutrition (preferably enteral) as soon as is feasible—ideally within 48 hours.
- Account for calorie provision outside of nutrition products (particularly in patients receiving propofol).
- Individualize caloric needs and account for hypercatabolism after TBI.
- Salt-free water and other hypotonic fluids may increase intracranial pressure or cerebral edema—avoid these in the acute phases of injury whenever possible.

STUDY QUESTIONS

1. A 24-year-old man is admitted to your intensive care unit (ICU) with severe TBI and is intubated at time of admission with an initial GCS of 7. It is 18 hours since admission; which of the following statements is most correct?
   a. The patient should be initiated on early PN due to mechanical intubation.
   b. The patient should be initiated on early EN as soon as possible, but no later than 72 hours after injury.
   c. The patient should undergo surgical G-tube placement by day 4 of ICU admission as long-term EN is likely necessary.
   d. The patient should be initiated on both EN and PN within 48 hours of injury.

2. A 65-year-old man is admitted to your ICU after being struck by a falling tree limb with resulting subarachnoid hemorrhage. A nasojejunal feeding tube is placed and the staff requests recommendations and orders for EN. Which of the following is not an accurate consideration when formulating or reviewing an EN plan for this patient?

    a. The patient likely has increased metabolic requirements when compared to basal metabolic expenditure calculations.

    b. The patient's caloric requirement will be typically in the range of 25 to 35 kcal/kg/day.

    c. Avoid over-feeding by keeping protein less than 1.2 g/kg/day.

    d. Large volumes of salt-free water or hypotonic fluids may exacerbate cerebral edema or hyponatremia.

3. A 55-year-old man is hospital day 2 in your ICU with severe TBI. He is mechanically intubated and requiring continuous sedation with propofol 30 mcg/kg/min. He weighs 80 kg and you wish to provide EN with a goal kcal of 25 kcal/kg/day. Does his propofol infusion clinically affect your EN calculation? What amount of kcal/day does propofol provide?

    a. No, propofol does not affect EN calculations.

    b. Propofol does provide some kcal/day but the amount is negligible and the EN calculation is unaffected.

    c. Yes, propofol does affect EN calculation, providing an additional 691 kcal/day.

    d. Yes, propofol does affect EN calculation, providing an additional 380 kcal/day.

4. A 64-year-old woman is admitted to your ICU with severe TBI after a motor vehicle collision. Her past medical history is significant for hypertension, hypothyroidism, obesity, and type 2 diabetes mellitus. Her glucose on admission is 197 mg/dL and after initiation of EN has ranged from 221 to 267 mg/dL. Which of the following is most correct with respect to glycemic control for this patient?

    a. The patient has a known history of diabetes mellitus; thus, elevated glucose is expected and hyperglycemia will not affect the patient.

    b. The patient should be started on an insulin infusion with a goal glucose range of 80 to 110 mg/dL.

    c. Insulin therapy should be initiated to maintain glucose range of 140 to 180 mg/dL to avoid both extreme hypo- and hyperglycemia.

    d. EN should be held due to hyperglycemia and not reinitiated until glucose is below 180 mg/dL.

5. A 45-year-old man is in your ICU with a severe TBI after an unhelmeted motorcycle collision. He requires mechanical ventilation and deep sedation along with neuromuscular blockade. Which of the following is most correct regarding his enteral nutrition?

    a. The patient will require increased protein to 2.5 g/kg.

    b. The patient's enteral nutrition should be decreased by half with initiation of neuromuscular blockade.

    c. The patient should receive gastric feeding and not jejunal feeding while on neuromuscular blockade.

    d. Indirect calorimetry should be used where available, as nutrition requirements may be decreased by 10% to 20%.

ADDITIONAL READING

Critical Care Nutrition Website: https://www.criticalcarenutrition.com/

American Society of Parenteral and Enteral Nutrition: http://www.nutritioncare.org

Cook AM, Peppard A, Magnuson B. Nutrition considerations in traumatic brain injury. *Nutr Clin Pract.* 2008;23:608–620. doi:10.1177/0884533608326060

Marik PE, Zaloga GP. Immunonutrition in critically ill patients: a systematic review and analysis of the literature. *Intensive Care Med.* 2008;34:1980–1990. doi:10.1007/s00134-008-1213-6

Rhoney DH, Parker D Jr. Considerations in fluids and electrolytes after traumatic brain injury. *Nutr Clin Pract.* 2006;21:462–478. doi:10.1177/0115426506021005462

ANSWERS TO STUDY QUESTIONS

1. Correct Answer: b

   While the patient may indeed require G-tube placement, it is not required that it be done immediately upon admission. According to ASPEN. guidelines, mechanical ventilation is not an indication for PN. While a combination of both EN and PN may be considered in some cases, current evidence does not support use of early/supplemental PN to improve mortality, length of ventilation, or length of stay. Additionally the potential for harm of PN needs to be factored into decision-making, and therefore an attempt at early EN should be made, reserving PN for patients in which EN is not tolerated or is contraindicated.

   Further Reading:

   McClave SA, Taylor BE, Martindale RG, et al. Guidelines for the provision and assessment of nutrition support therapy in the adult critically ill patient: Society of Critical Care Medicine (SCCM) and American Society for Parenteral and Enteral Nutrition (ASPEN). *JPEN J Parenter Enteral Nutr.* 2016;40(2):159–211. doi:10.1177/0148607115621863

2. Correct Answer: c

   Protein requirements are elevated in patients with brain injury, thus selection (c) is incorrect: Protein requirements range from 1.2 to 2 g/kg/day. It is true that patients with brain injury have increased metabolic demands compared to basal requirements. Providing calories at 120% to 140% of resting metabolic expenditure, or 25 to 35 kcal/kg/day will meet caloric requirements, though indirect calorimetry may be used to more precisely identify caloric needs. Hypotonic enteral fluids may exacerbate cerebral edema or hyponatremia if given in excess.

   Further Reading:

   Hurt RT, McClave SA, Martindale RG, et al. Summary points and consensus recommendations from the international protein summit. *Nutr Clin Pract.* 2017;32(1_suppl):142s–151s. doi:10.1177/0884533617693610

3. Correct Answer: c

   Medications prepared in a lipid emulsion (such as propofol or clevidipine) can provide a significant source of calories depending on dose/amount infused. In this example the patient's current rate of propofol will yield an infusion rate of 14.4 mL/hr or 345.6 mL/day. Propofol is in a 10% lipid emulsion, containing 1.1 kcal/mL, and provides the patient with 380 kcal/day. Lipid formulations for parenteral nutrition are commonly a 20% lipid emulsion, containing 2 kcal/mL. The initial EN recommendation should take this 380 kcal into account as part of the overall goal of 25 kcal/kg/day. As propofol is decreased/discontinued, the EN should be re-assessed to provide adequate caloric intake.

   Further Reading:

   Diprivan (propofol) [package insert]. Fresenius Kabi. 2017.

4. Correct Answer: c

It is generally recommended to maintain a more permissive glucose goal range of 140 to 180 mg/dL for this patient population. While intensive insulin therapy has shown benefit in some populations, the intensive goal of glucose 80 to 110 mg/dL does carry a higher risk for hypoglycemic episodes. The patient has a known history of diabetes mellitus, thus hyperglycemia in response to both her acute injury and enteral feeding is expected—she should still receive both EN and glycemic control to avoid the possibly deleterious effects of untreated hypertension.

Further Reading:

Finfer S, Chittock D, Li Y, et al. Intensive versus conventional glucose control in critically ill patients with traumatic brain injury: long-term follow-up of a subgroup of patients from the NICE-SUGAR study. *Intensive Care Med.* 2015;41(6):1037–1047. doi:10.1007/s00134-015-3757-6

American Diabetes Association. 15. Diabetes care in the hospital: standards of medical care in diabetes-2020. *Diabetes Care.* 2020;43(Suppl 1):S193–s202. doi:10.2337/dc20-S015

5. Correct Answer: d

Neuromuscular blockade, along with pharmacologically induced coma with agents such as pentobarbital, can decrease a patient's metabolic rate. The rate of metabolic depression may vary from patient to patient but a decrease of 50% will underfeed these critically ill patients. Indirect calorimetry can provide patient-specific nutrition requirements; however, a more conservative decrease in nutrition may be used where indirect calorimetry is not available.

Further Reading:

Hurt RT, McClave SA, Martindale RG, et al. Summary points and consensus recommendations from the International Protein Summit. *Nutr Clin Pract.* 2017;32(1_suppl):142s–151s. doi:10.1177/0884533617693610

REFERENCES

The full reference list appears in the digital product found on http://connect.springer-pub.com/content/book/978-0-8261-4768-4/part/part03/chapter/ch26

27 INITIAL REHABILITATION INTERVENTIONS IN THE ACUTE HOSPITAL SETTING AND TRANSITIONING TO THE NEXT LEVEL OF CARE

BRIAN D. GREENWALD, CHRISTINE GREISS, AND
MINA GAYED

INTRODUCTION

Moderate to severe traumatic brain injury (TBI) carries an overall mortality of 20% to 50% with 85% of those deaths occurring within the first 2 weeks of injury.[1,2] For those who survive, significant risk of disability remains. Initial TBI treatment goals are focused on decreasing its significant mortality and prevention of negative sequelae and disability.

Initial rehabilitation interventions in the acute hospital setting involve shifting focus from life-saving measures and medical stabilization to optimization of the medical milieu in the context of central nervous system (CNS) recovery and preservation or restoration of function. One mechanism to achieve neuroprotection is through pharmacological management, employing medications that are thought to promote neuro-recovery and minimize neural depression. Optimal trauma care should include rehabilitation considerations from the first day of injury.[3] A physiatrist may be actively involved in more specialized treatment including evaluating and treating disorders of consciousness, arousal, attention, memory, executive function, and agitation.[3] Family education and engagement is crucial in the rehabilitation process, and physiatrists are well versed in the continuum of recovery for this patient population. Early rehabilitation or physiatry consultation and formal intervention programs are associated with decreased acute hospital length of stay and improved functional outcomes.[3] The following topic areas represent commonly encountered acute hospital considerations for patients with TBI.

AGITATION

- Agitation occurs in 33% to 50% of moderate to severe TBI patients at some point during the acute hospital course.[4–6]
  - Search for the cause of agitation, which may include seizures, pain, hypoxia, recent medication changes, or infection.
  - Implement environmental modifications—dim lights, turn off TV and radio, decrease visitations and/or number of visitors in the room.

The full reference list appears in the digital product found on http://connect.springerpub.com/content/book/978-0-8261-4768-4/part/part03/chapter/ch27

- Minimize use of restraints because they can increase agitation and cause harm.
- Pharmacological treatment should be kept to a minimum; use the lowest dose possible to address symptoms, and taper as tolerated (see also Chapters 36 and 37).[5,7]
  - For restlessness, consider trazodone, carbamazepine, or valproate.[7]
  - For aggression, consider beta-blockers (metoprolol and other beta selective agents are preferred) or valproate.[7,8]
  - For emotional lability, consider selective serotonin reuptake inhibitors, dextromethorphan/quinidine, or valproate.[7]
  - To manage psychotic features, consider quetiapine, risperidone, olanzapine, or other atypical antipsychotics. Typical neuroleptics should be avoided due to dopamine blockade.[5]
  - Use of Ativan or other benzodiazepines should be discouraged to the extent possible, because they cause sedation and amnesia, are associated with risk of paradoxical agitation, and delay cognitive recovery by causing adverse effects on neuroplasticity.[5]

CONTRACTURES AND SPASTICITY (SEE ALSO CHAPTER 51)

- The first stage of treatment involves aggressive range of motion, stretching, and exercise.[9] Initial interventions should be initiated in the intensive care unit. Repeatedly reassess and modify approach as warranted based on evolving clinical condition.
- Treatment should be geared toward functional improvement and pain relief.
- Splinting or serial casting of extremities should be considered whenever appropriate.[5]
- Pharmacological therapies (e.g., dantrolene, baclofen) may be considered. Close patient monitoring is required, because tone-lowering medications can have negative effects on cognition and arousal.

NUTRITION/SWALLOWING STATUS (SEE ALSO CHAPTER 26)

- TBI results in catecholamine excess acutely, leading to hypermetabolism, increased energy expenditure, and increased protein loss; as a result, TBI patients have increased caloric requirements.[9–12]
- Early nutritional support decreases morbidity and mortality, shortens hospital length of stay, and may decrease disability.[9]
- Brain Trauma Foundation (BTF) Guidelines for the Management of Severe TBI recommend that patient's feeding requirements be met by the first week after TBI.[12]
- Swallow mechanism may be impaired in up to 82% of TBI patients.[13] Note that 12% of patients with swallowing disorders may have normal gag reflex and 77% have good voluntary cough reflex.[14] In other words, bedside swallow evaluations can produce false negatives.
- TBI patients may have impaired gastric emptying secondary to vagal nerve damage, elevated levels of endogenous opioids, or use of medications such as narcotics.
  - If using enteral nutrition, check feeding residuals periodically.
  - Promotility agents such as erythromycin may be considered.
  - Metoclopramide should be used sparingly if at all because of its dopamine antagonist activity.

BOWEL AND BLADDER (SEE ALSO CHAPTER 30)

- Injury to frontal lobes can cause loss of cortical control over bowel and bladder.
- Incidence of urinary incontinence is 62%[15] and that of urinary retention is 9%.[9] Note associated increased risk of urinary tract infection and skin ulcer development.
  - Urinary incontinence treatment options include timed voiding programs and use of anticholinergic agents; close monitoring is required because of potentially negative effects on cognition.
  - Urinary retention treatment may include intermittent catheterization or Foley catheter placement.
- Constipation can also be present secondary to immobility and medications.
  - Bowel treatment options include use of a timed bowel program, fiber supplementation, maintenance of adequate hydration, and selected medication use (e.g., stool softeners, stimulant suppositories).

PAIN (SEE ALSO CHAPTER 38)

Pain is a common cause of agitation; evaluating for etiology may be difficult due to confusion or altered consciousness.

- Management guidelines:
  - Whenever possible, use mechanical interventions to prevent exacerbation of pain (e.g., positioning, splinting).
  - Use long-acting or around-the-clock dosing for patients unable to effectively communicate pain medication needs.
  - Use opiates or other sedating pain medications with caution. If started, monitor and assess for continued need. Take note of arousal and cognition.
  - Scheduled use of non-sedating pain relievers such as acetaminophen can be highly effective in many instances.
  - For localized pain, lidocaine patches should be considered.

SEIZURE PROPHYLAXIS (SEE ALSO CHAPTER 46)

- Posttraumatic seizures are classified as immediate (first 24 hours), early (≤7 days after TBI), or late (>7 days after TBI).[10,16]
- BTF Guidelines suggest the use of phenytoin as prophylaxis for the first 7 days after TBI to prevent early seizures in high-risk patients, defined as those with Glasgow Coma Scale score less than 10, cortical contusion, depressed skull fracture, hematoma, penetrating head wound, or seizure within 24 hours of head injury.[10]
- Phenytoin trials demonstrate efficacy in preventing early seizures but no impact on incidence of late seizures.[17]
- Anticonvulsants have been associated with adverse side effects, including hematological abnormalities, ataxia, and neurobehavioral side effects; they may also impair neural plasticity. Levetiracetam has recently been favored due to fewer adverse side effects. Prophylaxis is not recommended beyond 7 days post injury.[17,18]
- Monitor use of anticonvulsants, and discontinue after the first week unless there is a specific indication for ongoing use.

DEEP VEIN THROMBOSIS PROPHYLAXIS

■ There is a reported 20% incidence of deep vein thrombosis (DVT) in TBI patients upon admission to inpatient rehab.[19–21]
■ High-risk patients are those older than 40, with severe injury, clotting disorders, prolonged immobilization, and/or multiple transfusions.[21]
■ General guidelines for DVT prophylaxis:
  ● Pharmacological intervention has been shown to be efficacious. Early use must be weighed against the risk of expansion of hemorrhage. Subcutaneous heparin (or a low-molecular-weight heparinoid [LMWH]) can generally be started 36 hours after trauma.[19]
  ● Mechanical compression stockings, aspirin, and lose-dose warfarin may reduce risk, but data do not suggest equivalent efficacy.
  ● Discuss timing of initiation with primary service.
■ Very high-risk patients with contraindications for other methods of prophylaxis can be considered for inferior vena cava filter placement. Consider use of a retrievable filter with removal soon after clinical indication for placement resolves.
■ DVT prophylaxis should be continued until the patient is ambulatory, or sufficient time has passed, given the comorbidities and clinical status. The time frame for stopping DVT prophylaxis in a patient who is medically stable but still immobilized is not well defined in the literature, but 3 months is generally considered reasonable.[21]

ENDOCRINE ABNORMALITIES (SEE ALSO CHAPTER 48)

The signs and symptoms of hypothalamopituitarism may be subtle and may overlap with the neurological and psychiatric sequelae of TBI.[22] Maintain a low threshold for suggesting or initiating an endocrine work-up when clinically indicated, as described in the following section.

■ Acute corticosteroid deficiency—adrenal crisis
  ● Symptoms—weakness, nausea, vomiting, abdominal or flank pain, hyperthermia or hypothermia, and hypovolemic shock.
  ● Clinical and laboratory findings—hypotension, hypoglycemia, hyponatremia, myopathy, anemia, eosinophilia, QT prolongation, or deep T waves on electrocardiogram.
  ● Adrenal crisis is life-threatening and should be treated immediately with glucocorticoid replacement.
■ Syndrome of inappropriate antidiuretic hormone secretion (SIADH)
  ● Symptoms—anorexia, vomiting, worsening cognitive function, agitation, headache, and seizures.
  ● Clinical and laboratory findings—hyponatremia; fractional excretion of sodium is greater than 1%
  ● May be precipitated by medications such as amitriptyline, carbamazepine, and phenobarbital.
  ● Treatment—fluid restriction, saline infusion. Correct no more than 12 mEq/L in first 24 hours and no more than 6 mEq/L on subsequent days.
■ Neurogenic diabetes insipidus
  ● Associated with basilar skull fractures.
  ● Treat with increased oral fluid intake, IV hypotonic fluid, and/or vasopressin.

MEDICATIONS TO BE AVOIDED

Regardless of clinical condition, certain medications should be avoided in TBI because of the risk of increased sedation, worsening cognitive, behavioral, or affective impairments, and/or adverse effects on neural plasticity. Some common examples are as follows:

- Anticholinergics (e.g., Benadryl, some tricyclic antidepressants)—can cause delirium and worsen sedation.
- Dopamine blockers (e.g., metoclopramide, haloperidol), particularly typical antipsychotics. Dopamine blockade is associated with worse motor recovery in animal studies and prolonged posttraumatic confusion in human trials.[23,24]
- Central-acting α-1 antagonists (prazosin) and α-2 agonists (clonidine)—can increase sedation.
- H2 blockers (e.g., famotidine)—can increase confusion and sedation.

KEY POINTS

- Early interdisciplinary rehabilitation should be considered for all patients after moderate to severe TBI.
- Agitation comes in many forms and treatment should consider possible causes and nonpharmacological treatment before considering pharmacological treatment.
- Knowledge of medical conditions that are common after TBI is critical for effective treatment.
- Familiarity with medications to avoid after TBI is important in treating this patient population.

STUDY QUESTIONS

1. A 36-year-old right-handed woman with recent traumatic subarachnoid hemorrhage is under your care in acute rehab. She is receiving boluses four times daily through her percutaneous endoscopic gastrostomy (PEG) tube and is experiencing intermittent bouts of vomiting. Out of the following options, which would NOT be advised?
   a. Check feeding residuals routinely
   b. Place the patient on erythromycin 250 mg orally every 8 hours
   c. Assess for constipation and treat if necessary
   d. Initiate twice daily metoclopramide

2. You are told by the nurse that your patient, a 59-year-old left-handed man with severe TBI, is urinating excessively. The liquid is clear without any significant odor. Which of the following is associated with his disease process?
   a. Can be treated by restricting fluid intake
   b. Carbamazepine can contribute to worsening this disease process
   c. Fractional excretion of sodium is greater than 1%
   d. Can be seen in patients with basilar skull fractures

3. In your brain trauma unit, a 24-year-old right-handed woman with moderate TBI is found to have an elevated heart rate of 120 bpm at rest. Upon examination, you find that she is restless and fidgeting. There are no adverse environmental factors. You assess her for sources of pain or infection. An electrocardiogram shows sinus tachycardia without any other abnormalities. All other testing is negative. What would be an appropriate pharmacologic treatment option?
   a. Fluoxetine
   b. Quetiapine
   c. Propranolol
   d. Trazodone

4. A 34-year-old man is being admitted to your rehab unit. Due to a motor vehicle collision, he suffered traumatic subarachnoid hemorrhage with diffuse axonal injury and is in a minimally conscious state. You note multiple pelvic fractures in your intake history and physical. What would be an appropriate pain regimen for this patient?
   a. Ibuprofen 600 mg every 8 hours scheduled
   b. Oxycodone/acetaminophen 5/325 mg every 4 hours as needed for severe pain
   c. Lidoderm 5% patch once daily
   d. Tylenol 650 mg every 6 hours scheduled

5. You are asked to prescribe a sleep aid for a 67-year-old man who suffered from a left-sided subdural hemorrhage after slipping and falling on ice. Which of the following would be an appropriate medication to consider?
   a. Temazepam 15 mg before bed
   b. Trazodone 25 mg before bed
   c. Clonidine 0.2 mg before bed
   d. Diphenhydramine 25 mg before bed

ADDITIONAL READING

CHEST—recommendations for DVT prophylaxis: http://www.chestnet.org/Guidelines-and-Resources/Guidelines-and-Consensus-Statements/Antithrombotic-Guidelines-9th-Ed

Brain injury rehabilitation outcomes: https://www.biausa.org/wp-content/uploads/PA.Media-2015-Brain-Injury-Outcomes.pdf

Wortzel HS, Silver JM. Behavioral dyscontrol. In: Silver JM, McAllister TW, Yudofsky, eds. *Textbook of Traumatic Brain Injury*. 3rd ed. American Psychiatric Association Publishing; 2019:395–413.

Mackay LE, Bernstein BA, Chapman P, et al. Early intervention in severe head injury: long-term benefits of a formalized program. *Arch Phys Med Rehabil*. 1992;73:635–641.

Yablon SA, Rock WA, Jr, Nick TG, et al. Deep vein thrombosis: prevalence and risk factors in rehabilitation admissions with brain injury. *Neurology*. 2004;63:485–491. doi:10.1212/01.WNL.0000133009.24727.9F

ANSWERS TO STUDY QUESTIONS

1. Correct Answer: d
   When assessing vomiting in the setting of traumatic brain injury, one should also assess for constipation. If the patient is on opiates, consider tapering off to minimize opiate-induced constipation. Residual feeds will need to be monitored. Promotility agents

such as erythromycin can be used. Metoclopramide as a dopamine antagonist is not ideal as it could theoretically delay motor recovery or prolong posttraumatic confusion.

Further Reading:
Krakau K, Omne-Pontén M, Karlsson T, Borg J. Metabolism and nutrition in patients with moderate and severe traumatic brain injury: a systematic review. *Brain Inj.* 2006;20(4):345–367. doi:10.1080/02699050500487571
Chiang YH, Chao DP, Chu SF. Early enteral nutrition and clinical outcomes of severe traumatic brain injury patients in the acute stage: a multi-center cohort study. *J Neurotrauma.* 2012;29(1): 75–80. doi:10.1089/neu.2011.1801

2. Correct Answer: d
Answer choices (a), (b), and (c) pertain to syndrome of inappropriate antidiuretic hormone (SIADH). The patient in this scenario suffers from diabetes insipidus which is treated by increasing fluid intake and with vasopressin in severe cases. Neurogenic diabetes insipidus is associated with basilar skull fractures.

Further Reading:
Greenwald BD, Park MJ, Levine JM, Watanabe TK. The utility of routine screening for deep vein thrombosis upon admission to an inpatient brain injury rehabilitation unit. *PMR.* 2013;5(4):340–347. doi:10.1016/j.pmrj.2013.03.006

3. Correct Answer: c
Fluoxetine, a selective serotonin reuptake inhibitor, would be preferred in cases of emotional lability. Quetiapine, an atypical antipsychotic, may be of benefit to manage psychotic characteristics. Trazodone may help to promote length of sleep. Propranolol, a beta blocker, may be used in this case to treat the patient's restlessness. As a lipophilic drug, it can pass through the blood–brain barrier and also manage the patient's tachycardia. Care must be taken to monitor the patient's vitals upon initiation.

Further Reading:
Zheng R-Z, Lei Z-Q, Yang R-Z, et al. Identification and management of paroxysmal sympathetic hyperactivity after traumatic brain injury. *Front Neurol.* 2020;11:81. doi:10.3389/fneur.2020.00081
Tateno A, Jorge RE, Robinson RG. Clinical correlates of aggressive behavior after traumatic brain injury. *J Neuropsychiatry Clin Neurosci.* 2003;15(2):155–160. doi:10.1176/jnp.15.2.155

4. Correct Answer: d
It may be prudent to avoid nonsteroidal antiinflammatory medications due to the recent hemorrhage. Opiate pain medications may have a negative impact on arousal and cognition. Lidoderm patches are best used for localized pain. A scheduled nonsedating pain reliever such as acetaminophen may be a good first step in his pain regimen. Scheduled medications would be indicated in a patient with impaired communication ability.

Further Reading:
Wortzel HS, Silver JM. Behavioral dyscontrol. In: Silver JM, McAllister TW, Yudofsky, eds. *Textbook of Traumatic Brain Injury.* 3rd ed. American Psychiatric Association Publishing; 2019:395–413.

5. Correct Answer: b
Benzodiazepines such as temazepam can cause cognitive slowing. Clonidine is a centrally acting alpha-2 agonist which is associated with sedation. Diphenhydramine can also interfere with cognitive recovery. Out of the listed options, trazodone has a relatively safe side effect profile in comparison with the rest of the medications.

Further Reading:
Williamson D, Frenette AJ, Burry LD, et al. Pharmacological interventions for agitated behaviours in patients with traumatic brain injury: a systematic review. *BMJ Open*. 2019;9:e029604. doi:10.1136/bmjopen-2019-029604

REFERENCES

The full reference list appears in the digital product found on http://connect.springer-pub.com/content/book/978-0-8261-4768-4/part/part03/chapter/ch27

DISORDERS OF CONSCIOUSNESS

BRIAN D. GREENWALD AND MATTHEW D. MOORE

BACKGROUND AND GENERAL PRINCIPLES

Definition

States of altered consciousness, referred to as disorders of consciousness (DOC), can be categorized as follows: coma, vegetative state (VS; also referred to as unresponsive wakefulness syndrome [UWS]), and minimally conscious state (MCS). This classification is based on published DOC guidelines.[1]

Pathophysiology

The etiology of DOC can be broadly categorized into traumatic versus nontraumatic brain injuries. Coma results from severe diffuse dysfunction of cerebral cortices, underlying white matter, or brainstem structures. The most common acute causes of VS are traumatic brain injury (TBI) and hypoxic-ischemic encephalopathy. After an initial severe TBI, a patient may enter the comatose stage, which can last from several days to weeks. Thereafter, the brainstem and lower diencephalon resume function and the patient transitions into the VS. In a minority of patients, the VS occurs immediately after the insult, without an initial period of coma. The two most common neuropathological changes noted in patients in VS are diffuse laminar cortical necrosis and diffuse axonal injury (DAI).

Differential Diagnosis

Other causes of altered mental status—including subclinical seizures; toxic, metabolic, and infectious encephalopathies; and structural changes such as hydrocephalus—should be considered and ruled out.

Evaluation of the Patient

A thorough bedside neurological examination should be performed to evaluate a patient with altered consciousness. The examination must be repeated to avoid misdiagnosis. The neurological examination should evaluate the integrity of the brainstem and presence of higher cortical functions. Findings on physical exam should be correlated with radiological findings.

The full reference list appears in the digital product found on http://connect.springerpub.com/content/book/978-0-8261-4768-4/part/part03/chapter/ch28

SPECIFIC STATES OF ALTERED CONSCIOUSNESS

Coma

Coma is a state of pathological unconsciousness in which the eyes remain closed and the patient cannot be aroused. The defining feature is absence of sleep–wake cycles.

Evaluation

- Glasgow Coma Scale (GCS)—Measures the best eye, motor, and verbal responses, and is a widely used and accepted severity score for TBI. GCS is commonly administered at initial presentation and in the acute care setting. Higher initial scores tend to predict better recovery.
- JFK Coma Recovery Scale–Revised (CRS–R)—CRS–R is considered the most accurate objective clinical evaluation measure of DOC.[2] CRS–R was developed to help characterize and monitor patients with DOC, and has been used widely in both clinical and research settings within the United States and Europe. The CRS–R assesses auditory, visual, verbal, and motor functions as well as communication and arousal level.

Vegetative State/Unresponsive Wakefulness Syndrome

VS/UWS is characterized by the absence of behavioral evidence of awareness of self or the environment in the context of evidence of functional restoration of the reticular activating system (e.g., eye opening or wakefulness).

Evaluation

This diagnosis is made when there is no evidence of sustained or reproducible purposeful behavioral response to visual, auditory, tactile, or noxious stimuli, and no evidence of language comprehension or expression. VS is usually preceded by a period of coma.[3]

Prognosis for Emergence From VS/UWS

Published guidelines suggest using the term "chronic VS" rather than "permanent VS" to describe patients with VS of duration greater than 3 months in nontraumatic injury and 12 months in traumatic injury. The term "permanent" is not justified as it implies irreversibility. Chronic VS should be further characterized based on length of time since onset.[4]

- Prognosis—Better prognosis is associated with disability rating scale (DRS) scores of <26 at 2 to 3 months post injury.[1] For posttraumatic VS, cumulative recovery of consciousness is 38%, 67%, and 78% at 3, 6, and 12 months, respectively.[1] In contrast, for nontraumatic VS, recovery of consciousness at 6 months is 17%.[1] Nontraumatic VSS lasting for more than 6 months is associated with only a 7.5% recovery of consciousness at 24 months.[1]
- Outcomes—Clinicians must avoid statements that suggest patients have a universally poor prognosis during the first 28 days post injury.[4] Studies have shown substantial recovery in DOC patients admitted to acute inpatient rehabilitation.[5] For example, in one study, of the patients admitted to rehabilitation after TBI who were unable to follow commands, two thirds regained command-following abilities and one fourth emerged from posttraumatic amnesia (PTA) by time of discharge.[5] Approximately 20% of participants were found to be capable of living without in-house supervision and 19% demonstrated employment potential in a long-term follow-up study.[5] More broadly, significant recovery may be seen during the first 2 years post-injury and modest recovery may continue to be observed between years 2 and 5 post injury.[5]
- Neuroimaging—Functional neuroimaging studies suggest conscious awareness in some patients with DOC. Activation studies have the potential to demonstrate distinct and

specific physiological responses to environmental stimuli, such as changes in regional blood flow or changes in regional cerebral hemodynamics.[6,7] For example, one study assessed subjects in VS and MCS[8]: 22 subjects were enrolled, 10 in VS and 12 in MCS. Participants performed a mental imagery functional magnetic resonance imaging (fMRI) paradigm in which they were asked to alternatively imagine playing tennis and navigating through their homes. In 14 of the 22 examined subjects (VS, $n = 5$; MCS, $n = 9$), a significant activation of the regions of interest (ROIs) of the mental imagery paradigm could be found. All five subjects with significant activation in ROIs who were in a VS at the time of the fMRI examination reached at least a MCS at the end of the observation period. In contrast, five participants in a VS who failed to show activation in ROIs, did not. Six of nine subjects in an MCS with activation in ROIs emerged from an MCS. Note that imagery fMRI has not been adequately studied at this point to be used as a clinically valid prognostic tool.

Minimally Conscious State

MCS is a condition of severely altered consciousness in which minimal but definite behavioral evidence of self or environmental awareness is demonstrated. In MCS, cognitively mediated behavior occurs inconsistently, but is reproducible or sustained long enough to be differentiated from reflexive behavior. A patient must demonstrate awareness of self and environment on a sustained basis by one or more of the following: simple command following, gestural or verbal yes/no responses, intelligible verbalization, or purposeful behavior.[9]

Emergence From Minimally Conscious State

Emergence from MCS to a higher state of consciousness is characterized by *reliable and consistent* demonstration of functional interactive communication and/or functional use of two different objects[9] as demonstrated by:

- Functional interactive communication may occur through verbalization, writing, yes/no signals, use of augmentative communication devices, or following commands.
- Functional use of objects requires that the patient demonstrate behavioral evidence of object discrimination; the patient should be able to use two different objects appropriately.[9]
- Two consecutive evaluations demonstrating six out of six correct verbal responses to basic orientation or situational questions, or functional manipulation of two objects (e.g., brush, toothbrush, pen), marks the transition from MCS to recovery of full consciousness.[9]

Avoiding Misdiagnosis

MCS can be differentiated from coma and VS by documenting the presence of specific behavioral features not found in either of these conditions. The distinction is important because overall prognosis for patients in MCS is more favorable than it is for those in VS. Misdiagnosis can be minimized by use of a structured clinical evaluation, performed by a clinician with experience in this field (Table 28.1). In contrast, reliance on nonstandardized protocols and clinician inexperience contribute to a diagnostic error rate of about 40%.[10]

Prognosis for Recovery Following Minimally Conscious State

When comparing patients in MCS to those in VS, functional outcome is better for the group of patients in MCS. Individuals in MCS show more rapid improvement, a longer period of recovery, and significantly less functional disability at 12 months.[11] A study that sought to characterize outcomes of an etiologically heterogeneous population of patients in VS and MCS for greater than 1 year found that 30% of patients in MCS regained consciousness between 1 and 5 years after injury, though all were severely disabled. None of the patients in VS improved during the follow-up period.[12]

TABLE 28.1 Comparison of Clinical Features Associated With Coma, Vegetative State, and Minimally Conscious State

Condition	Consciousness	Sleep/Wake	Motor Function	Auditory Function	Visual Function	Communication	Emotion
Coma	None	Absent	Reflex and postural responses	None	None	None	None
Vegetative state	None	Present	Postures/withdraws to noxious stimuli Nonpurposeful movement	Startle Brief orienting to sound	Startle Brief visual fixation	None	None Reflexive crying or smiling
Minimally conscious state*	Inconsistent	Present	Localizes to noxious stimuli Reaches for objects Holds objects Automatic movements	Localizes to sound Inconsistent command following	Sustained visual fixation and pursuit	Conditional vocalization Inconsistent but intelligible verbalization or gesture	Conditional smiling or crying

*For all clinical features, MCS is characterized by inconsistent responses to stimuli.

Source: Adapted with permission from Giacino JT, Ashwal S, Childs N, et al. The minimally conscious state: definition and diagnostic criteria. *Neurology.* 2002;58(3):349–353. doi:10.1212/WNL.58.3.506

TREATMENT

Pharmacological

The mainstay of pharmacological management in DOC is minimization of use of medication that may exacerbate central nervous system depression or sedation (e.g., opiates, benzodiazepines, beta-blockers, and anticonvulsants). That said, one neurostimulant in particular deserves further mention due to its wide use in TBI and potential benefit in DOC: amantadine.

Amantadine is a tricyclic water-soluble amine salt that affects the synthesis, accumulation, release, and reuptake of catecholamines in the central nervous system. Amantadine has been hypothesized to facilitate brain recovery through effects on dopamine and N-methyl-D-aspartate (NMDA) receptors. Amantadine is thought to increase the availability of dopamine by blocking reuptake and increasing synthesis.[13] It also works postsynaptically by increasing the density of dopamine receptor availability and altering receptor conformation.[13] Amantadine is one of the most commonly prescribed medications for patients with prolonged DOC after TBI. In a randomized, double-blinded, placebo-controlled, multicenter study, amantadine accelerated the pace of functional recovery during active treatment in patients with posttraumatic DOC. In this study, 184 patients who were in either VS or MCS 4 to 16 weeks after TBI were enrolled while in inpatient rehabilitation.[14] Subjects were randomly assigned to receive amantadine or placebo for 4 weeks and were followed for 2 weeks after the treatment was discontinued. The rate of functional recovery on the DRS was compared over the 4 weeks of treatment and during the 2-week washout period. During the 4-week treatment period, recovery was significantly faster in the amantadine group than in the placebo group, as measured by the rate of improvement in the DRS score.

A paradoxical wakening effect has been reported with use of the pharmaceutical *Zolpidem* in patients with DOC. In a placebo-controlled, double-blinded study, 4.8% of participants responded to a single dose of Zolpidem. Further research is needed to explore the mechanism and define a role for this agent in treatment of DOC.[15]

Nonpharmacological

Supportive care is key in the management of DOC. Maintaining skin integrity, preventing or treating infections, assessing or providing for adequate splinting and equipment needs, and educating family or caregivers about the nature of this condition are core components of management for these patients. Programs that provide services to DOC patients should assess cognitive function utilizing standardized instruments/processes to reduce misdiagnosis, monitor rate of functional change, identify and treat comorbidities, prevent complications, and provide caregiver training.[16]

Transcranial direct current stimulation (tDCS) is an experimental technique through which cortical excitability is achieved via passage of direct current between external electrodes.[17] A few studies suggest benefit for MCS patients but not those in a VS.[18–20] This remains an investigative tool at this time.

Deep brain stimulation (DBS) is an invasive implantation of brain electrodes that carry current to a specific area of the brain.[17] No large sham-controlled double-blinded study has been performed looking at the effects of DBS on DOC. One small (three-subject) prospective cohort study showed thalamic stimulation can improve the clinical status of DOC patients. It should be noted that effects of DBS are difficult to distinguish from spontaneous recovery.[21] DBS remains an investigative intervention and not a clinical treatment option at this juncture.

KEY POINTS

■ DOC can be classified into three categories: coma, VS, or MCS.

■ Patients in MCS have better outcomes than patients in VS, and patients in VS or MCS due to TBI have better outcomes than when caused by anoxic brain injury.

■ Amantadine has been shown to hasten functional recovery during inpatient rehabilitation in patients who sustained a TBI and are in either VS or MCS, and its use should be routinely considered in this population.

STUDY QUESTIONS

1. A 45-year-old man presented to the acute care hospital after suffering a TBI. He was in an altered state of consciousness until finally regaining consciousness while in acute rehabilitation. Which of the following is not considered a state of altered consciousness?
   a. Minimally conscious state
   b. Vegetative state
   c. Posttraumatic amnesia
   d. Coma

2. A 63-year-old woman who was found unconscious, with no obvious signs of trauma, was admitted to the acute care hospital. She has no discernable command following or purposeful actions. She is determined to be in a vegetative state. Which of the following terms can be used in place of vegetative state?
   a. Minimally conscious state
   b. Minimally responsive state
   c. Diffuse axonal injury
   d. Unresponsive wakefulness syndrome

3. A 63-year-old woman involved in an automobile accident was found to have multiple areas of subarachnoid hemorrhage, a large right subdural hemorrhage, and midline shift. Her physical exam findings support the diagnosis of coma. Which of the following is true regarding coma?
   a. Sleep–wake cycles are present
   b. The patient cannot be aroused
   c. Prognosis is better than VS
   d. Diffuse axonal injury must be present

4. A 24-year-old man is admitted to acute inpatient rehabilitation after suffering a TBI. He does not open his eyes or follow commands. Which of the following is the most appropriate objective clinical evaluation tool for this patient?
   a. Glasgow Coma Scale
   b. Disability rating scale
   c. Greenwald Consciousness scale
   d. JFK Coma Recovery Scale–Revised

5. A 55-year-old woman admitted to an acute care hospital is in a minimally conscious state. The family agrees to send the patient to acute inpatient rehabilitation. Programs that provide services to DOC patients should be able to do which of the following?
   a. Assess cognitive function utilizing standardized tools and protocols to reduce misdiagnosis
   b. Monitor rate of functional change
   c. Prevent complications
   d. All of the above

ADDITIONAL READING

JFK Coma Recovery Scale. http://www.tbims.org/combi/crs/index.html

Giacino JT, Katz DI, Schiff ND, et al. Comprehensive systematic review update summary: disorders of consciousness: report of the Guideline Development, Dissemination, and Implementation Subcommittee of the American Academy of Neurology; the American Congress of Rehabilitation Medicine; and the National Institute on Disability, Independent Living, and Rehabilitation Research. *Neurology.* 2018;91(10):461–470.

Practice guideline update recommendations summary: disorders of consciousness: report of the Guideline Development, Dissemination, and Implementation Subcommittee of the American Academy of Neurology; the American Congress of Rehabilitation Medicine; and the National Institute on Disability, Independent Living, and Rehabilitation Research. *Neurology.* 2019;93(3):135. doi:10.1212/WNL.0000000000007382

Jennett B, Plum F. Persistent vegetative state after brain damage: a syndrome in search of a name. *Lancet.* 1972;1:734–737. doi:10.1016/S0140-6736(72)90242-5

Jennett B, Teasdale G. Aspects of coma after severe head injury. *Lancet.* 1977;1(8017):878–881. doi:10.1016/S0140-6736(77)91201-6

ANSWERS TO STUDY QUESTIONS

1. Correct Answer: c
   Posttraumatic amnesia refers to memory loss related to TBI. MCS, VS, and coma are the stages of DOC.

   Further Reading:
   Giacino JT, Katz DI, Schiff N. Assessment and rehabilitative management of individuals with disorders of consciousness. In: Zasler ND, Katz DI, Zafonte RD, eds. *Brain Injury Medicine: Principles and Practice*. Demos Medical Publishing; 2013:517–535. doi:10.1891/9781617050572.0032

2. Correct Answer: d
   Unresponsive wakefulness syndrome (UWS) and vegetative state (VS) can be used interchangeably when referring to this patient population.

   Further Reading:
   Giacino JT, Katz DI, Schiff ND, et al. Comprehensive systematic review update summary: Disorders of consciousness: Report of the Guideline Development, Dissemination, and Implementation Subcommittee of the American Academy of Neurology; the American Congress of Rehabilitation Medicine; and the National Institute on Disability, Independent Living, and Rehabilitation Research. *Neurology.* 2018;91(10):461–470. doi:10.1212/WNL.0000000000005928

3. Correct Answer: b

The patient cannot be aroused. Sleep wake cycles are not present in coma. Prognosis is better in VS than coma. DAI in not necessary for the diagnosis of coma.

Further Reading:

Giacino JT, Katz DI, Schiff N. Assessment and rehabilitative management of individuals with disorders of consciousness. In: Zasler ND, Katz DI, Zafonte RD, eds. *Brain Injury Medicine: Principles and Practice*. Demos Medical Publishing; 2013:517–535. doi:10.1891/9781617050572.0032

4. Correct Answer: d

JFK Coma Recovery Scale–Revised is the best objective clinical measure of DOC patients. The GCS is useful for diagnosis and prognosis in the acute care setting. The Disability Rating Scale measures how disabled a patient is after injury. The Greenwald Consciousness Scale does not exist.

Further Reading:

Giacino JT, Kalmar K, Whyte J. The JFK Coma Recovery Scale–Revised: measurement characteristics and diagnostic utility. *Arch Phys Med Rehabil*. 2004;85(12):2020–2029. doi:10.1016/j.apmr.2004.02.033

5. Correct Answer: d

Recent publications recommend that programs that provide services to DOC patients should be able assess cognitive function to reduce misdiagnosis, monitor rate of functional change, identify and treat comorbidities, prevent complications, and provide caregiver training.

Further Reading:

Giacino JT, Whyte J, Nakase-Richardson R, et al. Minimum competency recommendations for programs that provide rehabilitation services for persons with disorders of consciousness: a position statement of the American Congress of Rehabilitation Medicine and the National Institute on Disability, Independent Living and Rehabilitation Research Traumatic Brain Injury Model Systems. *Arch Phys Med Rehabil*. 2020;101(6):1072–1089. doi:10.1016/j.apmr.2020.01.013

REFERENCES

The full reference list appears in the digital product found on http://connect.springer-pub.com/content/book/978-0-8261-4768-4/part/part03/chapter/ch28

29 THE ROLE OF SPECIALIZED BRAIN INJURY UNITS IN THE REHABILITATION PROCESS

BILLIE A. SCHULTZ

BACKGROUND: LONGITUDINAL CARE

- Consensus exists for providing a continuum of care to individuals and their families/ significant others after moderate to severe traumatic brain injury (TBI), from acute hospitalization to outpatient clinical care and community-based services.
- Ideally, inpatient rehabilitation brings into focus the comprehensive rehabilitation plan of care initiated by rehabilitation consultation and services provided during acute hospitalization, medical and surgical treatment, and stabilization.
- Inpatient brain injury rehabilitation provides comprehensive medical rehabilitation services as individuals emerge from trauma-induced alterations of consciousness and families/significant others begin adjusting to these changing circumstances.
- As the link between acute medical care and community-based services, specialized inpatient brain injury rehabilitation units are a crucial source of clinical data to define baseline injury severity, monitor progress, measure outcome and satisfaction, and to use for benchmarking and practice improvement.[1]
- Evidence exists showing that early rehabilitation intervention during the acute care stay can improve outcomes including rehabilitation length of stay.[2,3]

PRACTICE MODELS

Centralized Brain Injury Units

- Geographically smaller countries with nationalized health care, and states in the United States with single urban medical centers and large rural populations, often have trauma systems that direct individuals who experience catastrophic and polytraumatic injuries to designated accredited trauma centers for definitive care with treatment directed by consensus guidelines.[3,4]
- Regional brain injury rehabilitation hospital care, driven by a team-based model and treatment guidelines, has been shown to be associated with better outcomes after severe TBI when compared to historical controls.[5,6]
- A model of care that provides acute and rehabilitation services in a single location from admission to the acute hospital through discharge after rehabilitation is uncommon in the United States, and not as developed in Europe for TBI as it is for stroke.[7]

The full reference list appears in the digital product found on http://connect.springerpub.com/ content/book/978-0-8261-4768-4/part/part03/chapter/ch29

■ Whether care is provided in a rehabilitation hospital or a rehabilitation unit within an acute care hospital, effective communication between provider teams by handoff at care transitions is crucial to maintain continuity and minimize safety risks.[8]

Brain Injury Services in Rehabilitation Units

■ Most brain rehabilitation units in the United States exist either within acute hospitals or as freestanding rehabilitation hospitals.

■ Clinical services: Consensus exists about what clinical services should be provided during inpatient rehabilitation for TBI.[9]

● Rehabilitation services should be customized to individual needs and refined with clinical change.

● Services should be comprehensive and interdisciplinary.

● Cognitive and behavioral assessment should be included.

● Evaluation of and treatment for substance abuse should be a component of these rehabilitation programs.

● Persons with TBI, and their families/significant others should be involved in the rehabilitation process. Families and significant others should also be supported through the rehabilitation process.

● The use of medications for behavioral management and cognitive enhancement should be carefully considered.

● Specialized programming is necessary for individuals in pediatric and geriatric populations with TBI.

■ Admission guidelines: Many rehabilitation units in the United States use admission guidelines as set forth by the Centers for Medicare & Medicaid Services, although these guidelines may not apply to individuals not covered by government-funded health care.

● An individual should be able and willing to actively participate in an intensive rehabilitation program (recommended intensity and duration: 3 hours of daily therapy services, 5 out of each 7 days with the exception of carefully selected cases for which 15 hours of therapy over the course of a single week may be an appropriate alternative), and should be expected to make measurable improvement in functional capacity or adaptation to impairments within a reasonable period of time.

● Rehabilitation services should be ordered and coordinated by a rehabilitation physician with specialized training and experience in rehabilitation services and be administered by an interdisciplinary team.

● Specialized rehabilitation physician and nursing care is needed.

● Rehabilitation care should be provided by qualified personnel in rehabilitation nursing, physical therapy, occupational therapy, speech-language pathology, social services, psychological services, and prosthetic and orthotic services.

● Appropriate care cannot be provided in a less intensive medical setting, such as in a skilled care environment.

■ Rehabilitation treatment for individuals in coma or a minimally conscious state

● Rehabilitation care for individuals who remain in coma or who are minimally conscious after reaching medical stability is provided in specialized hospital-based rehabilitation settings, long-term acute care facilities, or in a skilled care environment.

● Treatment approaches are generally grouped into three types: sensory stimulation, physical management, and neuromodulation.[10]

- Variations in determining level of consciousness, small sample sizes, and poor study design have limited the application of existing research to develop clinical assessment and treatment guidelines.
- Effectiveness of treatment is monitored using common outcome tools.[11]
- Many interventions have shown some positive effects on increasing arousal, but more methodologically rigorous study has been recommended.[12] However, the use of amantadine has been shown to accelerate the rate of functional recovery in individuals who experienced trauma-related disorders of consciousness when compared to placebo, without difference in long-term outcomes.[13,14]
- Rehabilitation after TBI and polytrauma in the military (see also Chapters 66 and 67)
  - The Polytrauma System of Care is an integrated system of specialized care created by the Department of Veterans Affairs to manage patients with brain injury throughout all aspects of the rehabilitative process.[15]
  - It serves veterans and active duty service members who have TBI and polytrauma injuries through regional centers around the United States. Through the system, polytrauma is defined as "two or more injuries to physical regions or organ systems, one of which may be life-threatening, resulting in physical, cognitive, psychological, or psychosocial impairments and functional disability."[15]
  - Clinical trials in these centers have shown differential positive effects in subpopulations for cognitive and functional treatment approaches.[16]
  - To further advance research, the Department of Veterans Affairs polytrauma system of care has partnered with the National Institute on Disability and Rehabilitation research to establish a longitudinal data system similar to the TBI model system national database in the civilian world.[17]

BRAIN INJURY TREATMENT EFFECTIVENESS

- In an evidence-based review of randomized controlled trials, quasi-randomized and quasi-experimental designs—comparing multidisciplinary rehabilitation with either routinely available local services or lower levels of intervention; or trials comparing an intervention in different settings or at different levels of intensity—it was found that:[18]
  - For moderate to severe injury, there was "strong evidence" of benefit from formal intervention.
  - For patients with moderate to severe TBI already in rehabilitation, there was "strong evidence" that more intensive programs are associated with earlier functional gains.
  - There was "limited evidence" that specialized inpatient brain injury rehabilitation units may provide additional functional gains.
- In an assimilation of randomized controlled trials in the literature and a review of TBI rehabilitation trials chosen based on evaluation of research quality irrespective of study design, it was found that:[19]
  - Early intensive rehabilitation is recommended.
  - Specialized brain injury programs are recommended for individuals with complex needs.
  - Vocational programs are recommended for individuals with this potential.
- Further research is needed, and priorities have been defined, to further characterize the roles of cognitive rehabilitation and vocational programs.[20]

BRAIN INJURY REHABILITATION DATABASES

■ A national consortium of 16 academic rehabilitation research centers, the Traumatic Brain Injury Model System Centers (funded by the National Institute on Disability, Independent Living and Rehabilitation Research) has contributed data about individuals admitted to specialized brain injury inpatient rehabilitation units to a common database since 1989.
  • Data from acute care and inpatient rehabilitation are submitted, and outcome data are collected from subjects at 1, 2, and 5 years after injury and every 5 years thereafter.
  • This database is used for longitudinal analysis of data from people with TBI and supports research toward developing evidence-based TBI rehabilitation interventions.[21]
■ Other proprietary data sources (such as eRehabData.com and the Uniform Data System for Medical Rehabilitation) allow inpatient brain injury rehabilitation programs to monitor clinical metrics and outcomes for benchmarking and to support practice improvement.[22]
■ Uniform data collection methods are needed to allow comparison between studies. Much of the current body of published research is heterogeneous in metrics and outcomes. To develop more consistency, the National Institutes of Health (NIH) has developed recommendations for collection of standardized outcomes and demographics.[23,24]

KEY POINTS

■ Coordinated TBI care throughout the continuum of care including early rehabilitation intervention is recommended.
■ Clinical consensus for elements of TBI care in the inpatient rehabilitation setting exist and should be followed.
■ Future research should focus on use of consistent defined demographic/population data sets and outcomes.

STUDY QUESTIONS

1. Early rehabilitation intervention following traumatic brain injury contributes to:
   a. Improved functional outcomes at 12 months post injury
   b. Decreased pain
   c. Increased mortality
   d. Increased acute care length of stay

2. Which statement is true regarding use of amantadine following brain injury?
   a. Use of amantadine is correlated with improved outcomes in the acute and subacute periods
   b. Use of amantadine shows benefit in the acute recovery phase, but no change in subacute outcomes

    c. Use of amantadine shows no benefit in outcomes at any time after brain injury
    d. Use of amantadine slows brain injury recovery

3. Barriers to traumatic brain injury research:
    a. Do not exist
    b. Are primarily financial
    c. Are due to a small subject population
    d. Are due to a heterogeneous subject population and outcome measures

4. Consensus recommendations for acute inpatient rehabilitation do NOT include:
    a. Individualize rehabilitation plans
    b. Delay evaluation of and treatment of substance abuse until outpatient
    c. Carefully consider use of medications for agitation and inattention
    d. Involve family throughout the rehabilitation process

5. Treatment approaches to persons with disorders of consciousness include all of the following EXCEPT:
    a. Sensory stimulation
    b. Physical management
    c. Aggressive management of pain with narcotics
    d. Neuromodulation

ADDITIONAL READING

Model Systems Knowledge Translation Center. http://msktc.washington.edu/
The TBI Model System National Data and Statistical Center at Craig Hospital. http://www.tbindsc.org
Ivanhoe CB, Durand-Sanchez A, Spier ET. Acute rehabilitation. In: Zasler ND, Katz DI, Zafonte RD, eds. *Brain Injury Medicine: Principles and Practice.* Demos; 2013:385–405. doi:10.1891/9781617050572.0026
Prvu Bettger JA, Stineman MG. Effectiveness of multidisciplinary rehabilitation services in postacute care: state-of-the-science. A review. *Arch Phys Med Rehabil.* 2007;88(11):1526–1534. doi:10.1016/j.apmr.2007.06.768

ANSWERS TO STUDY QUESTIONS

1. Correct Answer: a
Research shows improved functional outcomes and decreased acute care length of stay with early rehabilitation intervention. No current research exists linking pain or mortality to early rehabilitation interventions after brain injury.

Further Reading:
Wagner AK, Fabio T, Zafonte RD, et al. Physical medicine and rehabilitation consultation: relationships with acute functional outcome, length of stay, and discharge planning after traumatic brain injury. *Am J Phys Med Rehabil.* 2003;82:526–536. doi:10.1097/00002060-200307000-00006 , doi:10.1097/01.PHM.0000073825.09942.8F

2. Correct Answer: b
Research has shown an increased rate of recovery in the acute stage; however, outcomes in the subacute stage are equivalent to no amantadine use. There is no current evidence that brain injury recovery is slowed with use of amantadine.

Further Reading:
Giacino JT, Whyte J, Bagiella E, et al. Placebo-controlled trial of amantadine for severe traumatic brain injury. *N Engl J Med*. 2012;366(9):819–826. doi:10.1056/NEJMoa1102609
Ghalaenovi H, Fattahi A, Koohpayehzadeh J, et al. The effects of amantadine on traumatic brain injury outcome: a double-blind, randomized, controlled, clinical trial. *Brain Inj*. 2018;32(8):1050-1055. doi:10.1080/02699052.2018.1476733

3. Correct Answer: d
It is well established that barriers exist to quality research about TBI outcomes despite a large sample size and reasonable financial resources. Barriers have included the heterogeneity of persons with brain injury but also a lack of consistency on best demographics and outcomes to assess. Thus the NIH has started work on Common Data Elements to homogenize research.

Further Reading:
Roe C, Tverdal C, Howe EI, et al. Randomized controlled trials of rehabilitation services in the post-acute phase of moderate and severe traumatic brain injury—a systematic review. *Front Neurol*. 2019;10:557. doi:10.3389/fneur.2019.00557

4. Correct Answer: b
According to recommendations made by the Consensus Conference for rehabilitation care patients following traumatic brain injury, published in 1999, rehabilitation services should be individualized, comprehensive, interdisciplinary, and inclusive of family members. Cognitive and behavioral assessments as well as evaluation of and treatment for substance abuse should also be components of these rehabilitation programs. Use of medications for behavioral management and/or cognitive enhancement should also be carefully considered.

Further Reading:
Brain Trauma Foundation; American Association of Neurological Surgeons; Congress of Neurological Surgeons. Guidelines for the management of severe traumatic brain injury. *J Neurotrauma*. 2007;24(S1):S1–S106.

5. Correct Answer: c
Recommendations include all of the above except aggressive management of pain with narcotic pain medication as this could have a negative impact on recovery.

Further Reading:
Giacino JT, Katz DI, Garber K, et al. Assessment and rehabilitative management of individuals with disorders of consciousness. In: Zasler ND, Katz DI, Zafonte RD, eds. *Brain Injury Medicine: Principles and Practice*. New York: Demos; 2013:517–535. doi:10.1891/9781617050572.0032

REFERENCES

The full reference list appears in the digital product found on http://connect.springer-pub.com/content/book/978-0-8261-4768-4/part/part03/chapter/ch29

REHABILITATION NURSING

ANN S. BINES AND LINDSAY HONG

DEFINITION

Rehabilitation nursing is a specialty that focuses on the diagnosis and treatment of individuals and/or groups relative to altered functional ability and lifestyle.[1] The goal of rehabilitation nursing is to assist individuals with disability and/or chronic illness in restoring, maintaining, and promoting maximal health.

- Major areas of focus with the inpatient traumatic brain injury (TBI) population:
  - Pain assessment and treatment
  - Maintenance/assessment of skin integrity
  - Promotion of a physiological sleep–wake pattern
  - Promotion of continence of bowel and bladder
  - Prevention of aspiration and promotion of oral health
  - Assessment/management of behavioral impairments
  - Providing for safety/promoting independence/restraint reduction
  - Promoting advocacy through education
  - Providing emotional/psychosocial support
  - Preparing and training family for a safe discharge

PAIN ASSESSMENT AND TREATMENT

- Incidence of pain in this patient population is significant.
  - Etiology is variable. In the acute-care phase, pain may be caused by fractures, intra-abdominal injuries, soft tissue injuries, and/or associated with invasive procedures. In the chronic stage, pain may be due to spasticity, hypertonicity, contractures, pressure sores, soft tissue injuries, peripheral nerve injuries, or headache. Assessment is inherently difficult in this patient population as a result of cognitive/communication and/or behavioral challenges. Few conventional tools have been validated in the cognitively impaired TBI population. Pain assessment in patients who cannot reliably verbalize their pain should include subjective assessment of pain behaviors.[2,3]
  - It is important to note that behaviors such as agitation and vocalizations may be due to something other than pain in the setting of TBI.[4]
  - Cognitive impairment does not exclude a patient from use of a self-report tool. When possible, this should be attempted first, and escalated to an observational tool if necessary.
  - Change in vital signs is not the best indicator of pain in this population, as this can also be due to dysautonomia, infection, or other comorbid conditions.[5]

The full reference list appears in the digital product found on http://connect.springerpub.com/content/book/978-0-8261-4768-4/part/part03/chapter/ch30

- Validated tools (primarily validated in elderly patients with dementia) include:
  - *Checklist of Nonverbal Pain Indicators*: scoring of six behaviors—vocalization, grimaces, bracing, rubbing, restlessness, and verbal complaints.[6]
  - *Critical Care Pain Observation Tool*: facial expression, body movements, muscle tension, vocalization, or compliance with ventilator.[7]
  - *Face, Legs, Activity, Cry, Consolability Scale*: facial expression, leg movement, body activity, cry/vocalization, and consolability.[8]
  - *Nociception Coma Scale (NCS)*: Was recently validated in patients with disorders of consciousness (minimally conscious state / vegetative state). This scale includes the observation of motor, verbal, and visual responses as well as facial expression. The total score varies from 0 to 12.[9]
- Treatment
  - Use multimodal therapy to provide pain relief while limiting drug side effects, thereby minimizing their effects on cognitive recovery.
  - Nonpharmacological therapies include heat, cold, repositioning, diversion, relaxation techniques, acupuncture, massage, and behavioral management. Maximize use of these modalities.[10]
  - Use analgesics for analgesia, not to control behavior. Taper or discontinue drugs that are not effective.
  - Consistency of caregivers (nurses, unlicensed personnel, and family) is very beneficial in identification of signs of pain in cognitively impaired patients.

ASSESSMENT AND PREVENTION OF SKIN BREAKDOWN

Assessment

- According to the Agency for Healthcare Research & Quality (AHRQ), pressure ulcers cost the U.S. healthcare system an estimated $9.1 to $11.6 billion annually.[11] Acquired pressure injuries may result in longer hospital stays and increased morbidity and mortality.[12]
- The brain-injured population is at high risk for development of pressure ulcers. Risk factors include decreased sensation/movement, agitation/nonpurposeful movement (e.g., spasticity/dystonia), nutritional impairment, and incontinence.
- Extrinsic factors causing pressure ulcers include pressure, shear, friction, moisture, and equipment/orthotics/positioning devices.
- Most frequently used risk assessment tools are the Braden and Norton scales. Risk for skin breakdown should be initially assessed on admission and then on a routine frequency; minimum once daily.
  - *Norton*: Five parameters are scored/assessed: physical condition, mental state, activity, mobility, and incontinence. Lower scores indicate high risk. Risk onset begins at 12 or less.
  - *Braden*: Six parameters are scored/assessed: sensory perception, skin moisture, physical activity, nutritional status, friction/shear, and ability to change body position. Lower scores indicate high risk. Risk onset begins at 16 or less.[13]

Interventions

- Pressure ulcer prevention, or prompt treatment if identified, is crucial for improved patient outcomes and reduced healthcare costs.
- Early identification: Inspect skin for areas of redness at least once daily, more frequently for high-risk patients and with the use of new devices

▨ Reduce/limit moisture: Establish a program to enhance continence. Use pH-balanced soaps/cleansers. Use moisture barrier as needed to prevent skin breakdown. Leave perineal areas open to air when in bed.[14]

▨ Optimize nutrition/hydration: Calorie counts, mineral/vitamin/protein supplements.[14]

▨ Shear/friction prevention: Use of lifting aids/equipment when repositioning. Raise knee gatch of bed when the head of the bed is elevated to decrease shear/friction forces from additional sliding.[14]

▨ Pressure relief aids: Bed surfaces, chair cushions, adequate padding of orthotics, and padding of rigid surfaces in bed and wheelchair. Specialized chairs such as tilt-in-space chairs also relieve pressure in immobilized patients.

▨ Repositioning/pressure relief programs: Establish an individualized turning program when patient is in bed, use of log to track. Prone positioning, when appropriate, can be very useful to off-load pressure points when patient is in bed. The use of timers with an alarm can be used to establish a repositioning program for wheelchair-bound patients who cannot weight shift independently to off-load bony prominences (due to immobility or cognitive impairments). The timers can be placed on wheelchair. Timer set for 20 to 30 minutes based on patient need for repositioning. When timer alarms, it signals patient/caregivers to reposition in chair.

▨ Pressure mapping: A computerized clinical tool that involves using sensors to assess pressure distribution between two contacting objects, such as a person and their support surface. It is commonly used by clinicians to determine the suitability of a wheelchair cushion or other support surfaces, and optimal positioning (when sitting or lying) to off-load pressure.[15,16]

PROMOTION OF SLEEP–WAKE PATTERN

▨ Sleep disturbances are common following a TBI, including complications such as insomnia, excessive daytime sleepiness and fatigue.[17]

▨ Assessment: A log maintained by caregivers is a common method of recording sleep patterns due to limited ability of patients to self-report. Document sleep onset and duration of sleep periods. Include patient/family assessment of quality of sleep. Actigraphs provide another means of assessing sleep duration.[18]

▨ Interventions
  ● Promote sleep hygiene through the following non-pharmacological means:
    ■ Control environmental factors such as noise, light, and temperature.
    ■ Employ sleep aids such as music, evening showers, soothing scents, or TV (may assist with promoting onset of sleep, not to be left on after sleep is established).[19]
    ■ Establish a "bedtime routine;" this can be advantageous in promoting sleep onset. Waking at the same time daily can also help to restore consistent sleep patterns.
    ■ Limit time in bed during the day, and at night if unable to sleep.
    ■ Avoid use of phones, tablets, and other electronic devices in bed and when preparing for sleep.
    ■ Be aware of patient's preinjury sleep behavior—hours of sleep per night, bedtime, and usual time of awakening and shift work. Do not force sleep.
    ■ Schedule nursing care so as not to interfere with sleep.
  ● Use of pharmacological agents. Timing of administration is important. Medications should be given early enough to enhance sleep but not affect ability to actively participate in therapy. Use sleep aids to promote sleep—not to control behavior.
  ● Regulation of the patient's sleep–wake cycle has been shown to have a positive impact on agitation, length of time in posttraumatic amnesia and other negative

behaviors. (See Chapter 54 for a more detailed discussion of management of insomnia in TBI.)

CONTINENCE OF BOWEL AND BLADDER

Continence is a major area of nursing focus. Continence is also a primary goal for families/caregivers. Incontinence may present a burden of care that prevents home discharge. Incontinence can also increase agitation in TBI patients.

- Bladder incontinence
  - *Causes*:
    - Incontinence is most often due to uninhibited neurogenic bladder. Signs and symptoms include reduced bladder capacity, frequency/urgency, nocturia, and voiding as soon as urge is perceived. Sensation and the bulbocavernosus and micturition reflex arcs are intact. The bladder empties completely.[20]
    - Transient, acute functional incontinence, often of precipitous onset, is typically reversible. It is related to impaired physical/cognitive/communication/behavioral function.
  - *Assessment*: Monitor post void residual; review medications, consider age, presence of premorbid incontinence issues, and urinary tract infection.
  - *Interventions to reestablish continence:*
    - Prior to initiating any program, assess patient's behavior, core strength, balance, and level of assistance with transfers. Continence can be achieved using bedpans, urinals, commodes, or condom catheters. Consistency of caregiver adherence to the continence program is very important. Regulate fluid intake. Ensure privacy. Provide positive reinforcement.[21]
    - *Scheduled/timed voids:* Assess patient's voiding patterns and replicate (usually every 2–4 hours). Patients are often unaware of the need/urge to void.
    - *Prompted voiding:* It is useful when the patient recognizes the need/urge to void. It requires intense caregiver intervention. There are three steps to the program: (a) monitor the patient for incontinence at regular, pre-established intervals, (b) prompt the patient to toilet if dry, and (c) provide positive reinforcement for successful toileting.
- Bowel incontinence
  - *Cause*: Uninhibited neurogenic bowel: reflexes, spinal reflex arc, and bowel and saddle sensation are typically intact. Decreased awareness of the need to defecate and decreased control of external sphincter result in inability to inhibit defecation. May have a sense of urgency (perceived).[21]
  - *Assessment:* Consider preinjury bowel habits. Identify date of last bowel movement. Review current diet, hydration status.
  - *Interventions to promote bowel continence:* Assess the patient's ability to transfer to/use the toilet. Be consistent in administering a bowel program. Promote an upright sitting position, with knees bent for defecation. Avoid use of a bedpan; utilize shower or toileting chair. Consider an abdominal binder to increase abdominal pressure. Ensure adequate hydration/fiber intake. Initiate program after food intake to activate gastrocolic reflex. Plan bowel program so as not to interfere with participation in therapy. Provide privacy.[21]
  - *Medications may include:*
    - Stool softeners (scheduled, not as needed) with or without a laxative component

- Bulk products
- Suppositories to stimulate the defecation reflex

BEHAVIOR MANAGEMENT

- Behavior dysfunction is directly related to injury in various regions of the brain, resulting in issues such as emotional lability, lack of initiation, poor insight into deficits, and low frustration tolerance.
- Management of negative behaviors exhibited during the acute recovery period post-TBI is one of the most challenging aspects of providing nursing care to this population.
- One such behavior is agitation, which is seen in up to 70% of rehabilitation TBI patients, and is defined as a heightened state of activity in which a patient is no longer capable of effectively processing information and responding in an appropriate way.[22,23]
- *Assessment:* Use of consistent tool(s) to assess behaviors and an understanding of the nature of the behavior by the entire team is important. The Agitated Behavior Scale (ABS) is one such assessment tool. This tool assesses the degree to which the behavior interferes with functional activities and the degree to which the behavior can be inhibited. It assesses 14 behaviors, characterizing presence and severity. Total score correlates with the severity of agitation. Subscores can be calculated, identifying correlated factors: aggression, lability, and disinhibition.[24]
- *Interventions:*
  - The success of interventions (medications, behavior management plans) in lessening the agitation can be assessed using the ABS.[25] Frequent, thorough assessment and documentation, regardless of the assessment tool utilized, are essential to track changes in behaviors.
  - Document behaviors, factors that provoke undesirable behaviors, and response to interventions. Medications should be used in conjunction with a consistent approach to management of adverse behaviors.
  - Staff training in early identification and de-escalation of behaviors facilitates maintaining a safe environment for the patient and staff. Certification of staff in nonviolent crisis intervention techniques can reduce staff and patient injuries, reduce staff fear/hesitation in caring for patients, and instill confidence. (See Chapter 36 for a more detailed discussion of behavior management.)

PROVIDING FOR SAFETY/PROMOTING INDEPENDENCE/ RESTRAINT REDUCTION

- Safety is an important area of focus for the rehabilitation nurse. Falls are a main concern in the rehabilitation setting, especially among patients with cognitive impairment[26]; therefore, clinicians must balance the risk against the benefits of encouraging patient autonomy.
- Any manual method, physical or mechanical device, material, or equipment that immobilizes or reduces the ability of a patient to move their arms, legs, body, or head freely is considered a restraint. Medications can also be considered a form of restraint.

■ The Joint Commission and other regulating bodies have developed standards for the use of restraints. The overriding premise is to reduce/limit the use of restraints. Institutions must have policies which govern the use of restraints. The policies should define what types of restraints can be used, who can apply restraints, how often the patient must be assessed while in a restraint and by whom, the time frame within which an order for restraint must be written, and how often the order must be renewed. There are specific criteria that define why a restraint can be used, and these criteria must be documented and consistent among the caregivers. Also required is documentation of alternatives tried prior to initiating a restraint. The standards also speak to the patient/ family education that must be provided when restraints are used. It is imperative that clinicians consider alternatives to restraints and reassess the need for the restraint often; restraints, regardless of the type, should generally not be the first intervention implemented.

Restraint orders cannot be written as "prn" or standing orders.[27]

■ Common restraints include limb restraints, side rails (not when used to facilitate repositioning in bed by patient), mittens, wrap-around seat belts (any belt that cannot be easily removed by the patient), and bed enclosures.
■ It is important to note that restraints have not been proven to decrease falls and have been implicated in increasing injuries associated with falls.[28]
■ An alternative approach is to use devices that do not restrict movement but either alert staff to egress or "slow down" a patient's ability to engage in an unsafe behavior. Examples of restraint alternatives include bed exit alarm systems, wheelchair alarm systems ("talking" seat belts), abdominal binders, wheelchair lap trays, upper limb orthotic devices for functional positioning, Velcro straps for positioning in wheel chairs, video observation areas/rooms, and 1:1 caregivers/sitters.[29]
■ Most institutions have Continuous Quality Improvement programs that monitor fall rates and restraint usage. At minimum, daily assessment should be made by the entire team of the need to continue use of restraints. Interventions that can be used as alternatives to restraints, to maintain patient safety, should be explored.

KEY POINTS

Pressure Ulcer Prevention

■ The Centers for Medicare & Medicaid Services guidelines have increased the requirements for reporting acquired pressure ulcers.
■ Thorough initial skin assessment and development of an individualized multidisciplinary plan of care, incorporating scheduled ongoing assessments and interventions to maintain skin integrity, are imperative to prevent skin breakdown.

Promoting Continence

■ Achieving continence can decrease lost therapy units and decrease caregiver burden, which can impact discharge destination (home vs. facility). Continence can help to maintain skin integrity and have a positive effect on behavior.

Behavior Management

■ A consistent method of assessing/describing behavior will promote the development of more effective interventions to control behavior. Use of a validated tool will also allow the team to more accurately assess the effectiveness of the interventions.

■ Effective management of negative behaviors can positively affect length of stay, decrease lost therapy units, and increase participation in therapy, thereby increasing therapeutic goal attainment.

STUDY QUESTIONS

1. Which statement regarding pain/pain assessment in the TBI patient is true?
   a. Vital sign changes in the nonverbal TBI patient are very reliable indicators of pain
   b. Several validated assessment tools exist for the assessment of pain in the cognitively impaired TBI patient
   c. The use of subjective pain assessments are never accurate in the cognitively impaired TBI patient
   d. Leg movement and body activity are among the objective assessments in validated tools for assessment of pain in the nonverbal patient

2. Which statement is true regarding risk assessment tools used to evaluate patients for skin breakdown?
   a. Risk assessment should be done minimally every 48 hours throughout hospitalization
   b. Activity level and ability to change body position are indicators common to both the Braden and Norton risk assessment tools
   c. The Norton risk assessment tool uses six parameters to evaluate for the risk of skin breakdown
   d. The higher the Braden score the greater the risk of skin breakdown

3. Which statement regarding incontinence is true?
   a. The development of bladder incontinence in the TBI patient signals the presence of irreversible neurogenic paralysis
   b. Correction of possible neurogenic causes of bowel incontinence should take place before any other interventions are undertaken
   c. Pre-injury bowel habits are not a factor in developing a comprehensive post-injury bowel program
   d. Incontinence can increase agitation in the TBI patient

4. Which statement regarding restraint use is true?
   a. A restraint is anything that restricts a patient's freedom of movement
   b. Restraints include the use of bed exit alarms
   c. The use of medication is not considered a form of restraint
   d. Restraints have been proven to reduce falls and injury

5. Which statement is true regarding assessment and prevention of pressure injury?
   a. Pressure reduction measures should be focused on measures a TBI patient can perform independently
   b. Prone positioning is contraindicated in TBI patients
   c. Skin should be kept moist to prevent the accumulation of dry skin under pressure points
   d. Reduction of shear and friction are important components of pressure injury prevention programs

ADDITIONAL READING

Jacelon CS, ed. *The Specialty Practice of Rehabilitation Nursing: A Core Curriculum.* 8th ed. Rehabilitation Nursing Foundation; 2019.

Amaot S, Resan M, Mion L. The feasibility, reliability and clinical utility of the Agitated Behavior Scale in brain injured rehabilitation patients. *Rehabil Nurs.* 2012;37(1):19–24. doi:10.1002/rnj.251

Aadal, L, Mortensen, J., & Feldbaek, J. Monitoring agitated behavior after acquired brain injury: onset, duration, intensity and nursing shift variation. *Rehabil Nurs.* 2015;41(5):289–297. doi:10.1111/jocn.14298

Oyesanya TO, Bowers BJ, Royer HR, Turkstra LS. Nurses' Concerns About Caring for patients with acute and chronic traumatic brain injury. *J Clin Nurs.* 2018;27(7–8):1408–1419. doi:10.1111/jocn.14298

Pryor J. What cues do nurses use to predict aggression in people with acquired brain injury? *J Neurosci Nurs.* 2005;37(2):117–121. doi:10.1097/01376517-200504000-00010

ANSWERS TO STUDY QUESTIONS

1. Correct Answer: d
   While the gold standard in pain assessment remains self-report, this may be difficult in the setting of cognitive impairment. The literature provides little direction as to a validated scale to use in the cognitively impaired population when the patient is unable to self-report pain. A change in vital signs as an indicator for pain has not been backed by evidence. Body and extremity movement as well as facial expression have been validated as indicators of pain in the nonverbal patient.

   Further Reading:
   Feldt KS. The checklist of nonverbal pain indicators (CNPI). *Pain Manag Nurs.* 2000;1(1):13–21. doi:10.1053/jpmn.2000.5831
   Schnakers C, Chatelle C, Demertzi A, et al. What about pain in disorders of consciousness? *AAPS J.* 2012;14(3):437–444. doi:10.1208/s12248-012-9346-5

2. Correct Answer: b
   The Braden and Norton scales are the most commonly used risk assessment tools. A risk assessment should be done at least once every 24 hours to ensure that if there is a change in the patient's risk for skin breakdown, interventions can be instituted quickly to address it. Two of the most important predictors of risk for skin breakdown are activity level/mobility and the ability to independently change position; therefore, they are key indicators in both risk assessment tools. A Braden scale score of 15 or less is considered high risk for skin breakdown.

Further Reading:
Braden B, Bergstrom S. A conceptual scheme for the study and etiology of pressure sores. *Rehabil Nurs*. 1989;14(5):258.

3. Correct Answer: d
Incontinence in the TBI population is most commonly due physiological not functional causes. Designing a bowel/bladder retraining program that incorporates pre-injury elimination patterns has the best chance of success. Incontinence can have many negative effects, including skin breakdown, falls, and agitation.

Further Reading:
Jacelon CS, ed. *The Specialty Practice of Rehabilitation Nursing: A Core Curriculum*. 8th ed. Rehabilitation Nursing Foundation; 2019.
Doughty DB, ed. *Urinary and Fecal Incontinence. Nursing Management*. 3rd ed. Mosby; 2006.

4. Correct Answer: a
Anything that restricts a patient's freedom of movement is considered a restraint. A bed exit alarm does not restrict a patient's ability to move; it alerts staff when a patient exits the bed. Restraints can be physical or chemical. Restraints do not reduce the number of falls; rather, they can result in injury. For example, wrist restraints can cause injury such as skin breakdown.

Further Reading:
Joint Commission on Accreditation of Healthcare Organizations. Alternatives to restraint and seclusion (Chapter 3). In: *Complying With Joint Commission Standards*. Joint Commission Standards; 2020.
Dunn K. The effects of physical restraints on fall rates in older adults who are institutionalized. *J Gerontol Nurs*. 2001;27(1):40–48. doi:10.3928/0098-9134-20011001-10
Cohen C, Neufeld R, Dunbar J, et al. Old problem, different approach: alternatives to physical restraints. *J Gerontol Nurs*. 1996;22(2):23–29. doi:10.3928/0098-9134-19960201-08

5. Correct Answer: d
Shear and friction are two of the main contributors to pressure injuries; reducing these can reduce the occurrence of skin breakdown. It is the care team's responsibility to assist with and/or provide pressure relief strategies for dependent patients. Prone positioning is not contraindicated solely based on TBI diagnosis. In fact, prone positioning can be a great pressure injury prevention strategy. Skin should be kept dry as moisture contributes to skin breakdown.

Further Reading:
Arnold MC. Pressure ulcer prevention and management: the current evidence for care. *AACN Clin Issues*. 2003;14(4):411–428. doi:10.1097/00044067-200311000-00003

REFERENCES

The full reference list appears in the digital product found on http://connect.springer-pub.com/content/book/978-0-8261-4768-4/part/part03/chapter/ch30

PHYSICAL THERAPY: MOBILITY, TRANSFERS, AND AMBULATION; VESTIBULAR REHABILITATION

CATHERINE BURRESS KESTNER

DEFINITIONS

- Physical therapists (PTs): "Health care professionals who help individuals maintain, restore, and improve movement, activity, and functioning, thereby enabling optimal performance and enhancing health, well-being, and quality of life. Their services prevent, minimize, or eliminate impairments of body functions and structures, activity limitations, and participation restrictions ... [due to] conditions of the musculoskeletal, neuromuscular, cardiovascular, pulmonary and/or integumentary system."[1]
- Functional mobility: Movements required to fully participate in activities of daily living, vocations, recreational, and leisure tasks. Includes, but is not limited to, bed mobility, transfers, sitting and standing balance, ambulation, and stair negotiation.
- Balance: The ability to maintain an upright position by keeping the body's center of gravity over the base of support as the body performs static or dynamic activity.[2] In a structurally healthy system, the central nervous system integrates information from the visual, somatosensory, and vestibular systems to maintain balance, and the vestibular system resolves conflict between somatosensation and vision. Patients with traumatic brain injury (TBI) demonstrate an increased reliance on vision and decreased ability of the vestibular system to resolve conflict between somatosensation and vision.[3,4]
- Vestibular system: Senses linear and rotary acceleration for orientation to upright. Includes the semicircular canals, otolith organs, vestibular nerve (cranial nerve VIII), vestibular nuclei, vestibular cortex, and cerebellum.
- Spasticity: "A motor disorder characterized by a velocity-dependent increase in tonic stretch reflexes ... resulting from hyperexcitability of the stretch reflex, as one component of the upper motoneuron syndrome."[5]
- Dystonia: "Tonic contraction of a muscle or muscle group when the subject is at rest."[5]

PRESENTATION AND EVALUATION

Physical therapy management of the patient with TBI is challenging due to the population's heterogeneous presentation without clear patterns of physical impairment. This requires the PT to have a thorough understanding of all systems that require examination. Often the evaluation will be incomplete and observational due to the patient's inability to fully participate in the examination.

The full reference list appears in the digital product found on http://connect.springerpub.com/content/book/978-0-8261-4768-4/part/part03/chapter/ch31

- Sensory impairments may include deficits in light touch, temperature sensation, deep pressure, pain sensation, proprioception, and vibratory sensation. Testing may be limited by communication and cognitive impairments. When due to a peripheral process, distribution may follow dermatomal patterns or peripheral nerve distribution.
- Decreased range of motion (ROM) or contracture may develop secondary to decreased mobility, suboptimal positioning, and spasticity. Evaluation includes the use of goniometry and visual observation.
- Motor control impairments present as weakness, decreased coordination, impaired initiation, and movement disorders. Evaluation includes use of manual muscle testing and observation of antigravity movement and assessment of rapid alternating movements. When possible, based on physical function and ability to follow commands, use of standardized assessments as recommended by the American Physical Therapy Association's (APTA) TBI Evaluation Database to Guide Effectiveness (EDGE) group should be included, such as the 10-m walk test or 6-minute walk.[6]
- Changes in tone may present in a hemiparetic pattern or tetraparetic pattern or may be localized. This may manifest as spasticity, spasms, or localized dystonia. Objective assessment of spasticity uses the Modified Ashworth Scale or the Tardieu Scale.[6,7]
- Balance impairments will be present in 30% to 60% of patients with TBI and require specific assessment by the PT.[2,8] Highly reliable and valid assessments have been identified by the APTA TBI EDGE group and should be selected as appropriate to the patient's abilities, such as the Berg Balance Scale or Community Balance and Mobility Scale.[6] When the exam is limited by cognitive deficits, observation and description using assist levels should be utilized.
- Up to 80% of TBI patients will present with some variety of vestibular pathology, including benign paroxysmal positional vertigo (BPPV), peripheral hypofunction, impaired central function, or a combination of deficits.[9,10] Symptoms may include dizziness, vertigo, nausea, disequilibrium, imbalance, visual disturbances, headache, and hearing loss. Assessments include use of positional testing and examination of oculomotor control and vestibular reflexes, and are best completed with use of Frenzel lenses or video goggles when available. Temporal bone fractures may cause damage to cranial nerve VIII and indicate the need for examination of peripheral vestibular function. The examination will often be incomplete due to physical and cognitive deficits, limiting it to observation of postural and oculomotor control. Examination should include specific outcome measures as appropriate to the patient's cognitive and physical abilities, including the Functional Gait Assessment or Dizziness Handicap Inventory.[6,9]
- Fractures and soft tissue injuries are often comorbid diagnoses that the therapist must consider and that may impact treatment.
- Functional mobility is often the area of greatest focus with TBI patients. Recommended outcome measures from the APTA TBI EDGE group should be utilized to objectively assess function when patients are reasonably able to follow instructions and achieve minimal mobility to participate in assessment.[6]
  - Bed mobility assessment should include rolling and supine to-and-from sit transitions. Rolling assessment will provide the PT with information on possible vestibular deficits, trunk ROM, and strength. Supine to-and-from sit transitions may provide information on trunk ROM and strength, as well as general upper- and lower-extremity ROM and strength.
  - Transfer assessment, including assist level, may incorporate use of mechanical lifts, squat pivot transfer, lateral or sliding board transfers, and stand pivot, stand step, or sit-to-stand transfers. Choosing the appropriate transfer requires the clinical assessment, observation, and judgment of the PT. This assessment provides the therapist with further insight into strength, ROM, coordination, spasticity, and balance skills.

- Ambulation assessment is not always appropriate with moderate to severe TBI patients. The PT's evaluation will dictate whether to proceed with this activity. Gait assessment may be limited to standing or, if appropriate, may be progressed in a highly supported environment, such as the parallel bars or a body weight-supported system. The assessment can provide further observational evidence of strength, ROM, balance, spasticity, and coordination.

TREATMENT

A systematic review found high-level evidence that more intensive rehabilitation programs for TBI patients lead to greater functional outcomes and that patients with moderate to severe brain injuries benefit from formal therapeutic intervention.[11]

- Sensory stimulation within the context of physical therapy will include weight-bearing activities in sitting and standing and change of position. Equipment such as a tilt table, tilt table with robotic stepping, and standing frame will be beneficial for the patient with significant mobility restrictions or disordered state of consciousness. Upright training has demonstrated improved neurobehavioral and functional outcomes and can be applied early in the rehabilitation process safely when hemodynamic and respiratory functions are stable.[12]
- ROM, stretching, and positioning programs have been considered a standard of care in physical therapy; however, evidence does not support improvements in ROM secondary to these interventions.[13] Clinicians must carefully consider the amount of treatment time that is spent in these interventions in the context of lack of evidence for short-term improvement in ROM, although clear evidence related to effects on quality of life, pain, and activity and participation restrictions are lacking.[13] Education for families and caregivers to perform these skills outside of therapy is appropriate; note that long-term use of these interventions has not been proven to be effective.
- Static or dynamic positioning orthoses are available commercially, or custom devices may be fabricated by an orthotist. Prescription of orthoses may facilitate positioning, prevent skin breakdown, and be used to address ROM goals, although evidence is sparse.[14,15]
- Spasticity may cause pain and contribute to skin breakdown, impact positioning in bed and wheelchairs, limit setup and positioning for transfers, and contribute to motor control impairments. When left untreated, spasticity may lead to muscle and soft tissue shortening and eventual contractures.[7] Physical therapy management may include stretching and ROM programs, strengthening of the antagonist muscles, recommendations for orthoses, serial casting, and functional mobility training. An effective program to treat spasticity requires the PT to work closely with the medical team for comprehensive management, including monitoring for pain, skin injury, nerve compression, or impaired blood flow.[7]
- Serial casting utilizes plaster or fiberglass casting material to position joints in submaximal stretch to facilitate improved joint ROM. Casts are applied every 1 to 7 days, while progressing joint positioning and monitoring for adverse effects such as skin breakdown, nerve injury, and compression of vascular structures. Evidence does not support reduced spasticity due to serial casting; however, there is good evidence to support ROM gains from serial casting. Average gains in the ankle ranged from 10° to 26°, and at the knee improvements of 15° to 27° were demonstrated.[16,17]
  - PTs should consider how ROM gains will be maintained and determine a strategy for ongoing spasticity management when casting is discontinued. Orthoses, motor

training, and ongoing collaboration with the medical team for spasticity management all may contribute to maintaining ROM improvements.[17] The functional goals that may be achieved following casting should be weighed against the risks inherent to casting when considering a serial casting protocol.

- Strengthening programs are important to allow progression of functional mobility skills. Patients with TBI are often not able to participate in traditionally structured progressive resistive strengthening programs. In these instances, patients can benefit from strengthening within the context of functional mobility.

- Fitness training can be initiated through appropriate aerobic modalities (e.g., biking, aquatics, walking) for participants who are first screened for cardiorespiratory stability and should follow American College of Sports Medicine recommendations for intensity. Further research is needed to support the benefits of fitness training, but positive results have been noted for improved power and gait speed.[18]

- Balance training will likely start in sitting, initially working on static sitting balance and head control, progressing as appropriate to dynamic standing balance. Therapists may include use of compliant and mobile surfaces, altered base of support, altered sensory inputs, distracting environments, visual cues, and dual tasking to progress balance training dependent on patient-specific impairments and goals. Limited high-quality studies have addressed balance training in TBI populations and have utilized varying interventions; however, it appears that a wide range of approaches including the use of virtual reality training may facilitate improvements in balance.[2,8,19] To achieve goals for ambulation, evidence suggests that balance training is only effective when it is paired with use of virtual reality or augmented visual feedback.[20]

- Vestibular rehabilitation programs will incorporate the use of adaptation exercises including gaze stabilization, habituation exercises, repositioning maneuvers for BPPV, compensatory training, or progressing functional mobility as appropriate.[9] Patients with TBI will often require modifications to the vestibular rehabilitation program, including hand-over-hand assist for cervical rotation when performing gaze stabilization exercises, using modified positioning for the canalith repositioning maneuver, or utilizing position changes and mobility training as habituation for patients who are unable to participate in a formalized treatment program.
  - Patients with central dysfunction can make improvements with vestibular rehabilitation, although full resolution of symptoms and balance impairments may not be achieved.[21]
  - As many as 20% of cases of BPPV are due to trauma. Posttraumatic BPPV required significantly more repositioning maneuvers compared to idiopathic BPPV for resolution, and recurrence of BPPV is more common following trauma.[20–22]

- Functional mobility training should include bed mobility, transfers, and sitting, and progress to standing and ambulation as appropriate. Current literature supports the use of task-specific training for improved skill acquisition: A systematic review of the literature found high-level evidence to support the use of task-oriented and repetitive training.[11] This supports performing specific functional mobility skills multiple times sequentially during a session. However, this may be challenging for patients with poor attention or problems with agitation; therefore, therapists may need to consider the use of varied practice throughout their sessions.
  - Recovery of ambulation is frequently a goal for patients and family members. Traditional gait training is often initiated in the parallel bars and progresses to an assistive device such as a walker or cane as patients improve their balance and strength. Recent evidence supports that early intensive, body weight-supported gait training may yield improved Functional Independence Measure (FIM) gains compared to traditional approaches.[23] In chronic TBI, there is increasing evidence to support the use of body weight-supported or robotic training systems to facilitate

improved outcomes, including improved self-selected and fastest gait speed.[24] Body weight-supported treadmill training (BWSTT) has been demonstrated to be better than non-gait interventions (e.g., strengthening, stretching, no intervention) for improving walking speed.[20] Robotic training systems may also be considered to facilitate gait training for nonambulatory patients, although they do not provide additional training benefit to the individual that is already ambulatory.[20]

- In clinical practice, BWSTT may be useful with TBI patients who are not following commands or who may have poor attention; for initiation of ambulation training; for those with impaired safety awareness, poor balance, or coordination; or for those who require a significant amount of physical assistance. BWSTT can be a safer, more successful, and earlier intervention to initiate gait training and increase intensity and volume of training. A variety of body weight-supported gait training systems are available commercially to assist over-ground or treadmill-based training.

- Orthoses are used by many clinicians to improve ambulation, although others avoid it because of concerns that an orthosis may disrupt normal gait kinematics and lead to disuse atrophy of the muscles that control the joint.[25]
  - Systematic reviews on the use of ankle-foot orthoses (AFOs) to improve ambulation have concluded there is good evidence that AFOs increase walking speed, increase step and stride length, decrease energy expenditure, and improve functional measures of ambulation.[25–27]
  - Conflicting evidence was found on effects on muscle activation of the anterior tibialis and gastrocnemius/soleus complex with use of traditional AFOs, but use of functional electrical stimulation (FES) orthoses may facilitate improved muscle function.[25,27]
  - The use of AFOs is often beneficial to facilitate early ambulation in brain injury patients. Clinicians should consider custom AFOs, off-the-shelf devices, and FES devices. Timing, appropriateness, and type of device prescribed must be based on clinical judgment and evaluation of patient-specific impairments and goals.

- Custom seating and positioning is recommended to prevent skin breakdown, decrease risk of secondary complications, maintain patient safety, optimize positioning, and allow patient mobility when ambulation is not an appropriate goal. Power wheelchair mobility should be considered for TBI patients with very low-level mobility but minimal cognitive deficits.

KEY POINTS

- Heterogeneous presentation of patient deficits will require an interdisciplinary approach with clinicians with a wide range of skills.
- Evaluation and treatment may be informal and unstructured due to cognitive and communication deficits; however, an evidence-based approach is recommended.
- Cognitive deficits will be a limiting factor in physical progress, but can be overcome with an effective behavior management plan and a team approach.
- Due to the high incidence of vestibular deficits in TBI populations, all patients should be screened for vestibular dysfunction.
- Tracking progress with reliable and valid outcome measures is important to guide the plan of care and ensure effective care is provided.
- Patients with moderate to severe TBI can make significant and functional gains with intensive and appropriate therapeutic intervention.

STUDY QUESTIONS

1. Patients should be referred to physical therapy following TBI for which of the following programs/goals?
   a. Stretching to be performed for 1 hour per day to improve ROM
   b. Improving attention skills for safe utilization of a walker
   c. Initiating upright tolerance training once hemodynamically stable
   d. Physical therapy should not be initiated if patients are demonstrating agitation

2. What is the role of standardized outcome measures in PT practice with patients following TBI?
   a. Standardized outcome measures cannot be utilized in a patient population with cognitive impairments
   b. Only one standard outcome measure should be selected to identify progress toward goals
   c. Valid and reliable outcome measures assist in guiding decision-making for interventions and objectively measuring progress toward goals
   d. Outcome measures utilized by PTs primarily measure constructs of gait

3. What type of injury puts the patient with TBI at a high risk for vestibular impairment and indicates the need for a vestibular evaluation?
   a. Temporal bone fracture
   b. Musculocutaneous nerve injury
   c. C6 transverse process fracture
   d. Liver laceration

4. Outcomes for recovery of ambulation are optimized when:
   a. Gait training is deferred until a patient is following commands to effectively utilize an assistive device
   b. Physical therapy interventions focus on strengthening and stretching
   c. Standing balance is addressed via weight-shifting activities
   d. Early intensive gait training is initiated in body weight-supported systems

5. Evidence-based treatment of BPPV following TBI includes:
   a. Brandt Daroff exercises to induce habituation of dizziness symptoms
   b. Positional testing to identify the involved canal, and repetition of repositioning maneuvers for resolution
   c. Bedrest to allow resolution of symptoms
   d. Gaze stabilization exercises to improve the gain of the vestibular ocular reflex

ADDITIONAL READING

Neurology Section Outcome Measures Recommendations: Traumatic Brain Injury. http://www.neuropt.org/professional-resources/neurology-section-outcome-measures-recommendations/traumatic-brain-injury

Herdman SJ, Clendaniel RA. *Vestibular Rehabilitation*. 4th ed. FA Davis Company; 2014.

Bhattacharyya N, Gubbels SP, Schwartz SR, et al. Clinical practice guideline: benign paroxysmal positional vertigo (update). *Otolaryngol Head Neck Surg.* 2017;16(3_suppl):S1–S47. doi:10.1177/0194599816689667

Harvey LA, Katalinic OM, Herbert RD, et al. Stretch for the treatment and prevention of contractures (Review). *Cochrane Database Syst Rev.* 2017;1(1):CD007455. doi:10.1002/14651858.CD007455.pub3

Hornby TG, Reisman DS, Ward IG, et al. Clinical practice guideline to improve locomotor function following chronic stroke, incomplete spinal cord injury, and brain injury. *J Neurol Phys Ther.* 2020;44(1):49–100. doi:10.1097/NPT.0000000000000303

ANSWERS TO STUDY QUESTIONS

1. Correct Answer: c
Evidence does not support the use of stretching for short-term improvements in ROM. Attention training is outside the scope of practice for a PT; however, assessment of whether a walker is the best assistive device is within a PT's scope. Upright tolerance training through use of tilt tables, tilt tables with robotic stepping, or standing frames have been shown to improve neurobehavioral and functional outcomes.

Further Reading:
Frazzitta G, Zivi I, Valsecchi R, et al. Effectiveness of a very early stepping verticalization protocol in severe acquired brain injured patients: a randomized pilot study in ICU. *PLoS One.* 2016;11(7): e0158030. doi:10.1371/journal.pone.0158030

2. Correct Answer: c
A wide variety of valid and reliable outcome measures have been identified for use in PT practice to measure impairment, activity, and participation restrictions. The PT should select assessments that are appropriate to a patient's cognitive function and goal areas, and utilize information from these measures to design focused interventions and assess progress toward goals.

Further Reading:
Neurology Section. *Neurology Section Outcome Measures Recommendations: Traumatic Brain Injury.* http://www.neuropt.org/professional-resources/neurology-section-outcome-measures-recommendations/traumatic-brain-injury

3. Correct Answer: a
Cranial nerve VIII passes through the internal auditory canal within the temporal bone. Fracture of the temporal bone may damage this nerve causing a unilateral peripheral hypofunction. This deficit can be identified during a vestibular evaluation and treated with adaptation exercises.

Further Reading:
Herdman SJ, Clendaniel RA. *Vestibular Rehabilitation.* 4th ed. FA Davis Company; 2014.

4. Correct Answer: d
Evidence does not support a direct connection between utilization of interventions such as stretching, strengthening, or balance activities without augmented visual feedback to significantly improve ambulation. Intensive gait training has demonstrated improved outcomes in FIM gains and gait speed and may be best implemented in body weight-supported systems to facilitate early initiation.

Further Reading:
Hornby TG, Reisman DS, Ward IG, et al. Clinical practice guideline to improve locomotor function following chronic stroke, incomplete spinal cord injury, and brain injury. *J Neurol Phys Ther.* 2020;44(1):49–100. doi:10.1097/NPT.0000000000000303

5. Correct Answer: b
   Although BPPV can resolve spontaneously, bedrest is not recommended for resolution of symptoms. Brandt Daroff exercises and gaze stabilization exercises are not specific to BPPV. Positional testing will allow the PT to identify which canal is impaired and perform repositioning maneuvers specific to that canal.

   Further Reading:
   Bhattacharyya N, Gubbels SP, Schwartz SR, et al. Clinical practice guideline: benign paroxysmal positional vertigo (update). *Otolaryngol Head Neck Surg.* 2017;16(3_suppl):S1–S47. doi:10.1177/0194599816689667

REFERENCES

The full reference list appears in the digital product found on http://connect.springerpub.com/content/book/978-0-8261-4768-4/part/part03/chapter/ch31

OCCUPATIONAL THERAPY: ACTIVITIES OF DAILY LIVING, DRIVING, AND COMMUNITY REINTEGRATION

ANNE W. HUNT AND JENNIFER FLEMING

BACKGROUND

Definitions

- *Occupation:* Activity that gives structure, value, and meaning and encompasses work (paid and unpaid), leisure, and self-care[1]—includes activities of daily living (ADLs).
- *Occupational performance:* The doing of activities in the environment in which they need to be done, for example, cooking a meal at home for the family.
- *Occupational therapist (OT):* Per the World Federation of Occupational Therapy, an OT is a therapist trained to enable people to participate in everyday life by enhancing their abilities and/or by modifying the environment to better support participation.
- *Activities of daily living:* Functional daily activities generally divided into basic (BADL, self-care tasks) and instrumental (IADL, everyday activities necessary for interacting with the environment, more complex than BADLs). Examples of the latter include using public transport, managing personal finances, meal preparation, and home management. Instrumental activities of daily living are generally understood to exclude work-related activities.
- *Driving:* The control and operation of a motor vehicle. By law, medical clearance is required following the onset of a medical condition or disability that could affect driving.
- *Community integration:* "Something to do, somewhere to live, someone to love."[2] Has three primary constructs: independent living, social support, and productive occupation.[3]

Epidemiology

More than 5 million Americans are estimated to have long-term disability resulting from traumatic brain injury (TBI).[4] After moderate to severe TBI, most people (95%) regain independence in BADLs; 20% to 30% require assistance for IADLs including domestic activities, shopping, using public transport and financial management; 30% to 50% are unable to drive; and approximately 50% are unable to return to leisure activities, employment, or study.[5] The estimated prevalence of TBI of all severities among offender individuals is 60% and among the homeless is up to 53%.[6,7]

The full reference list appears in the digital product found on http://connect.springer-pub.com/content/book/978-0-8261-4768-4/part/part03/chapter/ch32

ASSESSMENT AND EVALUATION

Step 1

Client-centered goal setting: Collaborative goal setting is critical to identifying key occupational performance issues for each client.[8] It may be necessary, useful, and/or relevant to involve a family member or other caregiver in this interview process.[9]

Step 2

Assessment of specific areas of occupation: Select assessments based on client-centered goals and whether you need an "outcome" measure (for evaluation) or a measure to describe client's abilities.[10] Important considerations: Do informant and self-reports concur with each other and with actual performance? Does the client use strategies to compensate for impairments in physical and cognitive functions? Consider the ecological validity of the assessments selected. (How well does the assessment capture the client's performance in the real world?)

- Performance-based measures involve direct observation and provide a comprehensive and accurate picture of strengths and weaknesses in everyday life. Performance is influenced by the environment and determining performance is best achieved in the client's own environment.[11] This will provide more ecological validity (i.e., performance on the test corresponds to an everyday situation).
- Consider the ADL and IADL Profile,[12,13] which provides comprehensive measures of ADLs and the impact of executive dysfunction on everyday life, or the Multiple Errands Test (MET),[14] which allows observation of strategies employed while shopping and collecting information. Different versions of the MET have been developed to address the need for ecological validity in assessment of performance of everyday life activity (e.g., home, hospital, Big-Store versions).[15,16]
- Questionnaires typically provide information about capability but not performance.[17]
  - BADL and IADL—Many available.[17]
  - Community integration: Self-report or informant report. The Community Integration Questionnaire (www.tbims.org/combi), Reintegration to Normal Living Index,[18] and Sydney Psychosocial Reintegration Scale[19] are psychometrically sound and clinically useful.

Step 3

Special areas for consideration:

- *Cognition* (see also Chapters 33 and 35): OTs assess cognition particularly as it relates to everyday life (e.g., safety with household ADLs, planning daily activities, remembering to take medication and attend appointments, navigating in the community).
- *Driving assessment:* A comprehensive multidisciplinary assessment—inclusive of an off-road assessment of visual, sensory, cognitive, and physical function and an on-road test—is critical in moderate to severe TBI.[20,21] Decisions regarding driving ability are based upon not only medical fitness but the functional abilities required for safe driving, which are determined using a combination of off-road and on-road assessment. Cognitive performance alone does not predict driving capacity.[22] A comprehensive driving evaluation is considered the gold standard to assess fitness to drive[21] and is administered by a trained OT.[20] The timing of on-road assessment is individual and occurs when sufficient recovery has occurred for medical clearance to be a realistic

outcome. Conducted in a dual-control vehicle, it usually follows a standardized route and set of maneuvers. One measure used is the Driver Observation Scale (DOS), which records driver behavior in the traffic environment and appropriateness of maneuvers performed.[23] Off-road assessments may include self-report questionnaires, caregiver reports, and driving simulator testing.[24,25] Readiness to resume driving is determined on an individual basis by experienced clinicians and is generally not considered until at least 3 months post-injury to allow for recovery of physical and cognitive impairments.[25] The Association for Driving Rehabilitation Specialists provides information on specialized testing and training services across North America (www.driver-ed.org). The few studies investigating whether people with TBI who return to driving have more accidents than healthy controls have produced mixed results.[26] Driving is a complex IADL that is linked to autonomy, self-identity, and community access and is considered a rite of passage to adulthood, making it a focus for rehabilitation for many patients with TBI.

■ *Return to work and school:* See Chapter 69.
■ *Social support, social integration, and sexuality:* Reductions in social support, social isolation, relationship breakdown, and negative changes in perceived sexuality are frequent outcomes[27] and need to be considered in a comprehensive assessment of community integration. (See also Chapter 41.)

INTERVENTION

Five key areas to consider: regaining functional independence (BADLs and IADLs), social support and community integration, housing, driving and transportation, and ongoing community participation. Participation in meaningful life situations is the goal, and gains can be achieved many years post injury.[27]

■ Regaining functional independence:
  ● Comprehensive rehabilitation programs that focus on (a) integration of therapies, (b) metacognition (i.e., self-awareness and comprehension of one's thinking processes), (c) self-regulation, and (d) participating in personally meaningful life activities have better outcomes than neuropsychological rehabilitation alone.[28]
    ■ External strategies to compensate for cognitive impairments (schedules, checklists, routines, smartphone calendar and alarm functions, memory notebooks, whiteboards, and personal digital assistants) are recommended as effective for clients with severe TBI.[27]
    ■ Individualized strategies should be selected on the basis of client goals, preferences, and abilities, and taught using techniques such as errorless learning, spaced retrieval, and distributed practice with the involvement of family members.[29]
    ■ Internal strategies (e.g., visualization/visual imagery) are effective for clients with mild to moderate TBI.[29]
    ■ Metacognitive strategy instruction is recommended for adults with TBI with executive dysfunction[30,31] and "should be focused on everyday problems and functional outcomes."[29] Such instruction includes "acknowledging or generating goals, self-monitoring and self-recording of performance and strategy decisions based on performance-goal comparison."[32]
    ■ Direct feedback on occupational performance delivered in the context of a therapeutic program is effective for improving occupational performance and level of self-awareness.[30,33]
  ● For severely impaired survivors, improving performance on selected skills may be achieved by specific functional skills training[32,34] comprising task analysis, written

prompts, embedding retrained skills in programming, consistent practice, and fading cues. Independence in any particular skill can take months to achieve, and as benefits are often not generalizable, the cost versus benefit should be evaluated carefully.
- Addressing psychosocial issues:
  - There are currently limited social support, social integration opportunities, and interventions to enhance positive expressions of sexuality.
  - Multifaceted social support groups that focus on education, coping-skills training, and goal setting may reduce hopelessness and engender a greater sense of control.[27]
  - Social-skills training, including individualized goal setting, shaping of behaviors, and social perception training, may improve specific aspects of social behavior.[35-37]
  - Peer mentoring may improve social participation.[32]
  - Family support and education may be necessary to assist family members to manage neurobehavioral changes after brain injury and adjust to relationship changes.[32]
  - Interventions to support the development of perceived control of one's life (e.g., stress management programs) may be helpful in the development of resiliency, an important factor in successful engagement in meaningful activities in life following brain injury that may also protect against the negative impacts of changes in relationships and social supports following brain injury.[38,39]
- Housing: OTs should provide input to team members regarding level of independence so appropriate housing can be arranged. This may include the prescription of home modifications to increase safety and independence.
- Driving and transportation: Access to transportation is key for community integration. Driving rehabilitation may include on-road driver training, goal-directed on-road driving lessons, simulation and off-road skill-specific training and education.[25,40] Emerging evidence suggests that driver rehabilitation, including on-road lessons, can support return to independent driving for individuals with TBI.[25]
- Community participation: Emerging research evidence and considerable anecdotal data suggest the value of community-based support programs for enhancing community participation even many years post TBI.[41,42] Important components appear to be (a) a long-term approach, (b) individualized goal clarification, and (c) therapy in the person's own environment.
  - Treatment environment:
    - Multidisciplinary rehabilitation programs improve overall community integration.[41]
    - Participants in community-based day programs report long-term emotional, social, and cognitive benefits[43] and better social participation and quality of life than those who are assessed as eligible but do not attend.[44]

KEY POINTS

- Following moderate to severe TBI, the majority of people return to independence with BADLs but most will require assistance with IADLs.
- Occupational therapy assessment relies on client-centered goal setting and the use of capacity and/or performance-based measures.
- Consider regaining functional independence (BADLs and IADLs), social support and integration, housing, driving and transportation, and ongoing community participation as targets for intervention.

STUDY QUESTIONS

1. Collaborative, client-centered goal setting is shaped by all of the following except:
   a. The degree of clinician–client collaboration
   b. The client's impairments
   c. The environment where goal setting takes place
   d. Clinician self-awareness

2. Characteristics of the Multiple Errands Test (MET), an ecologically valid assessment, include all but which of the following:
   a. Administered in a real-world setting
   b. Provides an opportunity to observe an individual's ability to plan, problem-solve, initiate behaviors
   c. Provides an opportunity to observe an individual's use of strategies
   d. Evaluates an individual's level of depression and anxiety

3. Factors that are predictive of lower resilience in the post-acute brain injury population include all but which of the following:
   a. Less education
   b. Supportive social relationships
   c. History of pre-injury substance abuse
   d. Post-injury anxiety

4. Which of the following is *not* recommended as part of metacognitive strategy training for people with moderate to severe TBI?
   a. Goal setting and selection
   b. Complex activities that involve planning and adjusting to feedback
   c. Computerized brain-training activities or games
   d. Self-assessment following performance

5. What is considered the best basis on which to make decisions about fitness to drive after TBI?
   a. A comprehensive off- and on-road driving assessment
   b. Testing in a driving simulator
   c. Report from family members
   d. Neuropsychological testing

ADDITIONAL READING

Alderman N, Baker D. Beyond the shopping centre: using the Multiple Errands Test in the assessment and rehabilitation of multitasking disorders. In: Oddy M, Worthington A, eds. *Rehabilitation of Executive Disorders: A Guide to Theory and Practice.* Oxford University Press; 2009. doi:10.1093/med/9780198568056.003.0006

Fleming J, Schmidt J. Metacognitive occupation based training. In: Soderback I, ed. *International Handbook of Occupational Therapy Interventions.* Springer; 2015;225–231. doi:10.1007/978-0-387-75424-6_20

Dawson DR, Binns MA, Hunt A, et al. Occupation-based strategy training for adults with traumatic brain injury: a pilot study. *Arch Phys Med Rehabil.* 2013;94:1959–1963. doi:10.1016/j.apmr.2013.05.021

Doig E, Fleming J, Kuipers P, Cornwell P. Qualitative exploration of a client-centered goal-directed approach to community-based occupational therapy for adults with traumatic brain injury. *Am J Occup Ther.* 2009;63:599–568. doi:10.5014/ajot.63.5.559

Fleming J, Liddle J, Nalder E, et al. Return to driving in the first 6 months after acquired brain injury. *NeuroRehabilitation.* 2014;34:157–166. doi:10.3233/NRE-131012. doi:10.3233/NRE-131012

ANSWERS TO STUDY QUESTIONS

1. Correct Answer: b

   Conducting collaborative, client-centered goal setting is considered to be standard practice in occupational therapy and other rehabilitation professions. The therapist's self-awareness of their performance during the goal-setting process is thought to be critical in including the client's perspective. Goal setting often takes place in areas that lack privacy which may negatively impact client's participation. Client's impairments may be a factor in goal setting but is typically managed through involvement of significant others (e.g., family members).

   Further Reading:

   Cameron L, Somerville L, Naismith C, et al. A qualitative investigation into the patient-centred goal-setting practices of allied health clinicians working in rehabilitation. *Clin Rehabil.* 2018;32(6): 827–840. doi:10.1177/0269215517752488

2. Correct Answer: d

   The MET is a performance-based test that assesses executive function in a naturalistic setting. The MET enables clinicians to observe an individual's performance in a real-life context and provides context for how they adapt to novel situations and challenges in everyday life tasks. Measuring levels of depression and anxiety is not part of the assessment.

   Further Reading:

   Antoniak K, Clores J, Jensen D, et al. Developing and validating a big-store multiple errands test. *Front Psychol.* 2019;10:2575. doi: 10.3389/fpsyg.2019.02575

3. Correct Answer: b

   Resilience is defined as the ability to "bounce back" after adverse life events and is thought to play a role in overall health and well-being. Resilience has been found to be lower for individuals with moderate to severe TBI than the general population. Post-injury emotional distress, less education, and higher levels of pre-injury substance abuse were found to be associated with lower resilience in people with TBI. Conversely, supportive social relationships appear to be a protective factor and may support resilience in those with TBI.

   Further Reading:

   Kreutzer JS, Marwitz JH, Sima AP, et al. Resilience following traumatic brain injury: a traumatic brain injury model systems study. *Arch Phys Med Rehabil.* 2016;97(5):708–713. doi:10.1016/j.apmr.2015.12.003

4. Correct Answer: c

   Metacognitive strategy instruction focused on everyday problems and occupational performance is recommended for people with executive dysfunction following TBI. It involves goal setting and compensatory strategy selection, engagement in complex activities that require planning and responding to feedback, practicing strategy use during performance, self-monitoring and self-assessing, and adjusting goals. Restorative techniques such as computerized brain training have limited evidence of generalization to performance of everyday activities.

   Further Reading:

   Tate R, Kennedy M, Ponsford J, et al. INCOG recommendations for management of cognition following traumatic brain injury, Part III: executive function and self-awareness. *J Head Trauma Rehabil.* 2014:29(4):338–352. doi:10.1097/HTR.0000000000000068

5. Correct Answer: a

A comprehensive driving evaluation including an off- and on-road assessment conducted by a driver rehabilitation specialist who is typically a specially trained OT can determine readiness to return to driving following TBI.

Further Reading:

Ross PE, Di Stefano M, Charlton J, et al. Interventions for resuming driving after traumatic brain injury. *Disabil. Rehabil.* 2018;40(7):757–764. doi:10.1080/09638288.2016.12 74341

REFERENCES

The full reference list appears in the digital product found on http://connect.springer-pub.com/content/book/978-0-8261-4768-4/part/part03/chapter/ch32

33 SPEECH THERAPY: DYSPHAGIA AND COGNITIVE COMMUNICATION IMPAIRMENTS

SARAH TAYLOR

DYSPHAGIA

Background

Definition

Dysphagia is a condition characterized by abnormality in the transfer of a bolus from the mouth to the stomach. Dysphagia results in unsafe or inefficient oral intake, which can cause aspiration, pneumonia, discomfort, and/or poor caloric intake. Behaviors associated with traumatic brain injury (TBI) such as impulsivity and unawareness can affect the safety and efficiency of oral intake.[1]

Epidemiology

Dysphagia is a common complication following TBI, with an incidence as high as 93% in patients admitted to brain injury rehabilitation.[2] Incidence is as high as 61% in patients following severe TBI; there is a relationship between length of coma, presence of a tracheostomy tube and/or mechanical ventilation, and severity of dysphagia.[3]

Etiology

A delay in triggering the pharyngeal swallow is the most prevalent cause of dysphagia and aspiration in individuals following TBI. Other problems include structural injuries to the oral cavity, pharynx, and/or esophagus; atrophy/weakness due to prolonged intubation and cognitive deficits; or behaviors that interfere with oral intake.[4]

Pathophysiology

Swallowing is typically described in four phases[4]:

- The oral preparatory phase: liquid or food (the bolus) is chewed or otherwise manipulated in the mouth to ready it for the swallow.
- The oral phase: the tongue propels food back until the pharyngeal swallow is triggered.
- The pharyngeal phase: the pharyngeal swallow is triggered. The bolus traverses the pharynx.
- The esophageal phase: peristalsis carries the bolus through the esophagus and into the stomach.

When one or more of these phases is disrupted, this results in dysphagia.[4]

The full reference list appears in the digital product found on http://connect.springerpub.com/content/book/978-0-8261-4768-4/part/part03/chapter/ch33

Assessment

Risk Factors

Low Glasgow Coma Scale (GCS) scores and low scores on the Rancho Levels of Cognitive Functioning (RLOCF) are associated with aspiration. Additionally, low GCS scores, low levels on the RLOCF, the presence of a tracheostomy tube, and increased ventilation time are associated with impairments affecting oral intake.[5]

Signs and Symptoms

These include, but are not limited to:

- Poor secretion management and/or need for frequent suctioning
- Inability to recognize food
- Difficulty placing food in the mouth
- Holding or pocketing liquid/food in the mouth
- A delay in swallowing
- Throat clearing, coughing, or choking before, during, or after swallowing
- Wet, gurgly vocal quality, or audible respirations
- Pain/discomfort in throat or chest when swallowing
- Sensation of food stuck in the throat or chest[4]

Clinical Swallowing Evaluation

- Preparatory examination
  - Patient chart review
  - Observation of level of alertness and awareness
  - Observation of respiratory status and secretion management
  - Suction patient orally and/or via the tracheostomy tube, if applicable
  - Oral examination
  - Oral motor control examination
  - Laryngeal function examination
- *Initial swallowing examination:* The clinician determines if trial swallows are safe based on the information obtained from the preparatory examination. If the patient is acutely ill, has significant pulmonary complications, is not alert, has poor secretion management, and/or has an obvious pharyngeal swallowing disorder, trial swallows may not be indicated. The patient is then suctioned orally and through the tracheostomy tube, when applicable, and observations are made during trial swallows that lead to recommendations.

Instrumental Evaluation

The following instrumental swallow studies are commonly used to study various aspects of the swallow. Following the initial swallowing examination, a referral for an instrumental study is appropriate for any patient who is suspected to be aspirating or have a pharyngeal phase dysphagia.

- *Fluoroscopic Swallow Study:* a radiographic procedure that obtains real-time images of the oral, pharyngeal, and esophageal phases of the swallow
- *Fiberoptic Endoscopic Swallow Study:* an endoscopic procedure in which a flexible scope visualizes the pharyngeal phase of the swallow

Symptoms of Oropharyngeal Dysphagia That Might Be Observed During Assessment[4]

- *Aspiration:* food or liquid passes into the airway below the true vocal folds.
- *Penetration:* food or liquid enters the larynx but does not pass below the true vocal folds.
- *Residue:* food that is left over in the mouth or pharynx after the swallow.

■ *Backflow:* food from the esophagus flows up to the pharynx and/or from the pharynx up into the nasal cavity.[4]

Management

Compensatory Treatment Procedures

■ Postural techniques
  ● Chin tuck—patient puts chin to chest and pulls up; helpful for patients with a delayed swallow, reduced airway closure, and/or problems with residue in the valleculae
  ● Head rotation—turning the head to the affected side closes the pharynx on that side so that the bolus flows down the unaffected side: helpful for patients with a unilateral vocal fold paralysis or unilateral pharyngeal wall problem
  ● Head tilt—tilting head to the strong side allows food to drain down the strong side; helpful for patients with oral and pharyngeal problems on the same side
■ Techniques to improve oral sensory awareness: The following techniques may be utilized with patients with swallow apraxia, tactile agnosia of food, reduced oral sensation, and delayed onset of the oral and/or pharyngeal swallow:
  ● Thermal tactile stimulation: contacting the tongue or faucial arches with a cold laryngeal mirror or metal spoon
  ● Increasing downward pressure of the spoon against the tongue when presenting food
  ● Varying taste, volume, and/or texture of bolus (i.e., sour, cold, solid)
■ *Diet changes*: the diet should be changed only if other compensatory or therapy strategies are not effective or feasible given behavior, cognition, physical impairments, or other reasons.
  ● Liquids—thin, nectar thick, honey thick, pudding thick; initially thickened liquids are easier for a patient to control and manage, reducing the risk of aspiration.
  ● Foods—puree, ground minced, mechanical soft, solid.
  ● International Dysphagia Diet Standardisation Initiative (IDDSI):
    ■ Drinks: Thin, Slightly Thick, Moderately Thick, Extremely Thick
    ■ Food: Liquidised (moderately thick), Pureed (extremely thick), Minced & Moist, Soft & Bite-Sized, Easy to Chew/Regular.[6]

Swallowing Therapy

■ Direct therapy—involves presenting food or liquid to the patient and asking them to swallow while the therapist manipulates the bolus or the patient follows specific instructions.
■ Indirect therapy—involves exercise programs or swallows of saliva, but no food or liquid is given: typically used with patients who are at high risk of aspiration.
■ Types of direct and indirect therapy include exercises for oral manipulation, bolus propulsion, tongue base retraction, laryngeal elevation and/or vocal fold adduction, thermal tactile stimulation, and swallow maneuvers. Exercises and swallow maneuvers require good attention and ability to follow complex instructions and are not indicated for patients with significant cognitive or language impairments.

Other Modifications

When patients cannot follow instructions due to cognitive or language impairments, the following suggestions can help prevent aspiration and pneumonia in dysphagic patients.

■ Frequent and thorough oral care to reduce bacteria.
■ Elevate the head of the bed to decrease the risk of aspirating saliva and/or tube feeding.
■ Limit the number of items during meals to increase attention to safe intake.
■ Encourage individuals to set utensil, food, or cup down and swallow before taking another bite or sip.

- Encourage small, single cup sips and avoid straws if signs of aspiration increase with straw use.
- Encourage individuals to take a sip of liquid after every two to three bites.

COGNITIVE COMMUNICATION IMPAIRMENTS

Background

Definition

Communication results from a complex interaction among cognition, language, and speech. Cognitive communication impairments result from underlying deficits in cognitive processes such as awareness, attention, memory, organization, and reasoning that impact the efficiency and effectiveness of communication skills.[7] Posttraumatic amnesia (PTA) is a period of confusion, disorientation, impaired attention, and poor memory for day-to-day events resulting from inability to encode, and therefore learn, new information. Individuals who are experiencing PTA exhibit moderate to severe cognitive communication impairments.[8]

Epidemiology

Moderate and severe TBIs are typically associated with cognitive deficits 6 months or longer post injury. Factors that modify association include location of injury in the brain, intelligence pre-injury, and severity of injury.[9] PTA occurs in all individuals when they emerge from coma.[8]

Assessment

Clinical Signs and Symptoms of Cognitive Communication Impairments

The following signs and symptoms of cognitive communication impairments result in reduced effectiveness and efficiency of communication of wants, needs, and ideas. Perseveration and confabulation are frequently present.

- Poor arousal, alertness, and/or reaction to environmental stimuli
- Increased fatigue, decreased endurance
- Restlessness and/or agitation
- Anosognosia: denial or poor awareness of deficits, difficulties, and errors[10]
- Poor concentration in open or closed environments, reduced attention to detail
- Confusion, disorientation
- Perseveration: the repetition of a particular response, such as a word, phrase, or gesture, despite the absence or cessation of a stimulus[7]
- Verbal confabulation: the spontaneous narrative report of events that never happened due to memory impairment[7]
- Poor impulse control resulting in inappropriate comments and/or behavior during social exchanges
- Poor eye contact, inappropriate response length (long or short), poor topic maintenance
- Inability to verbally reason or solve basic problems in the environment

Diagnostic Evaluation

The aforementioned signs and symptoms are best detected via observation of patients during functional task completion. In addition, a number of formal and informal assessment tools will be discussed elsewhere in this book. Every patient who has suffered from a loss of consciousness should be assessed to determine the presence or absence of PTA. Tests sensitive to the detection of PTA typically assess orientation, immediate memory, and/or concentration. The two most frequently utilized tests include the Galveston Orientation and Amnesia Test (GOAT) and Orientation Log (O-Log). The GOAT (Table 33.1) is designed to be administered daily until a patient scores greater than 75 on two consecutive administrations. The scale measures orientation to person, place, and time, as well as memory for events preceding and following the injury.[11] The second test, the O-Log (Figure 33.1), also explores orientation to person, time, and place. A patient is considered out of PTA when they score greater than 24 over two consecutive administrations using this measure. Distinguishing differences between the GOAT and the O-Log are that the

TABLE 33.1   The Galveston Orientation and Amnesia (GOAT) Test

Question	Error Score	Notes
What is your name?	−2	Must give both first name and surname
When were you born?	−4	Must give day, month, and year
Where do you live?	−4	Town is sufficient
Where are you now?		
(a) City	−5	Must give actual town
(b) Building	−5	Usually in hospital or rehab center. Actual name necessary
When were you admitted to this hospital?	−5	Date
How did you get here?	−5	Mode of transport
What is the first event you can remember after the injury?	−5	Any plausible event is sufficient (record answer)
Can you give some detail?	−5	Must give relevant detail
Can you describe the last event you can recall before the accident?	−5	Any plausible event is sufficient (record answer)
What time is it now?	−5	−1 for each half-hour error
What day of the week is it?	−3	−1 for each day error
What day of the month is it (i.e., the date)?	−5	−1 for each day error
What is the month?	−15	−5 for each month error
What is the year?	−30	−10 for each year error
Total error		
Total actual score = 100 - total errors, i.e. 100 - ___.		Can be a negative number

76 – 100 = Normal
66 – 75 = Borderline
<66 = Impaired

Instructions: Can be administered daily. Score of 76 or more on three consecutive occasions is considered to indicate that patient is out of PTA.
Source From Levin HS, Vincent M, O'Donnell MA, Grossman RG. The Galveston Orientation and Amnesia Test. A practical scale to assess cognition after head injury. *J Nerv Ment Dis.* 1979;167(11):675–684. doi:10.1097/00005053-197911000-00004

Patient name:

KEY: 3=spon/free recall; 2=logical cuing;
1=MultChoice/phon cuing;
0=unable; incorr; inappro

Date	4/30	5/1	5/2		5/7	5/8	5/9		5/13	5/14	5/15	5/16		5/19	5/20	5/21	5/22	5/23	
Time	7:36	N/T	7:45		7:35	7:20	7:20		7:15	7:20	7:15	7:10		8:00	7:15	7:20	7:00	7:00	
City	O		O		2	3	3		3	3	3	3		2	3	3	3	3	
Kind of place			0		3	2	3		3	2	3	3		3	3	3	3	3	
Name of Hospital			O		1	1	1		1	1	1	1		2	3	3	3	1	
Month			3		3	2	2		3	3	3	3		3	3	3	3	3	
Date			O		O	2	2		2	2	2	3		2	1	2	2	3	
Year			1		1	3	3		2	3	3	3		3	3	3	3	3	
Day of week			1		2	2	3		3	3	2	2		2	3	3	3	3	
Clock time			1		2	1	3		3	0	2	3		2	3	2	3	3	
Etiology/event			1		3	3	3		3	3	3	3		3	3	3	3	3	
Pathology/deficits	O		1		2	3	3		3	3	3	3		3	3	3	3	3	

ORIENTATION INDEX: 0, 5, 10, 15, 20, 25, 30

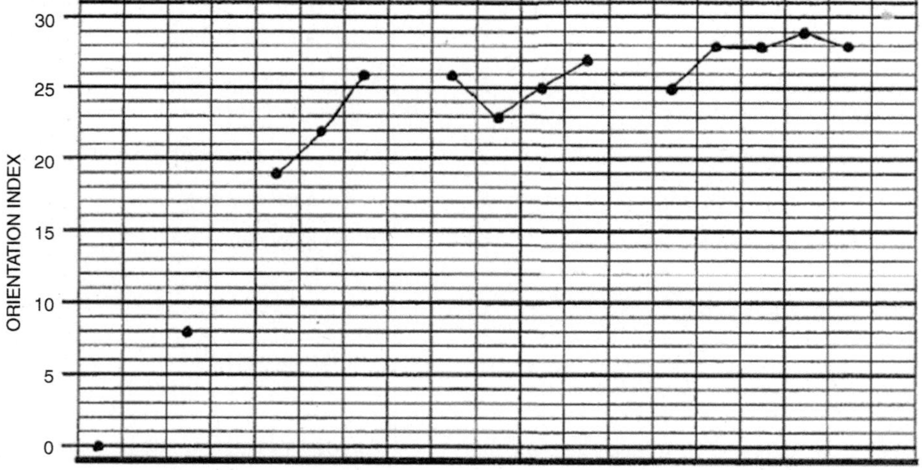

FIGURE 33.1   UAB Spain Rehabilitation Center: The Orientation Log (O-Log).

Source: From Jackson WT, Novack TA, Dowler RN. Effective serial measurement of cognitive orientation in rehabilitation: the Orientation Log. *Arch Phys Med Rehabil.* 1998;79:718–720. doi:10.1016/S0003-9993(98)90051-X

O-Log allows for a hierarchy of cuing, a focus on etiology and pathology rather than memory of events preceding and following injury, and equally weighted scores for each answer within the test.[12] Both tests have good concurrent validity.[13] Other frequently used assessments evaluate cognitive domains, including memory, attention, awareness, reasoning, auditory processing, and executive functioning. Such assessments may evaluate each domain independently, such as the California Verbal Learning Test[14] does with memory, or a number of domains simultaneously, such as the Cognitive Linguistic Quick Test.[15]

Management

Cognitive communication deficits can be managed by changing the patient's environment and/or behavior. Early in recovery, patients in PTA are not consistently able to modify their behavior. Techniques for modifying a patient's environment and/or behavior include:

- Eliminating, decreasing, or modifying stimuli and distractions.
- Allowing the patient sufficient time to respond.
- Gently allowing the patient to fail in a safe environment during functional task to promote deficit awareness.
- Providing frequent orientation; write the day and place for the individual to see and refer to frequently throughout the day.
- Verbally identifying perseveration or confabulation for the patient and educating and/or redirecting as appropriate.
- Providing specific, concrete feedback when a communication attempt is not successful or appropriate.
- Accepting all communication attempts including facial expression and gesture.
- Providing written and gesture cues when necessary.

KEY POINTS

- Dysphagia is a common impairment associated with TBI. All TBI survivors should complete an appropriate assessment and undergo treatment (if warranted) under the supervision of a speech-language pathologist.
- Cognitive communication impairments following TBI result from underlying deficits in cognitive processes such as awareness, attention, memory, organization, and reasoning. These impairments impact the efficiency and effectiveness of communication skills.
- Every patient who has suffered from a loss of consciousness should be assessed to determine the presence or absence of PTA. This is typically done utilizing either the GOAT or O-Log.

STUDY QUESTIONS

1. What is a behavior associated with TBI that can affect safety and efficiency of oral intake?
   a. Sustained attention
   b. Impulsivity
   c. Intact ability to inhibit responses in a social setting
   d. Lack of awareness of deficits

2. Low scores on what assessments are associated with aspiration?
   a. GCS
   b. The O-Log
   c. RLOCF
   d. a and c

3. What is the most prevalent cause of dysphagia and aspiration in individuals following TBI?
   a. Delay in triggering the pharyngeal swallow
   b. Esophageal stricture
   c. GERD
   d. Achalasia

4. What is posttraumatic amnesia (PTA)?
   a. The spontaneous narrative report of events that never happened due to memory impairment
   b. The repetition of a particular response, such as a word, phrase, or gesture, despite the absence or cessation of a stimulus
   c. A period of confusion, disorientation, impaired attention, and poor memory for day-to-day events
   d. Denial or poor awareness of deficits, difficulties, and errors

5. The Galveston Orientation and Amnesia Test (GOAT) and the Orientation Log (O-Log) are assessments that are used to monitor which of the following?
   a. Posttraumatic amnesia (PTA)
   b. Dysphagia
   c. Motor function
   d. Activities of daily living

ADDITIONAL READING

Halper A, Cherney L, Miller T. *A Framework for Clinical Management: Clinical Management of Communication Problems in Adults With Traumatic Brain Injury.* Aspen; 1991.

Logemann J. *Evaluation and Treatment of Swallowing Disorders.* Pro-Ed; 1998. doi:10.1097/00020840 -199812000-00008

Sohlberg M, Mateer C. *Cognitive Rehabilitation: An Integrative Neuropsychological Approach.* The Guilford Press; 2001.

Ward E, Green K, Morton A. Patterns and predictors of swallowing resolution following adult traumatic brain injury. *J Head Trauma Rehabil.* 2007;22(3):184–191. doi:10.1097/01.HTR.0000271119.96780.f5

ANSWERS TO STUDY QUESTIONS

1. Correct Answer: b
   Impulsivity can affect the rate at which a person eats/drinks; too fast and a person can choke. It can also affect the bite/sip size that a person takes. Large bites of food might be challenging for a person to chew thoroughly and therefore increase the chance of the food getting stuck, and large sips of liquids, especially consecutively, can increase the risk of the bolus entering the airway.

Further Reading:
Groher M. *Dysphagia: Diagnosis and Management*. Butterworth-Heinemann; 1997.

2. Correct Answer: d
Low GCS scores and low scores on the RLOCF are associated with aspiration. This is typically due to the fact that low scores indicate reduced consciousness. The O-Log is used after a person has regained consciousness and has started recovery, even if they are still in a confused state.

Further Reading:
Mackay LE, Morgan AS, Bernstein BA. Factors affecting oral feeding with severe traumatic brain injury. *J Head Trauma Rehabil*. 1999;14(5):435–447. doi:10.1097/00001199-199910000-00004

3. Correct Answer: a
All of these choices are causes of dysphagia for a variety of diagnoses; however, a delay in triggering the pharyngeal swallow is the most prevalent for the diagnosis of TBI.

Further Reading:
Logemann J. *Evaluation and Treatment of Swallowing Disorders*. Pro-Ed; 1998. doi:10.1097/00020840-199812000-00008

4. Correct Answer: c
PTA is a period of confusion, disorientation, impaired attention, and poor memory for day-to-day events resulting from inability to encode, and therefore learn, new information. Individuals who are experiencing PTA exhibit moderate to severe cognitive communication impairments.

Further Reading:
Horn LJ, Zasler ND. *Medical Rehabilitation of Traumatic Brain Injury*. Mosby; 1996.

5. Correct Answer: a
Tests sensitive to the detection of PTA typically assess orientation, immediate memory, and/or concentration. The two most frequently utilized tests include the GOAT and the O-Log.

Further Reading:
Levin HS, Vincent M, O'Donnell MA, Grossman RG. The Galveston Orientation and Amnesia Test. A practical scale to assess cognition after head injury. *J Nerv Ment Dis*. 1979;167(11):675–684. doi:10.1097/00005053-197911000-00004
Jackson WT, Novack TA, Dowler RN. Effective serial measurement of cognitive orientation in rehabilitation: the Orientation-Log. *Arch Phys Med Rehabil*. 1998;79:718–720. doi:10.1016/S0003-9993(98)90051-X
Novack TA, Dowler RN, Bush BA, et al. Validity of the Orientation-log relative to the Galveston Orientation and Amnesia Test. *J Head Trauma Rehabil*. 2000;15:957–961. doi:10.1097/00001199-200006000-00008

REFERENCES

The full reference list appears in the digital product found on http://connect.springer-pub.com/content/book/978-0-8261-4768-4/part/part03/chapter/ch33

34

NEURO-VISUAL PROCESSING REHABILITATION FOR VISUAL DYSFUNCTION

WILLIAM V. PADULA AND JONATHAN JENNESS

GENERAL PRINCIPLES

Definitions

- *Doctors of optometry* are "healthcare professionals concerned with the eyes and related structures, as well as vision, visual systems, and vision information processing in humans. Optometrists are trained to prescribe and fit lenses to improve vision, and trained to diagnose and treat various eye diseases."[1]
- *Doctors of ophthalmology* are "physicians who specialize in the medical and surgical care of the eyes and visual system and in the prevention of eye disease and injury."[2]
- *Neuro-Visual Processing Rehabilitation (NVPR)*, also referred to as *Neuro-Optometric Rehabilitation (NOR)*, refers to development of an individualized treatment regimen for patients with visual deficits as a direct result of physical disabilities due to traumatic brain injury (TBI) and other neurological insults.[3]
- *Vision therapy* can be provided by optometrists, ophthalmologists, and occupational therapists, each of whom utilize different professional approaches. Patient-specific needs will dictate which disciplines need to be involved in any particular case. The American Optometric Association defines *vision therapy and orthoptics* as "highly specific, sequential, sensory-motor-perceptual stimulation paradigms and regimens that are used to improve vision skills, such as eye movement control and eye coordination. This training procedure can be performed in both home and office settings, but always under the professional supervision of an optometrist."[4]
- *Neuro-Visual Postural Therapy* (NVPT): "Following a brain injury the spatial visual process is often compromised and this affects posture, balance and spatial orientation. NVPT is a series of therapeutic activities performed by a clinician in conjunction with prism lenses that facilitates visual-spatial organization affecting balance and binocularity in individuals who have had a neurological event. The weight shift movements in conjunction with the prisms organize and ground the visual-spatial process with the proprioceptive base of support (BOS). This stabilizes the bi-modal visual process (neuro-visual process) and supports organization of the vestibular and kinesthetic systems."[3]

Symptoms related to visual dysfunction following a TBI may include headache, diplopia, homonymous hemianopsia, vertigo, asthenopia, difficulty with focusing the eyes, movement of print when reading, tracking difficulty, photophobia, and blurred vision.[5]

The full reference list appears in the digital product found on http://connect.springerpub.com/content/book/978-0-8261-4768-4/part/part03/chapter/ch34

- *Diplopia*, typically due to binocular vision dysfunction, is quite prevalent following a TBI.[6,7] Binocular dysfunction may result in difficulties with balance, posture, and spatial orientation.[3]
- Visual field defect/visual neglect
  - *Homonymous hemianopsia*, field loss affecting either the entire left or right field, is often seen in the setting of TBI.[8,9]
  - *Visual neglect* is a lack of spatial conscious awareness in the absence of a homonymous hemianopsia.[10]
  - Homonymous hemianopsia or visual neglect can induce a shift in visual egocenter, resulting in Visual Midline Shift Syndrome (VMSS).[3,10,11]

Normal Visual Processing

The bimodal visual system is composed of two visual processes. The *focal visual process* is oriented toward detail, identification, attention, and concentration. It isolates figure from the ground, is conscious, and is related to the functioning of the occipital cortex and associated cortices. The *ambient* or *spatial-visual process* is oriented toward spatial orientation, balance, posture, and movement, and is preconscious. It is mediated primarily at the midbrain, although the occipital cortex also plays a role.[12,13] The ambient visual process integrates information with the sensorimotor system.[14]

Development of Posture

- Vision supports organization of balance and posture through the following processes:
  - The visual concept of egocenter (i.e., one's own midline) is a function of interaction between the ambient visual process and the sensorimotor system.[11,15]
  - Developmentally, vision matches information with the sensorimotor systems to organize the visual midline or egocenter to reinforce postural alignment with the proprioceptive system.[16]
  - Feed forward cooperation occurs between the ambient visual process and sensorimotor system. It is used to initiate movement within a closed-loop system between midbrain and the cortices. The closed-loop system depends upon the correction of errors and recognition from performance-related feedback.[12]
  - The ambient visual process is preconscious and serves as an anticipatory or readiness process following organization with the proprioceptive BOS. Following a brain injury, the spatial or ambient visual process can become compromised, affecting the component of vision that serves to establish the platform or base for higher conscious visual processing and perception. A compromise to the spatial-visual process affects child development. The compromise interferes with matching spatial-visual and proprioceptive information affecting postural alignment and weight shift.[3]

CLINICAL PRESENTATION

Visual Processing Dysfunction

Refers to visual compromise due to central pathology. Two clinical syndromes are recognized:

- Post-Trauma Vision Syndrome (PTVS)

- Following a neurological event, the spatial-visual process can become compromised, binding the focal process to the ambient or spatial-visual process. This has been termed *focal binding*.[3] The result causes a variety of symptoms and binocular dysfunctions that are characteristic of compromise in the spatial-visual process such as:
  - Exotropia and exophoria[17–19]
  - Diplopia[6]
  - Accommodative insufficiency[20]
  - Convergence insufficiency[20]
  - Deficiency in saccadic eye movements and pursuit tracking[20]
  - Photophobia[20]
  - Postural changes associated with compensation of vision dysfunction[11,15]
- Although symptoms and characteristics of binocular dysfunction are logically related to oculomotor nerve palsy, the mechanism for the cause of binocular dysfunction in the setting of PTVS appears to be related to trauma affecting the bimodal visual processing systems. Changes in visual evoked potential amplitude occur following treatment through use of base-in prisms and binasal occlusion. Following such treatment, a rapid decline in symptoms and syndrome characteristics may be seen. This condition has been termed PTVS.[21]
- VMSS—Bimodal visual processing dysfunction affecting posture, balance, and postural tone are common following a TBI.
  - TBI affects the balance of the bimodal visual process, which can alter the visual midline or egocenter.[17]
  - Common symptoms include perceived tilting of the floor, walls appearing to shift/move, drifting/leaning during ambulation, and abnormal weight shift.[17]

TREATMENT

Treatment of Centrally Mediated Visual Processing Dysfunction

Involves the discipline of NVPR. The following comprise the NVPR evaluation:

- Thorough review of history, visual acuities (near and far), visual field evaluation, sensorimotor evaluation, complex refraction, and refraction sequence evaluating state of binocular ranges and accommodative amplitudes for distance and near viewing, dynamic accommodation, binocularity, depth perception, color vision, visual midline assessment affecting posture and balance, and visual evoked potentials.[17]
- Lenses, prisms (compensatory and noncompensatory), and sectoral occlusion should be utilized to affect dysfunction in the bimodal visual process, and response to that intervention observed or recorded.[12,17]
  - Yoked prisms improve spatial orientation for visual neglect.[11,22,23]
  - Yoked prisms affect organization of the spatial-visual process with the proprioceptive BOS. Yoked or asymmetric yoked prisms can be used to realign displacement of the center of mass (CM) affecting balance and posture caused by VMSS.[24]
  - Binasal occlusion refers to a vertical opaque or translucent filter strip attached to the nasal border of each eyeglass lens. Its purpose is to provide a boundary or vertical line to support ambient visual processing for patients with PTVS.[25]

Neuro-Visual Postural Therapy

- NVPT emphasizes the analysis of the postural BOS and biomechanical alignment.[3]
- Unlike traditional vision therapy, NVPT facilitates organization of the spatial-visual process with the proprioceptive BOS to increase neuro-plasticity of the bimodal visual process, affecting posture and balance, and release of *focal binding* by enabling disassociation of the focal and ambient visual process.[3]
- The treatment approach should utilize yoked prisms as a facilitator for the organization of visual responses to match with body movements. The purpose of using the yoked prisms is to realign the visual midline or egocenter, which affects alignment of the CM. In turn, realignment engages the spatial-visual process with the BOS creating the anticipatory nature of vision prior to conscious perception. In other words, the spatial-visual process is the platform of higher vision and perception. When compromised it leaves the higher visual process functioning without the appropriate support.[3]
- A multidisciplinary approach is crucial and may include physical therapy, occupational therapy, and speech/language therapy.[17]

KEY POINTS

- The bimodal visual system is composed of two visual processes. The *focal visual process* is conscious and is oriented toward detail, attention, and concentration. The *ambient visual process* is preconscious and oriented toward spatial orientation, balance, posture, and movement.
- Following a TBI, VMSS and PTVS are common. Both of these conditions are consequences of an imbalance of the bimodal visual process. Thus, both conditions tend to occur together.
- Common signs and symptoms of PTVS following a TBI include diplopia, binocular vision dysfunction, accommodative dysfunction, and spatial disorientation. Common signs and symptoms of VMSS include abnormal weight shift, increase in postural tone, leaning or drifting during ambulation, and tilting of the floor.

STUDY QUESTIONS

1. Which of the following is not a characteristic of post-trauma vision syndrome (PTVS)?
   a. Exotropia and exophoria
   b. Convergence and accommodative insufficiency
   c. Oculomotor dysfunction
   d. Increased myopia
   e. Reduced best corrected visual acuity

2. Which of the following is not a symptom of PTVS?
   a. Diplopia and blurred vision
   b. Perceived movement of objects or patterns
   c. Headaches and asthenopia
   d. Hallucinations and photophobia
   e. Color blindness

3. The _____ visual process is oriented toward detail and the _____ visual process is oriented toward spatial orientation and posture.
   a. Ambient, focal
   b. Focal, ambient
   c. Spatial, focal
   d. Color, spatial

4. Which of the following is not a treatment for visual processing dysfunction following a TBI?
   a. Prism lenses
   b. NVPT
   c. Binasal occlusion
   d. Strabismus surgery

ADDITIONAL READING

Neuro-Optometric Rehabilitation Association (NORA). https://noravisionrehab.org
Cockerham G, Goodrich G, Weichel E, et al. Eye and visual function in traumatic brain injury. *J Rehabil Res Dev.* 2009;6:811–818. doi:10.1682/JRRD.2008.08.0109
Padula W, Argyris S, Ray J. Visual evoked potentials (VEP) evaluating treatment for post trauma vision syndrome in patients with traumatic brain injury. *Brain Inj.* 1994;8:125–133.
Padula W, Argyris S. Post trauma vision syndrome and visual midline shift syndrome. *J Neuro Rehabil.* 1996;6165–6171. doi:10.3109/02699059409150964
Sarno S, Erasmus G, Lippert M, et al. Electrophysiological correlates of visual impairment after traumatic brain injury. *Vision Res.* 2000;40:3029–3038. doi:10.1016/S0042-6989(00)00137-1

ANSWERS TO STUDY QUESTIONS

1. Correct Answer: e
   PTVS is caused by a compromise to the spatial-visual process causing disruption to binocularity.

   Further Reading:
   Padula W, Singman E, Magrum M, Munitz R. Evaluating and treating visual dysfunction. In: Zasler N, Katz D, Zafonte R, eds. *Brain Injury Medicine.* Demos Medical Publishing; 2013. doi:10.1891/9781617050572.0045

2. Correct Answer: e
   The symptoms of PTVS are caused by compromise of the spatial-visual process. This does not affect color vision.

   Further Reading:
   Padula WV, Argyris S, Ray J. Visual evoked potentials (VEP) evaluating treatment for post-trauma vision syndrome (PTVS) in patients with traumatic brain injuries (TBI). *Brain Inj.* 1994;8(2):125–133. doi:10.3109/02699059409150964

3. Correct Answer: b
   The bimodal visual process is composed of a "focal" visual process oriented to attention and concentration and an "ambient" visual process oriented toward supporting posture and balance upright against gravity.

Further Reading:
Padula W. *Neuro-Visual Processing: An Interdisciplinary Model for Neuro-Rehabilitation*. Optometric Extension Publishers; 2011.

4. Correct Answer: d
The ambient or spatial-visual process responds to changes produced by compression and expansion of visual space. Prisms, binasal occlusion, and NVPT provide options to establish rehabilitation of a spatial-visual processing compromise or dysfunction.

Further Reading:
Padula WV, Nelson CA, Padula WV, et al. Modifying postural adaptation following a CVA through prismatic shift of visuo-spatial egocenter. *Brain Inj*. 2009;23(6):566–576. doi:10.1080/02699050902926283

REFERENCES

The full reference list appears in the digital product found on http://connect.springer-pub.com/content/book/978-0-8261-4768-4/part/part03/chapter/ch34

COGNITIVE IMPAIRMENT: CHARACTERIZATION AND MANAGEMENT

ERIC B. LARSON

BACKGROUND

Formal structured assessment characterizes cognitive impairment relative to defined objective standards. In clinical settings, formal assessment identifies specific needs of the patient to inform management of care, including both treatment planning and patient education. It is an important complement to the bedside examination and neuroimaging since localization of a lesion and measurement of its size will not necessarily predict the impact on specific thinking abilities and on related function. This chapter focuses on implications for providers who work with patients who have moderate to severe traumatic brain injury (TBI).

Classification of Cognitive Impairment

Results of standardized assessment are reported in many different formats that vary by clinical setting. Although in some situations it is sufficient to limit reports to a terse qualitative summary that concludes with a diagnosis, in most settings it is necessary to document the details of test findings in a transparent format that explicitly states the quantitative basis of any conclusions and recommendations. Moreover, while citing test scores in documentation is helpful, it is also essential to recognize those quantitative data are useless and potentially harmful unless that documentation also includes interpretation in light of other clinical findings, as well as the patient's background and history. The following is a brief breakdown of parameters for reporting assessment results.

Approach

- *Dichotomous*: An aspect of cognition can be described with a brief qualitative label that indicates whether a problem is present or absent (e.g., "the patient was anomic" or "the patient remains in posttraumatic amnesia"). An advantage of this approach is that it does not require the reader of a report to know measurement theory to understand a finding.
- *Continuous*: Test performance can be described with a quantitative score which can be characterized in terms of deviation from a mean (e.g., "the patient scored 35 on the Boston Naming Test [<1st percentile for age and education], which was in the exceptionally low range"). An advantage of this approach is it communicates more information about the extent of the impairment and it specifies a criterion against which that impairment is measured.

Other parameters: Clinicians who choose to report assessment results in the form of continuous data will also need to consider the following when reporting those results: direction of scaling, selection of test norms, and range labels.

The full reference list appears in the digital product found on http://connect.springerpub.com/content/book/978-0-8261-4768-4/part/part03/chapter/ch35

- Direction of scaling
  - *Number correct*: large values indicate degree of strength.
  - *Number of errors*: large values indicate degree of weakness.
- Selection of test norms
  - Neurologically intact normative sample:
    - *Reference sample*: all examinees are measured against the same healthy reference group.
    - *Demographic-defined sample*: the examinee is measured against one of several different healthy cohorts matched on background characteristics (e.g., age and education).
  - Clinical normative sample:
    - To determine severity of a clinical condition, examinees are measured against others with that condition. For example, severity of aphasia in TBI may be characterized with percentiles relative to aphasics.
    - *Note*: A score corresponding to the 50th percentile relative to aphasics is much worse than a score that corresponds to the 50th percentile relative to a neurologically intact sample.
- Range labels
  - *Deviation-based labels*: describe how much a score differs from the mean.[1]

Exceptionally low score	<2nd percentile
Below average score	2nd to 8th percentile
Low average score	9th to 24th percentile
Average score	25th to 74th percentile
High average score	75th to 90th percentile
Above average score	91st to 97th percentile
Exceptionally high score	>98th percentile

  - *Impairment-based labels*: describe a score relative to a defined standard of impairment rather than deviation from a mean score, inherently implying a clinical conclusion. Some clinicians still use this approach, although it is falling out of favor since it oversimplifies interpretation of test scores (i.e., it implies impairment can be detected on the basis of an isolated test score).

Classification of Other Relevant Characteristics

- *Severity of injury* is rated by the Glasgow Coma Scale,[2] duration of loss of consciousness, and the duration of posttraumatic amnesia (PTA).
- *Stage of recovery* is described using the Rancho Los Amigos Scale of Cognitive Functioning[3] (see also Chapter 3).

DIAGNOSIS

Characterization of cognitive impairment involves different approaches to examination that evolve over the course of recovery. Regardless of the approach, responsible assessment does not begin and end with test scores. It involves analysis of contextual factors that impact those scores. It also incorporates complementary data from the patient's presentation.

Examination Approaches

Depending on what stage of recovery the patient has reached, any one of the following approaches may provide helpful quantitative data.

- *Assessment of level of arousal*—focuses on eye opening, visual tracking, responsiveness to commands, ability to answer questions. Standardized assessment can be performed with the JFK Coma Recovery Scale.[4]
- *Assessment of PTA*—addresses orientation, awareness of medical situation. Standardized assessment can be performed with the Galveston Orientation and Amnesia Test (GOAT)[5] or the Orientation Log (O-Log).[6] One accepted convention to establish emergence from PTA is to obtain GOAT scores of 78 and above for three consecutive days. (See also Chapter 33.)
- *Mental status exam*—screens for gross cognitive impairment by examining attention, recall, naming, auditory comprehension, reading, writing, simple construction ability. Standardized assessment can be performed with the Folstein Mini Mental State Examination[7] or the Montreal Cognitive Assessment (MOCA).[8]
- *Neuropsychological assessment*—provides detailed examination of cognitive domains. The typical time to refer inpatients for formal neuropsychological evaluation is after emergence from PTA. Examples of referral questions: Identify distinct areas of cognitive strengths and weaknesses. Assess severity of cognitive impairment. Determine if patient has independent decision-making ability. Assess need for supervision. Determine if patient is ready to attempt a return to work or school. Assess need for further cognitive rehabilitation. Determine impact of psychiatric factors on independent functioning.

Contextual Factors

An error that is common in clinical practice is a "test-bound" approach that treats an isolated test score as a sufficient basis for assessment of a cognitive domain. In contrast, thorough assessment recognizes the effects of multiple factors and weighs them into interpretation. Most cognitive constructs are complex and consequently the factors that affect measurement are very complicated. For example, interpretation of a score on a memory test should take the following into consideration.

- *Age and education*: This can usually be controlled by selecting the proper norm set (as described earlier). Most memory tests will allow you to compare a patient to others from the same demographic background.
- *Premorbid intelligence*: This can be estimated through a number of procedures. Demographic variables (e.g., years of education) are sometimes used by clinicians to form a rough estimate of cognitive ability. Since this is subject to substantial error, more precise estimates were developed using a combination of demographic variables and performance on standardized tests such as the Test of Premorbid Functioning.[9,10] The effects of intelligence on memory can then be controlled through analysis of the discrepancy of an actual memory score versus an expected memory score.
- *Level of effort:* Symptom validity testing can help assess whether patients may be exhibiting symptom magnification.
- *Fatigue*: Observation of a patient's level of arousal is an essential component of formal evaluation. When a patient shows evidence of somnolence during a particular test, the resulting score should be interpreted with caution.
- *Sensory or motor impairment*: Patients who are cognitively intact can appear impaired when physical impairment interferes with testing. For example, patients with intact capacity to learn and retain new information might appear impaired on a visual memory task if they do not wear corrective lenses that need during assessment.
- *Other cognitive abilities*: Impairment in one domain often exerts secondary effects in other domains. For example, attention deficits can affect initial encoding of information on memory testing. Language impairment can confound memory assessment when it interferes with comprehension of test items or expression of responses.

Clinical Presentation

- *Subjective complaints:* Moderate and severe TBI are associated with poor recall of diagnosis and limited awareness of disability. Depression or other psychological factors can result in magnification of symptoms and a failure to recognize progress.
- *Behavioral observation:*The following characteristic behaviors noted in conversation can be used to corroborate findings from other sources.
  - Attention impairment—distraction followed by a request for repetition or explanation of questions
  - Executive dysfunction—tangential thought or perseveration, impulsivity, and/or disinhibition
  - Language impairment—word-finding problems, word-substitution errors, irrelevant responses to questions because of poor understanding
  - Memory impairment—inability to recall important personal information (phone number, Social Security number) or to remember recent events (e.g., circumstances of referral for evaluation or treatment)

Assessment Controversies

- Computerized versions of standard neuropsychological tests are now available to users who do not have advanced psychometric training.
- The reliability of computer-administered neuropsychological tests was below acceptable levels in the majority of analyses reported in a recent literature review.[11]
- Innovative approaches to neuropsychological assessment, including computer-administered tests such as the battery designed by the National Institutes of Health (NIH Toolbox), show excellent psychometric properties that far exceed those of other applications currently available, although formal training is required to interpret the data they provide.[12]
- Although computer applications that administer and score neuropsychological tests may provide a narrative analysis of the results, it must again be emphasized that patients may be harmed when users fail to interpret those results in light of history, other neuropsychological measures, and data from other disciplines.[13]

TREATMENT

Guiding Principles

- Assess cost of therapeutic interventions (not just financial): For example, neurostimulant medication can cause or exacerbate psychosis. Cognitive remediation can cause frustration and fatigue.
- Assess potential benefit of interventions: Treatments that have not undergone randomized clinical trials should be recommended sparingly, if at all. Prescribing experimental interventions may provide false hope or divert patient resources away from validated treatment.
- Assess capacity of patients to participate: For example, psychotherapy may be of limited benefit in patients with marked cognitive impairment unless a neurologically intact family member joins treatment sessions.

Initial Management

In the early stages of recovery, treatment of cognitive impairment can include the following: neurostimulant medications, interaction with family members (verbal or nonverbal), early patient/family education, and orientation to medical situation. Some recommend withholding distressing news (e.g., recent deaths of loved ones) until the patient has emerged from PTA.

Ongoing Care

Later in recovery, treatment can include cognitive remediation, retraining in independent living skills, training in home exercises that can continue after therapy concludes, and gradual resumption of previously enjoyed activities. Psychotherapy may be beneficial if the family is involved and/or if the patient has emerged from PTA.

Treatment Controversies

- There is disagreement about the relative merits of direct remediation of cognitive impairment versus training in compensatory strategies to work around permanent deficits.[14]
- Computer-administered cognitive remediation applications are widely available and their developers claim their efficacy is well established. In contrast, peer-reviewed research has found more equivocal evidence of efficacy of such applications in people with TBI. A comprehensive review concluded such applications may have value as an adjunct to treatment with a therapist, but sole reliance on computer-administered remediation without care by a therapist was ineffective and is not recommended.[14] These findings and recommendations are consistent with those of a large review of similar applications in a nonclinical population, which concluded unsupervised at-home training is ineffective.[15]
- Innovative interventions are in development, including computer applications that incorporate new virtual reality technology, although evidence of efficacy is mixed, and unsupervised at-home training is specifically of questionable value.[16]

Prognosis

- In both moderate and severe injury, more diffuse cognitive impairment (affecting many areas of function) is observed in the early stages of recovery, and more specific impairment is observed by 12 months post injury.[17]
- By 6 years post-injury, memory is the most common persisting cognitive impairment (observed in more than 50% of severe TBI survivors).[18]

KEY POINTS

- Characterization of cognitive impairment is based on formal structured assessment that allows findings to be described relative to an objective standard.
- Assessment data are interpreted within the context of a patient's history and must be integrated with clinical information from other sources.
- Impairment is managed by identifying patient needs via assessment and tailoring treatment accordingly.
- Other factors to be considered in treatment planning include the patient's capacity to participate, cost, and potential benefit (as established by the research literature rather than by product marketing materials).

STUDY QUESTIONS

1. Which of the following is used to assess level of arousal?
   a. Galveston Orientation and Amnesia Test

    b. Orientation Log
    c. JFK Coma Recovery Scale
    d. Montreal Cognitive Assessment

2. Which of the following is a common source of error in assessment?
    a. A "test-bound" approach
    b. A dichotomous approach
    c. A continuous approach
    d. Scaling based on number correct

3. Which of the following is NOT a neurobehavioral correlate of executive dysfunction?
    a. Tangential thought or perseveration
    b. Impulsivity
    c. Disinhibition
    d. Anomia

4. Careful selection of test norms can control for the effects of which of the following?
    a. Inadequate effort
    b. Age and education
    c. Fatigue
    d. Sensory impairment

5. By 6 years after injury, which of the following is observed in more than 50% of severe TBI survivors?
    a. Memory impairment
    b. Fluent aphasia
    c. Hemispatial neglect
    d. Motor restlessness

ADDITIONAL READING

National Academy of Neuropsychology. Cognitive rehabilitation: official statement of the national academy of neuropsychology. http://www.nanonline.org/NAN/Files/PAIC/PDFs/NANPositionCogRehab.pdf.

Roebuck-Spencer T, Sherer M. Moderate and severe traumatic brain injury. In: Morgan JE, Ricker JH, eds. *Textbook of Clinical Neuropsychology.* 2nd ed. Taylor and Francis; 2018:387–410. doi:10.4324/9781315271743-17

Dikmen SS, Machamer JE, Powell JM, Temmkin NR. Outcome 3 to 5 years after moderate to severe traumatic brain injury. *Arch Phys Med Rehabil.* 2003;84:1449–1457. doi:10.1016/S0003-9993(03)00287-9

Dreer L, DeVivo M, Novack T, et al. Cognitive predictors of medical decision making in traumatic brain injury. *Rehabil Psychol.* 2008;53:486–497. doi:10.1037/a0013798

Hanks RA, Millis SR, Ricker JH, et al. The predictive validity of a brief inpatient neuropsychologic battery for persons with traumatic brain injury. *Arch Phys Med Rehabil.* 2008;89:950957. doi:10.1016/j.apmr.2008.01.011

ANSWERS TO STUDY QUESTIONS

1. Correct Answer: c
    The JFK Coma Recovery Scale provides standardized assessment of level of arousal, including eye opening, visual tracking, responsiveness to commands, and ability to answer questions.

Further Reading:
Giacino JT, Kalmar K, Whyte J. The JFK Coma Recovery Scale-Revised: measurement characteristics and diagnostic utility. *Arch Phys Med Rehabil.* 2004;85(12):2020–2029. doi:10.1016/j.apmr.2004.02.033

2. Correct Answer: a
A "test-bound" approach treats a test score in isolation as a sufficient basis for assessing a cognitive domain. In contrast, thorough assessment recognizes the effects of multiple factors and weighs them into interpretation.

Further Reading:
Sbordone RJ. Ecological validity: Some critical issues for the neuropsychologist. In RJ Sbordone, CJ Long, eds. *Ecological Validity of Neuropsychological Testing.* Gr Press/St Lucie Press, Inc.; 1996:15–41.

3. Correct Answer: d
Executive dysfunction is an abnormality of complex mental processes and cognitive abilities that control the skills required for goal-directed behavior. Perseveration, impulsivity, and disinhibition are all neurobehavioral problems associated with executive dysfunction, while anomia is a language problem.

Further Reading:
Wood RL, Worthington A. Neurobehavioral abnormalities associated with executive dysfunction after traumatic brain injury. *Front Behav Neurosci.* 2017;11:195. doi:10.3389/fnbeh.2017.00195

4. Correct Answer: b
Many tests have norms that control for the effects of age and education on performance.

Further Reading:
Lezak MD, Howieson DB, Loring DW. The rationale of deficit measurement. In: Lezak MD, ed. *Neuropsychological Assessment.* 4. Oxford University Press; 2004: 86–99.

5. Correct Answer: a
By 6 years post-injury, memory is the most common impairment (observed in more than 50% of severe TBI survivors).

Further Reading:
Tate RL, Fenelon B, Manning ML, Hunter M. Patterns of neuropsychological impairment after severe blunt head injury. *J Nerv Ment Dis.* 1991;179(3):117–126. doi:10.1097/00005053-199103000-00001

REFERENCES

The full reference list appears in the digital product found on http://connect.springer-pub.com/content/book/978-0-8261-4768-4/part/part03/chapter/ch35

BEHAVIORAL IMPAIRMENT: RECOGNITION AND MANAGEMENT

CYNTHIA L. BEAULIEU, TRACY SHANNON, AND JENNIFER BOGNER

GENERAL PRINCIPLES

Definition

Self-regulation is the ability to identify and produce a needed behavioral response. Deficits in regulation occur from either an inability to express behavior (initiation) or an inability to prevent expression of behavior (disinhibition) within the social context of the individual. Both types of deficits in self-regulation are often observed following moderate to severe traumatic brain injury (TBI). The following are common behavioral sequelae.

Impairments in Inhibition

- *Agitation*: "An excess of one or more behaviors that occurs during an altered state of consciousness."[1] Any excessive behavior can be classified as agitation, including but not limited to behaviors associated with restlessness, lability, disinhibition, or aggression. Agitation is observed in people with a range of disorders who experience an altered state of consciousness; following TBI, agitation is observed during posttraumatic amnesia/confusion.
- *Irritability, anger, and aggression*: Irritability is used to describe both the internal state (i.e., easily aggravated) and the external state (i.e., verbal or physical expressions of anger).[2] Aggression may be verbal or physical, and can be directed toward persons or objects.
- *Impulsivity and disinhibition*: Terms used to describe the tendency to behave without taking into consideration alternative actions or consequences. While both behaviors often run counter to social conventions, the two terms are distinct and can be individually defined.[3] *Impulsivity* refers to the behavioral tendencies (inability to suppress an action or verbalization) while disinhibition refers to the cognitive processes underlying the impulsivity.[4] *Social disinhibition* is defined as "socially inappropriate verbal, physical, or sexual acts which reflect a loss of inhibition or an inability to conform to social or cultural behavioral norms," which combines both behavior and cognition.[3,5]

Impairments in Initiation

- *Lack of initiation (inertia)*: Difficulties with starting an action despite the desire to do so.
- *Lack of empathy*: Loss or lack of remorse for actions or concern for others. May be observed as shallow or muted emotional reactivity in the context of distress in others.

The full reference list appears in the digital product found on http://connect.springerpub.com/content/book/978-0-8261-4768-4/part/part03/chapter/ch36

- *Apathy*: Loss or lack of interest, enthusiasm, or concern. May be observed as a lack of caring for or dismissal of goals and achievements.
- *Alexithymia*: Difficulty recognizing, identifying, or describing feelings or the subjective emotional experience.

Epidemiology

- Approximately one quarter to one third of patients receiving inpatient TBI rehabilitation in the United States display agitation during their inpatient hospitalization.[6-8] In the context of disorientation and confusion on acute care units and prior to rehabilitation, concomitant agitation has been reported in up to 70% of patients with TBI.[9]
- Reports of the incidence or prevalence of post-acute maladaptive behaviors have been wide-ranging due to differences in definitions and settings. A review of referrals to a behavior consult service suggested that 90% of maladaptive behaviors fall into approximately nine categories, including: physical aggression, verbal aggression, aggression toward self, aggression toward objects, sexually inappropriate/disinhibited behavior, socially inappropriate behavior, repetitive behavior, lack of initiation, and wandering behavior.[10] In one assessment of 514 community-based rehabilitation patients in Australia, a maladaptive behavior prevalence rate of approximately 54% was observed.[11] Aggression, inappropriate social behavior, and lack of initiation were the three most common types of maladaptive behaviors reported.
- Reports of the incidence and prevalence of reduced behavioral initiation and responsivity indicate up to 71% of persons with TBI will exhibit apathy,[12] up to 67% will exhibit impairments in empathy,[13-15] and up to 61% will exhibit alexithymia.[14]

Etiology and Pathophysiology

Following TBI, many individuals exhibit maladaptive behaviors that either did not exist prior to the injury or are exacerbations of pre-injury behaviors. While the environment, co-occurring disorders, and other person-related factors can contribute to the behavioral presentation, damage to the frontal and temporal regions and to connections of these regions to subcortical regions is frequently associated with changes in behavioral self-regulation.[16,17] The prefrontal cortex (PFC) is comprised of three major subdivisions—ventromedial (vmPFC), dorsolateral (dlPFC), and superior medial (mPFC). Collectively, these interconnected regions are responsible for behavioral integrity through feedback loops and pathways with subcortical structures such as the thalamus. Diffuse axonal injury occurring in these pathways can therefore result in loss of behavioral integrity. For example:

- vmPFC injury can lead to a decrease in impulse control, maintaining a consistent goal-directed response, and in regulating ongoing behavioral output.[18-21] Deficits in social conduct such as anger outbursts, impulsive actions, and sexual promiscuity have been reported following injury to this region.
- dlPFC injury can lead to difficulties in responding to unfamiliar or novel situations. While day-to-day routines may become rudimentary, any shift in the routine can create difficulty in problem-solving a needed or effective behavioral response.
- mPFC injury can lead to difficulties in drive and motivation, observed as a lack of responsiveness. Injuries to this area can result in akinetic mutism as well as behaviors and emotions described as muted or absent. Initiation to seek and maintain interactions with others may also be reduced. In severe cases, individuals may lack the capacity to initiate self-sustaining behaviors such as seeking out food and drink.

DIAGNOSIS

Risk Factors

▪ Post-TBI agitation is associated with lower cognitive functioning and the presence of factors that might decrease one's abilities to use cognitive and executive functions (e.g., medications that suppress cognition, presence of infection).[6] Otherwise, attempts to predict agitation have met with limited success.

▪ Predictors of aggression include age of onset (younger age at time of injury is associated with higher risk of developing aggression), communication deficits, and depression.[22,23]

▪ Identifying risk factors for the emergence of other maladaptive behaviors is extremely difficult. Multiple maladaptive behaviors may co-occur at any point in time. Nuanced features of any one behavior may be difficult to differentiate or isolate as a target for treatment. For example, apathy has been shown to impact outcome as it can interfere with rehabilitation, social/interpersonal functioning, and cognition. Apathy is commonly associated with depression, but apathy can also occur in the absence of depression. Predicting the emergence of apathy is challenging as it is not associated with severity of injury (e.g., duration of coma or posttraumatic amnesia), with time since injury, or with individual demographic characteristics such as age or education.[24] Careful clinical observation and diagnostic assessment are needed to determine factors driving maladaptive behavior.

Clinical Presentation

▪ Initially following injury, individuals may demonstrate periods of agitation associated with posttraumatic confusion. Agitation is characterized by a range of excessive behaviors that can be exacerbated by internal (e.g., disorientation, pain) and external (e.g., overstimulation) triggers. In the initial stages of recovery, agitation tends to be transient.[25]

▪ As individuals progress through the initial stages of recovery and orientation improves, difficulties with agitation often decrease; however, more specific problems with behavioral regulation can emerge.[26] (See Chapter 55 for a more detailed discussion of this topic.)

▪ Management of acute agitation and long-term behavioral changes associated with TBI is necessary to assist with treatment engagement, maintain patient and caregiver safety, and maximize the rehabilitation process and outcomes.[27–29]

Assessment

The assessment method should be chosen based on the nature of the target behavior(s). Rating scales have utility when the target is a cluster of behaviors that characterize one construct, such as agitation or irritability. If the target is a more specific behavior, such as physical aggression toward others, then functional behavioral analysis (FBA) will be more effective.

Rating Scales

Rating scales used to evaluate the effectiveness of interventions should provide more information than simply the presence or absence of the behavioral construct. The severity, frequency, and/or intensity should be measured serially on a continuous scale to evaluate changes from baseline to postintervention. Numerous rating scales have been developed for clinical and research purposes.[30] The few outlined here are those that have been frequently used to monitor the effectiveness of behavioral interventions.

- Given that agitation is comprised of a complex of excessive behaviors that can range in intensity, the *Agitated Behavior Scale* (ABS)[31] was developed to provide a method for quantifying the intensity of agitation by the extent that it interferes with functional activities. The ABS allows for serial assessments of agitation across observational periods (e.g., shifts, therapy sessions). The 14 behavioral items are rated on a scale of 1 through 4, with higher ratings indicating greater interference with functional activity and decreased responsiveness to redirection. The psychometrics of the ABS have been well established, indicating sound interrater reliability, internal consistency, concurrent validity, and construct validity.[31–34] Rating scale and factor analyses indicated that agitation as measured by the ABS is best represented as a unitary construct, though three correlated factors are present that may provide important clinical information (aggression, disinhibition, lability).[32,34]

- The *Neuropsychiatric Inventory*[35] was originally developed to evaluate behavioral disorders in persons with dementia. It has come into increased use with multiple neurological diagnoses, including TBI, as a means for assessing the effects of interventions on a range of psychiatric and behavioral disorders (e.g., thought disorders, agitation and aggression, irritability, disinhibition, depressed mood). Informants report on the presence, severity, and frequency of behaviors. Reliability, content, and concurrent validity have been established. Reports have been mixed regarding responsiveness to change.[36]

- The *Overt Aggression Scale*[37] is an observational scale involving the rating of aggressive behavior and the interventions that follow. It was adapted for use in neurorehabilitation settings by adding the ability to record information about antecedents as well as expanding information on interventions.[38] The scale provides information similar to that obtained using applied behavioral analysis (ABA) observational techniques. The measure has been used to report on the prevalence of aggressive behaviors as well as on the effectiveness of interventions.[30,37–39]

- The *Apathy Evaluation Scale* (AES)[40] is an 18-item scale that assesses features of apathy over the preceding 4 weeks. The AES has been validated for use with the TBI population, and has been found to discriminate effectively from features of depression and fatigue. The 14-item *Apathy* subscale of the *Frontal Systems Behavior Scale* (FrSBe-A)[41] has also demonstrated the ability to effectively assess apathy following TBI. The AES and the FrSBe-A differ in assessing apathy, with the AES assessing the emotional-affective features of apathy and the FrSBe-A assessing the cognitive-behavioral and goal-directed behaviors affected by apathy.[42]

Functional Behavioral Analysis

For the promotion of effective self-regulation of behavior, including initiation of adaptive behaviors and management of maladaptive behaviors in the post-acute stages of recovery, one needs to gain an understanding of the factors that influence current behavior through an FBA.

- FBA assists with informing the behavior treatment plan as it allows the treatment team to form interventions that specifically target the behavior.[43–45] Understanding the function of the individual's maladaptive behavior (e.g., task avoidance, social reinforcement, self-stimulation) and the context in which the behavior emerges allows for a more efficacious treatment plan. Continued data collection to assess the individual's response to the intervention (e.g., decrease in frequency, intensity) is necessary, as modification to the plan may be needed.

- FBA methods differ slightly depending on whether the approach is ABA or positive behavior interventions and supports (PBISs; see the Treatment section for details on these methods).[46] ABA utilizes a controlled environment that simulates potential conditions in the natural environment (usually four conditions: social negative reinforcement [task avoidance]; social positive reinforcement [attention, tangible items]; automatic reinforcement [self-stimulation]; and a control condition [access to play or preferred stimuli]).[38,39,43] PBIS functional analysis occurs within the natural environment, focusing on internal states and environmental factors that contribute to or impede positive behaviors.[46] For both approaches, once the function(s) of the behavior has been determined, an intervention can then be selected and a behavior plan implemented.

Adjunctive Assessments

Rating scales of behavior should be accompanied by serial assessments of cognition and level of confusion, pain, sleep, and any other patient-specific factors that may either be influencing the behavior or may be impacted by the intervention.

TREATMENT

Overview

Treatment can be categorized into one of two approaches—treatment designed for reduction of unwanted behavior or treatment designed for production of desired behavior. The former seeks to reduce, eliminate, or replace a generally high rate of behavior while the latter is designed to create or increase a generally low rate of behavior. In many cases, both types of treatment may be needed. Keep in mind that "maladaptive" behavior may be adaptive in select social contexts. The treatment goal for behavioral self-regulation is therefore to identify when the behavior is not needed, when the behavior is needed, and to adjust the intensity of the behavior within the context of the moment. Use of antecedent management, environmental management, reinforcements, consequences, shaping, contingencies, and other staples of behavior modification are employed to achieve the desired behavior.

Guiding Principles

- *Antecedent management can help foster positive behaviors and minimize maladaptive, undesired behaviors.* The control of antecedents (both internal and external, recent as well as remote) is required to facilitate positive behaviors in general.[46] Internal events can include the individual's sense of subjective well-being, level of physical discomfort, and clarity of thinking, among other factors. These factors can influence how the person is able to respond in accordance with goals and environmental demands. Ideally, the environment should facilitate positive behaviors by increasing the individual's ability to successfully meet demands. Environmental management of external triggers and barriers to positive behaviors is essential to shaping behavior, especially for those who are unable to self-monitor.[47] When manipulating the environment, the goal is to "establish external, situation and contextual influences on behavior" in order to shape behavior without placing an increased demand on the patient.[26] Individuals are more likely to respond with aggression or other maladaptive behaviors when they are confused, afraid, or are being asked to complete a task that is beyond their abilities. Provide a highly structured and consistent routine to assist with reducing these factors.[26]
- Identifying signs of escalating maladaptive behavior is also important (e.g., does the person appear to be tensing their muscles, breathing more heavily, does their face appear flushed). If such signs are identified early, redirection/distraction or a brief break may prevent a maladaptive behavior from fully emerging.[26] Additionally, if the maladaptive behavior is prevented, this can allow positive reinforcement for prosocial behavior (e.g., praising the individual for "walking away" when they needed a break).

■ *The consequences that follow the behavior can influence whether the behavior will occur again in the future.* Just as a maladaptive behavior is often a form of communication (e.g., I want your attention, this is too hard for me), it can also be maintained or extinguished by the caregiver or treatment team's response. Identifying contingencies that maintain, reduce, or increase the positive or negative behavior often inform the treatment process. For example, if an individual engages in a maladaptive behavior in order to gain attention, attending to prosocial behaviors and ignoring the maladaptive behavior (if the behavior does not place an individual at substantial risk) is recommended. In contrast, if an individual engages in a maladaptive behavior in order to escape from the task demand, structuring the task demands such that demands decrease only with prosocial behavior will be more effective.

■ *Treatment should, at best, enhance cognitive functioning; at worst, treatment should have no effect on cognition.* Deficits in cognitive and executive functioning are thought to often underlie agitation as well as later-occurring behavioral impairments. Based on this premise, treatment should work to maximize orientation and cognition, or at the minimum, not have any deleterious effects. This guiding principle is most applicable to pharmacological treatments that can vary according to whether they work to enhance cognition versus suppress excessive behavior through sedation. Animal studies have demonstrated that the use of antipsychotic agents to suppress behavior at the expense of cognition has a negative impact on short- and long-term outcomes.[48] Human studies have been limited and often based on observational rather than experimental designs; however, they lend support to the need to carefully assess the positive and negative effects of a pharmacological intervention on cognition, due to the potential deleterious impact on both short- and long-term outcomes.[6,7,49,50] For example, the use of antipsychotic agents or benzodiazepines to control agitation may suppress cognition and increase sedation, which can not only have a paradoxical effect on the behavior but can also impact short- and long-term outcomes.[49]

In addition to considering pharmacological agents that enhance rather than suppress cognition, treatment should focus on other internal factors that can impact cognition. Studies of small clinical samples have indicated that stabilization of the sleep/wake cycle is needed for improvement in cognition and agitation.[51] It has also been recommended that treatment of underlying disorders that can increase discomfort or confusion (e.g., infections, respiratory distress, constipation) be one of the first considerations for reducing agitation.[6,52] If changes in behavior occur rapidly, additional laboratory studies and radiographic assessment may be recommended to rule out metabolic disturbance, infection process, emergence of a new hemorrhage, and so on.

Acute Management

■ Agitation during the early stages of recovery from TBI is typically managed in a structured, predictable environment. Staff should be trained in how to skillfully redirect agitated behaviors. Families should be assisted in understanding that agitation is not willful or under the control of the patient, and provided with guidance regarding the avoidance of triggers that may exacerbate agitation.

■ As recommended by the International Traumatic Brain Injury Cognitive Rehabilitation Guidelines (INCOG),[53] some of the key components to an environment that provides the best opportunities for socially acceptable, adaptive behaviors include: consistency in staff, schedule, physical environment, and expectations; free, supervised movement without physical restraint; control of triggers (people, places, activities) that are associated with maladaptive behaviors; family and staff training to assist in understanding the behavioral impairments and management; and a means for the individual to communicate needs effectively.

■ Treatment plans for later-occurring behavioral impairments are best developed through direct observation, to determine the antecedents that may be triggering the behavior, the functions that the behaviors may serve, and the consequences that are maintaining the undesired behavior. Trained mental health professionals can develop plans to alter factors that trigger or maintain the behavior. Staff and family members can be trained to institute the plans, though ongoing assistance may be needed from the plan designer to monitor and troubleshoot.

■ The two primary approaches to increasing positive behaviors and decreasing maladaptive behavior include ABA and PBISs.[46] ABA is ideally implemented in environments where it is possible to exert consistent control over antecedents and consequences. The focus tends to be on the progressive shaping of specific behaviors. PBIS has its roots in classical ABA, but places a greater emphasis on the improvement of one's overall environment and quality of life. Adaptive behavior is encouraged (and undesired behavior discouraged) by identifying and modifying factors that can enhance the person's lifestyle, well-being, and overall functioning. The program is focused on antecedents, including environmental barriers and supports to adaptive behavior, as well as internal events (e.g., pain, frustration). Treatment is ideally provided within the person's natural setting to allow for ease in generalization.

■ Some of the techniques used with PBIS and ABA are as follows:

● Tasks can be adjusted to help to ensure early success and create behavioral momentum. Behavioral momentum strategies have been found helpful in obtaining and increasing treatment compliance/participation as it allows the individual to complete more basic tasks and build up confidence/momentum to complete more difficult/frustrating tasks.[54]

● Structuring the day and the environment to ensure routine in the context of meaningful activities and social exchanges.[46]

● Utilization of verbal cues (sometimes combined with physical cues) can be of benefit with regard to management of poor initiation. Using the same verbal cues or prompts is recommended to reduce confusion. Eventually, visual or external cues (e.g., lists, signs, wall calendars, phone alarms) can be used and verbal prompts can be faded out.

● Role playing and practice with various difficult social interactions following TBI may be of benefit in teaching individuals strategies for how to start conversations, avoid sexually inappropriate comments, and so on.

● For management of sexually inappropriate behavior, utilization of behavioral strategies may be warranted, in addition to providing the individual with feedback regarding the appropriateness of the behavior. It is recommended that when this feedback is provided, the caregiver must remain calm, straight-faced, and refrain from scolding or otherwise reinforcing the behavior (e.g., avoid laughing at the comment or behavior).

Ongoing Management

Individuals who are experiencing success in achieving their goals are more likely to maintain positive behaviors. With greater recovery and improved insight, the individual may be able to exert greater control of their behavior through the avoidance or management of triggers. Family and others within the environment can also support positive behaviors by monitoring their own behavior. Mental health professionals can assist the individual and family with identifying elements in their interactions that might trigger undesired behaviors.

Treatment Uncertainties

To date, there is minimal evidence to support the use of any one pharmacological intervention over another to reduce agitation or other undesired behaviors. Randomized controlled studies are difficult to conduct due to the heterogeneity of the population and the urgency to control maladaptive behaviors. Single-subject experimental designs are most often used to evaluate the effectiveness of behavioral interventions for individuals, and elements of these designs should be incorporated into clinical practice to assess effectiveness of a given intervention.

KEY POINTS

- Conduct a thorough assessment of the antecedents associated with the behavior, including both internal factors and external triggers.
- Collect information regarding function of the behavior (analyze the antecedents, behaviors, and consequence) when formulating a plan.
- Consider the patient's cognitive status and ensure that interventions serve to enhance cognitive functioning, or at a minimum do not impede cognitive functions.
- When possible, make modifications to the environment including reducing chaotic stimuli, providing breaks, and maintaining structure and routine.
- Continue to monitor after implementing an intervention to ensure the intervention is effective, or consider modifying the plan.

STUDY QUESTIONS

1. Which variables are most critical to include in assessment of maladaptive behaviors?
   a. Nutrition, supplements, and vitamins
   b. Opioids, SSRIs, and antipsychotics
   c. Personality, values, and beliefs
   d. Injury, individual, and environment

2. For severely maladaptive behavior such as physical aggression, what approach should be the default approach when considering treatment selection?
   a. Least restriction
   b. Variable restriction
   c. Consistent restriction
   d. Most restriction

3. What considerations should be given to the use of pharmacological intervention for severe maladaptive behavior?
   a. Pharmacological intervention should only be considered in lieu of behavioral intervention.
   b. Behavioral intervention should only be considered in lieu of pharmacological intervention.
   c. The potential for negative effects on cognition warrants careful monitoring of pharmacological interventions that target maladaptive behavior.
   d. Behavioral interventions are the treatment of choice for all maladaptive behavior.

4. What is the most common method to study the effectiveness of behavioral interventions?
   a. Single-subject experimental designs

   b. Randomized controlled trials
   c. Clinical medication trials
   d. None of the above

5. Which of the following is good practice for a caregiver struggling at home with caring for a person with TBI and maladaptive behavior?
   a. Prescribe medication(s) for the caregiver to ensure symptoms they may be experiencing are treated.
   b. Routinely assess the caregiver during patient office visits, encourage the caregiver to seek and accept assistance, and provide education for accessing support and resources.
   c. TBI rarely affects caregivers and therefore rarely requires action by a TBI provider.
   d. TBI always affects caregivers and therefore caregivers should be treated simultaneously with persons with TBI.

ADDITIONAL READING

The Agitated Behavior Scale: https://wexnermedical.osu.edu/-/media/files/wexnermedical/patient-care/healthcare-services/neurological-institute/departments-and-centers/research-centers/ohio-valley/for-professionals/agitation/abs_scale.pdf?la=en&hash=649ED35754A81D13277BF3891AD70A0F-057D4A4B

Accommodating Symptoms of TBI: https://wexnermedical.osu.edu/-/media/files/wexnermedical/patient-care/healthcare-services/neurological-institute/departments-and-centers/research-centers/ohio-valley/for-professionals/accommodating-symptoms/accommodating-tbi-booklet-1-14.pdf?la=en&hash=175F7559BA27362695DDBC8121A89C85F794F4D0

Ponsford J, Sloan S, Snow P. *Traumatic Brain Injury: Rehabilitation for Everyday Adaptive Living.* 2nd ed. Psychology Press; 2013. doi:10.4324/9780203082805

Baguley IJ, Cooper J, Felmingham K. Aggressive behavior following traumatic brain injury: how common is common? *J Head Trauma Rehabil.* 2006;21(1):45–56. doi:10.1097/00001199-200601000-00005

Hicks AJ, Clay FJ, Hopwood M, et al. The efficacy and harms of pharmacological interventions for aggression after traumatic brain injury: systematic review. *Front Neurol.* 2019;10:1169. doi:10.3389/fneur.2019.01169

Ylvisaker M, Turkstra L, Coehlo C, et al. Behavioral interventions for children and adults with behavior disorders after TBI: a systematic review of the evidence. *Brain Inj.* 2007;21(8):769–805. doi:10.1080/02699050701482470

ANSWERS TO STUDY QUESTIONS

1. Correct Answer: d
The location and extent of structural damage to the brain, individual pre-injury and post-injury behavioral repertoires and interpersonal skills, and environmental context can contribute adaptively or maladaptively to behavior. Assessment of these variables allows for a more thorough understanding of factors that play a role in creating or sustaining maladaptive behavior.

Further Reading:
Ponsford J, Sloan S, Snow P. *Traumatic Brain Injury: Rehabilitation for Everyday Adaptive Living,* 2nd ed. Psychology Press; 2013.

2. Correct Answer: a
Behavioral treatments are guided by the principle of "least restrictive" approach. Treatment that is likely to be the most effective while maintaining the most normative

context is the treatment of choice. The most positive and least depriving intervention is the ideal starting point.

Further Reading:
Jacobs HE. *Behavior Analysis Guidelines and Brain Injury Rehabilitation: People, Principles and Programs.* Aspen Publishers; 1993.

3. Correct Answer: c
Treatment of behavior with behavioral interventions versus pharmacological interventions is not an "either/or" situation. Both can be appropriate depending on case-specific needs. While pharmacological agents can be swift in their effectiveness, they can also produce negative side effects for cognition and long-term recovery. Cognition should be carefully monitored along with the target behavior to ensure that cognition is not sacrificed in service to behavioral control. The least restrictive principle applies across all interventions for maladaptive behavior.

Further Reading:
Ponsford J, Sloan S, Snow P. *Traumatic Brain Injury: Rehabilitation for Everyday Adaptive Living,* 2nd ed. Psychology Press; 2013.
Hicks AJ, Clay FJ, Hopwood M, et al. The efficacy and harms of pharmacological interventions for aggression after traumatic brain injury: systematic review. *Front Neurol.* 2019;10:1169. doi:10.3389/fneur.2019.01169

4. Correct Answer: a
Minimal evidence exists for the effectiveness of medications to induce behavior change. The heterogeneity of individual behaviors and the generally urgent need to change maladaptive behaviors precludes ease of study through randomized controlled trials. Single-subject experimental designs are often used to study the effects of behavioral interventions and these designs can be easily incorporated into clinical practice.

Further Reading:
Heinicke, MR, Carr, JE. Applied behaviour analysis in acquired brain injury rehabilitation: a meta-analysis of single-case design intervention research. *Behav Interv.* 2014;29:77–105. doi:10.1002/bin.1380

5. Correct Answer: b
TBI can significantly increase burden of care for families. Providers should familiarize themselves with common struggles experienced by persons with TBI and by their loved ones. Caregiver well-being should be routinely assessed. Caregivers should be encouraged to seek assistance when needed. Refer to the BIAA website and to Chapter 9 in the following Further Reading entry

Further Reading:
Ponsford J, Sloan S, Snow P. Traumatic Brain Injury: Rehabilitation for Everyday Adaptive Living. 2nd ed. New York, NY: Psychology Press; 2013.

REFERENCES

The full reference list appears in the digital product found on http://connect.springer-pub.com/content/book/978-0-8261-4768-4/part/part03/chapter/ch36

RATIONAL NEUROPHARMACOLOGY IN TRAUMATIC BRAIN INJURY

DURGA ROY, SANDEEP VAISHNAVI, AND VANI A. RAO

BACKGROUND

Neuropsychiatric impairments are common after traumatic brain injury (TBI). These include cognitive impairment, mood and anxiety disorders, psychosis, behavioral problems, apathy, and sleep disturbance. It is important to remember that most medications used for neuropsychiatric symptoms after TBI are off-label. More detailed descriptions of various disorders and their management, including less commonly used medications not mentioned in this chapter, can be found elsewhere.[1-3] This chapter provides a brief overview of only the pharmacological treatment of common neuropsychiatric problems after TBI. Management of these conditions should be multidisciplinary and include both pharmacological and nonpharmacological interventions.

The two tables that follow highlight the prevalence, core features of neuropsychiatric symptoms and syndromes following TBI (Table 37.1)[2,4,5] and the first-line pharmacological agents the authors recommend using for treatment (Table 37.2)[3,6]

GENERAL GUIDELINES FOR MANAGEMENT

Choose a Medication

In general, pharmacotherapy for neuropsychiatric problems after TBI is similar to that for primary psychiatric disorders but with extra caution, as persons with TBI may be more vulnerable to side effects.[7-9] The following are a few treatment guidelines.

Start low, go slow but do not stop until clinically therapeutic levels are attained. In other words, "Start low, go slow, but go."

A typical starting point would be one third to one half of the usually recommended dose. Increase the dose slowly. Persons with TBI are very sensitive to side effects of medications. Medications with known adverse central nervous system (CNS) effects, such as sedatives or anticholinergic drugs, should be avoided whenever possible as they have the potential to impair cognition and impede neural plasticity.

Minimize the Number of Medications

Treat at an adequate dose and for an appropriate length of time with a single agent before switching medications. If there is a partial response, consider augmenting with another

---

The full reference list appears in the digital product found on http://connect.springerpub.com/content/book/978-0-8261-4768-4/part/part03/chapter/ch37

TABLE 37.1   Prevalence, Core Features, and First-Line Treatment of Posttraumatic Brain Injury Neuropsychiatric Presentations

Symptoms and Conditions	Prevalence (All Injury Severities)	Core Features
Cognitive deficits	5%–60%	Disturbances of (a) memory, (b) attention/processing speed, and/or (c) executive function
Depression	6%–77%	Low mood, loss of pleasure, hopelessness, reduced self-attitude, suicidal ideation
Mania	1%–9%	Elated mood and/or irritability, increased energy, impulsivity
Anxiety	11%–70%	Persistent worry, tension, dread or apprehension; autonomic arousal
Psychosis	2%–20%	Hallucinations, delusions, thought disorder
Behavioral dyscontrol	11%–70%	Agitation, aggression, mood lability, disinhibition, impulsivity
Apathy	10%	Lack of motivation or drive, loss of initiative (euthymic mood)
Sleep disorders	30%–70%	(a) Insomnia (early or middle) (b) Hypersomnia and fatigue (c) Parasomnia

Sources: Data from Vaishnavi S, Rao V, Fann JR. Neuropsychiatric problems after traumatic brain injury: Unraveling the silent epidemic. *Psychosomatics*. 2009;50(3):198–205. doi:10.1176/appi. psy.50.3.198; Warden DL, Gordon B, McAllister TW. Guidelines for the pharmacologic treatment of neurobehavioral sequelae of traumatic brain injury. *J Neurotrauma*. 2006;23(10):1468–1501. doi:10.1089/neu.2006.23.1468; Rao V, Koliatsos V, Ahmed F, et al. Neuropsychiatric disturbances associated with traumatic brain injury: a practical approach to evaluation and management. *Semin Neurol*. 2015;35(1):64–82. doi:10.1055/s-0035-1544241

agent. Because CNS side effects are additive, use caution when prescribing more than one psychotropic agent. Watch for drug–drug interactions and monitor serum levels of medications if available.

Consider Coexisting Medical Problems

As seizure disorders are more common in TBI patients than in the general population, drugs that lower the seizure threshold—for example, clozapine and clomipramine—should be used with caution.

Caution

Avoid anticonvulsants such as phenytoin, benzodiazepines, and first-generation antipsychotics such as haloperidol in the acute post-TBI period, as there is strong evidence that they can worsen cognitive functioning[10] and adversely impact neural plasticity.[11] Anticholinergics (e.g., hydroxyzine) and antihistamines (e.g., diphenhydramine) should also be avoided due to their adverse effects on the CNS. Monoamine oxidase inhibitors (MAOIs) should be avoided due to their extensive food and drug interactions.

TABLE 37.2 First-Line Agents in the Management of Psychiatric Aspects Following Traumatic Brain Injury

Psychiatric Problems	First-Line Medications	Mechanism of Action	Standard Dosage	Common Adverse Effects	Precautions
Depression	Sertraline	Inhibits reuptake of serotonin	50–150 mg/d	Gastrointestinal side effects—e.g., nausea, diarrhea; sexual dysfunction	In persons at risk for bipolar disorder can cause switch to mania/hypomania
	Escitalopram	As in the preceding case	5–20 mg/d	As in the preceding case	
Mania: acute	Quetiapine	Antagonist activity at dopamine and serotonin receptors	25–300 mg/d	Parkinsonism; sedation, metabolic syndrome	Caution in older adults, those with cerebrovascular disease, dementia. Monitor weight, blood sugar, and lipids
Mania: maintenance	Valproate	Blocks voltage-gated sodium channels and increased levels of gamma-aminobutyric acid (GABA)	250–1,500 mg/d; in two divided doses	Nausea, abnormal liver functions, weight gain, tremor. hair thinning	Can increase levels of other anticonvulsants secondary to inhibiting their metabolism
Anxiety	Similar to depression				
PTSD	Sertraline	See Depression			Avoid benzodiazepines
Psychosis	Risperidone	Reduces dopaminergic neurotransmission in the mesolimbic pathway	0.25–4 mg/d	Parkinsonism; sedation, metabolic syndrome	Caution in older adults, those with cerebrovascular disease, dementia. Monitor weight, blood sugar, and lipids
	Quetiapine	See Mania			
	Lurasidone	Central dopamine type 2 (D) and serotonin type 2 (5HT2A) receptor antagonism	20–80 mg/d	Drowsiness, akathisia, parkinsonism	To be taken with 360 calories; avoid grapefruit/juice

(continued)

TABLE 37.2   First-Line Agents in the Management of Psychiatric Aspects Following Traumatic Brain Injury (continued)

Psychiatric Problems	First-Line Medications	Mechanism of Action	Standard Dosage	Common Adverse Effects	Precautions
Insomnia	Ramelteon	Melatonin agonist	8 mg	Dizziness, tiredness, daytime drowsiness	To be taken within 30 minutes of going to bed
	Trazodone	Inhibits reuptake of serotonin; blocks histamine and alpha-1 adrenergic receptors	50–200mg	Nausea, lightheadedness, orthostasis, daytime drowsiness	To prevent falls related to orthostasis, have the person rise slowly from a sitting or a lying down position
Apathy	Methylphenidate	Inhibits reuptake of dopamine	5–40 mg/d; divided doses	Agitation, insomnia, palpitations	Second dose to be given early afternoon
Memory deficits	Donepezil	Central reversible acetyl cholinesterase inhibitor	5–10 mg at night	Nausea, diarrhea, insomnia	Can cause bradycardia and syncope
Executive function deficits	Amantadine	Noncompetitive antagonism at NMDA receptor; enhances dopaminergic transmission	100–400 mg; divided doses	Headache, nausea, diarrhea, orthostasis; psychosis at high doses	Avoid in patients with history of seizures. Avoid or use lower doses in persons with kidney failure
Inattention	Methylphenidate	See Apathy			

NMDA, N-methyl-D-aspartate; PTSD, posttraumatic stress disorder.

Sources: Data from Vaishnavi S, Rao V, Fann JR. Neuropsychiatric problems after traumatic brain injury: Unraveling the silent epidemic. *Psychosomatics.* 2009;50(3):198–205. doi:10.1176/appi.psy.50.3.198; Polich G, Iaccarino MA, Zafonte R, Psychopharmacology of traumatic brain injury. *Handb Clin Neurol.* 2019;165:253–267. doi:10.1016/B978-0-444-64012-3.00015-0; Warden DL, Gordon B, McAllister TW. Guidelines for the pharmacologic treatment of neurobehavioral sequelae of traumatic brain injury. *J Neurotrauma.* 2006;23(10):1468–1501. doi:10.1089/neu.2006.23.1468; Rao V, Koliatsos V, Ahmed F, et al. Neuropsychiatric disturbances associated with traumatic brain injury: a practical approach to evaluation and management. *Semin Neurol.* 2015;35(1):64–82. doi:10.1055/s-0035-1544241

TREATMENT OF SPECIFIC POSTTRAUMATIC BRAIN INJURY DISORDERS

Cognitive Impairment

- *Arousal*: Psychostimulants and dopaminergic agonists have been used in the treatment of decreased arousal after TBI. Amantadine has been shown to increase arousal post-injury in a review, several case reports, retrospective studies, and randomized controlled trials with initiation from 3 days to 5 months post injury.[12–14] Methylphenidate has also been shown to improve decreased arousal during rehabilitation following TBI.[15,16]

- *Memory impairment:* Cholinergic augmentation with cholinesterase inhibitors is a reasonable first-line treatment for memory impairment. Possible benefits with donepezil have been noted in small case studies and in a systematic review.[17–19] Rivastigmine has been demonstrated to be safe, well tolerated, and effective in patients with moderate to severe TBI.[20,21] Galantamine was also found to be superior to placebo for improvement in episodic memory.[22]

- *Impaired attention and slow processing speed:* Psychostimulants are the mainstay of treatment for impaired attention and processing speed. Commonly used psychostimulants include methylphenidate, amphetamine, dextroamphetamine, and amphetamine sulfate. Often, symptoms consistent with dysexecutive syndrome including deficits in attention, focus, and goal-directed thinking are targets of these agents. A few studies have demonstrated the effectiveness of methylphenidate on various attentional tasks.[23,24] Other agents such as amantadine and acetylcholinesterase inhibitors (physostigmine, donepezil, and galantamine) can also be considered.

- *Executive dysfunction:* Stimulants such as methylphenidate, bromocriptine, lisdexamfetamine, noradrenergic agonist agents such as atomoxetine, which increase norepinephrine (and to a lesser extent, dopamine), and amantadine can be used to treat executive dysfunction.[24,25] However, it is important to remember that all these agents probably exert an effect via improving the attentional component of the dysexecutive syndrome.

Depression (See Also Chapter 53)

- *Selective serotonin reuptake inhibitors (SSRIs):* SSRIs are the first-line treatment for post-TBI depression because of their safety and tolerability.[26] Sertraline, the most dopaminergic of the SSRIs, has the best evidence supporting its use. However, the data are mixed.[27–30] Sertraline has also been found to be effective as a prophylactic agent for the prevention of depression following TBI.[31] Other commonly used SSRIs include citalopram and escitalopram. Citalopram has been shown to increase rates of remission from episodes of major depression in open label studies.[32] The use of SSRIs such as fluoxetine and paroxetine has a higher potential for drug–drug interactions due to inhibition of various enzymes in the cytochrome P450 system.[33] (Note that there is some concern about use of SSRIs and bleeding secondary to its platelet activating effects; however, the relative risk of intracranial bleeding is small.[34])

- *Serotonin–norepinephrine reuptake inhibitors (SNRIs):* SNRIs, dual reuptake inhibitors of both serotonin and norepinephrine (e.g., venlafaxine, duloxetine), may also be effective. SNRIs can be considered as first-line agents in persons with depression and chronic pain.

- *Tricyclic antidepressants (TCAs):* TCAs, which block reuptake of norepinephrine and serotonin, can be quite effective for depression in some TBI patients. Desipramine has been shown to be effective in treating patients with depression who suffered severe TBI.[35] Nortriptyline is considered to be the least anticholinergic and antihistaminergic among the TCAs and has demonstrated efficacy in the treatment of depression following stroke.[36] Although amitriptyline is recommended by certain groups,[4] the authors recommend use with caution secondary to its severe anticholinergic side effects. In general, due to the unfavorable side effect profile of TCAs (i.e., anticholinergic effects, antihistaminergic effects, weight gain, risk for seizures, and cardiac side effects such as orthostasis and arrhythmias), most clinicians use TCAs only if an initial trial of SSRIs has been unsuccessful.

- *Mirtazapine:* Mirtazapine, a presynaptic alpha-2 adrenergic and serotonin receptor antagonist, can be especially useful when insomnia or anorexia is a presenting comorbid symptom.
- *Dopamine–norepinephrine reuptake inhibitors (DNRI):* Bupropion, which facilitates dopamine transmission and has effects on norepinephrine, is known to lower the seizure threshold. When it must be used, the long-acting XL form is preferred with a daily dosage not to exceed 300 mg.
- Monoamine oxidase inhibitors (MAOIs): MAOIs may be used in persons with recalcitrant depression. However, the adherence to an MAOI appropriate diet can be difficult for persons with TBI. Further, there are no studies in the TBI population to support MAOI use.
- *Neuroleptics:* In cases of major depression with psychotic features, or in cases of depression with severe agitation or aggression, atypical antipsychotics (e.g., risperidone, olanzapine) may be used in conjunction with antidepressants. First-generation antipsychotics such as haloperidol should be avoided, as they can increase neuronal toxicity[37] and impede neural plasticity.[11] Further, dopamine blockade is relatively contraindicated after TBI, as these patients are typically dopamine-deficient.
- *Psychostimulants:* Methylphenidate might also have antidepressant effects comparable to those observed with sertraline.[38,39]
- *Brain stimulation therapies:* Electroconvulsive therapy (ECT) was found to be safe and effective in a retrospective chart review of a small group of 11 TBI subjects.[40] More research is needed in this area before its use can be recommended in a clinical context.

Suicidal Ideation Following Traumatic Brain Injury

- The most important factor in the management of suicidal ideation is to maintain safety. Immediate hospitalization should be considered for patients with active suicidal thoughts with intent or plan to die. Management of suicidal thoughts associated with psychiatric disturbances after TBI should focus on the primary psychiatric disturbances.

Mania

- *Anticonvulsants:* Anticonvulsants such as valproate[41] are the first-line treatment for post-TBI mania and bipolar disorder. Close monitoring of serum levels, liver function, and blood counts is recommended. Carbamazepine has also been studied in individual cases and shown to be effective in treating symptoms of post-TBI mania.[42]
- *Lithium:* Anecdotal reports[43] and animal studies[44] suggest efficacy, but clinical trials are needed. As TBI patients are particularly prone to its neurotoxic side effects, lithium should be used with caution and is usually reserved for patients with a prior history of mania. Serum levels of lithium and kidney and thyroid functions should be regularly monitored.
- *Neuroleptics:* While data in the TBI population are scant, there are a few case studies documenting the effectiveness of quetiapine.[45,46] Quetiapine has lower D2 binding affinity, making it less likely to induce extrapyramidal symptoms in patients with TBI. We recommend use of quetiapine as a first-line and risperidone or olanzapine as a second-line agent for acute mania or when psychosis, agitation, or restlessness is present.

Anxiety

- *SSRIs:* Sertraline is the first-line option for treating anxiety disorders following TBI. Citalopram may be a reasonable second choice, but caution is recommended above 20 mg daily because of potential cardiac adverse effects.
- *SNRIs:* SNRIs may also be a good option for anxiety in TBI patients.
- *Buspirone:* Buspirone is a partial 5-HT1A receptor agonist and alpha-2 antagonist that can be used safely as an anxiolytic in patients with TBI, though studies are lacking. Buspirone can be considered as a first-line agent because of its benign side effect profile and lack of significant drug–drug interactions.[47]
- *Other agents:*
  - Mirtazapine or tricyclic agents may also be considered, but there are no clinical trials to support their effectiveness.
  - Benzodiazepines should be used with extreme caution because their adverse effects can amplify TBI-related impairments. Animal studies also indicate that benzodiazepines may delay or impede neuronal recovery.[48] If they have to be used, they should only be prescribed for a short period until an SSRI or SNRI takes effect. Under such circumstances, preferable benzodiazepines include lorazepam secondary to milder side effects or clonazepam secondary to reduced risk of abuse/dependence.

Psychosis

- *Neuroleptics:* Atypical antipsychotics are the drugs of choice for psychosis following TBI. They are preferred over the older "typical" antipsychotics because of the lower incidence of neurological side effects such as extrapyramidal side effects and because they do not inhibit dopamine release to the same degree. The authors recommend use of risperidone, quetiapine, or lurasidone because of their favorable risk-to-benefit ratio. There are case reports on the effectiveness of olanzapine[49,50] and aripiprazole;[51] however, these scant data are not sufficient to formulate a formal recommendation for their use.
- *Anticonvulsants:* If there is no improvement on neuroleptics, anticonvulsants such as valproate or carbamazepine may be a reasonable alternative, and may specifically aid with management of agitation.

Behavioral Dyscontrol

A syndrome of behavioral dyscontrol characterized by mood lability, agitation, aggression, impulsivity, disinhibition, or apathy can often be seen in TBI. Patients can act impulsively in response to certain stimuli. For the treatment of behavior dyscontrol, it is important to determine if the behavioral symptoms are secondary to an affective disorder, psychosis, or cognitive deficits and then choose medications accordingly.[52]

- *Antidepressants:* In general, the authors tend to use low-dose SSRIs as a first-line treatment for chronic agitation and aggression, especially if comorbid depressive symptoms exist. Antidepressants have also been shown to be effective in cases of affective lability and syndromes of impulsivity or disinhibition related to TBI, such as pathological laughter and crying (PLAC) also known as pseudobulbar affect (PBA). Dextromethorphan/ quinidine in combination has been approved by the Food and Drug Administration for use in PBA. Dextromethorphan is an uncompetitive N-methyl-D-aspartate (NMDA) receptor antagonist, sigma-1 receptor agonist, and an SNRI; quinidine increases bioavailability of dextromethorphan by blocking its hepatic metabolism.[53] There are specifically also a few studies in the TBI population supporting use.[54-56]

- *Mood stabilizers:* Mood stabilizers such as anticonvulsants are routinely used in the treatment of post-TBI lability, impulsivity, or disinhibition.
- *Beta-blockers:* Small randomized controlled trials have demonstrated the efficacy of beta-adrenergic receptor blocker agents for the treatment of post-TBI aggression,[57] and guidelines have been established for their use.[4] Beta-blockers selective for the beta-1 subtype (e.g., metoprolol) are generally preferred because they tend to result in less CNS depression.
- Amantadine has also been evaluated as a treatment for behavioral problems following TBI. Amantadine is a noncompetitive antagonist at the NMDA receptor, which also indirectly enhances dopaminergic neurotransmission. Its effectiveness for treatment of chronic aggression after TBI has been documented,[58] but not for treatment of acute post-TBI irritability.[59] It is best to avoid amantadine in people at risk for seizures.[60]
- *Neuroleptics:* Acutely, if the patient is getting increasingly agitated, low-dose atypical antipsychotics can be used. Note, however, that antipsychotic medications do not help with chronic nonpsychotic aggression.
- *Psychostimulants:* Stimulants may be useful for impulsivity and disinhibition, especially if the symptoms are part of a dysexecutive syndrome.
- *Other agents:* Gabapentin has also been studied in postconcussion syndrome. In a retrospective study with longitudinal analysis of 277 patients diagnosed with concussion, Cushman et al. compared gabapentin versus TCA versus no medication to determine their effects on improving symptoms after concussion.[61] The two medications appeared to have an immediate effect on improving symptom burden but in the long term there were no differences between medications versus no medication. It is also not clear whether the immediate benefit was secondary to a decrease in headache-related pain, or an independent effect.

Apathy

Apathy refers to a syndrome of disinterest, disengagement, inertia, lack of motivation, and absence of emotional responsivity. Apathy can be a symptom of depression, which is the most common presentation, or occur as an isolated syndrome. Drugs of choice include the following:

- *Psychostimulants:* Stimulants (e.g., methylphenidate) and dopaminergic agents (e.g., amantadine[62,63]) may be beneficial in the treatment of post-TBI apathy.
- Cholinesterase inhibitors: These agents may also be useful if there is an associated post-TBI dementia.
- Antidepressants may also be used in the treatment of apathy, especially if it is a manifestation of major depression. A note of caution: SSRIs, especially in high doses, can worsen apathy and amotivational syndromes.[64]

Sleep Disturbances

- A variety of sleep disturbances are seen after TBI. They include insomnia (see Chapter 54), hypersomnia, circadian rhythm sleep–wake cycle disorders, and parasomnias. In patients with TBI who have excessive daytime sleepiness, sleep apnea should first be ruled out. Modafinil (100–400 mg) or armodafinil (150–300 mg) can be considered in patients with obstructive sleep apnea and excessive daytime sleepiness, though evidence of efficacy is conflicting.[4,65]
- Prazosin may be used as adjunctive treatment for persistent nightmares. However, a 10-week study comparing prazosin to placebo revealed no statistically significant differences in sleep quality between the two.[66]

■ For complex or unusual or persisting sleep disturbances, it is best to refer patients to sleep specialists. Whenever sleep disturbance is associated with other psychiatric disorders such as major depression, anxiety disorders, or psychotic disorders, it is important to treat the underlying psychiatric disorder.

SUMMARY

When assessing patients with neuropsychiatric symptoms that develop after TBI, it is critical to ascertain whether these symptoms originate in behavioral, psychotic, affective, or cognitive domains, as this can often guide treatment. As patients with brain injury are susceptible to side effects and adverse reactions to medication, polypharmacy should be avoided, and doses should be started low and titrated incrementally. As such, choosing the ideal treatment regimen may be challenging; an approach targeting specific symptoms is likely to prove most beneficial.

KEY POINTS

■ Neuropsychiatric syndromes are common after TBI and are treatable.
■ It is important to identify the predominant syndrome present (affective, psychotic, behavioral, cognitive) and associated comorbidities, which can guide choosing the appropriate agent.
■ Individuals with TBI are more susceptible to medication side effects, and thus the fewest medications at the lowest effective doses are safest.
■ In dosing medications in this population, it is recommended to start at low doses and go slowly in titrating doses.
■ It is important to avoid classes of agents that can impair neuronal growth and cognitive ability such as benzodiazepines and first-generation antipsychotics.
■ Regular monitoring and cognizance about drug–drug interactions are key.

STUDY QUESTIONS

1. Of the following medications, which should be avoided in the acute post-TBI phase?
   a. Quetiapine
   b. Olanzapine
   c. Clozapine
   d. Haloperidol
   e. Both c and d

2. Which of the following would not be a recommended medication for anxiety after TBI?
   a. Citalopram
   b. Bupropion
   c. Buspirone
   d. Quetiapine
   e. Lorazepam

3. Which of the following statements are NOT true about psychopharmacology after TBI?
   a. You should start at a lower dose for persons with TBI than what is typical with other persons
   b. You should not go to the maximum dose of a psychotropic in persons with TBI
   c. You should increase dosing more slowly for persons with TBI than with other persons
   d. You should go to the lowest dose that is effective and tolerable in persons with TBI
   e. b and c.

4. Which of the following medications would not be recommended for a person with TBI and comorbid seizures?
   a. Sertraline
   b. Citalopram
   c. Venlafaxine
   d. Clomipramine
   e. Mirtazapine

5. What would be a first-line medication for apathy after TBI?
   a. Mirtazapine
   b. Clozapine
   c. Trazodone
   d. Methylphenidate
   e. Vilazodone

ADDITIONAL READING

Neuropsychiatry of Traumatic Brain Injury: https://psychscenehub.com/psychinsights/neuropsychiatry-of-traumatic-brain-injury

Polich G, Iaccarino MA, Zafonte R. Psychopharmacology of traumatic brain injury. Chapter 15; In: Reus VI, Lindqvist D, eds. *Handbook of Clinical Neurology*; 2019; Vol. 165 (3rd series). Psychopharmacology of neurologic diseases. doi:10.1016/B978-0-444-64012-3.00015-0

Ponsford J, Always Y, Gould KR. Epidemiology and natural history of psychiatric disorders after TBI. *J Neuropsychiatry Clin Neurosci*. 2018. doi:10.1176/appi.neuropsych.18040093

Arciniegas DB, Wortzel HS. Emotional and behavioral dyscontrol after traumatic brain injury. *Psychiatr Clin North Am*. 2014;37(1):31–53. doi:10.1016/j.psc.2013.12.001

Perry DC, Sturm VE, Peterson MJ, et al. Association of traumatic brain injury with subsequent neurological and psychiatric disease: a meta-analysis. *J Neurosurg*. 2016;124(2):511–526. doi:10.3171/2015.2.JNS14503

ANSWERS TO STUDY QUESTIONS

1. Correct Answer: e
   Clozapine should be avoided due to increased risk of seizures, and haloperidol should be avoided due to data suggesting that it can impair cognition and neural plasticity.

   Further Reading:
   Dikmen SS, Temkin NR, Miller B, et al. Neurobehavioral effects of phenytoin prophylaxis of posttraumatic seizures. *JAMA*. 1991;265(10):1271–1277. doi:10.1007/s11940-012-0193-6
   Hoffman A, Cheng J, Zafonte R et al. Administration of haloperidol and risperidone after neurobehavioral testing hinders the recovery of traumatic brain injury-induced deficits. *Life Sci*. 2008; 83: 602–607. doi:10.1016/j.lfs.2008.08.007

2. Correct Answer: e
Benzodiazepines such as lorazepam should be avoided because their adverse effects can increase TBI-related impairments. Animal studies also indicate that benzodiazepines may slow or impede neuronal recovery.

Further Reading:
Schallert T, Hernandez T, Barth T. Recovery of function after brain damage: severe and chronic disruption by diazepam. *Brain Res.* 1986;379:104–111. doi:10.1016/0006-8993(86)90261-1

3. Correct Answer: b
It may be necessary to go to a maximum dose in TBI patients, but one should start at a low dose and go up slowly.

Further Reading:
Vaishnavi S, Rao V, Fann JR. Neuropsychiatric problems after traumatic brain injury: Unraveling the silent epidemic. *Psychosomatics.* 2009;50(3):198–205. doi:10.1176/appi. psy.50.3.198

4. Correct Answer: d
Clomipramine, a TCA, has a greater seizure risk than the other medications.

Further Reading:
Arciniegas D, Anderson C, Topkoff J, et al.: Mild traumatic brain injury: a neuropsychiatric approach to diagnosis, evaluation, and treatment. *Neuropsychiatr Dis Treat.* 2005;1(4):311–327.

5. Correct Answer: d
Psychostimulants like methylphenidate are first-line medications for apathy based on current research.

Further Reading:
Polich G, Iaccarino MA, Zafonte R, Psychopharmacology of traumatic brain injury. *Handb Clin Neurol.* 2019;165:253–267. doi:10.1016/B978-0-444-64012-3.00015-0
Gualtieri C, Evans R . Stimulant treatment for the neurobehavioural sequelae of traumatic brain injury. *Brain Inj.* 1988;2:273–290. doi:10.3109/02699058809150936, doi:10.3109/02699058809150898

REFERENCES

The full reference list appears in the digital product found on http://connect.springer-pub.com/content/book/978-0-8261-4768-4/part/part03/chapter/ch37

38 PAIN MANAGEMENT IN PERSONS WITH TRAUMATIC BRAIN INJURY

NATHAN D. ZASLER

INTRODUCTION

Pain, as defined by the International Association for the Study of Pain, is "an unpleasant sensory and emotional experience associated with actual or potential tissue damage or described in terms of such damage."[1,2] Pain should be considered as a multidimensional subjective experience mediated by cultural, emotional, biologic, and perceptual influences. Pain should not be confused with nociception.[1,2] Pain is a subjective experience; by definition, it exists only in the person who feels it (first-person perspective). Nociception is defined as observable nervous system activity in response to an adequate stimulus (third-person perspective). Characterological factors, prior experiences with pain, affective status, trauma history, and cultural beliefs, among other factors, may impact pain and suffering.

The problem of pain is quite common in persons with traumatic brain injury (TBI). On average, approximately 50% of civilians with TBI experience chronic pain.[3–5] Chronic pain among veterans may occur at a somewhat lower rate.[3,6,7] Chronic pain complaints following TBI, in particular headache, have been noted to generally be more common in persons following mild compared to moderate to severe TBI.[8]

PAIN GENERATORS IN PERSONS WITH TRAUMATIC BRAIN INJURY

There are often challenges with regard to accurately determining primary pain generators, or sources of pain, particularly in patients early after severe brain injury and/or polytrauma. Frequently, multiple pain generators can be identified following TBI and associated polytrauma. In the acute care phase, the primary pain generators are more likely to involve such phenomena as fractures, intra-abdominal injuries, peripheral nerve injuries, postsurgical pain, soft tissue injuries, and pain associated with invasive medical procedures.[9,10] In the chronic phase, spasticity/hypertonicity, contracture, myofascial pain, fibromyalgia, complex regional pain syndrome, shoulder subluxation, neuromusculoskeletal scoliosis, dystonia, central pain, central sensitization, skin breakdown, asymmetric joint wear, and tissue hypoxemia, among other phenomena, may be causes of pain.[9,11–14]

Headache is probably one of the most common of all posttraumatic complaints in persons with TBI; it is often related to other factors than the brain injury itself.[15,16] A good understanding of the differential diagnosis of posttraumatic headache or cephalalgia is essential to guide both assessment and treatment of this condition. Practitioners should strive to identify the specific causes of the headache disorder, which may often have multiple

The full reference list appears in the digital product found on http://connect.springerpub.com/content/book/978-0-8261-4768-4/part/part03/chapter/ch38

contributors including tension, cervicogenic dysfunction, neuralgia, and migraine, among others. It should be noted that there are no Food and Drug Administration approved drugs specific to posttraumatic headache,[17,18] and that treatment normally is guided by approaches used for primary headache disorders such as tension and migraine headache.

Given the wide spectrum of causes for pain after TBI, exams should be thorough yet problem focused. Understanding of the pathophysiology and mechanisms underlying the causes of posttraumatic pain after TBI and/or polytrauma is also of critical importance.[4,19] Appropriate and careful differential diagnosis needs to occur to assist in identifying the specific pain generators in each individual and then understand what interventions may be most appropriate.

PAIN ASSESSMENT

Pain assessment can be challenging, particularly in patients with moderate to severe TBI, where such assessments may be compromised by cognitive, behavioral, language, or insight capacities.[9,11] Such assessments are more challenging when the patient has significant impairments that impede conveyance of consciously mediated pain experiences. There is no general consensus about methodologies to assess these patients acutely after injury.

Pain History

In patients who are able to communicate their pain experiences, appropriate lines of questioning should examine the character, onset, location, exacerbating and relieving factors, and the duration of the pain complaint(s).[9-11] Pain severity, frequency, and evolution over time should be explored. Any pre-injury pain disorders/complaints should be noted. There are a plethora of measures that provide better biopsychosocially complex information regarding pain than do historically utilized unidimensional pain scales. Examples include PQRST (provocation or palliation, quality or quantity, region or radiation, severity scale, and timing), SOCRATES (site, onset, character, radiation, associations, time course, exacerbations/relief, and severity), COLDER (character, onset, location, exacerbation, and relief), and QISS-TAPED (quality, impact, site, severity/temporal characteristics, aggravating and alleviating factors, past response/preferences, expectations/goals/meaning, diagnostics, and physical exam) protocol.[20] Family history should be assessed for similar pain complaints in the setting of migraine. Information should be gathered regarding how the pain impacts the person's day-to-day function and whether it limits them from particular activities. Information should also be solicited from corroboratory sources including family and significant others who may have insights as to pain behaviors.[21]

In noncommunicative patients, the aforementioned methods of assessment are not feasible. In this context, indirect measurements such as behavioral observations or physiological measurements are needed. To facilitate the assessment of pain in noncommunicative patients, including those with disorders of consciousness (DoC), numerous standardized behavioral scales have been developed. Controversies remain regarding the methods for assessment and management of pain in persons with DoC, including differentiation between reflex and conscious pain responses.[22] There are now assessment measures specifically designed to assess for evidence of conscious pain responses in persons with DoC, which can be utilized in this context,[23-26] and which should be part of any assessment battery in such patients.

Obtaining a comprehensive, multimodal, biopsychosocial history is critical, particularly when pain is chronic.[20,27] Such assessment should include pre-injury pain disorders, personality factors that may impact pain chronification (such as anxiety, harm avoidance, catastrophization, and hypochondriasis), how an individual is coping with their pain, psychological adjustment, sexual trauma history, and perceptions regarding quality of life and pain-related disability. Pain appraisals, beliefs, and expectations should be queried.

Pain medication use history, inclusive of the dosing and duration of treatment and the overall efficacy of the intervention, should also be reviewed.[9] Historical compliance with pain medication and any substance abuse history should also be addressed, the latter to ensure that an at-risk patient is not being prescribed inappropriate medication.[28]

Pain Examination

Abnormal pain exam findings include not only pertinent positives but also pertinent negatives. In patients where communication is limited or absent, practitioners must rely to a great extent on observation of pain-related behaviors including grimacing, agitation, and tearfulness on nociceptive stimulus application; however, even these behaviors cannot be assumed to always be indicative of conscious pain experience. Vital sign fluctuations may also be a marker in the context of pain assessment.[29]

The practitioner should conduct a holistic evaluation including inspection, palpation, and appropriate neuromusculoskeletal examination. The physical examination should be guided by the results of the pain history.[30] Adequate time must be taken to assess the likely pain sources.[28] Peripheral nerve examination should include assessment for craniofacial neuralgias, occipital neuralgia, and/or peripheral neuropathies or radiculopathies where indicated based on pain history.[31,32] In any patient with craniocervical pain, there should be a detailed palpatory exam of the cranium/face, cranial adnexal structures, and the cervical spine.[16,33]

Diagnostic Assessment

Self-report remains the gold standard for pain measurement. There are measures that tap sensory and affective qualities of pain, temporal characteristics of pain, pain magnification, and coping, as well as other pain features including location, provocation of pain, and pain behaviors. Multidimensional scales tend to be the most helpful.[21,34]

Pain-specific measures that tap pain adjustment, coping, magnification, and/or functional impact of pain that practitioners should familiarize themselves with include the Pain Catastrophizing Scale (PCS) and Multidimensional Pain Inventory (MPI), the Pain Patient Profile (P3), Chronic Pain Coping Index (CPCI), Pain Disability Index (PDI), Tampa Scale of Kinesiophobia, and the McGill Pain Questionnaire (MPQ).[21,30] Evaluation for pain response bias, symptom and sign validity as well as performance validity should be conducted. Such testing is even more relevant when there are secondary gain incentives for maintaining subjective complaints of pain such as personal injury litigation, disability benefits, or workers' compensation.[35] Clinicians should keep in mind that reporting biases go both ways and some patients may underreport pain symptoms due to stoicism, desire to be cleared to return to pre-injury activities or employment, or being "macho."

PAIN MANAGEMENT

Primary Goals

It is paramount that the treating pain clinician maintain ongoing communication with other clinicians involved with the patient's health management to adequately coordinate clinical care.

In the acute care setting, emphasis should be on modulating physical and psychological signs and symptoms associated with the pain condition. In the post-acute care setting, efforts should also include prevention of secondary and tertiary complications including chronification and central sensitization, chronic affective and maladjustment issues, dyssomnia, cognitive impairment, and neurohormonal adverse consequences.

One should establish realistic treatment end points for the specific pain disorder as early as possible with both the injured person and other stakeholders. As part of this educational process, discussion regarding treatment options including risks versus benefits is crucial. Practitioners should use the simplest, least invasive, lowest risk, and most cost-effective management approaches that allow for optimization of patient compliance and maximal functional restoration whenever possible.

Where physical modalities can be used to ameliorate pain conditions, they should be attempted first, before utilizing pharmacological agents; however, when pain is moderate to severe, concurrent pharmacological management should be considered.

Pharmacological Treatment

Pharmacological approaches should be hierarchically divided based on the intensity and type of pain being treated and where the patient is in the continuum of care. Some of the agents discussed in the following should only be used with close, ongoing medical monitoring.[4,28]

Mild

Mild pain medicines that should be considered typically include aspirin, acetaminophen, and nonsteroidal anti-inflammatory drugs (NSAIDs).

Moderate

Moderate pain medications include high-dose aspirin or acetaminophen, high-dose standard NSAIDs, newer generation NSAIDs such as cyclooxygenase-II inhibitors, injectable nonsteroidal anti-inflammatories, mixed opiate analgesics with aspirin or acetaminophen (with or without caffeine), compounded topical medications, whether trademark or compounded, and tramadol.

Severe

Medications to consider would include parenteral opiates, with morphine sulfate being considered the standard; mixed agonist antagonists such as pentazocine; partial opiate agonists such as buprenorphine; ketamine; antidepressants; anticonvulsants; continuous local anesthetic; peripheral nerve block; and/or atypical agents including cannabinoids. Other agents can be considered as adjuvants including atypical antipsychotic agents and N-methyl-D-aspartate antagonists such as memantine.[36]

Medications that have been used for opioid insensitive pain (e.g., neuropathic pain, centrally mediated pain) include NSAIDs, tricyclic antidepressants, newer generation antidepressants such as venlafaxine or duloxetine, anticonvulsants including carbamazepine derivatives, gabapentin, pregabalin, levetiracetam, and lamotrigine, as well as less commonly used agents such as mexiletine. Other agents that have been recognized as potential adjuvants in the pharmacological management of pain include tizanidine and sodium amobarbital.[28,36]

Attempts should be made to minimize polypharmacy as this will improve compliance, decrease drug–drug interactions, and improve quality of life at the same time as decreasing cost to the patient. In addition, whenever possible, use of medications that may impede neural plasticity (e.g., opiates, barbiturates, certain anticonvulsants) should be minimized or ideally avoided.[37-39] Additionally, and particularly true for patients with posttraumatic headache, practitioners should be aware of medication overuse headache

(MOH; older term: rebound headache) and avoid prescribing medications that may cause MOH if used too frequently, or alternatively provide strict guidelines and monitoring if deemed apropos for prescription.

Practitioners should err on the side of providing pain modulating interventions including pharmacotherapy[22] in persons with DoC, given the unknowns regarding determination of degree of pain perception, if any, and/or suffering.

Nonpharmacological Treatment Methods

There are a number of nonpharmacological approaches that can be used in pain management. The efficacy of these approaches varies significantly. Much of the clinical response of these techniques correlates with pain chronicity, patient incentives for maintaining pain behaviors, and technical prowess of the clinician as well as the potential role of both placebo and nocebo effects. Of all physical approaches, exercise may be one of the least prescribed yet most beneficial intervention for chronic pain.[40]

Physical Approaches

There are a multitude of physical modalities that may be appropriate in the management of posttraumatic pain disorders after TBI. *Physical* modalities may include cryotherapy, heating modalities including superficial and deep heat, electrotherapy including transcutaneous electrical nerve stimulation and neuromuscular electrical stimulation, and techniques involving mechanical force including traction and massage as well as light therapy such as low-level energy lasers.[41] Other techniques that can be used for pain management include phonophoresis and iontophoresis, short wave as well as microwave diathermy, and vapocoolant sprays. Evidence for efficacy varies, with the literature generally supporting short-term benefit, but lacking as regards sustained pain modulation.

Appropriate prescription of adaptive equipment and durable medical equipment (e.g., bracing and orthotics), as well as ergonomically modifying the work environment, may also add to overall management of posttraumatic pain conditions and optimize work performance.

Injection therapies, including intra-articular, periarticular, peritendinous, ligamentous/fibrous tissue, and trigger point injections all have a potential role in the management of certain posttraumatic pain generators[42] and can be used therapeutically, diagnostically, prognostically, and/or prophylactically.

Acupuncture may provide pain modulation benefits in general and specific to persons with TBI. Evidence supports its efficacy in posttraumatic headache,[43] migraine, fibromyalgia, low back pain, cervicalgia, and abdominal pain.[44]

Neuromodulation is a relatively new pain management option. A variety of techniques are available, some with better evidence than others and hardly any with good evidence in persons with TBI. Techniques include vagal nerve stimulation, sphenopalatine ganglion neuromodulation, pulsed radiofrequency (PRF), occipital nerve stimulation, trigeminal system stimulation, and optogenetics.[45] These technologies can be implanted or applied externally depending on the specific intervention.

Psychological Approaches

A variety of psychological methods may be appropriate to consider in the context of pain management, either in conjunction with other interventions or as the sole intervention. Psychological interventions are underutilized treatment options for patients with chronic posttraumatic pain disorders, in part because clinicians are poorly informed on the efficacy of these interventions in pain management, in part due to the dearth of psychological services that are specialized to address pain concerns and, lastly, due to the historical reticence of commercial payers to cover psychological services because of the fear of transitioning into treatment of a more chronic "mental health" diagnosis.[21] Behavioral treatment interventions for pain in persons with TBI should focus on improved pain coping and stress management skills, modulation of affective responses to chronic pain and associated disability, and interventions to decrease somatic focus. Behavioral interventional techniques including biofeedback, relaxation training, operant treatments, cognitive behavioral interventions, as well as social and assertiveness skills and training, imagery and hypnosis, and habit reversal should also be considered.[21]

IMPAIRMENT ASSESSMENT

Although often requested of clinicians, the area of impairment rating associated with pain is wrought with controversy. Some of the challenges include the subjectivity of pain, the importance of rating pain from the whole person perspective rather than from the level of the specific organ or body part, the challenge of evaluating pain in isolation from the medical condition underlying the pain disorder etiologically, and the challenges associated with response biases both negative and positive regarding pain reporting, among other issues. In the context of rating pain-related impairment, it is important to look at the consistency and natural history of the complaint over time and situation, its congruency with known anatomy and physiology of the injury, the presentation's consistency with parallel conditions in other patients, and behavioral observations across observer/examiners including presence of nonorganic signs and/or symptoms. Clinicians should also be familiar with nonorganic indicators on interview and/or examination that may suggest the need for further assessment of functional contributors to the pain presentation, just as they should be attuned to response biases in pain reporting including both under- and overreporting.[21,35]

Rating Impairment

The American Medical Association Guides to Evaluation of Permanent Impairment assigns a percentage of loss due to injury relative to whole body function. Many clinicians would take the position that rating pain based on current science is not possible in the context of traditional percentage values based on the whole person model as dictated using this paradigm.[46]

Functional Capacity Evaluation

- A functional capacity evaluation (FCE) involves administering questionnaires, obtaining relevant history, and administering physical assessments, and then using these to make a determination regarding a person's ability, typically in the context of the ability to perform work-related tasks. FCE questionnaires as well as corroboratory interviews serve as useful sources of information. The aforementioned data are compared to physical performance in determining whether a specific set of occupational demands can be met. One particular limitation of FCEs is that they are traditionally time-limited and as a result do not tap work tolerance particularly well.

CONCLUSION

Pain is a common biopsychosocial problem after TBI across the severity spectrum. Clinicians need to be prepared to understand the array of pain generators that are possible in this patient population and provide sufficient examination time to take an adequate history and perform a relevant physical examination for the pain complaints in question. Key elements of the pain history and pain physical exam should be common parlance for physicians working with this patient population. Additionally, practitioners should understand the multidimensionality of pain, particularly when chronic, and the armamentarium of both assessment and treatment approaches that exists for pain in general as well as for persons post-TBI.

KEY POINTS

- Posttraumatic pain is a multidimensional condition and should be assessed and treated with that as a core foundation to optimize treatment outcomes.
- Adequate history taking and hands-on physical assessment are key to gaining a better understanding of all potential pain generators.
- Pharmacological treatment decisions must be guided by an understanding of pain etiology and treatment goals, as well as drug mechanisms, side effects, and interactions.
- Behavioral and psychological interventions can be very helpful in modulating posttraumatic pain symptoms, particularly when chronic, but are generally underutilized.
- The role of exercise as a chronic pain intervention should not be undervalued by either clinicians or those with chronic pain disorders.
- Further research is needed to develop appropriate methodologies for objectively assessing pain and pain-related impairment.

STUDY QUESTIONS

1. In persons with DoC, pain assessment may be complicated by all the following except:
   a. Cognitive limitations
   b. Lack of arousal
   c. The lack of pain measures specific to DoC
   d. Communication limitations
   e. All of the above

2. Headache is a common cause of pain following TBI and:
   a. Can cause work disability
   b. Can adversely impact cognition
   c. Can drive symptoms of behavioral irritability
   d. Can be due to a variety of causes associated with extracerebral trauma
   e. All of the above

3. Common descriptors used in the pain literature include:
   a. Allodynia
   b. Synesthesia
   c. Dipathia
   d. a and b
   e. All of the above

4. When getting a medication use history, the following are important elements to inquire about:
   a. Prior medications used to treat the pain disorder
   b. History of tobacco use
   c. Compliance with prescribed interventions
   d. a and c
   e. All of the above

5. The following provides an objective metric for documentation of an underlying experience of the pain condition:
   a. Results of the PCS
   b. Functional magnetic resonance imaging
   c. Quantitative electroencephalogram (EEG)
   d. Pain evoked potentials
   e. None of the above

ADDITIONAL READING

Inter-Agency Task Force Report: Pain Management Best Practices. https://www.hhs.gov/sites/default/files/pmtf-final-report-2019-05-23.pdf

Devlin JW, Skrobik Y, Gelinas C, et al. Clinical practice guidelines for the prevention and management of pain, agitation/sedation, delirium, immobility, and sleep disruption in adult patients in the ICU. *Crit Care Med.* 2018;46(9):e825–e873.

Irvine K, Clark JD. Chronic pain after traumatic brain injury: pathophysiology and pain mechanisms. *Pain Medicine.* 2018;19:1315–1333. doi:10.1093/pm/pnx153

Schnakers C, Zasler ND. Assessment and management of pain in patients with disorders of consciousness. *PMR.* 2015;7(11S):S270–S277. doi:10.1016/j.pmrj.2015.09.016

ANSWERS TO STUDY QUESTIONS

1. Correct Answer: c
   Answers (a), (b), and (d) can confound the pain assessment in persons with DoC. Answer (c) is incorrect since there are pain measures that have been developed specific to persons with DoC.

   Further Reading:
   Schnakers C, Zasler ND. Assessment and management of pain in patients with disorders of consciousness. *PMR.* 2015;7(11S):S270–S277.
   Zasler N, Martelli MF, Clanton S. Post-traumatic pain disorders: medical assessment and management. In: Zasler N, Katz D, Zafonte R, eds. *Brain Injury Medicine: Principles and Practice.* 3rd ed. Demos Medical. Pending publication; 2021.

2. Correct Answer: e
   Headache whether due to TBI or extracerebral injury can produce all the listed consequences.

   Further Reading:
   Zasler ND, Leddy JJ, Etheredge S, Martelli MF. Post-traumatic headache. In: Silver JM, McAllister TW, Arciniegas D, eds. *Textbook of Traumatic Brain Injury.* 3rd ed. American Psychiatric Publishing, Inc; 2019:471–490.

3. **Correct Answer: a**
   The correct answer is (a) as the other choices are either nonsensical or not relevant and not used as pain descriptors.

   Further Reading:
   https://www.iasp-pain.org/Education/Content.aspx?ItemNumber=1698. 2020.

4. **Correct Answer: d**
   The correct answer is (d) as tobacco use is not a relevant line of inquiry in this context.

   Further Reading:
   Zasler N, Martelli MF. Post-traumatic pain disorders: medical assessment and management. In: Zasler N, Katz D, Zafonte R, eds. *Brain Injury Medicine: Principles and Practice.* 2nd ed. Demos Medical. Pending publication; 2021.

5. **Correct Answer: e**
   None of the noted techniques objectively document the underlying experience of pain as it is subjective. Pain perception is influenced to varying degrees by biological, psychological, and social factors. Pain and nociception are different phenomena: The experience of pain cannot be reduced to activity in sensory pathways.

   Further Reading:
   IASP's proposed new definition of pain released for comment. 2020. https://www.iasp-pain.org/PublicationsNews/NewsDetail.aspx?ItemNumber=9218

REFERENCES

The full reference list appears in the digital product found on http://connect.springer-pub.com/content/book/978-0-8261-4768-4/part/part03/chapter/ch38

ASSISTIVE TECHNOLOGY IN TRAUMATIC BRAIN INJURY

KURT L. JOHNSON AND MARK HARNISS

GENERAL PRINCIPLES

Assistive technologies (AT) may serve important roles in rehabilitation, community living, education, and employment for people who have survived traumatic brain injuries (TBIs). AT is defined in the Assistive Technology Act of 2004 as ". . . any item, piece of equipment, or product system, whether acquired commercially, modified, or customized, that is used to increase, maintain, or improve functional capabilities of individuals with disabilities (29 U.S.C. Sec 2202(2))," and includes "any service that directly assists an individual with a disability in the selection, acquisition, or use of an AT device." AT can include a wide range of high-tech and low-tech devices and services. Variations in this definition of AT are found in federal laws related to vocational rehabilitation and special education and are relevant in terms of funding AT.

For AT to be adapted successfully, it is important that the user be actively involved in making decisions about AT selection. Not only should the needs of the individual with TBI be considered, but also the needs and preferences of family members or caregivers; the "unit" of consideration should be the dyad or even the family.[1] Other key considerations are the cognitive and motor prerequisites for use of AT, fatigue, access to technical assistance and repair after the AT is deployed, and access to funding.

AT needs should be evaluated at differing stages of recovery, ranging from inpatient rehabilitation to outpatient rehabilitation to community reentry to long-term living. Not only do individual needs change, but options for funding the AT change as well.

In considering AT solutions, we strongly recommend an interdisciplinary approach. Without careful consideration, AT can actually decrease performance on targeted tasks. Thinking through the AT carefully with the interdisciplinary team and individual with TBI is crucial. For example, in considering compensatory strategies in the workplace for memory deficits, a speech pathologist and rehabilitation counselor might consider the advantages and disadvantages of low-tech solutions such as memory books versus more complex AT systems including electronic calendaring.

FUNCTIONAL DOMAINS AND ASSISTIVE TECHNOLOGIES

Mobility

Many people who have survived TBI may require mobility aids. We do not discuss these here since the topic is addressed elsewhere (see Chapter 31).

The full reference list appears in the digital product found on http://connect.springerpub.com/content/book/978-0-8261-4768-4/part/part03/chapter/ch39

Navigation

People with TBI may have difficulty navigating independently.[2] There are systems in place in many larger communities to provide training in using public transportation, door-to-door transit, and other options, which people with TBI may use to navigate independently. The Global Positioning System (GPS) on handheld devices may be useful, although some people with TBI find the map interfaces to be too complex and difficult to use in community navigation.[3] Some GPS devices, including those on some smartphones, give voice output related to upcoming landmarks that may be more useful. It is important to not have individuals relying on systems such as looking at screens while walking, which may put them at risk for missing important environmental events and/or cues.

Caregiver Assurance

Some caregivers may be willing to negotiate more community independence for people with TBI if there is a way that they can monitor individuals' locations. Although there are clearly ethical and privacy issues associated with this, we have found that people with TBI are often willing to agree to this, especially if they can turn off the tracking devices. There are a number of commercial systems available, many of which use a standard mobile phone as a location device. Consideration of a backup plan in case the device is lost or loses power is critical; a plan should be in place to ensure a way for an individual to "call for help."

Note Taking

For students in K–12 or postsecondary education, or for employees in a work setting, taking notes is often critical. Unfortunately, because of difficulties with divided attention, people with TBI often say that they cannot take notes and listen at the same time and that they have difficulty taking notes because they cannot discern the salient points in real time. Individuals may audio-record lectures or meetings, but audio recordings themselves require a lot of effort to review. A low-tech option is to request a note taker as a reasonable accommodation in class, but even with this, individuals often want to be able to annotate as they go. One option that has been very useful for a number of individuals is a smart pen (e.g., Livescribe). These systems use a pen to record audio and sync it with handwritten notes. The individual can take very general notes, and then when reviewing the notes, can listen to audio playback corresponding to the time the notes were taken.

Memory/Memory Aids

Sometimes the "old way" is the "best way," and memory books ranging from calendars to daily planners to more complex paper and pencil systems have been successfully used for years. The disadvantages of these systems are that users may misplace or lose them, forget to record events or tasks, forget to check the memory book, or may create information overload by inserting numerous "yellow stickies," loose pieces of paper, and so on, so that they are overwhelmed by data. Electronic devices such as smartphones, tablets, and computers may be useful. Using electronic devices is easiest for people who already have experience with them since less new learning is required. It is important to fit the use of any memory device into the day-to-day routine of the individual, and to the extent possible, the context of their memory needs. Key considerations are the following:

- What functions does it perform? Calendar, task list, phone, text, email?
- Is the visual display easily readable? Is it too cluttered or distracting?
- Is there speech output?
- Is the keyboard/text entry usable?
- Is there voice to text input?
- Is it compatible with what family members, friends, or others use at home or at work?

- How difficult is it to learn to use?
- Is it redundant—that is, is there backup in case it gets lost, is not charged, or breaks?
- Is there technical assistance when the user runs into problems?

Although many smartphones or even "feature phones" include software calendars, we strongly recommend using cloud-based calendars and task lists instead, such as iCloud, Google, or Outlook Exchange. There are several significant advantages. First, if the phone or tablet or other primary device gets lost, the information remains in the "cloud." Second, the calendar and task lists can be shared with others. This can be a tremendous advantage because trusted family members, teachers, or others can be given access to the calendars/task lists and can ensure that key events or scheduled alarms are set, tasks are broken down into components, and so on.

Note that in many calendar systems, appointments, events, and even steps in tasks that need to be completed may be entered into the calendar and alarms can be enabled. One feature useful for some people is to have alarms set to send a text message reminder to the phone or voice output saying, for example, "appointment with Dr. Gray in 15 minutes" or "transfer to Bus #2 to hospital in 5 minutes."

There are also a number of dedicated memory aids, such as key fobs to help remember where one's car is parked and medisets for storing pills that remind the user to take meds.

Many people use email or text messages as a form of memory aid. They email or text themselves, or keep email in their inboxes as reminders. The difficulty with SMS texts is that they typically reside on the phone only, whereas email can be retrieved from multiple devices and there are more options for organizing and storing email. The problem with emailed reminders for TBI survivors is that they may be overwhelmed with email inbox chaos. We use the features associated with Microsoft Office Outlook as examples here, but many email products have similar features. Rules can be set for incoming email. For example, a rule can be established that codes all incoming email from certain people or domains by color, such as "all email from my boss is colored red in my inbox." Alternatively, incoming email can be sorted into different folders. For example, "All email from my instructor is filed in the folder, 'Professor J.'" We recommend that decisions about managing complex email systems be done in consultation with a specialist, such as a speech pathologist or psychologist, so that a balance is struck between reducing the inbox chaos and manageable efficiency.

SOCIAL PARTICIPATION

TBI survivors may find that they are socially isolated and/or that their social networks change as they recover. Social media, such as Facebook, Instagram, and Twitter, may offer valuable options for social participation. Although there is not a great deal of evidence to support the benefits of participation in social media, there have been efforts to organize TBI support groups on social media, and there are numerous anecdotal reports from people with TBI about the benefits of using social media.[4] Assistance may be needed to navigate details about computer access and contextually appropriate online social interactions.

COMPUTER ACCESS

The whole construct about computer access has changed as the lines between desktop computing, tablets, and mobile devices have blurred. Access to computers includes issues around cognition, vision, seating and positioning, voice, and motor control. We begin by addressing standard desktop computers or tablets/notebooks set up for use as desktop computers. iOS, Android, and Windows environments include extensive accessibility features, which may be enabled. These include features such as reducing the sensitivity of touch for keys/online keyboards to minimize error from unintended strikes, screen enlargement, spelling correction, text to speech, and so on.

Seating and Positioning

Ensuring appropriate seating and access to the computing tasks is critical to minimize fatigue and maximize ability to focus and concentrate, especially for anyone who may have had concurrent orthopedic trauma and/or chronic musculoskeletal pain and fatigue. There are a number of adjustable work surfaces that can be matched with seating schemes, and/or attached to power chairs. Mobile arm supports may be useful to reduce fatigue and improve accuracy of positioning of arm(s). These can be mounted on a power chair or desktop.

Keyboards

There are a wide variety of off-the-shelf keyboards; individuals may find some easier to use than others. Many people needing accommodations find that they prefer compressed keyboards, which require less movement to strike keys and can easily be mounted on power chairs, or custom mounted on desktops. Note that standard keyboards on notebook computers typically are in the format of compressed desktop keyboards. For people with difficulty striking a single key, software settings may be set in the "accessibility" settings of the operating system to require that an individual dwell on a key before the stroke registers, or that brief unintentional keystrokes are not recorded. Also, within word processing programs, macros can be enabled so that if a person habitually types "rhe" instead of "the," the correct word will be substituted. Alternatively, there are Lucite keyboard covers that have holes through which fingers or pointing devices are inserted to reach keys.

Word prediction may help with text entry as well on several fronts. As one begins to enter the text, the software predicts the intended word and, rather than continuing to type, one can accept and move on. Users of mobile phones are familiar with this type of software. On desktop, notebook, or tablet devices, when phonetic spelling is entered, the software will predict the correct spelling. Word prediction software can turn writing into a "multiple choice" task and can be paired with keyboarding.

Voice Commands

Text may also be entered using voice commands with software built into the operating system (e.g., in Apple, Android, and Windows devices) or via stand-alone programs such as Naturally Speaking. Voice recognition built into the operating system is often "user independent," but more sophisticated systems such as Naturally Speaking require that the user train the system to have the best results and, without adequate training and consultation, voice recognition software may not be adequately integrated and used. With Naturally Speaking, the individual can speak into a digital recorder and then transcribe that audio using the software. This is sometimes an advantage because the user is not viewing the text as it is generated, which can be confusing and distracting.

Modern voice recognition software requires that text be entered as continuous speech for best recognition. To attain this, it is necessary to dictate at least whole phrases without pauses or incidental sounds such as "uhmmm." People with dysarthria or accented English often get very poor recognition. That said, voice recognition on smartphones has improved dramatically over the past few years and is a viable option for text entry for many people. Although one can use voice recognition software to manage computing "hands free," many people find that they are much more efficient if they can combine voice recognition with some keystrokes or use of pointing devices.

Pointing Devices

Pointing devices, such as the computer mouse, can be challenging for people with motor deficits. It may be difficult to reach the target, and/or to click once the target is acquired. It may also be difficult to see and/or follow the tracking motion on the display. In the settings of the operating system, the sensitivity of the pointer may be set to either speed it up or slow it down. The image of the pointing device can also be changed to make it bigger and easier to see, and to provide a "tail" so that one can view the movement more easily. Alternatives to conventional mouse pointers include joysticks. The advantage of a joystick is that when the user stops applying pressure, the pointer stops, as opposed to devices like a trackball where the pointer often moves off target. The disadvantage is that use is considerably slower. Touch pads may also be preferable for some users. In general, mouse clicks may be separated from pointers or used independently of pointers with independent switches, such as "big red" switches or microswitches activated by electro-myographic input (EMG). Individuals can also use a variety of pointing devices, such as mouth-operated joysticks or even eye gaze, to enter text using on-screen keyboards and to manipulate computer actions.

Viewing the Screen

People may have difficulties with vision, including converging on the image, double vision, and field cuts. Some of these may be addressed by manipulating the size of the display, positioning the display to maximize vision, increasing image size, or using software for people with reading disabilities (see Reading Software in the section that follows). Displays come in all different sizes, and LCD displays are light enough to allow for creative mounting and positioning. Tablets and some notebook computers can be mounted to a variety of devices using Velcro, although it can sometimes be difficult to maximize both visual access and text/data entry. Screen enlargement options and changes in contrast can be found in the accessibility features or general display settings of operating systems. Alternatively, there are dedicated software packages such as ZoomText, which enlarge all images on the screen, read the text to the user, and have advanced features. One point to keep in mind is that using these features may increase cognitive load. For example, as one increases the size of text, one reduces the amount of information available on the screen, and for people with cognitive difficulties, it may be difficult to keep track of where text is, and to move to text that is now off screen due to enlargement.

Reading Software

Reading text from a computer screen can be difficult for people with TBI. For some, having concurrent text to speech can help. There are "lightweight" options such as ReadPlease, which will read highlighted text to the user. There are more sophisticated packages designed for people with reading disabilities such as Kurzweil, which import text in a variety of formats including PDF, highlight a portion of the text, such as a sentence, in one color, and the word being read in another color, and provide a selection of reading voices. These more elaborate systems may be useful for people with field cuts that are resolving, or difficulties sustaining attention. For example, we have had professionals use these systems to read professional journals while they were still in the healing process.

Mobile Phones

A significant portion of the population use mobile phones as their primary means of accessing the Internet, communicating through SMS/text, and so on. Mobile phones present opportunities because they may be relatively affordable and are easy to transport, but they may also present barriers to access because of their small size, reliance on online keyboards, general reliance on pointing with fingers, and so on. Some phones can be accessed using add-on keyboards and/or pointing devices, but many cannot. As noted earlier for computers and tablets, both iOS and Android operating systems on phones have a variety of built-in accessibility features, which may improve access for people with disabilities, including TBI. These features are typically located in Settings and may be enabled by users. There are also a wide variety of add-on apps, which may be downloaded and enabled. These add-ons change frequently; users must aim to inform themselves about features, costs, company support/customer service, and so on when considering use of add-on "apps."

ENVIRONMENTAL CONTROL AND HOME AUTOMATION SYSTEMS

Managing the environment at home and at work may increase independence. Ensuring that a path from the bedroom to the bath or living quarters is lighted can reduce risk of falls and is easy to automate. Integrated environmental control systems have become ubiquitous and can be purchased at many big box stores and online. These systems can control heating, lighting, audio–video entertainment, and so on, and the interfaces can be voice-activated or switched. Many can be managed through smartphone or tabletop smart-speaker interfaces. Devices such as robotic vacuum cleaners should not be ignored either since they may provide additional independence.

KEY POINTS

- Technology should be considered as an adjunct to other interventions for people with TBI.
- The relative value of technology should be weighed against potential negative consequences since technology may add to cognitive load.
- An interdisciplinary approach to technology and TBI is strongly advised.
- Consider physical/built environment and social context in which technology will be deployed.

STUDY QUESTIONS

1. What are potential negative consequences of using AT for people with TBI?
   a. Dependence on the device
   b. Unwillingness to learn new approaches
   c. Increased cognitive load/cognitive demands
   d. Screen fatigue

2. What are the risks of aided navigation?
   a. The user may not learn the route independently
   b. The user may focus on the device rather than their environment, raising safety concerns

    c. The user may leave home without adequate support
    d. Loss of the GPS device

3. All of the following are examples of off-the-shelf commercial devices that may improve independence in the home except:
    a. GPS devices
    b. Robotic vacuum cleaners
    c. Reading software
    d. Pointing devices

4. What are examples of alternative pointing devices?
    a. Medisets
    b. Smart pens
    c. Word prediction
    d. Joysticks, trackballs

5. What is often key to successful use of voice recognition software?
    a. A loud voice
    b. Training
    c. Adequate breath control
    d. A computer with a large monitor

ADDITIONAL READING

National Assistive Technology Act Technical Assistance and Training Center provides a comprehensive set of resources: https://www.at3center.net/home
Alternative finance programs provide low-cost loans for the purchase of AT: http://www.resnaprojects.org/allcontacts/allafpcontacts.html
Statewide AT Act Programs provide demonstration and loan of AT: https://www.ataporg.org
O'Neill B, Gillespie A (eds.). *Assistive Technologies for Cognition.* Psychology Press; 2014.
Rispoli M, Machalicek W, Lang R. Assistive technology for people with acquired brain injury. In: Lancioni GE, Singh NN, eds. *Assistive Technologies for People With Diverse Abilities, Autism and Child Psychopathology Series.* Springer Science+Business Media. 2014. doi:10.1007/978-1-4899-8029-8_2
Gillespie A, Best C, O'Neill B. Cognitive function and assistive technology for cognition: a systematic review. *J Int Neuropsychol Soc.* 2012;18(1):1–19. doi:10.1017/S1355617711001548

ANSWERS TO STUDY QUESTIONS

1. Correct Answer: c
Increased cognitive load/cognitive demands. Unless AT is carefully assessed for appropriateness and adequate training is provided, the demands of learning and using new AT may increase the cognitive demands of a task for a while. Sometimes people with TBI may abandon AT before developing the proficiency to use it with efficiency.

Further Reading:
Lewis C. Simplicity in cognitive assistive technology: a framework and agenda for research. *Univers Access Inform Soc.* 2006;5(4):351–361. doi:10.1007/s10209-006-0063-7
Liu AL, Hile H, Borriello G, et al. Informing the design of an automated wayfinding system for individuals with cognitive impairments. In *Proceedings of the International*

Conference on Pervasive Computing Technologies for Healthcare. 2009:1–8. doi:10.4108/
ICST.PERVASIVEHEALTH2009.6018

2. Correct Answer: b
Focusing on device rather than environment/safety concerns. Navigation systems may draw the user's attention away from the environment to focus on the device. When this happens, they may respond slowly to hazards in the environment.

Further Reading:
Liu AL, Hile H, Borriello G, et al. Informing the design of an automated wayfinding system for individuals with cognitive impairments. In *Proceedings of the International Conference on Pervasive Computing Technologies for Healthcare.* 2009:1–8. doi:10.4108/
ICST.PERVASIVEHEALTH2009.6018

3. Correct Answer: a
GPS requires a connection to satellites and therefore does not work well indoors. A number of other technologies are available to support indoor positioning, including sensors, cameras, and radio-based technologies.

Further Reading:
Samama N. *Indoor Positioning: Technologies and Performance.* John Wiley & Sons, Inc.; 2019. doi:10.1002/9781119421887

4. Correct Answer: d
Alternative pointing devices replace a standard computer mouse or laptop touch pad. There are many different ways to acquire a target on a screen. Two broad categories of devices include those that are moved directly (e.g., by hand) and those that connect with software (e.g., eye recognition, speech, switch technology).

Further Reading:
Washington Assistive Technology Act Program. *Computer Access–Motor Dexterity;* 2020. http://watap.org/tourofat/computer-access-motor-dexterity

5. Correct Answer: b
Training refers to both the training of the system by reading a preset narrative script and training of the user to ensure that they understand how to control the system. Although some systems can manage reasonable accuracy with limited training of the system, all users benefit from training and education in how to use the system and reasonable expectations about the time it will take to become fluent.

Further Reading:
AbilityNet. *Voice Recognition—An Overview;* 2019. https://abilitynet.org.uk/factsheets/
voice-recognition-overview
National Center for Technology Innovation. *Speech Recognition for Learning;* 2010. www.ldonline.org/article/38655

REFERENCES

The full reference list appears in the digital product found on http://connect.springer-pub.com/content/book/978-0-8261-4768-4/part/part03/chapter/ch39

40 PRACTICAL GUIDELINES FOR PROGNOSTICATION AFTER TRAUMATIC BRAIN INJURY

SUNIL KOTHARI AND BEI ZHANG

INTRODUCTION

- Families report that they rarely receive the prognostic information they desire after traumatic brain injuries (TBIs).[1-4]
- Subjective estimates of prognosis based solely on a clinician's personal experience vary widely and are far less accurate than evidence-based prognoses derived from well-designed studies.[5,6]
- Evidence-based guidelines on prognosis after severe TBI[7] are summarized in this chapter. Additional details about the methodology used are available elsewhere.[7]
- These guidelines are designed to facilitate prognostication in individual patients by using readily available information (*predictor variables*) to predict the likelihood of long-term outcomes.

EVIDENCE-BASED GUIDELINES: BACKGROUND

- The guidelines are meant for *adults with severe TBI*. Information on both mild TBI and pediatric TBI is found in Chapters 8 and 59, respectively.
- The primary *outcomes* include classification according to the Glasgow Outcome Scale (GOS) or Glasgow Outcome Scale-Extended (GOS-E), independent living, and/or vocational reentry, all assessed at 6 months or later.
- The *GOS and GOS-E* are the most widely used measures of outcome after TBI; the guidelines assume a basic familiarity with their main categories (Tables 40.1 and 40.2).
- The primary *predictor variables* include age, initial Glasgow Coma Scale (GCS) score, time to follow commands (TTFC), early neuroimaging (both computed tomography [CT] and magnetic resonance imaging [MRI]), and duration of posttraumatic amnesia (PTA).
- Several of the predictor variables have *threshold values*, which are values above or below which a particular outcome is especially unlikely. For example:
  - If PTA lasts *more* than 3 months, a person is very unlikely to achieve a "good recovery" as defined by the GOS.
  - If PTA lasts *less* than 2 months, a person is very unlikely to be "severely disabled" as defined by the GOS.
- Clinicians can use these *threshold values as milestones* in a patient's recovery. For instance, as the length of a patient's PTA extends beyond 3 months, rehabilitation clinicians can

---

The full reference list appears in the digital product found on http://connect.springerpub.com/content/book/978-0-8261-4768-4/part/part03/chapter/ch40

TABLE 40.1   Glasgow Outcome Scale

1 = Dead
2 = Vegetative state ("alive but unconscious")
3 = Severe disability ("conscious but dependent")
  ○ Unable to live alone for more than 24 hours: the daily assistance of another person at home is essential as a result of physical and/or cognitive impairments
4 = Moderate disability ("independent but disabled")
  ○ Independent at home; able to utilize public transportation; able to work in a supported environment
5 = Good recovery ("mild to no residual deficits")
  ○ Capacity to resume normal occupational and social activities, although there may be minor residual physical or mental deficits

TABLE 40.2   Glasgow Outcome Scale-Extended

1 = Dead
2 = Vegetative state
3 = Lower severe disability ("dependent at home")
  ○ Cannot be left alone at home for more than 8 hours due to physical and/or cognitive impairments
4 = Upper severe disability ("dependent at home")
  ○ Cannot be left alone at home for more than 24 hours due to physical and/or cognitive impairments
5 = Lower moderate disability ("dependent in the community")
  ○ Independent at home; unable to return to work/school or most social/leisure activities
6 = Upper moderate disability ("dependent in the community")
  ○ Able to resume work/school at a reduced capacity
7 = Lower good recovery ("minimal residual deficits")
  ○ Resumption of normal vocational and avocational activities, even if not at pre-injury status; minimally disabling physical and/or cognitive deficits
8 = Upper good recovery ("minimal residual deficits")
  ○ Any residual physical and/or cognitive deficits are nondisabling

counsel family members about realistic expectations for the future. On the other hand, if 2 months have not yet elapsed since the injury, clinicians can give hope to families, even if the patient is still in PTA.

■ Although they are well supported by research, these *threshold values are not absolute*; there is a degree of clinical and statistical uncertainty in their use. In particular, the upper limit of the confidence interval averaged approximately 10%. This means that approximately 10% of individuals will prove to be exceptions to the guidelines.

EVIDENCE-BASED GUIDELINES: RESULTS

■ The results of the studies reviewed are summarized in Table 40.3. The final guidelines are presented in Table 40.4.
■ The duration of PTA is the most powerful single predictor of outcome after TBI. Even when other variables are available (e.g., TTFC), one should rely most on the duration of PTA, if it is available.[7]

TABLE 40.3   Summary of Findings From Studies of Nonpenetrating Traumatic Brain Injury

Glasgow Coma Scale
- Lower scores associated with worse outcomes
- No threshold values

Time to follow commands
- Longer duration associated with worse outcomes
- Threshold values:
  - Severe disability unlikely* when less than 2 weeks
  - Good recovery unlikely* when more than 4 weeks

Posttraumatic amnesia
- Longer duration associated with worse outcomes
- Threshold values:
  - Severe disability unlikely* when less than 2 months
  - Good recovery unlikely* when more than 3 months

Age
- Older age associated with worse outcomes
- Threshold values:
  - Good recovery is less likely† when older than 65 years

Neuroimaging
- Certain features (e.g., depth of lesions) associated with worse outcomes
- Threshold values:
  - Good recovery is less likely† when bilateral brainstem lesions present on early MRI*

*When used in this table and elsewhere, "unlikely" represents a very low likelihood of occurrence, approximately 10% or less.

†When used in this table and elsewhere, "less likely" represents a low likelihood of occurrence (although greater than 10%).

MRI, magnetic resonance imaging.

Source: From Kothari S, Zhang B, Darji N, Woo J. Prognosis after severe TBI: a practical, evidence-based approach. In: Zasler N, Katz D, Zafonte R, eds. *Brain Injury Medicine: Principles and Practice. 3rd ed.* Demos Medical Publishing; 2021.

TABLE 40.4   Summary of Evidence-Based Guidelines for Prognostication After Severe Nonpenetrating Traumatic Brain Injury

Severe disability (according to GOS) is unlikely when
- Time to follow commands is less than 2 weeks
- Duration of PTA is less than 2 months

Good recovery (according to the GOS) is unlikely when
- Time to follow commands is longer than 1 month
- Duration of PTA is more than 3 months

Good recovery (according to the GOS) is less likely* when
- Age is more than 65 years
- MRI indicates bilateral brainstem injury

*Although still possible for a significant minority of patients.

GOS, Glasgow Outcome Scale; MRI, magnetic resonance imaging; PTA, posttraumatic amnesia.

Source: From Kothari S, Zhang B, Darji N, Woo J. Prognosis after severe TBI: a practical, evidence-based approach. In: Zasler N, Katz D, Zafonte R, eds. *Brain Injury Medicine: Principles and Practice. 3rd ed.* Demos Medical Publishing; 2021.

PENETRATING INJURIES

- Although the mortality rate from penetrating injuries is much higher than with closed head injuries, survivors are less likely to be vegetative or severely disabled.
- In general, after penetrating missile injury, lower GCS scores and CT findings of bilaterality or transventricular injury are associated with worse outcomes. Moreover, patients with a post-resuscitation GCS score of 8 or less (and particularly 5 or less) are unlikely to achieve a good recovery.[7]

MODERATE TRAUMATIC BRAIN INJURY

- More than 90% of individuals with moderate TBI (GCS 9–12) will achieve either a moderate disability or good recovery.[8–10]
- Risk factors associated with poorer outcomes include GCS score of 9 or 10, older age (i.e., 65 or older), and abnormalities on CT scan. When these are present, patients are more likely to have a moderate disability (or, infrequently, severe disability) rather than good recovery.[8,9]

RECENT DEVELOPMENTS

- Our ability to prognosticate after TBI may improve as a result of recent advances in technology such as diffusion tensor imaging, magnetic resonance spectroscopy, serum markers (e.g., s100b), and neural networks. Although promising, there is not yet enough evidence to support the use of these modalities in routine clinical practice.[11,12]

COMMUNICATING PROGNOSES

- Formulating a prediction is only the first step in prognostication; this information must then be conveyed to the family. Tables 40.5 to 40.7 provide some suggestions for communicating prognostic information.

TABLE 40.5   General Guidelines for Communicating Prognostic Information

- Begin with the family's *desire for information* as well as their *current beliefs*.
- Ensure that the meaning and content of the *outcomes* are understood.
- Present *quantitative information* in a manner that can be understood (see Table 40.6).
- Foster *hope*.
- Pay attention to the *process* of communication (see Table 40.7).

Source: From Kothari S, Zhang B, Darji N, Woo J. Prognosis after severe TBI: a practical, evidence-based approach. In: Zasler N, Katz D, Zafonte R, eds. *Brain Injury Medicine: Principles and Practice. 3rd ed.* Demos Medical Publishing; 2021.

TABLE 40.6   Guidelines for the Communication of Quantitative Information

- Try to use "natural frequencies" when communicating probabilistic information (e.g., "Eight out of 10 people with this type of injury will make a good recovery").
- Present information both qualitatively as well as quantitatively (e.g., "There is a very good chance of a good recovery").
- Attempt to "frame" information in both a positive and negative manner (e.g., "That is the same as saying that 2 out of 10 people with this type of injury will not make a good recovery").
- When possible, consider presenting the information visually.
- Ask the person to restate, in their own words, their understanding of the information provided.

Source: From Kothari S, Zhang B, Darji N, Woo J. Prognosis after severe TBI: a practical, evidence-based approach. In: Zasler N, Katz D, Zafonte R, eds. *Brain Injury Medicine: Principles and Practice. 3rd ed*. Demos Medical Publishing; 2021.

TABLE 40.7   Guidelines for the Communication Process

- Find a quiet, comfortable room without interruptions.
- Sit close and speak face to face.
- Have the family member's support network present, if they desire.
- Present the information at a pace the family can follow.
- Periodically summarize the discussion to that point.
- Periodically ask family members to repeat or summarize what was said.
- Keep the language simple but direct, without euphemism or jargon.
- Allow time for questions.

Source: From Kothari S, Zhang B, Darji N, Woo J. Prognosis after severe TBI: a practical, evidence-based approach. In: Zasler N, Katz D, Zafonte R, eds. *Brain Injury Medicine: Principles and Practice. 3rd ed*. Demos Medical Publishing; 2021.

KEY POINTS

- Lower *GCS* scores are associated with worse outcomes, but there are no threshold values.
- *TTFC* is associated with worse outcomes.
  - Severe disability is *unlikely* when less than 2 weeks.
  - Good recovery is *unlikely* when greater than 4 weeks.
- *PTA* duration is associated with worse outcomes.
  - Severe disability is *unlikely* when less than 2 months.
  - Good recovery is *unlikely* when greater than 3 months.
- Older *age* is associated with worse outcomes.
  - Good recovery is *less likely* when older than 65 years of age.
- Deeper lesions on *MRI* are associated with worse outcomes.
  - Good recovery is *less likely* when bilateral brainstem lesions are present on an early MRI.

STUDY QUESTIONS

1. Which of the following is NOT true about the Glasgow Outcome Scale (GOS)?
   a. A patient with GOS 3 (severe disability) can be physically independent with basic mobility and activities of daily living even if cognitive deficits preclude independent living
   b. A patient with GOS 4 (moderate disability) can be left alone at home, but for no more than 8 hours
   c. A patient with GOS 4 (moderate disability) is able to work in a supported setting
   d. A patient with GOS 5 (good recovery) may still have residual neurological and/or psychological deficits

2. Severe disability (according to the GOS) is unlikely when:
   a. Initial GCS is above 6
   b. Duration of PTA is less than 2 months
   c. TTFC is less than 4 weeks
   d. Age is younger than 65 years ago
   e. MRI shows no brainstem injury

3. Good recovery (according to the GOS) is unlikely when:
   a. Initial GCS is less than 5.
   b. Duration of PTA is greater than 2 months.
   c. TTFC is greater than 4 weeks.
   d. Age is greater than 60 years ago.
   e. MRI shows unilateral brainstem injury.

4. Which of the following is NOT true about prognosis following a penetrating TBI?
   a. Relative to patients with nonpenetrating brain injuries, survivors of penetrating brain injuries are less likely to be severely disabled
   b. Relative to patients with nonpenetrating brain injuries, patients with penetrating brain injuries have higher mortality rates
   c. Lower GCS scores are associated with worse outcomes
   d. Subarachnoid hemorrhage seen on a CT scan is associated with worse outcomes
   e. Transventricular injury seen on a CT scan is associated with worse outcomes

5. Which of the following are considered preferred (i.e., more easily understandable) ways of communicating quantitative prognostic information to patients and families?
   ① "8 out of 10 people with this type of injury will make a good recovery in a year"
   ② "There is an 8 out of 10 chance of having a good recovery in a year"
   ③ "There is an 80% chance of having a good recovery in a year"
   ④ "This is the same as saying that 2 out of 10 people with this type of injury will not make a good recovery in a year"
   ⑤ "This is the same as saying that there is a 20% chance of not having a good recovery in a year"
   a. ①④
   b. ③⑤
   c. ②
   d. ①②③

ADDITIONAL READING

https://www.braintrauma.org/guidelines/prognosis#/
Maas AI, Lingsma HF, Roozenbeek B. Predicting outcome after traumatic brain injury. Handb Clin Neurol. 2015;128:455-474. doi:10.1016/B978-0-444-63521-1.00029-7

ANSWERS TO STUDY QUESTIONS

1. Correct Answer: b
GOS 4 (moderate disability) implies that a patient is independent at home and can work in a supported setting. In GOS 3 (severe disability), independent living is precluded by physical and/or cognitive deficits. Patients with a GOS 5 (good recovery) can still have residual deficits although they are considered nondisabling.

Further Reading:
Jennett B, Snoek J, Bond MR, Brooks N. Disability after severe head injury: observations on the use of the Glasgow Outcome Scale. *J Neurol, Neurosurg, Psychiat.* 1981;44:285-293. doi:10.1136/jnnp.44.4.285
https://www.tbims.org/gos/gossyl.html

2. Correct Answer: b
Based on recent evidence-based guidelines for prognostication after severe TBI, severe disability on the GOS is unlikely when (a) the TTFC is less than 2 weeks and/or (b) the duration of PTA is less than 2 months. GCS >6, age less than 65, or the lack of brainstem lesions on an MRI do not make severe disability unlikely.

Further Reading:
Kothari S, Zhang B, Darji N, Woo J. Prognosis after severe TBI: a practical, evidence-based approach. In: Zasler N, Katz D, Zafonte R, eds. *Brain Injury Medicine: Principles and Practice*. Demos Medical Publishing; 2021.

3. Correct Answer: c
Based on recent evidence-based guidelines for prognostication after severe TBI, good recovery on the GOS is unlikely when (a) the TTFC is greater than 4 weeks and/or (b) the duration of PTA is greater than 3 months. GCS <5, age greater than 60, or the presence of unilateral brainstem lesions on an MRI does not make a good recovery unlikely.

Further Reading:
Kothari S, Zhang B, Darji N, Woo J. Prognosis after severe TBI: a practical, evidence-based approach. In: Zasler N, Katz D, Zafonte R, eds. *Brain Injury Medicine: Principles and Practice*. Demos Medical Publishing; 2021.

4. Correct Answer: d
Although patients with penetrating brain injuries have higher mortality rates than patients with nonpenetrating injuries, they are less likely to be severely disabled. Both lower GCS scores and transventricular injury seen on CT are associated with worse outcomes. Studies have not identified an association between subarachnoid hemorrhage seen on a CT scan and outcome.

Further Reading:
Kothari S, Zhang B, Darji N, Woo J. Prognosis after severe TBI: a practical, evidence-based approach. In: Zasler N, Katz D, Zafonte R, eds. *Brain Injury Medicine: Principles and Practice*. Demos Medical Publishing; 2021.

5. Correct Answer: a

It is recommended that clinicians use "natural frequencies" when communicating probabilistic information, and to frame information in both a positive and negative manner. A natural frequency describes the number of people out of an easily comprehensible set (e.g., 10 or 100) who have the outcome of interest. Studies have demonstrated that most people have significant difficulties with percentages, odds, rates, risks, and so on.

Further Reading:
Kothari S, Zhang B, Darji N, Woo J. Prognosis after severe TBI: a practical, evidence-based approach. In: Zasler N, Katz D, Zafonte R, eds. *Brain Injury Medicine: Principles and Practice*. Demos Medical Publishing; 2021.

REFERENCES

The full reference list appears in the digital product found on http://connect.springer-pub.com/content/book/978-0-8261-4768-4/part/part03/chapter/ch40

41

SEXUALITY AFTER TRAUMATIC BRAIN INJURY

ANGELLE M. SANDER

GENERAL BACKGROUND

- A majority (>75%) of persons with complicated mild to severe traumatic brain injury (TBI) describe themselves as sexually active (including self-stimulation and/or activity with a partner) at 1 or more years post-injury, and 52% to 62% report having a sexual partner.[1,2]
- Sexual dysfunction is frequent after complicated mild to severe TBI, occurring in one -fourth to over one-half of persons at 1 or more years post injury.[1–4]
- Failure to address sexuality can lead to emotional difficulties, low self-esteem, and relationship problems.

COMMON TYPES OF SEXUAL PROBLEMS AFTER TRAUMATIC BRAIN INJURY

- Decreased desire or drive[1,2,5–7]
- Decreased arousal in men[5–9] and women[1,6] (e.g., difficulty obtaining or maintaining an erection in males and decreased vaginal lubrication in females)
- Decreased ability to achieve orgasm[1,2,6,7,9]
- Ejaculatory dysfunction in males[10,11]
- *Hypersexuality:* Drastic increase in sexual drive, accompanied by disinhibition and inappropriate sexual behaviors, or sexual behavior in inappropriate settings; occurs rarely (<10% of persons with TBI receiving rehabilitation services)[12] but can result in significant distress for rehabilitation staff and family members[10,13]
- *Qualitative problems with sexual functioning:* Overall dissatisfaction with sexual activity,[1,2,4] decreased frequency of sexual activity relative to pre-injury,[1,2] fewer opportunities for sexual activity,[1,2] and reduced ability to satisfy their partners[2]

CONTRIBUTORS TO SEXUAL DYSFUNCTION AFTER TRAUMATIC BRAIN INJURY

- Damage to neuroanatomic substrates
  - Frontal lobe damage or damage to related subcortical structures, including the thalamus and hypothalamus[14–16]
    - Dorsolateral frontal damage: apathy and decreased initiation and/or interest in sex
    - Orbitofrontal damage: disinhibited and impulsive sexual behavior

The full reference list appears in the digital product found on http://connect.springerpub.com/content/book/978-0-8261-4768-4/part/part03/chapter/ch41

- Damage to temporal lobe or related limbic structures, including amygdala[14,17,18]
- Damage to afferent (sensory) and efferent (motor) pathways in the brainstem[15,16]
- Disruption of neurochemical/neurotransmitter systems (dopamine, serotonin)[15,16]
- Neuroendocrine dysfunction (hypothalamic–pituitary–gonadal system)[19]
  - Hypopituitarism occurs in 20% of persons with TBI during the first year following TBI[20]
  - Deficient gonadotropin release in 10% to 15% of people following TBI; can impact hormone levels (testosterone, progesterone, and estrogen)[21]
  - For women, can lead to disruptions in menstrual cycle and decreased fertility, as well as to decreases in sex drive, lubrication, and orgasm[22]
  - For men, can lead to decreased sperm production and infertility, as well as to decreased sexual desire[23]
- Medication side effects[24,25]
  - Anticonvulsants: decreased desire; erectile dysfunction; painful, prolonged erections
  - Acetylcholinesterase inhibitors: increased sex drive; hypersexuality
  - Baclofen: erectile dysfunction
  - Stimulants: decreased desire; painful or frequent erections
  - Selective serotonin reuptake inhibitors (SSRIs) and noradrenaline–serotonin reuptake inhibitors (NSRIs): low sexual desire; difficulty achieving orgasm; erectile and/or ejaculatory dysfunction
  - Serotonin antagonist and reuptake inhibitors (SARIs): increased or decreased desire; erectile dysfunction; have also shown positive effects in reducing sexual dysfunction resulting from SSRIs
  - Dopamine agonists: erectile dysfunction; have also shown positive effects in reducing sexual dysfunction resulting from SSRIs
  - Opioids: decreased desire; erectile dysfunction; difficulty achieving orgasm
- Physical impairments[26]
  - Motor impairments (e.g., spasticity, hemiparesis, decreased balance): can lead to difficulty with positioning and to pain during sexual activity
  - Sensory impairments: can affect arousal and ability to achieve orgasm
- Cognitive impairments[26,27]
  - Impaired attention and concentration can impact sexual arousal and ability to sustain attention during a sexual encounter
  - Impaired memory can impact ability to recall sexual encounters and/or dates that can lead to sexual opportunity
  - Impaired initiation affects frequency of sexual activity and can be interpreted as disinterest by partner
  - Impaired social communication/pragmatics can result in: decreased awareness of the impact of actions on others; decreased ability to read nonverbal cues and gestures; decreased ability to interpret others' emotions; decreased empathy; decreased ability to initiate conversation
  - Impaired planning and goal-directed behavior may result in difficulty accomplishing social planning leading to opportunities for sexual relationships (e.g., cannot make a date, plan date activities, set up a romantic environment)
  - Impaired cognitive flexibility and abstract thinking limit the ability to fantasize, which is important for drive and arousal
- Emotional changes: including depression,[28] anxiety,[29] irritability,[30] low self-esteem and/or poor body image,[31] child-like and dependent behaviors, self-centeredness,[32] aggression, and impulsivity[26]

- Relationship issues: reduced relationship quality and quality of overall intimacy among partners,[32,33] with effects on partners' sexual function[34,35]
- Sleep disturbance[36]

TREATMENT

- The most important thing that you can do for your patients is to create an atmosphere of openness and comfort regarding the discussion of sexuality. Let them know that sexual problems are not infrequent after TBI. Emphasize that problems are treatable.
- Integrate one or two questions on sexuality into your intake or follow-up interview because, although they do not perceive such questions as inappropriate, many people will not bring up a sexual problem unless directly asked by the physician.[1,37]
  - "Are you sexually active and/or are you satisfied with your sexual functioning?"
  - "Do you have any questions or concerns about the impact of TBI on sex?"
- Conduct a comprehensive medical examination, referring out and/or treating as appropriate:
  - Screen for other medical illnesses that could contribute to sexual dysfunction (e.g., diabetes, heart disease, kidney disease, thyroid dysfunction).
  - Obtain hormone levels and investigate possibility of pituitary dysfunction.
  - Conduct or refer for urological exam and/or OB/GYN exam.
  - Review medications for side effects affecting sexual function.
  - Rule out pain as a cause of sexual problems.
  - Rule out sensory and motor problems as a contributor to sexual dysfunction.
- Provide specific suggestions to improve sexual functioning:
  - A change in positioning during sexual activity can reduce impact of motor problems, balance problems, and pain.
  - Assist men with investigating drugs to enhance sexual performance and/or prosthetic devices to compensate for erectile dysfunction. Familiarize yourself with the guidelines for treatment of erectile dysfunction and premature ejaculation in men.[38]
  - Assist women with investigating lubricants and/or dilators to compensate for lack of vaginal lubrication. Familiarize yourself with treatment options for the management of sexual dysfunction in women.[39]
  - Altering the environment during sexual encounters can reduce the impact of distractibility and other cognitive deficits (e.g., arranging a quiet environment, with minimal background noise).
  - Use of erotic movies or books to assist with arousal.
  - Investigation of ways to increase social networks can increase the opportunity to form intimate relationships (e.g., local YMCA, church groups, and other social organizations). Have a list of these available in your clinic.
  - Provide information on safe sex practices, including birth control and prevention of HIV and other sexually transmitted diseases.
- Refer for other services as appropriate:
  - Post-acute cognitive rehabilitation to address cognitive deficits, such as social communication, that can impact sexual functioning
  - Individual counseling/psychotherapy to address emotional issues
  - Marital or couples therapy to address relationship issues
  - Licensed sex therapy to directly address sexual problems

- Bibliotherapy: reading about sexuality and alternative ways for sexual fulfillment, books or Internet, including information on sexual prostheses
▪ In all aspects of assessment and treatment, remain sensitive to cultural issues that may impact willingness to provide intimate information and openness to certain recommendations for treatment. Seek permission for each phase of assessment and treatment, asking the patient to share concerns, including feelings of embarrassment or guilt.

KEY POINTS

▪ Sexual dysfunction is common after TBI and failure to address it can lead to low self-esteem, emotional distress, and decline in intimate relationships.
▪ Sexual dysfunction after TBI can be due to a variety of causes. A comprehensive medical evaluation, including hormone levels, gynecological examination for women, and urological examination for men is the best way to identify potential contributing factors and plan appropriate treatment and referrals.
▪ Many people will not spontaneously broach the topic of sexual difficulties with a physician, so it is important to integrate a question or two about sexual functioning into the clinical interview of persons with TBI.

STUDY QUESTIONS

1. Which of the following is not a potential contributor to sexual dysfunction after TBI?
   a. Changes in the relationship of the person with TBI and their partners
   b. An increase in gonadotropin release
   c. Emotional distress
   d. Motor impairments

2. Which of the following medications, typically used to treat persons with TBI, is least likely to contribute to sexual difficulties?
   a. Baclofen
   b. Prozac
   c. Trazodone
   d. Methylphenidate

3. Which is the least likely type of sexual difficulty to occur in a man with TBI?
   a. Hypersexual/impulsive sexual behavior
   b. Difficulty achieving orgasm
   c. Decreased sexual desire
   d. Ejaculatory dysfunction

4. Which of the following statements best describes the dynamic between physicians and patients with TBI regarding discussion of sexuality?
   a. The discussion of sexual concerns is fairly common during physician–patient follow-up appointments following TBI

   b. Most patients with TBI would prefer that physicians not talk with them about sexuality, as they are embarrassed and think it inappropriate

   c. Patients with TBI are unlikely to broach the topic of sexual difficulties unless directly asked by their physician, but they do not feel that it is inappropriate for their physician to raise the topic

   d. Sexuality is an important topic for persons with TBI, and it is one of the most frequent concerns raised during patient–physician discussions during follow-up appointments

5. Which of the following neuroanatomical substrates is least likely to contribute to sexual difficulties following TBI?

   a. Thalamus/hypothalamus

   b. Temporal lobe/amygdala

   c. Orbitofrontal lobe

   d. Cerebellum

ADDITIONAL READING

TBI Model Systems Fact Sheet on Sexuality After TBI: http://www.msktc.org/tbi/factsheets/Sexuality-After-Traumatic-Brain-Injury

Sexual Functioning and Satisfaction After Traumatic Brain Injury: An Educational Manual https://www.biausa.org/wp-content/uploads/Sexual-Functioning-and-Satisfaction-after-Traumatic-Brain-Injury-.pdf

Addressing sexuality in traumatic brain injury rehabilitation: A Guide for Rehabilitation Professionals. https://www.biausa.org/wp-content/uploads/Addressing-Sexuality-in-Traumatic-Brain-Injury-Rehabilitation.pdf

Moreno, JA, Arango-Lasprilla, JC, Gan, C, McKerral, M. Sexuality after traumatic brain injury: A critical review. *Neurorehabilitation.* 2013;32:69–85. doi:10.3233/NRE-130824

Moreno, A, Gan, C, Zasler, N. Neurosexuality: A transdisciplinary approach to sexuality in neurorehabilitation. *NeuroRehabilitation.* 2017;41(2):255–259. doi:10.3233/NRE-001480

ANSWERS TO STUDY QUESTIONS

1. Correct Answer: b

Gonadotropins are not increased, but rather decreased in about 10% to 15% of people after TBI, and the decrease can impact hormone levels.

Further Reading:

Agha A, Thompson CJ. Anterior pituitary dysfunction following traumatic brain injury (TBI). *Clin Endocrinol.* 2006;64:481–488. doi:10.1111/j.1365-2265.2006.02517.x

2. Correct Answer: c

While all of these medications can contribute to sexual difficulties, serotonin antagonist and reuptake inhibitors (SARIs) have also been found to improve sexual difficulties associated with selective serotonin reuptake inhibitors (SSRIs).

Further Reading:

Sander AM. Sexual functioning. In Silver JM, McAllister TW, Arciniegas DB, eds. *Textbook of Traumatic Brain Injury.* American Psychiatric Association Publishing; 2019:535–544. doi:10.1177/1363460718811225

3. Correct Answer: a

Hyposexuality is much more common than hypersexuality following TBI. Although rehabilitation staff and caregivers may verbalize more concerns about hypersexuality, it occurs in a small percentage of cases.

Further Reading:
Simpson GK, Sabaz M, Daher M. Prevalence, clinical features, and correlates of inappropriate sexual behavior after traumatic brain injury: a multicenter study. *J Head Trauma Rehabil.* 2013;28:202–210. doi:10.1097/HTR.0b013e31828dc5ae

4. Correct Answer: c

While the majority of healthcare professionals acknowledge that sexuality should be addressed in rehabilitation, only about one third report discussing it with their patients. Healthcare providers typically do not broach the topic of sexuality unless the patient spontaneously mentions it as a problem. Unfortunately, many persons with brain injury do not feel comfortable raising the topic of sexuality with healthcare providers. However, most do not feel that it is inappropriate for their physician to ask about sexual issues.

Further Reading:
Sander AM, Maestas KL, Pappadis MR, et al. Sexual functioning 1 year after traumatic brain injury: findings from a prospective traumatic brain injury model systems collaborative study. *Arch Phys Med Rehabil.* 2012;93(8):1331–1337. doi:10.1016/j. apmr.2012.03.037
Moreno A, Gan C, Zasler N, McKerral M. Experiences, attitudes, and needs related to sexuality and service delivery in individuals with traumatic brain injury. *NeuroRehabilitation.* 2015;37(1):99–116. doi:10.3233/NRE-151243
Arango-Lasprilla JC, Olabarrieta-Landa L, Ertl MM, et al. Provider perceptions of the assessment and rehabilitation of sexual functioning after traumatic brain injury. *Brain Inj.* 2017;31:1605–1611. doi:10.1080/02699052.2017.1332784

5. Correct Answer: d

The thalamus/hypothalamus, temporal lobe/amygdala, and orbitofrontal lobe are among the most common areas of the brain impacted by TBI, and are also involved in regulating sexual activity.

Further Reading:
Latella D, Maggio MG, De Luca R, et al. Changes in sexual functioning following traumatic brain injury: an overview on a neglected issue. *J Clin Neurosci.* 2018;58:1–6. doi:10.1016/j.jocn.2018.09.030

REFERENCES

The full reference list appears in the digital product found on http://connect.springer-pub.com/content/book/978-0-8261-4768-4/part/part03/chapter/ch41

ASSESSMENT OF DECISION-MAKING CAPACITY

ERIC S. SWIRSKY AND KRISTI L. KIRSCHNER

INTRODUCTION

The shared decision-making paradigm reflects the importance of patient autonomy in clinical encounters. Respect for patient autonomy (or the right of self-determination) requires that individuals have the right to accept or refuse recommended interventions, even those that are potentially lifesaving. The paradigm of informed consent is aimed at satisfying this clinical duty; however, a patient's capacity to evaluate complex information and communicate choices are both prerequisites. Adult patients are generally presumed to have decision-making capacity. Patients with brain injuries should be formally assessed. Decision-making capacity is not binary but exists on a continuum; it can be fluid, complex, informed by context, and the nature of the question at hand.

GENERAL PRINCIPLES

Definitions

- *Advance directive* is a statement of desired future medical treatment that allows an individual to preserve some level of autonomy surrounding such medical decisions in the event of incapacity. Examples include living wills and proxy documents such as durable powers of attorney for healthcare. Orders that require a clinician's signature to execute, such as do-not-resuscitate orders, are similar to advance directives in that they plan for a future medical decision, but they are unlike advance directives as they require a practitioner's signature.
- *Assent* refers to a person's expression of agreement to a care plan. Adults who do not have full capacity for decision-making and minor children who have not reached the age of majority should still be engaged to the greatest extent possible in making medical decisions. The legally authorized decision-maker in such situations is still responsible for the final decision, but obtaining assent ensures the respectful engagement of the person who has the most at stake.
- *Autonomy* represents a bundle of rights, both positive and negative, including an individual's right to make choices about their healthcare and take actions based on personal values and beliefs. The principle of autonomy requires that providers respect the patient's agency and liberty. This specifically necessitates disclosing adequate information to enable informed decision-making. Through shared decision-making, patients can express their values and preferences, and ultimately make authentic decisions— decisions that must be freely chosen within the range of realistic options (not wishes that are not possible).

The full reference list appears in the digital product found on http://connect.springerpub.com/content/book/978-0-8261-4768-4/part/part03/chapter/ch42

- *Capacity* is the term used in healthcare to describe a patient's functional ability to make decisions regarding their healthcare and to provide informed consent for treatment. Determinations of patient capacity are made by qualified clinicians. Patients are referred to as being "decisional," "incapacitated," or as having/lacking "decisional capacity" or "decision-making capacity." A court of law does not need to be involved for capacity decisions; these are clinical judgments for a specific medical decision.
- *Competency* is a global assessment that refers to the legal decision-making status of a patient, which is determined by a court of law. Patients adjudged to be incompetent by a court of law will have a court-appointed decision-maker (guardian). The person may be judged to be wholly incompetent or partially so (such as for medical or financial decisions), and will invariably lose certain rights, such as the right to vote, marry, or enter into contractual agreements. The U.S. court system has yet to articulate a universal standard for determining *competence,* as most states have their own statutory definitions.
- In colloquial parlance, the terms "capacity" and "competency" are often used interchangeably but we recommend that not be the case in a clinical context. The concepts involve different processes and have different implications for patients and providers.
- *Self-determination* refers to the inherent locus of control and right of decision-making that resides within the individual. Self-determination recognizes that no one is truly independent and able to live without a web of relationships and supports, taking into consideration the rights, needs, and responsibilities to others. People living with disabilities may have specific needs for physical assistance but be able to express authentic preferences and values that warrant respect and consideration.
- The need for physical assistance is a separate issue from the need for assistance in making decisions and should not be conflated. The language of self-determination can make it clear that one can be physically dependent, but able to direct one's care and make one's own decisions.
- *Supported decision-making* is an approach in which a person with cognitive disability has a person or team of people who assist in making decisions only to the extent such assistance is needed.[a]
- *Surrogate* is a healthcare decision-maker identified by the provider if the patient lacks capacity and has no advance directive. It is important to know your state's definitions: In some states, the power of attorney is referred to as the *agent* and the *surrogate* is the individual identified in state surrogate statutes. *Proxy* is another term that might be used for one or the other.

Fundamental Principles of Decision-Making Capacity

- Decision-making capacity is situation-specific and revolves around a particular question or decision at hand. It is not an all-or-none phenomenon. A person can have adequate capacity for making some decisions but not others. Thus, a capacity evaluation must be adapted to the complexity of decision-making required to answer the question.
- Healthcare decision-making requires a constellation of abilities. The four most commonly assessed are a patient's abilities to understand relevant information, appreciate the consequences of the situation, reason through treatment decisions, and communicate choices.[1] Another commonly cited factor is the possession and expression of a set of values and goals.[2]
- It is generally presumed that every adult patient has capacity unless proven otherwise.

---

[a] This approach is gaining traction for people with intellectual and developmental disabilities and mental health issues and is getting some attention for people with acquired brain injuries particularly in other countries such as Australia and England.

▪ Patients with decision-making capacity can provide informed consent for, or refuse to undergo, medical interventions. The right to refuse unwanted medical treatment is legally protected. Some jurisdictions may require "clear and convincing evidence" (often defined as an advance directive) when relying upon an incapacitated patient's previously stated wishes. This is particularly true when permanent harm or death can result from the treatment refusal.[3] In the absence of an advance directive, it is important for a physician to know the details of their state's surrogate statute, as individual states may limit the ability to withhold or withdraw life-sustaining treatment.

▪ Decision-making capacity is not static. A patient's capacity may wax and wane and can be influenced by mood, time of day, metabolic status, fatigue, pain, medications, infections, brain diseases, and psychosocial factors. If a patient is believed to not have adequate decisional capacity for the question at hand, reversible factors need to be optimized if time permits (i.e., removing sedating medications, treating infections or metabolic derangements), and then capacity should be reassessed.

▪ Refusal of treatment is not evidence of incapacity; however, patients who disagree with recommended interventions and are less adherent are more likely to have their capacity challenged by providers. In assessing capacity, providers should focus on the process—how patients arrive at a decision—rather than the decision itself.

ASSESSING CAPACITY

Background

▪ The ability to assess decision-making capacity is described as a "core competency" in brain injury rehabilitation[4]; however, it is not an area in which most clinicians are well-trained or experienced.[5]

▪ Evidence suggests that physicians routinely fail to recognize incapacity. A review of studies reporting physician recognition of capacity found that physicians correctly identified incapacity in about 42% of patients whose lack of capacity was independently judged.[6]

▪ Patients living with disabilities should not be deemed to lack capacity based solely on their medical diagnosis or condition, unless the person is in a state of unconsciousness.

▪ Unstructured evaluations of capacity are considered unreliable. Evaluation tools have been developed to help clinicians and researchers assess patient capacity. At a minimum, it is recommended that the practitioner use a structured interview, document the conversation with the patient, including the date and time, decision at hand, content of the discussion, and specific elements that were assessed in the conversation.[7]

▪ Capacity is decision-specific. A patient may have capacity to make some decisions but remain unable to make more complex decisions related to care. When assessing capacity, clinicians should explicitly state which decision is being tested (e.g., "this patient is being assessed for her ability to make decisions about having a shunt revision this week to relieve intracranial pressure").

▪ Capacity should be assessed on a sliding scale: The level of capacity required changes in proportion to the complexity and gravity of the decision and risk to the patient.[8]

▪ Most traumatic brain injuries (TBIs) are mild in degree, and these patients may regain capacity quickly. Patients with more severe TBIs may recover partial or full capacity over time, thus underscoring the importance of continual reassessment.[9]

Assessment Instruments and Protocols

There are assessment tools available to assist providers through the process of capacity assessment using oral and written vignettes, essays, questionnaires, and structured interviews. Though it is not necessary to use a formal tool, they can be used to ensure all the necessary elements are formally queried and the interview is structured. Examples include the Aid to Capacity Evaluation, the Capacity to Consent to Treatment Instrument, and the Hopkins Competency Assessment Test. It is important to note that instruments should be selected based on context of use, that each instrument has limitations, and that the various tools do not always agree in assessment of decisional capacity.[10]

The Structured Interview

The Decisional Capacity Structured Interview: Whether or not an assessment instrument is used to rate patient responses, assessing capacity involves a structured conversation or interview between a clinician and the patient. Brain injury physicians need to be comfortable with this process, be familiar with the nuances, and know when it is appropriate to postpone decisions (when possible) until the patient is in the best position to make a decision, and when to seek a legally authorized decision-maker to act on the patient's behalf. The following elements should be assessed:

- *Alertness*: Patients must have a level of alertness that allows for the assessment to take place. Patients who are unconscious are universally viewed as lacking capacity; however, recent advances in neuroimaging may provide for a novel approach for determining the awareness of neurologically impaired and behaviorally nonresponsive patients.[11]
- *Orientation*: What is their medical condition? What has happened to them? Where are they? Assessing their appreciation of their circumstance and the need to participate in decision-making is what is most critical. It is not as critical that people be oriented specifically to time as to place and situation.
- *Ability to communicate a choice*: Patients must be able to express a decision via verbal or nonverbal means. They cannot have a level of ambivalence so extreme that choices cannot be determined. Stability of choice is relevant and can be tested by asking the same questions at different times/days.
- *Understanding of relevant information*: Includes the ability to attend to, comprehend, store, recall, and interpret information. Deficits in intelligence, memory, and attention span can interfere with this element. Clinicians should test understanding by asking the patient to paraphrase what they have been told about the treatment or life decision, and the risks and benefits of the options (otherwise known as a "teach-back.").
- *Appreciation of the situation and its consequences*: Can the patient grasp the probable outcomes of the treatment and the consequences of refusal? Pathological denial, delusional perceptions, and affective/cognitive deficits may interfere with this ability.
- *Rational manipulation of information*: Can the patient engage in a balanced risk/benefit analysis? This involves the ability to reach conclusions that are logically consistent with the starting premise, as well as individual preferences and values. The chain of reasoning and not the conclusion should be the focus.

DECISION-MAKING AFTER TRAUMATIC BRAIN INJURY: ETHICAL AND LEGAL CONSIDERATIONS

Decision-Making for Incapacitated Patients

- Patients suffering from moderate to severe TBI are commonly confronted by medical decisions such as sustaining or removing artificial respiration, nutrition, and hydration support; cardiopulmonary resuscitation; neurosurgical and orthopedic intervention; managing medications; and execution of advance directives.[12]

▪ Patients who lack decisional capacity need to have the appropriate legally authorized decision-maker identified. For those who had a proxy appointed by a prior advance directive, the named agent is the appropriate decision-maker. For those who do not have such a directive, most states have surrogate acts or a priority list of "next of kin" to identify the authorized decision-maker. On rare occasions, for the unbefriended or unrepresented patient who has no family or friends to act on their behalf, a court-appointed guardian may be needed. Usually an ethics consult can be helpful in this circumstance.[13] The default stance in the absence of a decision-maker in such conditions is usually to continue treatment.

▪ When capacity to make treatment decisions is impaired, clinicians should make reasonable efforts to determine if the patient has the capacity to name a trusted supported decision-maker or healthcare agent. In some circumstances, it is possible to have sufficient decisional capacity to name a proxy decision-maker even when an individual does not have sufficient capacity for making medical decisions.

▪ Clinicians should actively seek patient assent despite the lack of decisional capacity whenever possible.

▪ Advance directives should be sought and utilized, as they have legal standing as an expression of patient autonomy. There are in general two types of documents; proxy, which names a trusted individual (i.e., power of attorney for healthcare), and instructional, which provides guidance for future care decisions (i.e., living will). These instruments are a recognized part of the decision-making process and are generally honored out of respect for patient autonomy. It should be noted, however, an old instructional advance directive may not represent the authentic self and perspective of a patient now living with TBI.[14] Instructional directives made prior to a disability may not be fully informed. Given this, durable powers of attorney for healthcare may be the most useful because they appoint a proxy decision-maker who can work with the patient and care team through the various nuanced decisions that must be made on the patient's behalf.

▪ Decision-making for those who lack capacity should be informed by substituted judgment or, in the absence thereof, the patient's best interests. Substituted judgment requires that decisions be made in accordance with a patient's preferences and goals of care when known. If not known, then surrogates and providers should be guided by what is in a patient's best interests; that is, after considering available options, the decision-makers should seek outcomes that provide the most benefit to the patient while keeping in mind the patient's values.[15]

▪ Approximately 60% of patients die after a decision to limit the intensity of medical interventions, rather than from the direct effects of TBI.[16] Early requests for withdrawal of life-sustaining treatment should be assessed with care, as there can be a great deal of prognostic uncertainty early after a brain injury, especially about the extent of disability and what their future life might be like.[17,18]

▪ Although intended to respect patient autonomy and preferences, clinical decision-making practices for TBI patients are not without controversy. For example, the healthcare system and society in general exhibit bias against people living with disabilities. Moreover, there are differing views on what it means to be healthy. Many people's views are negatively skewed regarding the reality of living with disability, and advance directives may reflect such. Disability advocates aim toward respect for the decisions made by competent patients; however, "in cases of terminal refusal of treatment, [clinicians] have a responsibility to correct misinformation about life with disability, a duty to counter the coercive influence of the stigma that has been attached to human dependency."[19]

▪ Ethics committees, ethics consultation services, spiritual care services, and social work departments can provide valuable guidance and insight to assist providers in these matters. Inclusion of peer support, and people with lived experience of brain injuries can also be invaluable.

Capacity to Consent to Research

■ Laws, policies, and guidelines for consent to research have developed separately from those related to treatment; accordingly, there are separate assessment protocols and instruments for determining capacity to consent to clinical research. Consent for research and consent for treatment are similar in that they provide for autonomous decision-making, represent a process that conveys the specifics of the intervention or research, and detail the potential risks involved to patients and research subjects. Nevertheless, there are major differences in the standards; for example, research consent forms must contain financial disclosures to identify conflicts of interest and require approval by Institutional Review Boards (IRBs). The U.S. Food and Drug Administration provides specific items to be included on consent forms in the Code of Federal Regulations.[20]
■ Capacity assessment for research for adults with TBI raises ethical questions including who should determine capacity, what conflicts of interest exist, and whether current definitions of capacity are adequate for subjects with TBI.[21]
■ There are no widely accepted and validated methods for assessing consent capacity for research with TBI populations. Adequate safeguards should be in place to ensure minimal risk to vulnerable research participants, including consulting with providers with relevant experience, use of independent participation monitors, and a process to reassess capacity when fluctuations are anticipated.[22] Other safeguards include outlining a specific plan to assess capacity when targeting subjects with decisional impairment, proxy consent, requiring assent from subjects who lack capacity, a process for reassessing capacity for those previously impaired, and enrolling subjects without capacity only when their participation is "scientifically necessary."[23]

Neuropsychological Testing and Decisional Capacity

■ Determination of decision-making capacity should not be made solely or primarily based on neuropsychological testing, but such testing can be used to support clinical judgment.[7,12]
■ Providers and courts traditionally rely on neuropsychological testing when making determinations about capacity and competency; however, research in this area suggests that no single or small grouping of neuropsychological functions is associated with decision-making capacity across conditions.[7]
■ At the time of inpatient hospitalization, impaired short-term verbal memory appears to be strongly associated with incapacity in patients suffering moderate to severe TBI; by 6 months post-injury improvements in working memory and executive function have been associated with improved capacity.[12]
■ During the early stages of recovery and emergence from coma, a patient's capacity may change rapidly. It is impractical to repeat full neuropsychological batteries while a patient's status is in flux.

Decisional Capacity Versus Performative Capacity

■ Many patients with TBI demonstrate discrepancies between decisional capacity and performative capacity.[24] They may be able to describe what they want to do in a particular situation, but they may not be able to act accordingly when that situation arises.
■ Most capacity tools focus on a patient's ability to provide consent for medical treatment while on brain injury units. It is often also necessary to assess a patient's capacity to make decisions about practical life situations—such as a decision to choose to live independently or a decision to drive a car.[25] This usually necessitates moving beyond a

structured interview to some type of simulated testing environment where observable behaviors can be incorporated into the assessment.[26]

Personhood and Family Matters

There are long-term effects of TBI not only for patients but for their families, who often relate that patients living with TBI seem like "different people" and demonstrate uncharacteristic behaviors or beliefs post injury. Patients may be impulsive, lack initiative, or be interpersonally provocative. Ethically, it may be difficult to know how to respond when a patient who appears to have some limited capacity makes decisions that their loved ones know to be profoundly different from those made prior to their injury.

- Many families experience a type of ambiguous loss in that their loved one is present physically but psychologically absent or different. This can have a detrimental impact upon relationships. Patients and families may require counseling and access to resources on loss and moving forward with new and unanticipated identities.[27]
- A tendency to minimize the severity of cognitive deficits, while not necessarily denying the fact that they sustained injuries—a hallmark of many patients with TBI—may be a reason to place greater weight on previously demonstrated preferences and life choices. That said, the decisions made by brain injury patients with decision-making capacity should be honored; they should not be forced to sacrifice present autonomy for their former selves or past attitudes.[4,19]
- TBI creates a host of decision-making responsibilities for the family and loved ones as well as the patient. The patient's role and status in the family may change, as patients with TBI may be more dependent on others and no longer have capacity to make decisions for dependent minor children, older adult parents, or a spouse. Family members may be unprepared for new decision-making roles, conflicts may arise regarding care, and relationships may be strained. Clinicians should perform a family assessment and be prepared to assist family members through the decision-making process.[28]

KEY POINTS

- There is no uniform definition of capacity or method for determining capacity.
- Decisional capacity, or lack thereof, cannot be assumed by virtue of diagnosis; individualized assessment is required.
- Capacity assessment is an essential skill for rehabilitation clinicians.
- Patients who lack capacity should still be involved in their healthcare decision-making processes to the extent they are capable of doing so, and with proper support.

STUDY QUESTIONS

1. A homeless 14-year-old was brought to the emergency department (ED) by a friend who said he had gotten into a fight with another person on the street, fell, and hit his head. She is not sure how long he was unconscious, but by the time she flagged down a police car he was "coming to." Initially in the ED, the patient appeared confused and disoriented, complaining of a painful headache. His head computed tomography (CT)

scan was negative for bleed; his drug screen was positive for marijuana use. He improves over the next hour and is alert, able to talk, and expresses a desire to immediately leave the hospital. Which of the following is the most appropriate response to this situation?

a. Inform law enforcement that the patient is ready to be discharged.

b. Seek a surrogate decision-maker; if none is available, discuss with your legal office about whether to initiate guardianship procedures

c. Discharge the patient as requested

d. Ask the patient to complete an advance directive so that their wishes can be known and followed

2. Edna is a single 89-year-old woman with moderate dementia and a history of falls. She was treated for a subdural hematoma requiring drainage a year ago. She was ultimately discharged to a nursing home where she has resided ever since. She has no known family or close friends. About a month ago, she was noted to become short of breath with minimal exertion. She was sent to the hospital and was diagnosed with metastatic lung cancer. Her doctor judges that she lacks capacity to understand her current condition and make health decisions. The doctor recommends a plan of care that would emphasize comfort measures and would also put in place a do-not-resuscitate order. What principle is the doctor employing to justify this recommendation?

a. Substituted judgment

b. Best interests

c. Surrogate decision-making

d. Informed consent

3. Fifteen years ago, Maria had a severe TBI caused by an improvised explosive device while deployed in the armed forces. She had a moderately severe brain injury, and partial amputation of one upper and lower limb, but is able to live in an apartment in an assisted living facility and get around with a power wheelchair. Maria's mother or sister visit weekly and help her with setting up her pill box and paying her bills. Maria does not have a guardian but relies on her mother and sister to help her make decisions when needed. They try to attend her doctor's appointments so that they can help her ask clarifying questions, debrief afterward about what information is discussed, and think about what is important to her when considering important decisions. This type of decision-making is best described as:

a. Informed consent

b. Best interests

c. Supported decision-making

d. Surrogate decision-making

4. Tisha is a 45-year-old married mother of three who sustained a TBI after a hit and run accident as she was crossing a busy intersection. An ambulance was called, and her husband was notified after her identification was found in her purse. There is increasing evidence of swelling of the brain and her neurosurgeon recommends that she be intubated and an intracranial pressure monitor be urgently placed. Tisha is intermittently able to state her name but appears to be confused and getting sleepy. The neurosurgeon asks her husband to consent to the surgical procedure. This scenario is an example of:

a. Informed consent

b. Substituted judgment

   c. Supported decision-making
   d. Surrogate decision-making

5. Steven is a 45-year-old with a history of paranoid schizophrenia who was struck by a taxi while in a crosswalk. He is brought to the ED by ambulance, and the examining doctor finds him to be angry, hostile, and guarded. His brain CT is negative, and he is diagnosed with multiple contusions but no serious injuries. He is admitted to the hospital for observation.

   Steven lives with his sister, who is his legal guardian, and her two young children. They have a good relationship, and his sister is a strong advocate for his care. His sister confides in the attending physician that while she wants to remain active in his care as guardian, she is concerned about taking him back home. She is feeling less able to care for Steven at home, due to her own failing health. She asks about whether Steven can be transferred to an assisted living facility. They have the means to pay for such care. Steven has no other siblings. When this option is discussed with Steven, he becomes enraged, states his refusal to enter such a facility, and demands that he be allowed to return to his sister's home immediately. Which is the most appropriate next response?
   a. Further problem-solving among trusted advisers and the care team to explore immediate, short-term options that are safe and supportive, and how to engage Steven in exploring these choices
   b. Begin discharge planning as suggested by Steven's sister
   c. Request Steven's sister to revoke guardianship and begin the process of finding a new guardian to make healthcare decisions
   d. Obtain psychiatry consult to evaluate Steven's decision-making capacity

ADDITIONAL READING

Stanford Encyclopedia of Philosophy. Decision-making capacity. http://plato.stanford.edu/entries/decision-capacity/#EleCap

Ganzini L, Volicer L, Nelson WA, et al. Ten myths about decision-making capacity. *J Am Med Dir Assoc.* 2005;6(3 suppl):S100–S104. doi:10.1016/j.jamda.2005.03.021

Knox L, Douglas J, Bigby C. Whose decision is it anyway? How clinicians support decision-making participation after acquired brain injury. *Disabil Rehabil.* 2013;35(22):1926–1932. doi:10.3109/09638288.2013.766270

Lazaridis C. Withdrawal of life-sustaining treatments in perceived devastating brain injury: the key role of uncertainty. *Neurocrit Care.* 2019;30(1):33–41. doi:10.1007/s12028-018-0595-8

Davidson G, Kelly B, MacDonald G, et al. Supported decision making: a review of the international literature. *Int J Law Psychiatry.* 2015;30:61–67. doi:10.1016/j.ijlp.2015.01.008

Vesney BA. A clinician's guide to decision making capacity and ethically sound medical decisions. *Am J Phys Med Rehabil.* 1994;73(3):219–226. doi:10.1097/00002060-199406000-00013

ANSWERS TO STUDY QUESTIONS

1. Correct Answer: b
   At 14 years of age, the patient is not of the age of majority to make healthcare decisions. According to law in the United States, minors are presumed to be incompetent.

Further Reading:
Buchanan AE, Brock DW. *Deciding for Others: The Ethics of Surrogate Decision Making.* Cambridge University Press; 1989. doi:10.1017/CBO9781139171946

2. Correct Answer: b
Unbefriended patients who lack capacity present unique challenges for providers. When it is not possible to honor the wishes of a patient because they are unknown, clinicians and surrogates are guided to follow the *Best Interests* standard of decision-making.

Further Reading:
Schweikart SJ. Who makes decisions for incapacitated patients who have no surrogate or advance directive? *AMA J Ethics.* 2019;21(7):E587–E593. doi:10.1001/amajethics.2019.587

3. Correct Answer: c
This scenario describes a process of supported decision-making for Maria. She is being assisted in problem-solving by trusted advisers and the care team to explore options that are safe and supportive of her needs and self-determination (Center for Public Representation. Legal Capacity, Supported Decision-making).

Further reading:
https://www.centerforpublicrep.org/initiative/supported-decision-making

4. Correct Answer: d
This scenario describes the process of surrogate decision-making. The patient lacks capacity and decisions must be made, and there does not seem to be an advance directive available. The team has identified the person with the highest priority for surrogate decisions—the patient's spouse—who should be contacted to make decisions for the care of his wife.

Further Reading:
Buchanan AE, Brock DW. *Deciding for Others: The Ethics of Surrogate Decision Making.* Cambridge University Press; 1989. doi:10.1017/CBO9781139171946

5. Correct Answer: a
Discussion is needed to find a solution that works for the patient, family, and the care team. Steven's sister has yet to indicate that she is disinterested in continuing as her brother's guardian, but he can no longer live with her. Steven needs to be involved in this process and an approach of supported decision-making is the appropriate next response.

Further Reading:
Knox L, Douglas J, Bigby C. Whose decision is it anyway? How clinicians support decision-making participation after acquired brain injury. *Disabil Rehabil.* 2013;35(22):1926–1932. doi:10.3109/09638288.2013.766270

REFERENCES

The full reference list appears in the digital product found on http://connect.springer-pub.com/content/book/978-0-8261-4768-4/part/part03/chapter/ch42

COMMUNITY INTEGRATION

DMITRY ESTEROV, JULIE WITKOWSKI, AND THOMAS BERGQUIST

GENERAL PRINCIPLES

Throughout this chapter, the term "brain injury" primarily refers to moderate to severe traumatic brain injury (TBI), although some of the discussed topics may also be applicable to other forms of acquired brain injury such as stroke, hypoxia/anoxia, mass lesions, and so on. This chapter defines community integration and the need for an individualized approach, discusses an assessment of participation and community integration within the context of the International Classification of Functioning, Disability and Health (ICF) Model, and highlights available community resources and post-acute rehabilitation interventions for this population.

Definition

Community integration following moderate to severe TBI can be defined as "the assumption or resumption of culturally and developmentally appropriate social roles following disability."[1] Community integration has been described as falling into one of three main areas: employment or other productive activity, independent living, and social activity.[2] Both of these descriptions emphasize the need to identify goals from the point of view of the individual who has sustained the TBI, as well as highlight the variability in perceptions of community integration among individuals with TBI. Factors such as age, race/ethnicity, sex/gender identity, community setting (rural vs. urban), regional differences, and level of functioning prior to injury can influence individual community integration goal setting.[3-6] In addition, the nature of one's familial and social relationships has been identified as a particularly important factor for individuals living with moderate to severe TBI, and is a key component of community integration. In a mixed qualitative and quantitative study of persons with TBI from diverse racial, ethnic, and socioeconomic backgrounds, having friends and family living nearby was cited as a factor that increased sense of belonging, as was feeling acknowledged in their surrounding community.[3] Maximizing community integration must take into account the diverse priorities, psychosocial settings, and cultural differences. An understanding of these individual and environmental factors allows for an individualized treatment approach.

Epidemiology

TBI is increasingly being recognized as a chronic condition.[7,8] Despite this recognition, research has shown continued gaps in optimal community integration as compared to the general population, persisting years after injury.[9,10] While functional trajectories vary, the majority of TBI survivors do return to the community.[11] Despite this, individuals living with sequelae of TBI continue to have difficulty with employment/productive activity, independent living, and in societal participation.[4,12]

The full reference list appears in the digital product found on http://connect.springerpub.com/content/book/978-0-8261-4768-4/part/part03/chapter/ch43

There are a number of individual characteristics or factors that influence successful community integration, including age, race, years of education at time of injury, prior employment, injury severity, and level of social support pre injury.[4,6,13–15] In addition, individual ratings of resiliency have been linked to higher perceived quality of life following disability, and thus evaluation of individualized resiliency patterns may contribute to identification of those particularly at risk for declining life satisfaction after TBI.[16]

DIAGNOSIS

Assessment With International Classification of Functioning, Disability, and Health Model

The World Health Organization (WHO) has developed the ICF Model as the standard for understanding and classifying the changes in functioning associated with health conditions for both clinical and research purposes.[17] This model has been used to investigate factors impacting social integration for adults with brain injury,[18–20] and classifies the sequelae of brain injury into body functions and structure, activity limitations, and participation restrictions. Figure 43.1 demonstrates the interplay of these factors.

Body functions and structure are characterized based on identification of normal structure/function versus impairments in physical or mental functioning. Activity is defined as the execution of a task by an individual. Activity limitations are defined by

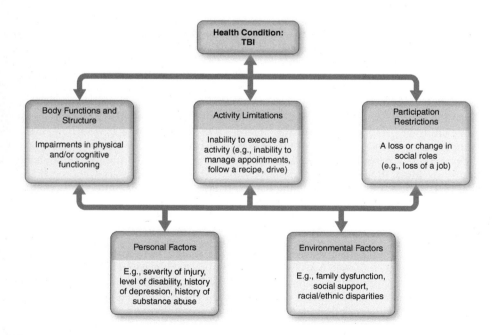

FIGURE 43.1 An adapted International Classification of Functioning, Disability and Health Model from a traumatic brain injury perspective.

Source: Adapted from the International Classification of Functioning, Disability, and Health: ICF. Version 1.0. World Health Organization© 2001.

an individual's inability to execute an activity (e.g., inability to recall appointments, to follow a recipe while cooking, recall a medication regimen, money management) due to impairments in body functions and structure. Participation restrictions represent a loss or change in social roles due to changes in body functioning and associated activity limitations (e.g., loss of a job or inability to attend college). Participation is typically assessed through patient or family report and measured by the degree to which an individual is (a) an active, productive member of society and (b) well integrated into family and community life. In other words, participation restrictions reflect community integration factors,[2] including the ability to run a household, maintain a network of friends and family, and be involved in productive activities such as employment, education, and volunteer activities. In the ICF model, there is a dynamic interplay among changes in body functions and structure (physical and cognitive), activity limitations, and the participation restrictions that impact the person's reintegration into the community.

According to the ICF model, individual and environmental/situational factors may obstruct or facilitate successful community integration. While understanding the severity and nature of TBI in a given individual is necessary to understand the challenges an individual will face as they move forward in recovery, this information alone is not sufficient. Understanding individual and environmental differences will lead to the person served receiving the most appropriate and effective rehabilitation, leading to the best possible recovery. Here are some examples of each.

Personal Factors

Injury severity and the extent of disability has been found to predict the variance in community integration.[21] History of depression and substance abuse, pre-injury chemical dependency and psychiatric history, unemployment, and limited education can all represent barriers to community integration.[22–25] Conversely, a strong work history and higher premorbid educational level can favorably impact outcome.

Environmental Factors

- Families commonly experience stress, which can be exacerbated after TBI, and is associated with poorer outcome.[26]
- There are health disparities related to race and health insurance coverage in the likelihood of admission to inpatient rehabilitation, which in turn can impact outcome post-TBI.[27]

Measures of Community Integration

There are several measures that assess community integration, and measure participation as described in the ICF Model. These and other measures of outcome are available at the Center for Outcome Measurement in Brain Injury (COMBI) at the following website: www.tbims.org/list.html. Many of these measures can be downloaded free of charge. Three of the more commonly administered measures are described in the following.

Community Integration Questionnaire-Revised

The original Community Integration Questionnaire (CIQ) is one of the most frequently used instruments to measure home, social, and productivity integration in the field of brain injury. The original CIQ consisted of 15 items measuring domains including home integration, social integration, and productive activities. The Community Integration Questionnaire-Revised (CIQ-R) has since been expanded to 18 items and also includes a measure of electronic social networking.[28]

Mayo-Portland Adaptability Inventory Participation Index

The Mayo-Portland Adaptability Inventory Participation Index (M2PI) is an eight-item scale, with items measuring behavioral initiation, social contact with friends and coworkers, leisure activities, self-care (eating, dressing, hygiene), independent living/homemaking, transportation, employment, and money management. [29]

Participation Assessment With Recombined Tools-Objective

The Participation Assessment With Recombined Tools-Objective (PART-O) consists of 24 items tapping a range of participation domains including those related to productivity, out and about, and social relations. [30]

TREATMENT

Early Intervention Versus Long-Term Follow-Up and Care

Early onset neurorehabilitation, ideally within days of injury onset, as well as intensive neurorehabilitation in a rehabilitation facility, promotes functional recovery of patients with moderate to severe TBI.[31] In light of the trend toward reduced rehabilitation lengths of stay over the past few decades,[32] the role of programs that provide ongoing, community-based treatment after hospitalization has taken on increasing importance.[33–35]

Two broad categories of post-acute rehabilitation have been described: intensive rehabilitation programs and supported living programs. The overarching goal of intensive rehabilitation programs is to *improve* the functional and adaptive abilities as well as community participation, whereas supported living programs aim to *maintain* stability in function, adaptation, and participation. Intensive post-acute rehabilitation programs include: (a) *neurobehavioral*—pharmacological and behavioral treatment for patients with severe behavioral disturbances in a highly restricted environment; (b) *residential*—rehabilitation and community services in an environment with professional supervision throughout the day; (c) *outpatient holistic day treatment*—intensive, integrated, interdisciplinary rehabilitation for those with severe and pervasive disabilities typically including impaired self-awareness; (d) *outpatient community integration*—focused rehabilitation for individuals with circumscribed and self-identified goals; and (e) *home- and community-based*—interdisciplinary rehabilitation to improve independent living and community reintegration provided in participant's homes and community settings. Most patients, even after severe TBI, are appropriate for one of the last three types of programs. Supported living programs include: (a) programs for patients who are *slow to recover*, (b) *long-term residential* programs, and (c) *long-term community-based supported living* programs.

Studies have shown that such intensive post-acute brain injury programs—particularly intensive residential and intensive outpatient and community-based rehabilitation— are effective in improving community integration by reducing disability and improving community participation.[33–35] See Chapters 27 and 29 for more information regarding post-acute care.

Coordinated Care by Specialized Providers

For patients with complex injuries, coordinated care provided by specialists encouraging return to community is essential.[36] Even as progress is made and successful community living with or without supports has been realized, a change in family status, health, work, external supports, or environment can result in renewed need for rehabilitation services. A system of care that allows for long-term follow-up is critical.

Resource facilitation (RF) refers to promoting access to services and coordinating care specific to the needs of a person with brain injury by bridging medical and community-based services.[37] The RF coordinator has been described as an extension of case management, assisting the individual with TBI to develop a self-directed plan for community reentry, identifying access to needed services and supports, and developing a sustainable network of these services and supports.[38] RF has a positive impact in improving productive community-based activity, competitive employment, and volunteering.[37] Resource facilitators can serve as continuous, knowledgeable, and accessible points of contact and ensure the patient receives services from well-qualified practitioners in specialized facilities. Examples of resource facilitators are staff at Brain Injury Association chapters or at a local Brain Injury Clubhouse. RF programs vary from state to state, and there is a need to develop standardized procedures and a common definition of RF.[38]

Community Partnerships

Connecting patients and families with community services, peers, and advocacy organizations is essential for successful community integration. Examples of traditional services include: social services, state department of vocational rehabilitation, public education, public health, health care funding (Medicaid, Medicare), subsidized accessible housing, and independent living centers, among others. These services are not available in all locales, particularly in rural communities. An individualized network of community supports may need to be constructed involving, for instance, family and friends and social and religious groups. Such social support networks promote positive outcomes after brain injury.[39] The Brain Injury Association of America is a national organization geared toward improving the quality of life for those affected by brain injury. State-specific Brain Injury Alliances exist in most states, offering services including RF services, case management, educational opportunities, and support groups.

Vocational Reentry

Successful vocational reentry is a critical component of overall community integration, and often requires specialized vocational rehabilitation services. Multiple models of vocational rehabilitation exist.[12] See Chapter 70 for more details.

Mental Health Services

Accessibility of mental health services is paramount in optimizing social integration, as the prevalence of major depression in persons with moderate to severe TBI has been shown to range from 26% to 36% and is associated with increased unemployment, decreased social participation, and reduced quality of life.[40] See Chapters 52, 53, and 55 for more details regarding screening, diagnosis, and treatment of neuropsychiatric sequelae after TBI.[40]

Family Education/Caregiver Support

Families may be the sole providers of community-based care for individuals with TBI, and they play a critical role in facilitating recovery and integration into the community. It is important to communicate a long-term perspective regarding recovery to families, highlighting TBI as a chronic disease as individuals with TBI return to the community.[7,10] Studies have shown that caregivers identify need for accurate information about the consequences of TBI as being important, and some evidence suggests that increased knowledge can improve self-efficacy and engagement in one's rehabilitative efforts.[7,10,41]

Behavioral, cognitive, and emotional sequelae following TBI can significantly interfere with successful community living. Teaching families about these and other common issues, and imparting problem-solving and advocacy skills, fosters successful coping and integration. Education for families in formal settings, such as structured classes, or more informally, via support groups, can be helpful, as can use of multimedia and web-based education approaches.[42] Caregivers often require ongoing support due to the high burden experienced by caregivers, which can itself have effect on TBI outcomes.[43,44] Interventions for caregivers have been found to improve their emotional well-being.[43] See Chapter 71 for additional resources for families and caregivers.

Telemedicine Interventions

In discussion of community integration, technological advancement has caused rehabilitation programs to increasingly move toward interventions aimed at delivering rehabilitation care remotely through the use of telemedicine. There is a high potential for improving care by providing interdisciplinary treatment, care coordination, and social support remotely to underserved areas and to those with limited mobility; however, more research is needed to determine efficacy. [42,45-47]

KEY POINTS

- Community integration can be defined with respect to three main areas: employment or other productive activity, independent living, and social activity.
- In assessing community integration, it is essential to account for the diverse priorities, psychosocial settings, and cultural differences of persons living with TBI.
- The ICF Model offers a framework for understanding how an individual's unique biopsychosocial factors impact development of an appropriate and effective rehabilitation program, leading to the best possible recovery.
- Successful community reintegration requires coordinated and ongoing care provided by medical, therapy, and vocational specialists across the continuum of care.

STUDY QUESTIONS

1. A 47-year-old male sustained a TBI following a motor vehicle collision. His initial Glasgow Coma Scale score was 10. Galveston Orientation and Amnesia Test (GOAT) scores were 77 and 81 on days 13 and 14 post-injury, respectively. You are evaluating the patient during an outpatient 6-month follow-up visit. What are the important screening tools to consider in assessing for the patient's community integration?
   a. Patient Health Questionnaire-9 (PHQ-9)
   b. Cut–Annoyed–Guilty–Eye (CAGE) Questionnaire
   c. Headache Impact Test (HIT-6)
   d. Community Integration Questionnaire-Revised (CIQ-R)
   e. All of the above

2. Which of the following is an example of a participation restriction in the ICF Model?
   a. Difficulty with short-term memory
   b. Inability to follow a recipe

    c. Losing a job
    d. Making errors with medication management
    e. Worsening of depression and anxiety after injury

3. Which of the following is correct regarding the CIQ-R?
    a. It is a rarely used community integration instrument used to measure home, social, and productive activity
    b. It consists of eight questions measuring behavioral initiation, social contacts, and leisure activities
    c. It is a 24-item questionnaire assessing productivity, community engagement, and social relations
    d. The original CIQ consisted of 12 items measuring integration in the workforce and social activity
    e. The CIQ-R is an 18-item questionnaire that includes a measure of electronic social networking

4. All of the following are correct regarding resource facilitation (RF) except:
    a. RF refers to promoting access to services and coordinating care specific to the needs of a person with brain injury by bridging medical and community-based services
    b. The RF coordinator has been described as an extension of case management, assisting the individual with TBI to develop a self-directed plan for community reentry
    c. RF has a positive impact in improving productive community-based activity, competitive employment, and volunteering
    d. RF programs are fairly consistent from state to state, with an existing set of standardized procedures across various RF programs
    e. All of the above are correct

ADDITIONAL READING

Community resources offered through the Brain Injury Alliance of America: https://www.biausa.org/brain-injury/community

Sander AM, Clark A, Pappadis MR. What is community integration anyway?: defining meaning following traumatic brain injury. *J Head Trauma Rehabil.* 2010;25:121–127. doi:10.1097/HTR.0b013e3181cd1635

Malec JF, Kean J. Post-inpatient brain injury rehabilitation outcomes: report from the National Outcome Info Database. *J Neurotrauma.* 2016;33:1371–1379. doi:10.1089/neu.2015.4080

Corrigan JD. Community integration following traumatic brain injury. *NeuroRehabilitation.* 1994;4(2):109–121. doi:10.3233/NRE-1994-4207

ANSWERS TO STUDY QUESTIONS

1. Correct Answer: e
Comprehensive follow-up for individuals living with moderate to severe TBI should include a focus on reintegration in terms of assessing independent activity, independent living, and social activity. While the CIQ-R is a measure specifically of community of integration, various factors are also critical to assess including neuropsychological disturbances, substance abuse, as well as other symptoms that limit optimal community integration.

Further Reading:
Sander AM, Pappadis MR, Clark AN, Struchen MA. Perceptions of community inte-gration in an ethnically diverse sample. *J Head Trauma Rehabil*. 2011;26(2):158–69. doi:10.1097/HTR.0b013e3181e7537e

2. Correct Answer: c
Body functions and structure are measured by the presence or absence of impairments in physical or mental functioning. Activity limitations are defined by an individual's inability to execute an activity due to impairments or changes in body functions and structure (e.g., inability to recall appointments, to follow a recipe while cooking, recall a medication regimen, money management). Participation restrictions represent a loss or change in social roles due to changes in body functioning and associated activity limitations (e.g., loss of a job or inability to attend college).

Further Reading:
Ditchman N, Sheehan L, Rafajko S, et. al. Predictors of social integration for individuals with brain injury: an application of the ICF Model. *Brain Inj*. 2016;30(13–14):1581–1589. doi:10.1080/02699052.2016.1199900

3. Correct Answer: e
The original CIQ is one of the most frequently used instruments to measure home, social, and productivity integration in the field of brain injury. The original CIQ con-sisted of 15 items measuring domains including home integration, social integration, and productive activities. The CIQ-R has since been expanded to 18 items and also includes a measure of electronic social networking.

Further Reading:
Callaway L, Winkler D, Tippett A, et al. The Community Integration Questionnaire-Revised: Australian normative data and measurement of electronic social networking. *Aust Occup Ther J*. 2016;63(3):143–153. doi:10.1111/1440-1630.12284

4. Correct Answer: d
All of the above are correct except for (d). RF programs vary from state to state, and there is a need to develop standardized procedures and a common definition of RF.

Further Reading:
Ibarra S, Parrott D, Waldman W, et al. Provision of resource facilitation services for indi-viduals with acquired brain injury across the United States: results of a 2018 resource facilitator provider survey. *Brain Inj*. 2020;34(6):732–740. doi:10.1080/02699052.2020.1 749931

REFERENCES

The full reference list appears in the digital product found on http://connect.springer-pub.com/content/book/978-0-8261-4768-4/part/part03/chapter/ch43

IV COMPLICATIONS AND LONG-TERM SEQUELAE

CRANIAL NERVE PALSIES

FLORA M. HAMMOND AND SHERYL D. KATTA-CHARLES

GENERAL PRINCIPLES

Definition

Cranial nerves (CNs) provide motor and sensory innervation to the head, neck, viscera, glands, and vasculature and are termed such since they arise from the brainstem and emerge through openings in the cranium to reach their peripheral targets.

Epidemiology

True incidence of CN injuries in traumatic brain injury (TBI) is not certain, but it is thought to be common and to occur even in mild TBI.[1]

- Most frequently injured—Olfactory (CN I), followed next by Facial (CN VII) and Vestibulocochlear (CN VIII)
- Less commonly injured—Optic (CN II) and Oculomotor (CN III) nerves
- Rarely injured—Trigeminal (CN V) and lower CNs

Etiology

Etiology includes acceleration–deceleration, shearing, skull fracture, intracranial hemorrhage, intracranial mass lesion, uncal herniation, infarct, and vascular occlusion.

Mechanism of Injury

- Mechanisms include compression, traction, transection, and ischemia.
- Central (nuclear) CN injury occurs from brainstem damage; peripheral CN injury results from fracture or local injury.
- CNs are at particular risk for injury, because they traverse over bony protuberances and canals, and because they may be directly injured due to skull fracture.

DIAGNOSIS

Risk Factors

Risk factors include skull fractures due to proximity to CN (especially CNs I, II, III, IV, V [first two branches], VII, and VIII); and increased intracranial pressure, causing compression (CN III).

The full reference list appears in the digital product found on http://connect.springerpub.com/content/book/978-0-8261-4768-4/part/part04/chapter/ch44

Clinical Presentation

- *Olfactory* (I)—altered sense of smell.
- *Optic* (II)—altered visual acuity and/or visual field defects.
- *Oculomotor* (III)—ptosis, lack of accommodation, dilated and fixed pupil, divergent strabismus, diplopia, and the eye only moving laterally. When looking straight ahead, the affected eye turns outward and slightly down. When looking inward, the affected eye can move only to the middle and cannot look up or down. Because the pupillary fibers of CN III run at the periphery of the nerve, whereas the fibers responsible for extraocular movements are located centrally, mechanical trauma or compression tends to cause pupillary abnormalities before causing extraocular movement abnormalities, while the converse is true for ischemic lesions to CN III.
- *Trochlear* (IV)—diplopia (especially when descending stairs); affected eye rotated out with inability to turn the eye in and down, compensatory head tilt away from the affected side.
- *Trigeminal* (V)—scleral injection caused by corneal abrasions and drying, decreased facial sensation or neurogenic pain, and weakness with chewing.
- *Abducens* (VI)—impaired ability to move the affected eye outward along the horizontal plane, resulting in diplopia on lateral gaze toward the affected side, and when head is turned laterally toward the paretic side.
- *Facial* (VII)—weakness of the face and lid closure, inclusive of the forehead, and loss of taste sensation on anterior two thirds of the tongue. Facial muscle weakness may affect mastication with impaired oropharyngeal swallowing phase.
- *Vestibulocochlear* (VIII)—hearing loss, vertigo, nystagmus, or impaired balance; commonly associated with temporal bone fracture, mastoid fracture, Battle's sign, otorrhea, bleeding from the ear, and hemotympanum.
- *Glossopharyngeal* (IX)—loss of taste over the posterior third of the tongue, deviation of the uvula contralaterally, decreased salivation, and slight dysphagia.
- *Vagus* (X)—palate paralysis with loss of the gag reflex, dysphagia, and aphonia or hypophonia due to unilateral paralysis of the vocal fold. Bilateral vagal disruption is fatal.
- *Spinal* (XI)—inability to turn the head to the opposite side, and ipsilateral shoulder drooping, which may result in shoulder dysfunction and pain.
- *Hypoglossal* (XII)—inability to protrude tongue on the affected side; may lead to dysphagia.

Physical Examination

Generally, diagnosis is based on physical examination of CN functions. The examination may need to be repeated or completed as consciousness recovers.

- *Olfactory* (I)—Test detection of familiar, non-noxious smells with eyes closed. Giving the person choices may help overcome word-finding problems.
- *Optic* (II)—Assess visual acuity, visual fields, and pupillary reactivity, and perform ophthalmoscopic examination. Complete monocular blindness with preservation of normal pupillary reflexes is usually a sign of malingering or other types of functional (nonorganic) disorders.
- *Oculomotor* (III)—Assess tracking in the six cardinal positions, convergence on near targets, pursuit movements, saccades, pupillary reaction, and eyelid elevation. CN III palsy is indicated by difficulty moving the eye in, or up and down, with preserved outward movement, and may be associated with pupillary dilatation and ptosis. Doll's eye maneuver and pupillary light reflex are used for assessment if unconscious. A fixed

and dilated pupil signals herniation as the nerve runs medial to the temporal lobe at the tentorium edge.

- *Trochlear* (IV)—Assess adduction in conjunction with downward gaze of the involved eye. Individuals with CN IV palsy cannot look down when the eye is adducted.
- *Trigeminal* (V)—Test facial sensation, corneal reflex, and motor function of the jaw. Differentiation between deficits of the three divisions of CN V may facilitate more precise localization of injury.
- *Abducens* (VI)—Look for deficiency in lateral gaze when testing movement of the eyes through the full extent of the horizontal plane.
- *Facial* (VII)—Test the five main functions: facial expression (smile, wrinkle forehead, puff cheeks, close eyes tightly), taste identification on anterior two thirds of the tongue, external ear sensation, stapedius muscle function, and lacrimal and salivary gland function.
  - Upper motor neuron lesion—facial weakness contralateral to the lesion with sparing of forehead wrinkle because of the bilateral innervation of the frontalis muscle
  - Lower motor neuron lesion—ipsilateral facial weakness inclusive of flattened forehead wrinkle; inability to close eye
  - Pontine lesion (CN VII nucleus)—complete ipsilateral facial paralysis along with contralateral hemiparesis, and frequently accompanied by ipsilateral CN VI palsy
- *Vestibulocochlear* (VIII)—Examine tympanic membrane for tears, and test eye movement for nystagmus, postural responses, and hearing.
- *Glossopharyngeal* (IX)—Test sensation of posterior palate and gag reflex.
- *Vagus* (X)—Test palate elevation and gag reflex.
- *Spinal* (XI)—Test resisted head rotation to the opposite side and ipsilateral shoulder shrug.
- *Hypoglossal* (XII)—Look for ipsilateral atrophy, tongue fasciculations, and deviation with tongue protrusion. The tongue deviates to the side of the weak tongue muscles because of the unopposed, contralateral muscles. In lesions at or below the level of the hypoglossal nucleus in the brainstem, this deviation is toward the side of the lesion. (In cortical lesions, the tongue deviation is away from the side of the lesion.)

Diagnostic Evaluation

- *Olfactory* (I)—Evaluation may include imaging the anterior cranial structures, ethmoid tomography to detect basal skull fracture, and an electroencephalogram (EEG) in cases of parosmia.
- *Optic* (II)—Consider EEG to evaluate for occipital seizures. Visual evoked response may be considered to assess the integrity of the visual system from the eye to the occipital cortex.
- *Oculomotor* (III)—CN III palsy may be a sign of impending neurological compromise, and as such, diagnostic imaging studies (computed tomography [CT]/magnetic resonance imaging [MRI]) are needed emergently to evaluate the cause.
- *Trochlear* (IV) and *abducens* (VI)—CT or MRI may help assess the location of associated pathology, and to exclude structural pathology such as tumor.
- *Facial* (VII)—electromyography and nerve conduction can provide prognostic data. Brain imaging may be warranted to aid in distinguishing between central and peripheral lesions.
- *Vestibulocochlear* (VIII)—CT of the temporal bones may be indicated to assess for skull fracture in the region of the auditory canal. Audiometry helps detect, characterize, and quantify hearing loss and guide treatment decisions. Brainstem auditory evoked responses (BAERs) may be useful in those who are unable to cooperate with audiometry.

TREATMENT AND PROGNOSIS FOR RECOVERY

Measures are needed to prevent secondary injury, and a variety of treatments may be aimed at promoting recovery and improving function.

- *Olfactory* (I)—There are no established effective treatments. Safety measures and education are needed to include awareness of potential risks (e.g., inability to detect smoke, spoiled foods, or toxins), use of smoke alarms on all floors, labeling food, and need for hygiene routines. Reported prognosis is: 33% recovery, 27% worsened, and 40% no change.[2] Recovery owing to olfactory nerve regeneration usually occurs within the first 6 to 12 months post-injury,[3] with later recoveries (up to 5 years) occasionally reported.[4] Parosmia (sensation of smell in the absence of stimulus) may be the first sign of return.
- *Optic* (II)—Evaluation by a neuro-ophthalmologist or optometrist is warranted. Steroids and/or optic canal decompression may be beneficial in selected cases. Special optics may help visual field defects.[5] Visual training may help visuospatial disorders.[6] The optic nerve is a direct extension of the brain and does not regenerate.
- *Oculomotor* (III)—Occlusive therapy resolves diplopia during patching, but does not produce long-term effects. Strabismus surgery may be performed to correct cosmetic deformity, although it should be delayed for 6 to 12 months to allow for spontaneous recovery. The return of function is usually incomplete, with complete recovery in 40%.[4] Aberrant regeneration may occur.
- *Trochlear* (IV)—Treatment depends on the cause. Ocular exercises may help. Sometimes strabismus surgery is necessary.
- *Trigeminal* (V)—Decreased corneal sensation with resulting risk of corneal abrasions requires frequent eye irrigation, lubricating gel, and patching of the affected eye, especially at night. If irritation continues, lateral or complete tarsorrhaphy is needed to avoid development of corneal ulceration and opacities. If trigeminal neuralgia develops, consider nerve block, anticonvulsants, or other agents and modalities for neuropathic pain.[7] While carbamazepine provides more than 50% pain reduction in 60% to 70% of individuals, full dosage may not be reached due to side effects. In that case, another medication (e.g., lamotrigine, gabapentin, amitriptyline) may be considered.[8,9] Because CN V innervates the muscles of mastication, injury to CN V can result in difficulty with chewing, and oral dysphagia.
- *Abducens* (VI)—CN VI palsy due to TBI usually resolves over time.
- *Facial* (VII)—Treatment considerations for facial nerve swelling within the facial canal may include corticosteroid administration, otolaryngology consultation, and facial nerve decompression. Complete facial nerve disruption may be helped with surgical techniques. Inadequate lid closure requires frequent topical lubricant and may require an eye pad/taping or tarsorrhaphy. In cases of oral-motor weakness, speech therapy may be needed to assess swallowing safety and exercises for oral-motor strengthening should be administered. With delayed onset palsy, CN VII is usually structurally intact and recovers in 8 weeks.[3] During nerve regeneration, aberrant reinnervation may occur, resulting in synkinesis (e.g., "crocodile tears," in which tearing replaces salivation during eating).
- *Vestibulocochlear* (VIII)—Vestibular treatment is aimed at the system's capacity to habituate to stimuli.[3] Refer to a physical therapist well versed in vestibular rehabilitation. Labyrinthine exercises are used to decrease vestibular sensitivity.[10] Medications for vestibular dysfunction are discouraged because of potential sedation, cognitive side effects, and prevention of central adaptation.[3] Unilateral hearing loss may be helped with contralateral routing of signal (CROS) type hearing aid.[3] Sensorineural hearing loss is not amenable to surgery or hearing aids. Surgical repair may help conductive

hearing loss that fails to recover spontaneously.[11] Masking sound devices and biofeedback may help tinnitus.[3]

■ *Glossopharyngeal* (IX)—Treat symptomatically, and assess risk for aspiration. May need speech pathology to assist with oral-motor exercises.

■ *Vagus* (X)—Identify alternative feeding techniques for those at risk for aspiration. Pharyngeal exercises may improve mild dysarthria.[10] Glottic incompetence may be improved with procedures that augment vocal cord bulk. For high vagal lesions, aggressive surgical procedures (e.g., thyroplasty and arytenoid adduction) may be beneficial.[12]

■ *Spinal* (XI)—Aggressive physical therapy should be initiated as soon as possible. Surgical nerve repair after sectioning may be possible in selected cases.

■ *Hypoglossal* (XII)—Dysarthria exercises may improve coordination and strength. Assess for dysphagia, possible need for swallowing precautions, or oral-motor exercises.

KEY POINTS

■ CN injury is common with TBI, and can even be seen when the TBI is mild.

■ CN palsies may occur with TBI for several reasons, including acceleration–deceleration, shearing forces, skull fracture, intracranial hemorrhage, intracranial mass lesion, uncal herniation, infarct, or vascular occlusion.

■ CNs are particularly at risk for injury as they traverse over bony protuberances and through bony canals and because they may be directly injured due to skull fracture.

■ Injury to the CNs may result in significant consequences to the individual with TBI, as they may compound the deficits caused by a cortical injury. It is essential to identify any CN injuries so that the associated deficits may be addressed, optimizing clinical outcome and quality of life.

STUDY QUESTIONS

1. You are examining a 22-year-old with TBI resulting in diffuse axonal injury, grade 3, and facial fractures, caused by a motor vehicle collision. The patient's left eyelid is drooping. When the eyelid is lifted, the eyeball appears to be deviated laterally and slightly inferiorly and the pupil is fixed and dilated. What issues might this patient expect with their vision?
   a. Blurred vision
   b. Diplopia
   c. Monocular blindness
   d. Loss of outward gaze

2. A patient comes in with pain in the face, located over the medial cheek, episodic in nature but severe in intensity, electric in quality, which started around the time of a motor vehicle collision in which the patient suffered TBI and an orbital blowout fracture. He did not have any change in vision, so the fracture was managed nonoperatively. On physical exam, his extraocular muscles are full and he has no facial droop. He is reporting so much pain that the pain prevents him from working or sleeping. Pain is not relieved by over-the-counter medications. What is the diagnosis?

a. Malingering
b. Postconcussive syndrome
c. Trigeminal neuralgia
d. Bell's palsy

3. A 51-year-old presents with chief complaint of dizziness, which started shortly after a motor vehicle collision, in which the patient's vehicle was T-boned. The patient was restrained. The airbags deployed and hit him in the side of his head. He did not lose consciousness, but felt dazed, wobbly, and nauseated. Vertigo came on that evening and persisted. Now, he is dizzy only when he bends down to tie his shoes or when he gets into bed. What will your management consist of?
a. Meclizine
b. Physical therapy referral
c. MRI brain
d. Valium

4. Which special sensation is most frequently lost after a TBI?
a. Smell
b. Vision
c. Hearing
d. Touch

ADDITIONAL READING

Cranial nerve exam: http://library.med.utah.edu/neurologicexam/html/cranialnerve_normal.html
Blumenfeld H, Brainstem I. Surface anatomy and cranial nerves. In: *Neuroanatomy through Clinical Cases.* 2nd ed. Sinauer Associates, Inc.; 2010.
Azarmina M, Azarmina H. The six syndromes of the sixth cranial nerve. *J Ophthal Vis Res.* 2013;8(2):160–171.
Jin H, Wang S, Hou L, et al. Clinical treatment of traumatic brain injury complicated by cranial nerve injury. *Injury.* 2010;41(7):997–1002. doi:10.1016/j.injury.2010.03.007

ANSWERS TO STUDY QUESTIONS

1. Correct Answer: b
Down and out appearance of the eye and fixed and dilated pupil indicate an oculomotor palsy, which may result in diplopia. Visual acuity exam would need to be conducted to assess for blurring or loss of vision (a and c). Outward gaze (d) is lost with an abducens palsy and the eyeball would be deviated inwardly.

Further Reading:
Keane JR, Baloh RW. Posttraumatic cranial neuropathies. *Neurol Clin.* 1992;10(4):849–867. doi:10.1016/S0733-8619(18)30183-X

2. Correct Answer: c
The infraorbital nerve can be compressed in an orbital blowout fracture leading to neuralgiform pain in the maxillary distribution. Pain can be debilitating and responds to surgical decompression or other treatment options. Patients with postconcussive syndrome (b) may also present with pain, insomnia, mood disturbance, and inability

to work. However, the specific distribution of pain is indicative of traumatic trigeminal neuralgia and not postconcussive syndrome or malingering (a). Bell's palsy is a peripheral facial palsy (CN VII), which may present with facial pain, though typically associated with weakness.

Further Reading:
Katta-Charles, SD. Craniofacial neuralgias. *NeuroRehabilitation.* 2021;47(3):299–314. doi:10.3233/NRE-208004

3. Correct Answer: b
   The most frequent form of vertigo after head trauma is benign paroxysmal vertigo, due to unilateral canalolithiasis and responds well to canalith repositioning maneuvers by a trained vestibular therapist (b). Vestibular suppressant medications such as antihistamines (a) or benzodiazepines (d) are not recommended. Brain imaging (c) is not warranted for benign postural peripheral vertigo.

Further Reading:
Sismanis A. Post-concussive neurootological disorders. *Phys Med Rehabil: State Art Rev.* 1992;6(1):79–88.

4. Correct Answer: a
   The olfactory nerve is most frequently affected by TBI.

Further Reading:
Keane JR, Baloh RW. Posttraumatic cranial neuropathies. *Neurol Clin.* 1992;10(4):849–867. doi:10.1016/S0733-8619(18)30183-X

REFERENCES

The full reference list appears in the digital product found on http://connect.springer-pub.com/content/book/978-0-8261-4768-4/part/part04/chapter/ch44

45 HYDROCEPHALUS

DAVID F. LONG AND MITHRA B. MANEYAPANDA

GENERAL PRINCIPLES

Definition and Epidemiology

- Hydrocephalus is defined as "a dynamic imbalance between the formation and absorption of cerebrospinal fluid resulting (CSF) in accumulation of excess CSF associated with ventricular dilatation and/or enlargement of the subarachnoid space."[1]
- It is the most common treatable neurosurgical complication in traumatic brain injury (TBI) rehabilitation.[2]
- Hydrocephalus can be difficult to distinguish from ex vacuo ventriculomegaly, a hallmark of severe diffuse brain injury.[2,3]

Classification

- Communicating hydrocephalus—all ventricles are interconnected with free exit of CSF to subarachnoid space[2]; most posttraumatic hydrocephalus cases.
- Noncommunicating hydrocephalus—obstruction between ventricles or preventing outflow from ventricles; consider aqueductal stenosis decompensated by TBI when lateral and third ventricles are large but fourth ventricle is small or normal; lumbar puncture is contraindicated.[2]

Pathophysiology of Hydrocephalus

- The processes causing the development of hydrocephalus are complex. Hydrocephalus is not necessarily associated with increased pressure, because when ventricles enlarge, the expanding force is distributed over a larger area, reducing the pressure. Also, the size of the ventricles reflects the pressure within them relative to that of the surrounding tissues (just as the size of a balloon depends on the pressure inside compared with that outside).[2,3]

DIAGNOSIS

Clinical Presentation

- Risk factors—subarachnoid or intraventricular hemorrhage, meningitis, craniectomy.[1,4]

The full reference list appears in the digital product found on http://connect.springerpub.com/content/book/978-0-8261-4768-4/part/part04/chapter/ch45

■ Acute hydrocephalus may present with signs of increased intracranial pressure, including headache, nausea, vomiting, lethargy, papilledema, bulging craniectomy flap, and Cushing's triad (hypertension, bradycardia, and hypoventilation).[2]

■ Normal-pressure hydrocephalus (NPH) may present with triad of gait "apraxia" (shuffling magnetic quality with reduced cadence, decreased step height, loss of counter-rotation), "subcortical" cognitive impairment, and urinary incontinence.[2,5] Of these three symptoms, gait impairment is the most indicative of hydrocephalus and the most likely to respond to shunting.

■ Decompensated aqueductal stenosis may present with Parinaud's/pretectal syndrome (loss of upgaze, lid retraction, impaired pupillary reactivity, convergence retraction nystagmus).

■ Other presentations of hydrocephalus include akinetic mutism, bradykinesia, parkinsonian syndrome, and nonspecific deterioration in neurological status.[2,5]

Computerized Tomography and Magnetic Resonance Imaging

■ Typical appearance—progressive ventriculomegaly with convex frontal horns, enlarged temporal horns, and narrowing of the callosal angle.[6]

■ Sulci are typically less prominent than ventricles, especially in high convexity, but the presence of enlarged sulci does not exclude hydrocephalus.[2,5]

  • Disproportionately enlarged subarachnoid space hydrocephalus (DESH)—specific focal enlargement of Sylvian fissures and sometimes other major fissures along with ventriculomegaly, but with decrease of sulci at medial high convexity; these patients often respond well to shunting. The subtly different scan appearance of these patients from that of patients with diffuse atrophy may be most evident on coronal magnetic resonance imaging (MRI).[5–7]

■ Transependymal fluid may be present—smooth periventricular signal (MRI) or lucency (computed tomography [CT]); predictive of a good response to shunting. Differential considerations—frontal contusions, cerebral infarctions, or demyelination—are usually more irregular and asymmetric.[2,5–7]

Supplemental and Invasive Assessment

■ CSF tap—involves a lumbar puncture with removal of 40 to 50 mL of CSF.[8] Viewed as positive if patient shows improvement in neurological status, though no standard exists. Gait assessment (standardized and video) pre– and post–lumbar puncture is recommended and gait is the aspect most likely to respond.[9] Cognitive assessment pre and post can also be compared in evaluating responsiveness to a therapeutic tap.[8] To optimize reliability of testing, follow-up assessments should be performed within 30 minutes to 4 hours after lumbar puncture.[5,8,9] A recent systematic review reported an average sensitivity of only 58%[8] though some patients with a negative test may still improve with shunt surgery as it produces more sustained ventricular decompression.

■ External lumbar drain trial—placement of a continuous external lumbar drain for 3 to 5 days, if available in a specialized center, is more reliable for diagnosing NPH than CSF tap,[2,10,11] with positive predictive value in one series of 96%.[10] In one small series, patients who were shunted despite a negative lumbar drainage test did poorly ($p <$ .006).

■ Cisternography—does not have a current role as it does not add to accuracy of diagnosis of hydrocephalus and does not predict shunt responsiveness.[12,13]

TREATMENT

Initial Management

Surgical Options

- Ventriculoperitoneal shunt—CSF drains from a ventricular catheter, out of the skull through a burr hole, through a one-way valve. The catheter passes under the skin, terminating in the peritoneal space; the standard procedure for managing communicating hydrocephalus.[2,14]
- Other shunt types—include ventriculoatrial, ventriculopleural (often performed to get lower pressure or when an unrelated intra-abdominal process contraindicates a ventriculoperitoneal placement), and lumboperitoneal (for communicating hydrocephalus only).[2,14]
- Third ventriculostomy—For aqueductal stenosis: a hole created between the floor of the third ventricle and the adjacent cistern allows passage of CSF without requiring a shunt.[15]

Basic Shunt Concepts

- Shunts typically have a one-way valve, either with a fixed setting or programmable with an external magnet; very large ventricles may need a particularly low-pressure valve setting.[2]
- A palpable reservoir or pumping chamber will generate forward flow if there is a valve between it and the ventricle; if the valve is further downstream than the reservoir, pumping can generate retrograde flow into the ventricle, such as for intrathecal medication administration.[2,16]
- Clinical improvement and reduction in ventricular size after shunting do not correlate well. Recent efforts with combined programmable and gravitational shunts seem to indicate that good clinical results can sometimes be obtained from shunting with little associated reduction in ventricular size.[2]

Shunt Complications

Shunt Failure

- Incidence of shunt revision in adults is approximately 30%.[2]
- Shunt failure symptoms include irritability, confusion, lethargy, headache, or acute neurological change.
- Shunt palpation may show excessive resistance (distal occlusion) or inadequate refill (proximal obstruction). Unfortunately, one cannot determine with certainty whether a shunt is working by bedside palpation.[16]
- Perform CT or MRI and look for increased ventricular size compared with prior scan.
- Distal shunt occlusion may also be associated with fluid loculation or pseudocyst on abdominal CT.[17]
- Shuntogram is most definitive—A needle is inserted into a safely perforable part of shunt, pressure measured, and contrast or isotope injected and followed down into peritoneal space.[14,18]

Shunt Infection

- Insidious presentation—low-grade fever, malaise, irritability; erythema over shunt; 70% occur in the first 2 months after insertion; *Staphylococcus epidermidis* is most common; lumbar puncture is unreliable; diagnosis is by shunt tap.[2]

■ Treatment—IV antibiotics and either shunt removal or externalization.[2]
■ Prevention—antibiotic impregnated catheters have been shown to reduce overall incidence of shunt infection, but not for methicillin-resistant *Staphylococcus aureus* or gram-negative infections.[19]

Overdrainage

■ Gravitational pressure of the column of CSF between the valve and the distal end of the catheter in an upright position frequently causes siphoning of CSF, resulting in overdrainage.[2,14]
■ Acute overdrainage symptoms can include orthostatic headache, dizziness, vomiting, lethargy, and diplopia. Chronic overdrainage causes slit ventricle syndrome with nonpostural headache and intermittent proximal shunt malfunction.[2]
■ Overdrainage predisposes to development of subdural hematomas and hygromas—CSF drainage from ventricles creates increased potential subdural space. Subdural collections occur in 4.5% to 28% of shunted patients and are more likely with very large ventricles before shunting.[2]

Syndrome of the Trephined

■ Syndrome in patients with craniectomy where the flap becomes sunken, the CT shows mass effect, sulcal effacement, and midline shift away from craniectomy, and there are associated neurological impairments.[20–22]
■ Patients with concurrent shunts for hydrocephalus are more likely to develop the syndrome as CSF is drained internally, which decreases the outward force and allows external forces (atmospheric pressure, gravity) to push inward.[20]
■ Definitive treatment is with cranioplasty.[20,23]

Additional Considerations

Programmable Shunts—Concepts and Use

■ These allow bedside adjustment of the opening pressure of shunt valves by use of an external magnet to prevent underdrainage (poor clinical response) or overdrainage.[2,14,17,24,25]
■ Cost-effective (often avoids reoperation), and adjustments can improve clinical course.[16,26]
■ Inadvertent valve resetting by MRI, magnets, valve filliping, or transcranial magnetic stimulation may occur[2,27,28]; MRI scans are not contraindicated, but valve settings need to be rechecked after MRI (even with MRI-resistant valves); some valves require confirmatory x-ray to verify setting.[2,27,28]

Antisiphon Devices and Gravitational Shunts

■ Antisiphon devices are added to a shunt system in an attempt to prevent excessive CSF flow induced by siphoning.[2,29] Some of these work through a subcutaneous membrane; others have flow regulated or gravitational units. A programmable antisiphon device is also now available.[30]
■ A gravitational unit in series with a programmable valve can decrease siphoning and allow adjustment with an external magnet.[29] The incidence of overdrainage at 6 months was significantly decreased with valve systems including a gravitational valve component compared with those without.[31]

Specific Programmable Shunts

■ Codman Hakim Programmable Valve—first in the United States, multiple clinical trials, 18 settings at 10 mm increments from 30 to 200 mm H_2O; MRI can reset valve, and determination of setting requires x-ray.[2,24,27]

- Medtronic Strata Valve—multiple models with five settings from 0.5 to 2.5 for opening pressures ranging from 15 to 220 mm H_2O; MRI can reset, but valve can be read and adjusted at bedside.[2,27]
- Sophysa Programmable Valves—two models, Sophy and Polaris. Polaris has locking mechanism to prevent setting changes by MRI.[25,27,29]
- Aesculap-Miethke proGAV Programmable Shunt System—combines a gravitational unit in series with a programmable valve with a brake to prevent inadvertent MRI valve change; settings can be checked at bedside and verified by x-ray.[29]
- Codman Certas Adjustable Valve—seven settings for opening pressures from 26 to 247 mm H_2O plus a "virtual off" setting for treating shunt-associated subdural collections; designed to be resistant to MRI reprogramming even at 3 Tesla.[32]

KEY POINTS

- Differentiation of hydrocephalus from ex vacuo ventricular dilation/atrophy can be very difficult. Clinical decline and positive response to lumbar drainage can help identify shunt responsive hydrocephalus.
- The syndrome of DESH can have a scan appearance easily confused with atrophy. Look for focally dilated Sylvian fissures but lack of prominent sulci at medial high convexity to differentiate.
- Do a shuntogram to determine if a shunt is blocked, and, when looking for shunt infection, culture fluid from the shunt, not by lumbar puncture.
- The combination of craniectomy and shunt placement increases risk of developing the syndrome of the trephined. Cranioplasty is the definitive treatment.
- Programmable shunts can be adjusted to ensure adequate CSF drainage without overdrainage. Make sure to check programmable valve settings after MRI to detect inadvertent reprogramming.

STUDY QUESTIONS

1. Which of the following is true about programmable shunts?
   a. Programmable shunts can be turned to a lower setting at the bedside to drain more CSF if initial shunt response is inadequate
   b. Programmable shunts should have their settings rechecked after MRI
   c. A number of different programmable valves are available, and sometimes they are combined with antisiphon devices to prevent overdrainage
   d. Patients with programmable shunts are less likely to need surgery if they develop postoperative subdural hematomas compared to patients with fixed–opening-pressure shunts
   e. All are true

2. In performing a therapeutic CSF tap, what is most likely to improve, and how long after lumbar puncture should formal follow-up assessment be performed?
   a. Cognition, 1–2 days
   b. Equally cognition and gait, 1–2 days
   c. Gait, 6–8 hours
   d. Gait, 0.5–4 hours

3. In patients with shunts for hydrocephalus who develop the syndrome of the trephined, extracranial forces exceed intracranial forces. All of the following measures can raise intracranial pressure and counter external forces *except*:
   a. Trendelenburg position
   b. Hydration
   c. Increasing shunt valve setting
   d. Hyperosmolar therapy

ADDITIONAL READING

X-ray appearance for shunt valves:ˑ http://www.kinderneurochirurgie-leipzig.de/therapeuticfocus/hydrocephalus/radiologic-identification-of-vp-shunt-valves-and-adjustment

Damasceno BP. Neuroimaging in normal pressure hydrocephalus. *Dement Neuropsychol.* 2015;9(4):350–355. doi:10.1590/1980-57642015DN94000350

Graff-Radford R, Jones T. Normal pressure hydrocephalus. *Continuum: Lifelong Learning in Neurology.* 2019;25(1):165–186. doi:10.1212/CON.0000000000000689

Lollis SS, Mamourian AC, Vaccaro TJ, Duhaime AC. Programmable CSF shunt valves: radiographic identification and interpretation. AJNR Am J Neuroradiol. 2010;31(7):1343–1346. doi:10.3174/ajnr.A1997

Sundström N, Lagebrant M, Eklund A, Koskinen LD, Malm J. Subdural hematomas in 1846 patients with shunted idiopathic normal pressure hydrocephalus: treatment and long-term survival. *J Neurosurg.* 2018;129(3):797–804. doi: 10.3171/2017.5.JNS17481

Miyake H. Shunt devices for the treatment of adult hydrocephalus: recent progress and characteristics. *Neurol Med Chir (Tokyo).* 2016;56:274–283. doi:10.2176/nmc.ra.2015-0282

Williams MA, Malm J. Diagnosis and treatment of idiopathic normal pressure hydrocephalus. *Continuum (Minneap Minn).* 2016;22(2 Dementia):579–599. doi:10.1212/CON.0000000000000305

Akins PT, Guppy KH. Sinking skin flaps, paradoxical herniation, and external brain tamponade: a review of decompressive craniectomy management. *Neurocrit Care.* 2008;9(2):269–276. doi:10.1007/s12028-007-9033-z

ANSWERS TO STUDY QUESTIONS

1. Correct Answer: e
   All are true.

   Further Reading:
   Miyake H. Shunt devices for the treatment of adult hydrocephalus: recent progress and characteristics. *Neurol Med Chir (Tokyo).* 2016;56:274–283. doi:10.2176/nmc.ra.2015-0282
   Sundström N, Lagebrant M, Eklund A, Koskinen LD, Malm J. Subdural hematomas in 1846 patients with shunted idiopathic normal pressure hydrocephalus: treatment and long-term survival. *J Neurosurg.* 2018;129(3):797–804. doi: 10.3171/2017.5.JNS17481

2. Correct Answer: d
   Gait is the most likely thing to improve after a tap test. Given that CSF is made at a rate of 0.3 mL/min and 30 to 50 mL of CSF is removed during lumbar puncture, the volume removed will be replaced in a few hours. As such, follow-up assessments are recommended to be performed early, between 30 minutes and 4 hours after lumbar puncture.

Further Reading:
Graff-Radford R, Jones T. Normal pressure hydrocephalus. *Continuum: Lifelong Learning in Neurology.* 2019;25(1):165–186. doi:10.1212/CON.0000000000000689
Williams MA, Malm J. Diagnosis and treatment of idiopathic normal pressure hydrocephalus. *Continuum (Minneap Minn).* 2016;22(2 Dementia):579–599. doi:10.1212/CON.0000000000000305

3. Correct Answer: d
   Hyperosmolar therapy, such as hypertonic saline and mannitol, decreases intracranial pressure and would exacerbate the force imbalance in syndrome of the trephined.

   Further Reading:
   Akins PT, Guppy KH. Sinking skin flaps, paradoxical herniation, and external brain tamponade: a review of decompressive craniectomy management. *Neurocrit Care.* 2008;9(2):269–276. doi:10.1007/s12028-007-9033-z

REFERENCES

The full reference list appears in the digital product found on http://connect.springer-pub.com/content/book/978-0-8261-4768-4/part/part04/chapter/ch45

46 POSTTRAUMATIC SEIZURES

KAN DING AND RAMON DIAZ-ARRASTIA

GENERAL PRINCIPLES

Definition

A seizure is an abnormal excessive synchronous discharge of cortical neurons that can result in transient clinical manifestations such as sensations, alteration in behavior or consciousness, and/or body movements.[1,2]

- Subclinical seizure—"nonconvulsive seizure"; seizure activity seen on an electroencephalogram (EEG) with no overt clinical features.
- Focal seizure—seizure originates within a neuronal network limited to one hemisphere that may be discretely localized or more widely distributed. Based on clinical manifestation, focal seizures are classified according to the patient's level of awareness and whether they evolve to a bilateral tonic–clonic seizure.
- Generalized seizure—seizure rapidly engages bilateral distributed networks. Generalized seizures are also further classified according to motor or nonmotor manifestations.
- Epilepsy—at least two unprovoked seizures more than 24 hours apart or one unprovoked seizure but with high probability of recurrent seizures in the next 10 years based on history and abnormal imaging.[2] Broadly, "epilepsy" refers to the tendency to have a seizure, while the "seizure" refers to the ictal event itself.

A posttraumatic seizure (PTS) is a seizure which occurs after a traumatic brain injury (TBI), when the TBI is felt to be the proximate cause after other provoking factors (i.e., substance use, metabolic derangement) are excluded.

- Immediate seizures or "concussive convulsions" are acute symptomatic seizures that occur within 24 hours of TBI; they are not predictive of posttraumatic epilepsy (PTE).[3]
- Early PTS are acute symptomatic seizures occurring within 1 week after TBI. They are associated with increased risk of PTE.[4]
- Late PTS occur more than 1 week after TBI.

PTE refers to a disorder of recurrent, unprovoked, late PTS. The recurrence rate after a single late PTS is over 70%, so a single late PTS is sufficient for the diagnosis of PTE.[3]

Epidemiology

- The prevalence of PTS in the United States is 2% to more than 50% depending on cohort and injury severity.[5]

The full reference list appears in the digital product found on http://connect.springerpub.com/content/book/978-0-8261-4768-4/part/part04/chapter/ch46

- About 80% of first PTS occur within 2 years, 50% to 60% within 1 year, and 40% within 6 months of TBI.[6]
- Early PTS occur in 2% to 17% of all patients with brain injuries, are more common in children, and correlate with TBI severity.[5]
- For survivors of moderate to severe TBI, the cumulative incidence of late PTS is 12% at year 1 and 20% by year 5.[7] The cumulative incidence of late PTS in the first 30 years after TBI is 2% for mild injuries, 4% for moderate injuries, 20% for severe closed head injuries, and more than 50% if the dura is penetrated.[8] The cumulative incidence of epilepsy in the general population is approximately 1.5%.[6]

Pathophysiology

- Physiological mechanisms causing PTS are not completely understood.[9]
- Both focal and diffuse brain insults often coexist in TBI patients. Focal insults (contusions or intracranial hematomas) result in neighboring neural inflammation, gliosis, sprouting, and neurogenesis, which are felt to result in epileptogenesis.[10] Diffuse insults can result in injury to susceptible brain regions, such as the hippocampus. Injury can lead to atrophy and sclerosis; up to one third of PTE is of temporal lobe origin.[11]

DIAGNOSIS

Risk Factors

- For early PTS—younger age (especially less than 5 years), acute intracranial hemorrhage (ICH), acute subdural hematomas (SDH; in children), diffuse cerebral edema (in children), metal fragment retention, neurological deficits, depressed or linear skull fractures (in adults), and loss of consciousness or amnesia for greater than 30 minutes.[5]
- For late PTS—age greater than 65 years, early PTS (in adults), SDH, brain contusion, alcoholism, penetrating injury, retained metal fragments, depressed skull fracture, posttraumatic amnesia greater than 24 hours, neurological deficits, brain tissue loss, and severe TBI with initial Glasgow Coma Scale (GCS) of 8 or less.[5-7] (see Engel under Additional Reading).
- The relative risk (RR) of late PTS in moderate to severe TBI is 13% in the first year and decreases with time and reaches the baseline value for the population at 10 to 15 years after the injury.[6] In mild TBI, the RR reaches baseline for the population by 5 years post injury.[6]
- A single late PTS has a 65% to 90% chance of progressing to PTE.
- The likelihood that PTE will go into remission is lower if PTS are frequent in the first year after TBI, if PTS onset is greater than 4 years after TBI, or if there is ICH.[12,13] (See Engel under Additional Reading.)
- The effect of genetic variation is unclear in posttraumatic epileptogenesis.

Clinical Presentation

- PTS may present as subclinical seizures, focal seizures with or without impaired consciousness (majority), or even as generalized seizures (up to 5%) but not as generalized absence seizures. (See Diaz-Arrastia et al. under Additional Reading.)
- Any focal seizure (with or without impaired consciousness) can secondarily generalize; more common with frontal than temporal lobe origin seizures.
- Typical symptoms associated with focal seizures without impaired consciousness by location of seizure origin:

- Frontal lobe—rare auras; clonic or tonic posturing of body parts
- Temporal lobe—autonomic (abdominal discomfort, nausea, abdominal rising feeling), psychic (fear or sense of impending doom, anxiety, feelings of déjà vu or jamais vu), or olfactory and gustatory hallucinations (usually of an obnoxious smell or taste)
- Parietal lobe—vertiginous aura, elementary sensory symptoms (which can be painful)
- Occipital lobe—elementary visual hallucinations (bright lights, zig-zagging colored lines, or kaleidoscopic shapes), formed visual hallucinations

■ Typical symptoms associated with focal seizures with impaired consciousness by location of seizure origin:
- Frontal lobe—hyperkinetic motor movements, bicycling, hip thrusting, thrashing, and asymmetric tonic posturing
- Temporal lobe—staring, unresponsiveness, automatisms (i.e., stereotyped behaviors such as chewing, lip smacking, self-polishing movements or fumbling with their clothes), or dystonic posturing of the extremities

■ Generalized tonic–clonic seizures (GTCS) are characterized by tonic extensor posturing of the arms and legs, followed by rhythmic clonic movements of the arms, legs, and trunk. GTCS are often associated with transient apnea, vomiting, tongue biting, and sphincter incontinence.

■ After a focal seizure with impaired consciousness or GTCS, there may be a postictal period (typically lasting less than 10 minutes), during which the patient is obtunded and difficult to arouse. Even after regaining consciousness, patients are often confused and amnestic for up to several more hours. Patients often report headaches, dizziness, and sleepiness after a seizure, particularly GTCS.

■ Subclinical seizures are common after prolonged clinical convulsive seizures or in critically ill patients. Unexplained, prolonged, postictal confusion should raise the concern for subclinical seizures.

Physical Examination

■ Neurological findings, if present, may correlate with the epileptogenic zone.
■ Immediately after a seizure, transient focal neurological deficits (i.e., weakness that later resolves ["Todd's paralysis"] or aphasia) are often helpful in localizing seizure origin.

Diagnostic Evaluation

■ Differential diagnosis includes psychogenic nonepileptic seizures (PNES) (i.e., "pseudoseizures"), syncope (e.g., concussive syncope), confusional states (i.e., delirium), acute memory disorders (e.g., fugue state), dizziness, and imbalance.
■ In patients with moderate to severe TBI with refractory spells, about 30% were misdiagnosed as having PTE but actually had PNES.[14] Therefore, if atypical features are present and seizures continue despite treatment, the diagnosis of PTE should be verified by video electroencephalogram (vEEG).

Laboratory Studies

■ Serum tests: chemistry panel, liver function tests, urine drug screen, and antiepileptic drugs (AED) serum level, if appropriate.
■ Routine scalp EEG: A single 30-minute interictal (between seizures) EEG has a low sensitivity (30%–50%, which approaches 80%–85% with serial EEGs) for capturing epileptiform activity. However, if captured, epileptiform discharges (spikes or sharp waves)

are greater than 97% specific for epilepsy. An EEG after sleep deprivation or after a seizure may increase the yield of detecting epileptiform discharges.

- Inpatient Epilepsy Monitoring Unit (EMU) evaluation with vEEG monitoring should be considered if seizures are disabling and do not respond to appropriate AEDs.
- vEEG monitoring is required for the diagnosis of subclinical seizures. 24-hour vEEG recording is generally required to rule out subclinical seizures in noncomatose patients and 48-hour vEEG recording for comatose patients.[15]
- Prolonged ambulatory EEG monitoring is less expensive than inpatient vEEG and may be of value, but the lack of video recordings to correlate with EEG findings significantly limits the sensitivity and specificity.

Radiographic Assessment

- Patients who present with an acute TBI and a seizure should be imaged with a computed tomography (CT) scan immediately and the study should be repeated if the condition of the patient does not improve or worsens.
- Head CT is more accessible and cheaper than magnetic resonance imaging (MRI) and is usually better able to depict acute pathology (i.e., intracranial bleed) that needs urgent intervention.
- Brain MRI is the study of choice for nonurgent evaluation of PTS or PTE. Transient diffusion weighted imaging (DWI) and/or fluid-attenuated inversion recovery (FLAIR) imaging changes may occur with recent seizure activity and do not reflect structural injury.

TREATMENT

Guiding Principles

- Prophylaxis with AEDs is often initiated as soon as possible after moderate to severe TBI.[16] AEDs (i.e., phenytoin, levetiracetam) given within a day of injury prevent early PTS but not late PTS or PTE.[17–19] Chronic prophylactic use of AEDs is possibly associated with an increased risk for PTS. For these reasons, AEDs are widely recommended for use for only a short time after head trauma (7 days), to prevent early but not late PTS. (See Temkin under Additional Reading.)
- Late PTS or PTE worsens functional outcome after TBI significantly, and therefore prevention of PTS is an important goal. That said, there is no treatment which has been shown to prevent the development of epilepsy (e.g., antiepileptogenesis). AEDs may suppress seizures if late PTS or PTE do occur.
- In children, AEDs may be ineffective in preventing both early and late PTS.[20,21]
- Treatment of PTE does not require hospitalization, but admission may be needed for the treatment of status epilepticus or for vEEG to assist in the diagnosis.

Initial Management

- PTS prophylaxis—See Guiding Principles section.
- In those with a single unprovoked seizure, the decision whether or not to begin an AED depends on the risk of developing further seizures (see Risk Factors section).
- Early PTS
  - Early PTS should be treated promptly. Acutely, benzodiazepines (i.e., lorazepam, diazepam, and midazolam), phenytoin/fosphenytoin, sodium valproate, and levetiracetam are the drugs of choice and are usually effective in stopping an ongoing

seizure. There are few data to inform duration of therapy, but many continue AEDs for a few weeks to months, especially in those with moderate to severe TBI.[16]

● AED selection should be based on comorbidities and the side effect profile. Table 46.1 provides a summary of commonly used AEDs. No randomized controlled studies have been performed to prove that one is better than the other for PTS. Phenytoin probably should be avoided, because it increases the risk of impairing cognitive

TABLE 46.1 Summary of Antiepileptic Drugs

AED and Therapeutic Level	MOA	Adult Dosing	Pediatric Dosing
Carbamazepine 5–12	Na+	Initial: 200 mg bid Titration: 100 mg/day qwk, check level in q2wk Max: 1,600–2,400 mg/day	Maintenance: 10–30 mg/kg/day in bid–qid Titration: 10–30 mg/day qwk
Clobazam	GABA	Initial: 5–15 mg/day Titration:10–20 mg/day qwk Max: 80 mg/day	Initial: 5 mg daily Titration: 5–10 mg daily qwk Max: 20–40 mg daily
Ethosuximide 40–100	Ca++ L type	Initial: 500 mg/day Titration: 250 mg/day qwk Max: 1,500 mg/day	Initial: 250 mg/day Titration: 250 mg/day qwk Max: 1,500 mg/day
Ezogabine	K+	Initial: 50–100 mg tid Titration: ≤150 mg daily per wk Max: 1,200 mg daily	Data is unavailable
Felbamate 30–140	NMDA	Initial: 1,200 mg/day Titration: 600–1,200 mg/day per 1–2 wk Max: 3,600 mg/day	Initial: 15 mg/kg/day Titration: 15 mg/kg/day qwk
Gabapentin	Ca++ L-type	Initial: 300 mg tid Max: up to 1,200 mg tid	Maintenance: 15–45 mg/kg/day Titration: 25–40 mg/kg/3 days
Lacosamide	Na+ CRP-2	Initial: 50–100 mg bid Titration: 100 mg/day qwk Max: 200 mg bid	Initial: 50–100 mg bid Titration: 100 mg/day qwk Max: 100–200 mg bid
Lamotrigine 2–20	Na+	With VPA: 100–400 mg/day Initial: 25 mg qod Titration: 25 mg/day q2wk Max: 200 mg/day w VPA alone With enzyme inducer: 150–250 mg bid Initial: 50 mg qd Titration: 100 mg/day q2wk Max: 700 mg/day	Maintenance (with VPA): 0.15–3 mg/kg/day for 2 wk Titration: 0.3 mg/kg/1–2 wk to 1–5 mg/kd/day; if no VPA >0.6–15 mg/kg/day
Levetiracetam 30–60	SV2A	Initial dose: 500 mg bid Max: 3,000–5,000 mg/day	Maintenance: 10–60 mg/kg/day Titration: 10–20 mg/kg/2 wk

(continued)

TABLE 46.1 **Summary of Antiepileptic Drugs (*continued*)**

AED and Therapeutic Level	MOA	Adult Dosing	Pediatric Dosing
Oxcarbazepine 10–40	Na⁺	Initial: 300 mg bid Titration: 300 mg daily q3d Max: 2,400 mg daily	Initial: 8–10 mg/kg/day (not to exceed 600 mg daily) Titration: 8–20 mg/kg/day qwk Max: 900–1,800 mg/day based on the weight and age
Perampanel	AMPA	Initial: 2–4 mg daily Titration: 2 mg/day qwk Max: 8–12 mg qhs	Initial: 4 mg qhs Titration: 2 mg/day qwk Max: 8–12 mg qhs
Pregabalin	Ca⁺⁺ L-type	Initial: 150 mg daily in bid or tid Titration: 150 mg qwk or as tolerated Max: 600 mg daily	No dosing available
Rufinamide	Na⁺	Initial: 200–400 mg bid, or <400 mg/day with VPA Titration: 400–800 mg/day qod Max: 3,200 mg/day	Initial: 10 mg/kg/day Titration: 10 mg/kg qod to 45 mg/kg/day Max: 45 mg/kg/day up to 3200 mg/day
Tiagabine	GABA	Initial: 4 mg/day Titration: 4–8 mg/day qwk Max: 12–56 mg/day	Initial: 4 mg qd Titration: 4 mg/day qwk Maintenance: 4–32 mg/day For >12 yr same dosing as adult
Topiramate	Mixed	Initial: 25 mg daily Titration: 25–50 mg q2wk Max: 400 mg daily	Maintenance: 1–25 mg/kg/day Titration: 1–3 mg/kg/day qwk
Phenobarbital 20–40	Na⁺	Initial: 15–20 mg/kg Maintenance: 60 mg PO bid-tid and follow level	Initial: 15–20 mg/kg Titration: 10–30 mg/day qwk Maintenance: 3–6 mg/kg/day div BID
Phenytoin/ fosphenytoin 10–20	Na⁺	IV loading: 20 mg/kg Initial maintenance: 300 mg daily, then follow level	Initial loading: 20 mg/kg Titration: 25–30 mg/kg/day qwk
Vigabatrin	GABA	Initial: 500 mg bid Titration: 500 mg/day qwk Max: 1,500 mg bid	Maintenance: 40–100 mg/kg/day Titration: 10–20 mg/kg/day qwk
Valproic acid 50–150	Mixed	Initial: 10–15 mg/kg/day Titration: 5–10 mg/kg/day qwk Max: 60 mg/kg/day and follow level	Loading: 20 mg/kg/dose Titration: 5–10 mg/kg/day qwk Maintenance: 15–60 mg/kg/day
Zonisamide	Mixed	Initial: 100 mg daily Titration: 100 mg daily q2wk Max: 600 mg daily	Maintenance: 2–15 mg/kg/day Titration: 2–8 mg/kg/day q1–2 wk For >16 yrs same as adult

AMPA, α-amino-3-hydroxy-5-methyl-4-isoxazolepropionic acid receptor; AED, antiseizure medication; Ca++, calcium; GABA, ɣ-aminobutyric acid; MOA, mechanism of action; Na+, sodium; SV2A, synaptic vesicle protein A; therapeutic level, µg/L; qwk, every week; q2wk, every two weeks; qod, every other day.

function, and may adversely impact neural plasticity. Levetiracetam is better tolerated and just as effective as phenytoin in TBI.
- If seizure control is not achieved with one drug, changing to a second or even a third AED may be required to achieve seizure control.
- Late PTS
  - The risk of seizure recurrence after a first late PTS is high; chronic use of AEDs is recommended in these individuals. The choice of AEDs is the same as mentioned earlier.
- PTE—The choice of AEDs is the same as mentioned earlier.

Ongoing Care

- Regular follow-up (at least yearly) should be conducted.
- Once a therapeutic medication regimen is achieved, the individual is typically maintained on the same dosage for a period of 2 years. After a minimum 2-year seizure-free interval, the individual should be evaluated for the possibility of withdrawal from antiseizure therapy.
- Factors such as the presence of focal neurological deficits, CT or MRI evidence of structural brain disease, and persistent EEG abnormalities increase the risk of recurrence.
- If seizures become intractable, referral to an epilepsy specialist may be indicated, and consideration may need to be given to interventional approaches such as placement of a neurostimulator or epilepsy surgery.

Additional Considerations

- Patients must be warned to exercise safety precautions during swimming and climbing heights. They should never be alone during these activities. Tub baths are dangerous in patients with epilepsy, and showers are recommended.
- Patients must also be counseled about limitations in driving based on the laws in their states or countries of residence.
- Psychological problems related to social isolation and the stigma of epilepsy must be addressed. Depression is also a common comorbidity. Consultation with psychiatrists, counselors, and/or social workers should be considered when these issues are identified.

KEY POINTS

- PTE is a common consequence of TBI and is directly related to injury severity. Risk is highest after severe TBI.
- Prophylactic use of AEDs is common in most TBI centers. These should be discontinued at approximately 1 week after injury.
- The risk of recurrence after a single late PTS is high, and starting patients on an AED is recommended after only a single late PTS.

STUDY QUESTIONS

A 66-year-old man was referred to the neurology clinic for the evaluation of seizures. He started to have seizures about 6 months ago. He reports an aura of metallic taste in his mouth and being anxious. After that, he is noted to stare off with some repetitive movement of his right hand and lip smacking. During the seizures, he is not able to respond to external verbal stimulation. His seizures usually last less than 2 minutes. He is amnestic to the seizures. Occasionally, a seizure may evolve into bilateral tonic and clonic movements associated with tongue biting. The frequency of his seizures is about twice a month despite being on levetiractam 500 mg twice a day for the past 2 months. His past medical history is significant for a severe TBI secondary to a motor vehicle collision about 2 years ago. At that time, he underwent a surgical evacuation of subdural hematoma. His recent MRI was unremarkable other than mild atrophy of bilateral hippocampi.

1. Based on the history, what is the most likely classification of his seizures?
   a. Subclinical seizures
   b. Focal seizures without impaired consciousness
   c. Focal seizures with impaired consciousness
   d. Generalized seizures, likely absence seizures
   e. Not seizure activity

2. What kind of posttraumatic seizures (PTS) does this patient have?
   a. Immediate PTS
   b. Early PTS
   c. Late PTS
   d. Chronic PTS
   e. Posttraumatic epilepsy

3. What part of his TBI history makes him high risk for posttraumatic seizures?
   a. The severity of TBI
   b. Subdural hematoma
   c. Having undergone surgical evacuation
   d. Age
   e. All of the above

4. What would be the next step to manage his seizures?
   a. Increase levetiractam to 1,000 mg twice a day
   b. Add a new AED
   c. Refer to neurosurgery for epilepsy surgery
   d. Continue current treatment
   e. Refer to neuropsychology

5. The patient continues to have seizures on an optimized levetiracetam regimen and newly added lacosamide. What would be the next step in the management of his seizures?
   a. Add third AED
   b. Request a routine EEG
   c. Refer to Epilepsy Monitoring Unit for seizure characterization
   d. Repeat MRI brain
   e. All of the above

ADDITIONAL READING

AAN PTS Practice Guideline. https://n.neurology.org/content/60/1/10.full

Annegers JF, Hauser WA, Coan SP, Rocca WA. A population-based study of seizures after traumatic brain injuries. *N Engl J Med.* 1998;338(1):20–24. doi:10.1056/NEJM199801013380104

Diaz-Arrastia R, Agostini MA, Frol AB, et al. Neurophysiologic and neuroradiologic features of intractable epilepsy after traumatic brain injury in adults. *Arch Neurol.* 2000;57(11):1611–1616. doi:10.1001/archneur.57.11.1611

Engel J. Epileptogenesis. In: Engel J, ed. *Seizure and Epilepsy.* New York, NY: Oxford University Press; 2013:296–319.

Temkin NR, Dikmen SS, Wilensky AJ. A randomized, double-blind study of phenytoin for the prevention of post-traumatic seizures. *N Engl J Med.* 1990;323(8):497–502. doi:10.1056/NEJM199008233230801

Ritter AC, Wagner AK, Fabio A, et al. Incidence and risk factors of posttraumatic seizures following traumatic brain injury: a traumatic brain injury model systems study. *Epilepsia.* 2016;57:1968–1977. doi:10.1111/epi.13582

ANSWERS TO STUDY QUESTIONS

1. Correct Answer: c
Based on the International League Against Epilepsy (ILAE) 2017 seizure classification, the described seizure is mostly likely from one hemisphere at the onset. The patient is unresponsive during the seizures and amnestic to the seizures. Thus, it is a focal seizure with impaired consciousness.

Further Reading:
Pack AM. Epilepsy overview and revised classification of seizures and epilepsies. *Continuum (Minneap Minn).* 2019;25:306–321. doi:10.1212/CON.0000000000000707

2. Correct Answer: e
The seizures developed more than 1 week after the initial head injury; thus he meets the definition for late PTS. However, since he has had more than two seizures, he further meets the diagnosis of posttraumatic epilepsy.

Further Reading:
Lowenstein DH. Epilepsy after head injury: an overview. *Epilepsia.* 2009;50(Suppl 2):4–9. doi:10.1111/j.1528-1167.2008.02004.x

3. Correct Answer: e
Epidemiological studies have shown that the older age, severe TBI, subdural hematoma, subarachnoid hemorrhage, and history of surgical evacuation procedures at the acute stage after TBI are all associated with greater risk for late PTS and PTE.

Further Reading:
Frey LC. Epidemiology of posttraumatic epilepsy: a critical review. *Epilepsia.* 2003;44(Suppl 10):11–17. doi:10.1046/j.1528-1157.44.s10.4.x
Annegers JF, Hauser WA, Coan SP, Rocca WA. A population-based study of seizures after traumatic brain injuries. *N Engl J Med.* 1998;338:20–24. doi:10.1056/NEJM199801013380104

Ritter AC, Wagner AK, Fabio A, et al. Incidence and risk factors of posttraumatic sei-zures following traumatic brain injury: a traumatic brain injury model systems study. *Epilepsia*. 2016;57:1968–1977. doi:10.1111/epi.13582

4. Correct Answer: a
   The treatment of PTE follows the same guidelines used for other types of focal epilepsy. The dose of AED should be optimized before switching to a second AED or adding a second agent to the regimen. Neuropsychological evaluation and therapy are indicated for treatment for psychological nonepileptic seizures.

   Further Reading:
   Hudak AM, Trivedi K, Harper CR, et al. Evaluation of seizure-like episodes in survivors of moderate and severe traumatic brain injury. *J Head Trauma Rehabil*. 2004;19:290–295. doi:10.1097/00001199-200407000-00003

5. Correct Answer: c
   When PTE fails to respond to two AEDs with optimized doses, then it is considered to be pharmacologically resistant epilepsy. An evaluation for potential surgical treatment should be considered for pharmacologically resistant epilepsy. The first step in the pre-surgical evaluation is to capture habitual seizures in an Epilepsy Monitoring Unit in order to localize the seizure focus.

   Further Reading:
   Gupta PK, Sayed N, Ding K, et al. Subtypes of post-traumatic epilepsy: clinical, electro-physiological, and imaging features. *J Neurotrauma*. 2014;31:1439–1443. doi:10.1089/neu.2013.3221

REFERENCES

The full reference list appears in the digital product found on http://connect.springerpub.com/content/book/978-0-8261-4768-4/part/part04/chapter/ch46

HETEROTOPIC OSSIFICATION

NORA CULLEN

GENERAL PRINCIPLES

Heterotopic ossification (HO) is a common sequela of traumatic brain injury (TBI) that can lead to pain and restricted joint range of motion (ROM), limiting a patient's ability to participate in rehabilitation and further adding to disability by reducing mobility and function.

Definition

The abnormal formation of mature lamellar bone within soft tissues such as tendons, ligaments, and muscles.[1]

Epidemiology

The incidence of HO following TBI is 11% to 73.3%, reaching clinical significance in 10% to 20% of cases.[2]

Classification

After Brooker et al. 1973[3]:

- Class I—Islands of bone in the soft tissue
- Class II—Bone spurs leaving at least 1 cm between opposing surfaces
- Class III—Bone spurs leaving less than 1 cm between opposing surfaces
- Class IV – Ankylosis

Etiology

While HO is seen in rare genetic conditions, it is most prevalent after trauma (TBI, traumatic spinal cord injury, burns) and joint replacement surgery.[4]

Pathophysiology

Neurogenic Factors

Osteoblastic cells undergo inappropriate differentiation within soft tissues. They are likely stimulated by an osteogenic factor released by the injured brain[5-8] which affects prostaglandins (PG) and bone-morphogenetic proteins (BMPs), leading to abnormal regulation of bone metabolism.[9] Other contributing factors include hypercalcemia, hypoxia, sympathetic imbalance, and disequilibrium of parathyroid hormone and calcitonin.[10]

Enhanced Osteogenesis

Ectopic bone is highly metabolically active, with a rate of formation three times greater and an osteoclastic density twice that of normal age-matched bone.[11] *Timeline:* The ectopic

---

The full reference list appears in the digital product found on http://connect.springerpub.com/content/book/978-0-8261-4768-4/part/part04/chapter/ch47

organic osteoid matrix reaches full calcification within a matter of weeks. Osseous reorganization to mature trabecular bone occurs during subsequent months.[5]

DIAGNOSIS

Early detection is imperative in preventing the progression of HO.

Risk Factors

There is an increased risk with skeletal trauma, spasticity, immobilization, post-injury coma greater than 2 weeks, diffuse axonal injury, and a longer period of mechanical ventilation or intubation.[5,12–14]

Clinical Presentation

Restricted joint ROM, joint swelling and warmth, and joint pain.[15] The presence of a firm palpable mass is a late stage clinical sign.[5]

Timing
- HO formation precedes symptom onset; decreased ROM is often the earliest clinical sign.
- Symptoms generally begin 2 months post-injury, but range from 2 weeks to 12 months.[1]
- The condition may occur later with other, non-traumatic, precipitating circumstances (e.g., fracture, surgery).[16–18]

Location
HO can occur at any joint following TBI but most often develops at fracture sites or in bruised soft tissue. The most commonly affected joints in the absence of fracture are the hip, shoulder, elbow, and knee.[13,15] A single joint is affected in approximately 40% of patients; in another third, two joints are affected,[2] and in approximately 25% three or more joints are affected. Ankylosis is most likely to occur at the elbow.

Physical Examination

Clinical exam often reveals a swollen, warm, and tender joint, with decreased ROM. Other findings may include erythema, para-articular mass, and fever.

Differential Diagnosis

These clinical findings may be mistaken for deep vein thrombosis, infection, local trauma, or fracture,[19] all of which should be considered in the differential diagnosis of HO.

Bloodwork

- Elevated serum alkaline phosphatase (SAP) levels can occur from 7 weeks before[6] to 3 weeks after[19] appearance of clinical symptoms.
- Erythrocyte sedimentation rate (ESR) and C-reactive protein (CRP) may also become elevated early in the formation of HO.[20]

Radiography

- Triple-phase bone scan with increased uptake during first and second phases is the diagnostic gold standard. HO can be detected as soon as clinical features appear.[6]
- Plain radiographs may remain negative until 2 to 6 weeks after clinical symptoms begin.[21]

MANAGEMENT

The aim is prevention of progression, pain management, and maximization of joint mobility.

Physical Modalities

- *Physiotherapy* involving assisted ROM exercises and gentle stretching is of benefit in relieving pain, maintaining mobility, and preventing ankylosis.[6,22] The joint should not be moved beyond its pain-free range of movement.[23]
- Manipulation under anesthesia may help differentiate between spasticity and ankylosis and relax muscles enough to perform *forceful manipulation*, increasing ROM.[24]
- *Continuous passive motion* can increase and maintain joint ROM both during HO development and after surgical excision.[25]

Medical Management

Nonsteroidal Anti-Inflammatory Drugs[25]

Action: minimize HO formation and patient discomfort in early and intermediate stages.
Mechanism: most nonsteroidal anti-inflammatory drugs (NSAIDs) act as non-selective inhibitors of cyclooxygenase, thereby blocking the formation of PG.
Optimal Drug: indomethacin

- Indomethacin is the gold standard in the prevention of HO following total hip arthroplasty (THA). Other NSAIDs, such as naproxen and diclofenac, have been shown to be equally effective and are considered alternative first-line treatments.
- Cyclooxygenase-2 inhibitors, such as rofecoxib and celecoxib, can also be used.

Potential Side Effects of NSAIDs: gastrointestinal complications, cardiovascular side effects, delayed fracture healing.

Bisphosphonates[25]

Action: inhibitory effect on the formation of hydroxyapatite.
Mechanism: bisphosphonates block the aggregation, growth, and mineralization of hydroxyapatite, thereby retarding the ossification process.
Optimal Drug: disodium etidronate

- When used in conjunction with NSAIDs, etidronate affects the osteoblasts that escape the inhibitory action of NSAIDs. It may also reduce the number of osteoclasts and alter their cellular morphology.
- Etidronate may have an anti-inflammatory effect.

Dosing: should be started as early as possible post-injury at a dose of 10 to 20 mg/kg/day, before significant ectopic bone begins to form, and administered for at least 6 months.
Potential Side Effects: gastrointestinal symptoms, hyperphosphatemia, and possibly osteomalacia.
Caution: a Cochrane Review states: "There is insufficient evidence to recommend the use of disodium etidronate or other pharmacological agents for the treatment of acute HO."[26] It has been suggested that disodium etidronate acts by delaying, rather than preventing, the mineralization of ectopic bone, which may then occur after treatment cessation.

Surgical Intervention

General Principles: Surgical excision of HO is an option if conservative treatment has failed. It has been shown to significantly improve joint mobility, ambulation, and patient comfort, as well as to reduce spasticity.[20,27]

Timing: The optimal timing of surgical resection of HO following TBI is still controversial. Some evidence suggests waiting until 12 to 18 months after formation to reduce the likelihood of recurrence.[28] However, there is increasing evidence that timing of surgical intervention does not affect recurrence rates.[29–32] Further, late surgical intervention may result in poorer functional outcomes by leading to an increased risk of ankylosis, disuse osteopenia, and associated iatrogenic intraoperative fracture.[30] Thus, the optimal time has yet to be elucidated.

Potential Complications: HO has approximately a 20% to 36% recurrence rate, usually within 3 months of surgical excision.[33] Intraoperative fracture can also occur.[27,30] NSAIDs and etidronate may be useful in preventing HO recurrence following surgical excision.[23]

Other Treatment Options

- Local radiotherapy has been used successfully to prevent HO after total hip arthroplasty.[6] Its utility in TBI patients is less clear due to the difficulty in predicting the site of HO formation after a TBI. Radiotherapy has not been shown to be of benefit in reducing the volume of established ectopic bone in TBI patients.
- A case series ($N = 11$) has shown that application of high-energy extracorporeal shock wave therapy can significantly improve ROM (flexion) and functional reach of the affected knee, resulting in improved mobility and balance for patients with chronic neurogenic HO (NHO) post TBI.[34,35]

KEY POINTS

- Heterotopic ossification is a fairly common sequela of TBI.
- Spasticity, decreased ROM and inflammatory signs near a joint suggest the possibility of HO. Prior to the late-stage presence of a palpable mass, a definitive diagnosis can only be made with a bone scan.
- Etidronate disodium may prevent the development of heterotopic ossification in individuals with TBI.
- Forceful joint manipulation may prevent bony ankylosis post-TBI and may increase ROM in joints affected by heterotopic ossification.
- Radiotherapy and shock wave therapy may be effective for the treatment of pain and/or ROM associated with heterotopic ossification in TBI populations.
- Surgical excision of heterotopic ossification may improve ROM and functional ability.
- Earlier surgical excision may not increase the risk of further heterotopic ossification, and may decrease surgical complications and increase functional outcomes.

STUDY QUESTIONS

1. What is the difference in the rate of formation of ectopic bone in those with severe TBI when compared with normal age-matched bone?
   a. Three times greater
   b. Four times greater

   c. Six times greater
   d. Eight times greater

2. Who is at most risk of HO following TBI?
   a. Patients with spasticity
   b. Immobilized patients
   c. Patients with diffuse axonal injury
   d. Those requiring a longer period of mechanical ventilation
   e. All of the above

3. What are the early signs of HO following TBI?
   a. Presence of a firm mass
   b. Restricted joint ROM, joint swelling/warmth, and joint pain
   c. Fever and high alkaline phosphatase
   d. Abnormal shadow on muscles surrounding joint on x-ray

4. The diagnostic gold standard for HO is:
   a. Plain x-ray
   b. Serum alkaline phosphatase
   c. Decreased ROM
   d. Triple-phase bone scan

5. The action of bisphonates in conjunction with NSAIDs on heterotopic bone is:
   a. To augment osteoclastic activity
   b. To inhibit osteoblasts that escape the inhibitory action of NSAIDs
   c. To augment the anti-inflammatory effect of NSAIDs
   d. To inhibit the circulatory supply to the heterotopic bone

ADDITIONAL READING

Teasell R, Hilditch M, Marshall S, et al. Heterotopic ossification and venous thromboembolism. *Evidence-Based Review of Moderate to Severe Acquired Brain Injury.* 6th ed. Module 11. https://erabi.ca/modules/module-11

Garland DE, Varpetian A. Heterotopic ossification in traumatic brain injury. In: Ashley MJ, ed. *Traumatic Brain Injury: Rehabilitative Treatment and Case Management.* 2nd ed. CRC Press; 2003:119–132. doi:10.1201/NOE0849313622.ch4

Brady RD, Shultz SR, McDonald SJ, O'Brien, TJ. Neurological heterotopic ossification: current understanding and future directions. *Bone.* 2018;109:35–42. doi:10.1016/j.bone.2017.05.015

Cipriano CA, Pill SG, Keenan MA. Heterotopic ossification following traumatic brain injury and spinal cord injury. *J Am Acad Orthop Surg.* 2009;17:689–697. doi:10.5435/00124635-200911000-00003

Cullen N, Bayley M, Bayona N, et al. Management of heterotopic ossification and venous thromboembolism following acquired brain injury. *Brain Inj.* 2007;21:215–230. doi:10.1080/02699050701202027

ANSWERS TO STUDY QUESTIONS

1. Correct Answer: a
Ectopic bone is highly metabolically active, with a rate of formation three times greater than that of normal age-matched bone.

Further Reading:
Puzas JE, Brand JS, Evarts CM. The stimulus for bone formation. In: Brand RA, ed. *The Hip*. CV Mosby, St Louis; 1987:25–38.

2. Correct Answer: e
   There is an increased risk with skeletal trauma, spasticity, immobilization, post-injury coma greater than 2 weeks, diffuse axonal injury, and a longer period of mechanical ventilation or intubation.

   Further Reading:
   Pape HC, Lehmann U, van Griensven M, et al. Heterotopic ossifications in patients after severe blunt trauma with and without head trauma: incidence and patterns of distribution. *J Orthop Trauma*. 2001;15(4):229–237. doi:10.1097/00005131-200105000-00001
   van Kampen PJ, Martina JD, Vos PE, et al. Potential risk factors for developing heterotopic ossification in patients with severe traumatic brain injury. *J Head Trauma Rehabil*. 2011;26(5):384–391. doi:10.1097/HTR.0b013e3181f78a59
   Dizdar D, Tiftik T, Kara M, et al. Risk factors for developing heterotopic ossification in patients with traumatic brain injury. *Brain Inj*. 2013;27:807–811. doi:10.3109/02699052 .2013.775490
   Huang H, Cheng WX, Hu YP, et al. Relationship between heterotopic ossification and traumatic brain injury: why severe traumatic brain injury increases the risk of heterotopic ossification. *J Orthop Translat*. 2018;12:16–25. doi:10.1016/j.jot.2017.10.002

3. Correct Answer: b
   Restricted joint ROM, joint swelling and warmth, and joint pain. The presence of a firm palpable mass is a late-stage clinical sign.

   Further Reading:
   Garland DE, Blum CE, Waters RL. Periarticular heterotopic ossification in head-injured adults. Incidence and location. *J Bone Joint Surg Am*. 1980;62(7):1143–1146. doi:10.2106/00004623-198062070-00012

4. Correct Answer: d
   Triple-phase bone scan with increased uptake during first and second phases is the diagnostic gold standard. HO can be detected as soon as clinical features appear.

   Further Reading:
   Pape HC, Marsh S, Morley JR, et al. Current concepts in the development of heterotopic ossification. *J Bone Joint Surg Br*. 2004;86(6):783–787. doi:10.1302/0301-620X.86B6.15356

5. Correct Answer: b
   When used in conjunction with NSAIDs, etidronate affects the osteoblasts that escape the inhibitory action of NSAIDs. It may also reduce the number of osteoclasts and alter their cellular morphology.

   Further Reading:
   Linan E, O'Dell MW, Pierce JM. Continuous passive motion in the management of heterotopic ossification in a brain injured patient. *Am J Phys Med Rehabil*. 2001;80(8):614–617. doi:10.1097/00002060-200108000-00013

REFERENCES

The full reference list appears in the digital product found on http://connect.springer-pub.com/content/book/978-0-8261-4768-4/part/part04/chapter/ch47

48

THE MANAGEMENT OF ENDOCRINE DYSFUNCTION IN TRAUMATIC BRAIN INJURY

NIGEL GLYNN, LUCY-ANN BEHAN, AND AMAR AGHA

INTRODUCTION

Posttraumatic hypopituitarism (PTHP) refers to any abnormality of the hormonal hypothalamic-pituitary axis following traumatic brain injury (TBI). Research studies, over the last two decades in particular, have highlighted a significant burden of pituitary hormone deficiency in survivors of TBI. Symptoms of hypopituitarism including fatigue, muscle weakness, and neuropsychiatric disturbance may impair rehabilitation progress among survivors of TBI.

EPIDEMIOLOGY

The prevalence of chronic hypopituitarism after TBI is a matter of debate; several studies report variable rates due to differences in methodology and cut-off levels used to define hormone deficiency. However, two systematic reviews, one in 2007 and another in 2014, have estimated the pooled prevalence of 27.5% and 31.6%, respectively, following TBI.[1,2]

PITUITARY GLAND ANATOMY AND PHYSIOLOGY

The pituitary gland is located at the base of the skull within the sella turcica, and is joined to the hypothalamus by the infundibulum. The pituitary gland, measuring 8 mm by 10 mm, receives its blood supply from the internal carotid arteries, primarily via the superior hypophyseal artery and the long hypophyseal portal vessels, which arise above the diaphragma sella, while the inferior hypophyseal artery and short hypophyseal vessels enter below the diaphragma sella. The hormones produced by the pituitary and their peripheral targets are described in Table 48.1.

The full reference list appears in the digital product found on http://connect.springerpub.com/content/book/978-0-8261-4768-4/part/part04/chapter/ch48

TABLE 48.1   Pituitary Physiology

Pituitary Hormone	Target Gland	Result
Anterior		
Growth hormone	Various end organs, liver	Mainly acts via insulin-like growth factor-1
Adrenocorticotropin hormone	Adrenal gland	Cortisol, androgens
Gonadotropins (FSH/LH)	Ovaries/testes	Estrogen/testosterone
Thyroid stimulating hormone	Thyroid gland	Thyroid hormone
Prolactin	Mammary glands	Lactation and gonadal suppression
Posterior		
Antidiuretic hormone (arginine vasopressin)	Distal nephron	Fluid balance
Oxytocin	Uterus and breast in females	No known role in males. Contracts pregnant uterus and contributes to lactation. No confirmed adverse effects with deficiency of this hormone

FSH, follicle-stimulating hormone; LH, luteinizing hormone.

PATHOPHYSIOLOGY

The pathophysiology of PTHP is not completely understood. Current evidence suggests that multiple factors are involved in the development of PTHP including:

- Primary brain injury
  - Mechanical trauma may injure the gland, the infundibulum, and/or the hypothalamus.
  - Skull base fractures or rotational and shearing injuries may compromise the blood supply to the pituitary. The long hypophyseal vessels along the infundibulum are particularly vulnerable.
  - Hemorrhage into the sella turcica or into the pituitary gland may also result in direct structural injury.
- Secondary insults
  - Hypoxia, hypotension, cerebral edema, or anemia may all contribute to pituitary ischemia.
  - Medications used following TBI may also contribute to PTHP by both direct effects on the hypothalamic/pituitary axis or by direct effect on the adrenal glands or cortisol metabolism. Those at risk of PTHP may not be able to compensate for any adrenal insult or altered cortisol metabolism. Medication effects are usually transient and reversible. Agents to be aware of include opiate derivatives, phenytoin, etomidate, and high-dose pentobarbital and propofol, all of which can induce acute adrenal insufficiency.
  - Antibodies directed against pituitary and hypothalamic tissue have been detected at higher titers in the serum of survivors of TBI who have hypopituitarism in comparison to those with intact hypothalamic-pituitary hormonal axes.[3] The true role of these antibodies in the pathophysiology of hypopituitarism remains unclear.
- Note that severe brain injury is not required for the development of PTHP; several studies have demonstrated hypopituitarism following moderate TBI, mild TBI, and repetitive mild sport-related injury.[4]

ASSESSMENT AND MANAGEMENT OF ENDOCRINE STATUS FOLLOWING TRAUMATIC BRAIN INJURY

Identifying patients at risk of PTHP is clinically challenging. Some but not all studies in TBI survivors have identified severity of injury (as assessed by the Glasgow Coma Scale) as a risk factor for chronic hypopituitarism. Radiological features of the injury including base of skull fracture may also increase the risk of PTHP. More recently, detailed magnetic resonance imaging (MRI) has identified decreased apparent diffusion coefficient in pituitary tissue as a potential risk factor for PTHP.[5]

Anterior Pituitary Dysfunction in the Acute Phase (Hours to Days Post-TBI)

▪ Adrenocorticotropic hormone (ACTH) deficiency
   ● Glucocorticoid deficiency is potentially life-threatening.
   ● Suspicion should be high if any of the following are present: hypotension despite inotrope support, hypoglycemia, or hyponatremia.
   ● Morning serum (total) cortisol less than 300 nmol/L (11 μg/dL) in a subject in intensive care is inappropriately low and glucocorticoid replacement is recommended.[6]
   ● Morning serum (total) cortisol between 300 and 500 nmol/L in a subject following TBI must be interpreted in the clinical context. Replacement should be considered if any clinical features of hypocortisolism (i.e., hypotension despite inotrope support, hypoglycemia, or hyponatremia) are present.
   ● Confirm the subject has received no exogenous steroids that may alter the interpretation of serum cortisol results; for example, dexamethasone.
   ● The synthetic ACTH (Synacthen) test should not be used to diagnose adrenal insufficiency in the acute phase of TBI as adrenal atrophy has not yet developed and this test may give a falsely reassuring result. The diagnosis should be based on the aforementioned features.
▪ Assessment of the growth hormone (GH), gonadal, and thyroid axes is not necessary in the acute phase as there is currently no evidence to suggest replacement of these hormones is beneficial.

Posterior Pituitary Dysfunction in the Acute Phase

▪ Cranial diabetes insipidus (DI)
   ● Due to antidiuretic hormone, also known as arginine vasopressin (AVP), deficiency.
   ● Defined by production of greater than 3 L of dilute urine (urine osmolality less than 300 mOsm/kg) in 24 hours and plasma sodium greater than 145 mmol/L.
   ● May be transient in this phase of TBI.
   ● Urine output greater than 200 mL/hr for 2 consecutive hours may be suggestive.
   ● Electrolyte abnormalities in this setting may be life-threatening.
   ● Adequate fluid replacement and AVP replacement (desmopressin) may be required and should be adjusted according to hourly urine output response and plasma sodium.[7]
▪ Syndrome of antidiuretic hormone secretion (SIADH)
   ● Characterized by hyponatremia in an apparently euvolemic patient, in the absence of glucocorticoid deficiency or hypothyroidism.
   ● The biochemical diagnosis requires that a plasma osmolality less than 270 mOsm/kg, urine osmolality greater than 100 mOsm/kg, and spot urinary sodium concentration greater than 40 mmol/L are all present.

- Treat with fluid restriction to 500 mL to 1.5 L in 24 hours.
- Rarely, hypertonic saline infusion may be required. Note that rapid changes in plasma sodium increase the risk of cerebral pontine myelinolysis. Aim to correct sodium at a rate less than 0.5 mmol/L/hr.
- Cerebral salt wasting
  - A very rare differential diagnosis for hyponatremia in the setting of TBI.
  - Characterized by hypovolemic hyponatremia. Hypovolemic fluid status is the key differentiator from SIADH.
  - Plasma osmolality less than 270 mOsm/kg, urine osmolality greater than 100 mOsm/kg, and spot urinary sodium concentration greater than 40 mmol/L, low central venous pressure/hypotension.
  - This syndrome is responsive to salt and volume replacement. Fluid restriction is not utilized. Treat with isotonic saline administration to restore euvolemia. Aim to correct sodium at a rate less than 0.5 mmol/hr.

Pituitary Hormone Dysfunction in the Chronic Phase (Greater Than 3 Months) After Traumatic Brain Injury

Screen all patients with moderate (GCS 9–12) and severe (GCS ≤8) TBI; screen subjects with mild TBI (GCS 13–15) if indicated based on clinical symptoms and signs of pituitary hormone deficiency. It is noteworthy that there is considerable overlap between the post-concussive syndrome and symptoms of hypopituitarism. However, clinical features of gonadal dysfunction (gonadotropin deficiency)—for example erectile dysfunction in men, oligo/amenorrhea in women—may be more specific indicators of PTHP.

- Glucocorticoid deficiency
  - Characterized by life-threatening adrenal crisis, hypotension, fatigue, weight loss, and recurrent infections.
- GH deficiency
  - Impaired linear growth and abnormal body composition in children; in adults reduced lean body mass, decreased exercise capacity, reduced quality of life, impaired cardiac function, and reduced bone mineral density.
- Gonadotropin deficiency
  - In men, testosterone deficiency is associated with reduced lean body mass and bone mineral density, low libido, erectile dysfunction, and muscle weakness. Estrogen deficiency in pre-menopausal women leads to amenorrhea and reduced bone mineral density. Although 1.5% to 41% subjects following TBI (principally moderate to severe injury) will have chronic gonadotropin deficiency, there are no available data regarding fertility outcomes. These patients should be referred to an endocrinologist for fertility assessment.
- Thyroid-stimulating hormone (TSH) deficiency
  - Lethargy, fatigue, weight gain, and neuropsychiatric manifestations
- Diabetes insipidus (DI)
  - Polyuria, polydipsia, and excess thirst (in those with cognitive impairment clinicians must rely on urine output and biochemical markers to suggest this diagnosis)

All of these endocrine abnormalities may have a serious adverse impact on patients with TBI and may impair recovery and rehabilitation. Untreated hypopituitarism in any population is associated with premature mortality and increased morbidity.

Subjects with moderate or severe TBI should undergo endocrine evaluation between 3 and 6 months following TBI; hormone deficiencies should be replaced as appropriate (Figure 48.1). Evaluation during the chronic recovery phase should include[8]:

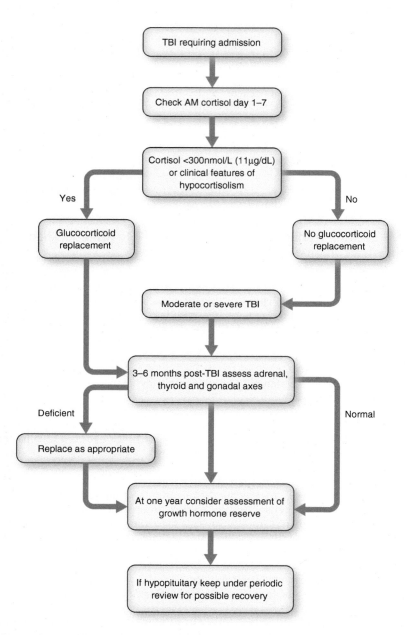

FIGURE 48.1 Algorithm for the endocrine assessment of patients following traumatic brain injury.

GH, growth hormone; TBI, traumatic brain injury.

- Synacthen (ACTH stimulation) test—adrenal reserve
- Basal serum free T4 and TSH
- Basal serum estrogen/testosterone and gonadotropins (menstrual diary in women)
- Serum sodium and clinical assessment of thirst, polyuria (greater than 3 L/24 hours), polydipsia, and nocturia. If abnormal, formal water deprivation testing should be carried out under the guidance of a pituitary endocrinologist
- The GH–insulin-like growth factor-1 axis should not be assessed until at least 1-year post-TBI, as changes before this time may be transient.[9] The reported prevalence of GH deficiency following TBI varies significantly depending on the type of dynamic test and cut-offs applied and whether a second confirmatory test is utilized.[10] In view of this variability, dynamic stimulation testing should be performed in specialist pituitary units. There is some evidence to suggest that GH replacement may improve quality of life and some metabolic parameters in this patient group; however, long-term prospective studies are lacking. GH replacement may be considered on an individual basis in conjunction with endocrine specialist advice.

CONCLUSION

PTHP may be an underdiagnosed complication of TBI and, in the case of resultant adrenal insufficiency, it may be life-threatening if overlooked. PTHP can contribute to the morbidity associated with TBI. An increased level of awareness among all disciplines caring for this patient group is vital in order to provide appropriate and timely hormone replacement. Subjects with moderate to severe TBI or those with clinical suggestion of hypopituitarism should be referred to a pituitary endocrinologist for evaluation.

KEY POINTS

- PTHP is not limited to those with severe TBI.
- Glucocorticoid deficiency is life-threatening, and in the acute intensive care setting a morning cortisol <300 nmol/L (11 µg/dL) is abnormal.
- Do not use the synthetic ACTH test to diagnose adrenal insufficiency in the acute phase.
- GH deficiency should be diagnosed utilizing an appropriate dynamic test by a pituitary endocrine center with established cut-offs and assays.

STUDY QUESTIONS

1. A previously healthy 25-year-old man is intubated and ventilated in the intensive care unit (ICU) after suffering a severe TBI during a motor vehicle collision. Twelve hours after the injury you are asked to review his urine output, which has ranged between 350 and 450 mL per hour for the preceding 3 hours. He has received only isotonic intravenous (IV) fluids since admission to the hospital and his blood pressure is elevated without inotropic support.

Serum urea and electrolytes are as follows:

Sodium 150 mEq/L

Potassium 3.8 mEq/L

BUN 32 mg/dL

Creatinine 0.68 mg/dL

Glucose 205 mg/dL

Urine osmolality 108 mOsm/kg

Which of the following answers is correct?
a. Inappropriate IV fluid management is the most likely cause of polyuria
b. Diabetes mellitus is the most likely cause of polyuria
c. Cerebral salt wasting is the most likely cause of polyuria
d. Cranial diabetes insipidus is the most likely cause of polyuria
e. Nephrogenic diabetes insipidus is the most likely cause of polyuria

2. A 27-year-old woman is 6 months status post moderate TBI due to a fall from a horse. She is making limited progress with rehabilitation and still has significant physical and cognitive complications of her injury. She has gained some weight (BMI 29 kg/m²) and she has had secondary amenorrhea since the accident. She does not suffer from polyuria. The rehabilitation team considers a diagnosis of posttraumatic hypopituitarism and obtains serum hormone levels.

Which of the following statements about chronic hypopituitarism is correct?
a. Chronic posttraumatic hypopituitarism is a rare disorder following moderate to severe TBI detectable in only 3% to 5% of long-term survivors
b. She should be evaluated for growth hormone deficiency (GHD) at this stage of her recovery as GHD may be impairing her recovery
c. Pituitary hormone deficiencies detected early following TBI may improve spontaneously over time
d. Amenorrhea following TBI always indicates posttraumatic hypopituitarism
e. The risk of chronic hypopituitarism is usually predictable based on clinical and radiological features of the TBI

3. In relation to the pathophysiology of posttraumatic hypopituitarism, which of the following statements is true? Select the most appropriate answer.
a. Postmortem pathology studies have detected infarction of the pituitary gland in some victims of TBI
b. Vascular injury to the pituitary area represents one plausible mechanism for hypopituitarism after TBI
c. Fracture of the bony sella turcica can result in pituitary damage
d. Survivors of TBI may have anti-pituitary antibodies in the serum
e. All the above

4. Which of the following statements in relation to evaluation of pituitary function after TBI is correct?
a. Pituitary function may subsequently recover in survivors of TBI who had evidence of hypopituitarism during the first 6 months following injury
b. Hormonal evaluation should be completed at 6 months in all cases

c. All patients who suffer concussion should be referred to an endocrinologist for formal evaluation of pituitary function

d. Prediction of chronic hypopituitarism on the basis of clinical and radiological features is highly precise in survivors of moderate to severe TBI

e. Hypopituitarism does not occur after TBI in childhood

ADDITIONAL READING

Glynn N, Agha A. Neuroendocrine dysfunction following concussion: a missed opportunity for enhancing recovery? In: Victoroff J, Bigler ED, eds. *Concussion and Traumatic Encephalopathy: Causes, Diagnosis and Management*. Cambridge University Press; 2019:767–779. doi:10.1017/9781139696432.028

Pavlovic D, Pekic S, Stojanovic M, Popovic V. Traumatic brain injury: neuropathological, neurocognitive and neurobehavioral sequelae. *Pituitary*. 2019;22(3):270–282. doi:10.1007/s11102-019-00957-9

Dassa Y, Crosnier H, Chevignard M, et al. Pituitary deficiency and precocious puberty after childhood severe traumatic brain injury: a long-term follow-up prospective study. *Eur J Endocrinol*. 2019;180(5):281–290. doi:10.1530/EJE-19-0034

ANSWERS TO STUDY QUESTIONS

1. Correct Answer: d
Cranial diabetes insipidus (DI) is common complication of moderate to severe TBI (16%–28%) and predicts a poor prognosis. It typically occurs early following injury, nearly always within the first 3 days, and is characterized by hypotonic polyuria. Intubated patients cannot respond to normal thirst mechanisms and, therefore, intravascular contraction and dehydration are common if the diagnosis is not recognized promptly. Cranial DI is easily treated with parenteral desmopressin and hypotonic fluid. It typically resolves within a few days in TBI survivors.

Further Reading:
Hannon MJ, Finucane FM, Sherlock M, et al. Clinical review: Disorders of water homeostasis in neurosurgical patients. *J Clin Endocrinol Metab*. 2012;97(5):1423–1433. doi:10.1210/jc.2011-3201

2. Correct Answer: c
There is a wide range in the reported prevalence of posttraumatic hypopituitarism, as different investigators have used a variable definition of hypopituitarism, have examined cohorts with different severity and mechanism of TBI and at variable time points following injury. However, systematic reviews suggest the prevalence to be between 27.5% and 31.6% following TBI. Prospective studies of TBI patients have shown that hypopituitarism is a dynamic process. While new deficiencies occasionally emerge during follow-up, the general trend is toward improvement in pituitary function over time.

Further Reading:
Schneider HJ, Kreitschmann-Andermahr I, Ghigo E, et al. Hypothalamopituitary dysfunction following traumatic brain injury and aneurysmal subarachnoid hemorrhage: a systematic review. *JAMA*. 2007;298(12):1429–38. doi:10.1001/jama.298.12.1429

Lauzier F, Turgeon AF, Boutin A, et al. Clinical outcomes, predictors, and prevalence of anterior pituitary disorders following traumatic brain injury: a systematic review. *Crit Care Med*. 2014;42(3):712–721. doi:10.1097/CCM.0000000000000046

3. Correct Answer: e

The pathophysiology of hypopituitarism after TBI is not fully understood. However, the combination of pituitary infarction and the complex blood supply of the pituitary gland makes vascular injury a plausible mechanism in many cases. GH and gonadotrophin deficiency are the most commonly reported hormone deficiencies after TBI. The cells secreting these hormones are supplied by the long hypophyseal portal arteries—delicate blood vessels susceptible to damage due to edema, shear forces, or raised intracranial pressure.

Further Reading:

De Bellis A, Bellastella G, Maiorino MI, et al. The role of autoimmunity in pituitary dysfunction due to traumatic brain injury. *Pituitary*. 2019;22(3):236–248. doi:10.1007/s11102-019-00953-z

4. Correct Answer: a

Several professional societies have suggested algorithms for the screening and assessment of posttraumatic hypopituitarism in adults after moderate to severe TBI. It is well recognized that hypopituitarism can be a dynamic process following TBI—early deficiencies can recover, and new deficiencies may emerge during the first year of recovery. In the setting of mild TBI, only patients with convincing symptoms of hypopituitarism after repeated concussion should be referred for specialist evaluation. Pituitary function can be affected in children following TBI; however, the prevalence may be lower than in adulthood.

Further Reading:

Tritos NA, Yuen KC, Kelly DF, AACE Neuroendocrine and Pituitary Scientific Committee. American Association of Clinical Endocrinologists and American College of Endocrinology Disease State clinical review: a neuroendocrine approach to patients with traumatic brain injury. *Endocr Pract*. 2015;21(7):823–831. doi:10.4158/EP14567. DSCR

REFERENCES

The full reference list appears in the digital product found on http://connect.springerpub.com/content/book/978-0-8261-4768-4/part/part04/chapter/ch48

49

AUTONOMIC DYSFUNCTION

CHERINA CYBORSKI

BACKGROUND

The autonomic nervous system (ANS) maintains homeostasis, without conscious direction, via a balance between two main subsystems: the parasympathetic and sympathetic nervous systems.

- Sympathetic nervous system (SNS): increases heart rate and cardiac ejection fraction, raises blood pressure, shunts blood to musculoskeletal system, dilates pupils.
- Parasympathetic nervous system (PNS): slows heart rate, shunts blood to the gastrointestinal tract, contracts pupils.

Peripherally, the ANS spans from the end organ integrating into the spinal cord, brainstem, hypothalamus, amygdala, hippocampus, insular cortex, cingulate cortex, dorsolateral prefrontal cortex, and middle temporal cortices. The "central autonomic network" integrates visceral perception and efferent autonomic responses with emotion and behavior.[1] The more damage to the central ANS pathways, the less refined the homeostatic response.[2] Additionally, there is emerging evidence that catecholaminergic surges after moderate to severe traumatic brain injury (TBI) affect the functions of the heart, lung, kidney, and lymphoid organs via the ANS, making TBI a systemic condition.[3,4]

AUTONOMIC NERVOUS SYSTEM DYSFUNCTION AFTER MILD TRAUMATIC BRAIN INJURY

- No Level I studies have investigated mild TBI (MTBI) and related ANS dysfunction. There are, however, emerging human studies evaluating physiologic measures of ANS post-MTBI (such as heart rate variability [HRV], pupillary dynamics, Valsalva, isometric hand grip, eye pressure, arterial pulse wave) and their dysfunction. One study found that more than 6 months after injury, MTBI patients' resting sympathetic modulation was higher and parasympathetic modulation was lower as compared to controls. (These measures were more pronounced in those after a moderate–severe TBI.[5])
- Headache, cognitive dysfunction, anxiety/depression, and sleep disturbance may in part be due to ANS dysfunction. ANS dysfunction post-MTBI may lead to increased neuroinflammation and oxidative stress contributing to neurodegeneration, blood–brain barrier disruption, and vascular dysfunction, which may cause the aforementioned symptoms.[6]
- There are no specific therapies targeting ANS dysregulation; most aim to alleviate resultant symptoms. Expert opinion, unsubstantiated by literature, addressing ANS

The full reference list appears in the digital product found on http://connect.springerpub.com/content/book/978-0-8261-4768-4/part/part04/chapter/ch49

dysfunction post-MTBI, suggests the following approaches: cognitive behavioral therapy, graded exercise, relaxation techniques, and beta-adrenergic blockade.[4,6]

AUTONOMIC NERVOUS SYSTEM DYSFUNCTION AFTER MODERATE TO SEVERE TRAUMATIC BRAIN INJURY: PAROXYSMAL SYMPATHETIC HYPERACTIVITY

Paroxysmal sympathetic hyperactivity (PSH) is a condition characterized by widespread autonomic dysregulation. It has been known by several other names including dysautonomia, paroxysmal autonomic instability with dystonia (PAID), sympathetic/autonomic storming, and autonomic dysfunction syndrome.[2]

Definition

- A syndrome characterized by paroxysmal transient increases in autonomic (specifically sympathetic, e.g., tachycardia, hypertension, diaphoresis, hyperthermia) and motor (typically posturing) activity in a subpopulation of those with an antecedent severe acquired brain injury.[7] This consensus term and the diagnostic criteria were published in 2014, leading to a more standardized clinical definition; earlier literature has a wide range of findings resulting from a previous lack of a unified definition or process to evaluate paroxysmal sympathetic hyperactivity (PSH) or its cause/effects.

Epidemiology

- 8% to 33% of patients with severe TBI develop prolonged PSH (greater than 7 days post injury). Most literature supports the lower end of the range, especially since the consensus guidelines have emerged as discussed.[2,8–11]
- PSH is associated with worse outcome, prolonged swallowing abnormalities, longer time to follow commands, longer posttraumatic amnesia, longer length of hospital stay, and greater healthcare cost.[2,8–10]

Risk Factors

- Younger age at time of injury,[1,8,10,12] although within the pediatric population specifically, older age (i.e., adolescence) is associated with higher risk[13]
- Male gender
- Tracheostomy[14]
- Lower Glasgow Coma Scale score [6,15]
- Longer coma duration [1,16]
- Concomitant fractures[16]

Etiology

- Though most commonly due to TBI, PSH can occur from many etiologies, including hypoxic–anoxic injury, subarachnoid hemorrhage, encephalitis (autoimmune, infectious), stroke, thalamic tumor, vasculitis, fulminant multiple sclerosis, postpartum vasoconstriction, cerebral fat embolism, leukemia, and acute disseminated encephalomyelitis.[17]

Pathophysiology

- Current theory is the excitatory:inhibitory ratio model. This proposes that PSH results from a lack of central inhibitory pathway control on regulation of afferent information with maladaptive dendritic spinal circuit formation, resulting in increased activation of the SNS, leading to excessive autonomic reactivity.[2,11,18]

- Elevated levels of catecholamines, in the range of 200% to 300% of normal, as well as a 40% increase in adrenocortical hormones, have been measured during PSH episodes.[19]
- It is likely that the mechanisms which underlie this phenomenon are heterogeneous. A patient-centric approach based on the dominant clinical presentation is recommended.[11]

Clinical Presentation

- PSH occurs across a spectrum of severity and not every patient has every feature. Tachycardia is almost universal, however.[17]
  - Fever within the first 72 hours post-injury may predict PSH development[15]
- Typical onset is within 7 to 10 days post-injury[12,17] but the first episode can happen up to 22 to 65 days after injury[16]
- Up to 80% of episodes appear to be triggered by and are more severe with noxious stimuli, including pain, suctioning, passive movements, bowel or bladder issues, or loud noise[2,11]
- Episodes can last 27.9 to 30.8 minutes (ranging from 15 to 50 minutes) for an average of 5.01 to 5.6 times per day.[12,20]
- Episodes become less severe, shorter, and less frequent over time[2]
  - In one study, 80% of PSH episodes resolved at 12 month follow-up.[12]
- Improvement often coincides with neurological recovery.[2]
- Earlier diagnosis, hence earlier treatment, may decrease pursuing costly negative evaluations[17]

Diagnosis

- PSH-Assessment Measure (PSH-AM), validated in the adult and pediatric populations (with age adjusted criteria),[13,21–23] has two components that are combined to give a PSH diagnostic likelihood, and can stratify PSH severity:
  - *Clinical Feature Scale*: grades the presence and severity of increased heart rate, respiratory rate, systolic blood pressure, temperature, sweating, and posturing during episodes
  - *Diagnosis Likelihood Tool*: assesses the presence and clinical context of 11 symptoms or phenomena known to be seen in PSH.[7] The higher the score (0–11), the greater the likelihood that the patient has PSH
    - Simultaneity of clinical features
    - Clinical features are paroxysmal
    - Sympathetic over-reactivity to normally nonpainful stimuli
    - Absence of intraparoxysmal parasympathetic features during episodes
    - Features persist greater than or equal to 3 consecutive days
    - Features persist greater than or equal to 2 weeks post injury
    - Features persist despite treatment of alternative differential diagnoses (e.g., infection)
    - Greater than or equal to two episodes daily
    - Medication administered to decrease sympathetic features
    - Lack of alternative explanations
    - Antecedent acquired brain injury
- Improved diagnosis based on the PSH-AM may decrease length of stay and hospital costs

- Assuming clinical assessment is the gold standard, PSH-AM yielded a sensitivity of 94% and specificity of 35%; those clinically diagnosed were discharged 5 days earlier in one study[23]
- Remember that PSH is a diagnosis of exclusion. Consider/rule out the following as appropriate: infection (most common cause of hyperthermia in TBI patients); seizures; acute hydrocephalus; increased intracranial pressure; neuroleptic malignant syndrome; serotonin syndrome; malignant hyperthermia; thyroid storm; venous thromboembolism; medication reaction; withdrawal from medications, illicit drug or alcohol ingestion; concomitant spinal cord injury/autonomic dysreflexia; acute coronary syndrome; pain (undiagnosed fractures, spasticity, constipation, pressure area, heterotopic ossification [HO]); and subarachnoid hemorrhage.

Radiological Findings

The current published medical literature offers a mixed and at times inconsistent picture:

- *Computed tomography (CT)*: no correlation between imaging findings and PSH[12]
- *Magnetic resonance imaging (MRI)*: one study showed an association with deep lesions, including periventricular white matter, corpus callosum, basal ganglia, and brainstem;[8,24] another showed that PSH was associated with DAI.[16]
- *Diffusion Tensor Imaging (DTI)*: PSH may be associated with damage to the right insular cortex[1]
- The variability in the above findings may be because of a lack of consensus diagnostic criteria (pre 2014), timing of imaging, different imaging techniques, different interpreters, and/or variability in anatomical lesions which can lead to development of PSH[11]

Treatment

- Given gaps in understanding pathophysiology of PSH, it is difficult to therapeutically target underlying etiology. There is a lack of high-quality evidence-based literature to guide management of symptoms.[2] The following is a clinical guide to management based on currently available evidence:
- Initiate treatment as early as possible because:
  - Core temperatures above 38°C to 39°C have produced neuronal death in animal models
  - An increased catabolic state may lead to loss of body weight
  - PSH is associated with an increased risk of developing critical illness polyneuropathy
  - Spasticity/dystonia can lead to contractures, pressure areas, and/or pain[25]
- Environmental management:
  - Assess for triggers
  - Decrease noxious stimuli: remove cervical collars as soon as possible, remove indwelling bladder catheters, prevent pressure areas, prevent constipation, use rubber tubes for suctioning, premedicate prior to known triggers
  - Minimize noise and activity around the patient
  - Be proactive and expeditious in adjusting hydration and caloric needs[16]
- Pharmacological treatment: Medication recommendations are anecdotal, not evidence-based.[2] That said, many patients need more than one medication for symptom control, especially acutely.[17,26]
- Medications should be used with caution as they can be sedating, potentially impair cognition, and/or affect recovery/neuroplasticity.
- Medications that modulate afferent spinal cord sensitization

- Gabapentin (voltage-dependent calcium channels)
  - Modifies reactivity of neurological circuits in brain and spinal cord[25]
  - Mitigates the autonomic symptoms and the dystonic posturing and may also be beneficial in treating neuropathic pain
- Baclofen (GABA B antagonist)
  - Oral route not typically used for this indication
  - Intrathecal baclofen (ITB)—Effective but invasive
    - ☐ Years long follow-up of TBI patients who received ITB for PSH symptoms shows that, on average, it was placed 6.6 months after injury, with an average baclofen dose of 232.6 µg/day, with higher doses and earlier placement in those with longer coma duration and lower pre-operative Glasgow Coma Scale (GCS) score.
    - ☐ Complication rate over 10-year follow-up was 90.7% and included overdose, withdrawal, battery failure, pain, infection, sedation, catheter migrations, and pump failures[27]
- Medications that modulate centrally mediated sympathetic outflow:
  - Propofol, diazepam, lorazepam, midazolam (GABA A antagonists)
    - Anecdotal reports favor midazolam and diazepam[28]
  - Bromocriptine (dopamine D2 agonist)
    - May be useful for centrally mediated fever and dystonia
    - Contraindicated in uncontrolled hypertension
  - Morphine (mu opioid receptor agonist): When it is effective, mechanism is believed to be modulation of central pathways, suppression of sympathetic outflow, and decreased pain[29,30]
  - Methadone[29]
- Medications that have a central and peripheral effect
  - Propranolol (nonselective beta antagonist) and labetalol (nonselective beta and alpha1 agonist)
    - Lipophilic, so crosses the blood–brain barrier
    - Decreases circulating catecholamines, reduces cardiac work and catabolic drive
      - ☐ Propranolol may decrease in-hospital mortality[31]
    - Decreases hypertension and hemodynamic abnormalities
    - Does not alter diaphoresis (mediated by sympathetic cholinergic neurons)
  - Clonidine (alpha-2 agonist)
    - Modulates blood pressure and heart rate (through decreased plasma catecholamines)
  - Dexmedetomidine (alpha-2 agonist)
    - Effective in intensive care unit (ICU) setting[32] and may attenuate development of PSH in those who have undergone neurosurgery[33]
- Medications that act peripherally
  - Dantrolene
    - Inhibits calcium release in sarcoplasmic reticulum
    - Treats extensor posturing/spasticity with minimal effect on other symptoms
  - Chemodenervation/lysis with alcohol or botulinum toxin: decreases noxious trigger (spasticity/pain) for PSH[34]
- Other treatment:
  - Hyperbaric oxygen therapy (HBOT): One case report of six TBI patients (30–70 days post-injury, pre-HBOT GCS 8-11) who were given HBOT with 100% oxygen up to 1.5 atm for 120 minutes once daily for 10 days, 5 days of rest, then another course of daily treatment for 10 days found that all PSH symptoms resolved after 3 to 10 treatments.[35] A subsequent review, looking at the role of HBOT in management of TBI did not recommend its use for any TBI-related indication.[36]

■ In the pediatric population, medications discussed in the literature include: acetaminophen ± codeine, benzodiazepines, and antihistaminergic antipsychotics; with clonazepam, delorazepam, and hydroxyzine found to be most efficacious in suppressing PSH episodes.[37]

Prognosis

■ Studies impact of PSH on prognosis; and the assessment of PSH's unique contribution to overall prognosis is challenging given that PSH tends to develop in the most severe/complicated injuries[11]
■ PSH increases risk for development of HO[11,38] and prolongs time to tracheostomy weaning[39]
■ Subclinical sympathetic over-responsiveness may persist indefinitely, both at rest, but especially in response to noxious stimuli as measured by heart rate variability[2,40-41]
■ Most studies show those with PSH have worse functional independence measures (FIM) scores, worse Glasgow Outcome Scale (GOS) scores, increased length of stay in the ICU, greater length of hospitalization, more infections, more tracheostomy placement, greater healthcare cost overall, worse disability rating scale (DRS), and lower modified Rankin scores at 6 and 12 months[1,12,13,15,16,22,28,25,42-44]

KEY POINTS

■ Though more common in the setting of severe injury, autonomic dysfunction can be seen across the spectrum of TBI. More studies are needed to further elucidate the pathophysiology, refine diagnostic criteria, guide treatment, and inform outcomes.
■ PSH is a syndrome, recognized in a subgroup of survivors of severe acquired brain injury, characterized by simultaneous, paroxysmal transient increases in sympathetic (elevated heart rate, blood pressure, respiratory rate, temperature, sweating), and motor (posturing) activity.
■ Treatment approaches are primarily based on anecdotal reports; there is a lack of robust evidence-based data to aid in therapeutic decision-making.

STUDY QUESTIONS

1. Which of the following beta-adrenergic blockers has the best support in the medical literature for management of PSH?
   a. labetalol
   b. propranolol
   c. metoprolol
   d. atenolol

2. A 24-year-old man who was in a motorcycle collision 4 days ago underwent a decompressive craniectomy. Upon arriving back to the ICU, what medication should be considered for post-operative sedation to attenuate PSH development?
   a. propofol
   b. midazolam

    c. morphine
    d. dexmedetomidine

3. A 21-year-old man with severe TBI is diagnosed with PSH after a thorough workup. Blood was drawn during one of the PSH episodes. What result would be expected?
    a. increased cortisol by 200%
    b. decreased cortisol by 200%
    c. increased epinephrine by 200%
    d. decreased epinephrine by 200%

4. While on an inpatient rehabilitation unit, a 30-year-old woman who had a severe TBI 10 days ago is diagnosed with PSH. With the diagnosis of PSH, which of the following is the patient at increased risk for developing?
    a. hydrocephalus
    b. heterotopic ossification
    c. seizures
    d. deep vein thrombosis

5. A 35-year-old man sustained a severe TBI 48 hours ago. Which of the following is most predictive of development of PSH based on current published evidence?
    a. temperature of 38.6°C
    b. respiratory rate of 25
    c. heart rate of 125
    d. systolic blood pressure of 142

ADDITIONAL READING

About Paroxysmal Sympathetic Hyperactivity: https://www.rainbowrehab.com/weathering-the-storm-storming

PSH Assessment Measure, in Identification and Management of Paroxysmal Sympathetic Hyperactivity After Traumatic Brain Injury: https://www.ncbi.nlm.nih.gov/pmc/articles/PMC7052349/pdf/fneur-11-00081.pdf

Baguley IJ, Perkes IE, Fernandez-Ortega JF, et al. Paroxysmal sympathetic hyperactivity after acquired brain injury: consensus on conceptual definition, nomenclature, and diagnostic criteria. *J Neurotrauma*. 2014;31(17):1515–1520. doi:10.1089/neu.2013.3301

Fernandez-Ortega JF, Prieto-Palomino MA, Gacia-Caballero M, et al. Paroxysmal sympathetic hyperactivity after traumatic brain injury: clinical and prognostic implications. *J Neurotrauma*. 2012;29:1364–1370. doi:10.1089/neu.2011.2033

Lv L, Hou L, Yu M, et al. Risk factors related to dysautonomia after severe traumatic brain injury. *J Trauma*. 2011;71(3):538–542. doi:10.1097/TA.0b013e31820ebee1

ANSWERS TO STUDY QUESTIONS

1. Correct Answer: b
Propranolol is a lipophilic nonselective beta blocker (central, cardiac, and peripheral) with consistent efficacy in the literature. Labetalol is a beta and alpha blocker with limited efficacy for PSH management. Metoprolol and Atenolol are cardioselective beta blockers and are ineffective in PSH management.

Further Reading:
Meyfroidt G, Baguley IJ, Menon DK. Paroxysmal sympathetic hyperactivity: the storm after acute brain injury. *Lancet Neurol.* 2017;16(9):721–729. doi:10.1016/S1474-4422(17)30259-4

2. Correct Answer: d
While all of the medications can assist with the management of PSH episodes, dexmedetomidine is the only medication shown to prevent PSH development in TBI patients after neurosurgical intervention.

Further Reading:
Tang Q, Wu X, Weng W, et al. The preventive effect of dexmedetomidine on paroxysmal sympathetic hyperactivity in severe traumatic brain injury patients who have undergone surgery: a retrospective study. *PeerJ.* 2017;5:e2986. doi:10.7717/peerj.2986

3. Correct Answer: c
A recent study demonstrated peripheral levels of catecholamines (norepinephrine, epinephrine, and dopamine) at the time of PSH episodes of up to 200% to 300% and a 40% increase in adrenocortical hormones.

Further Reading:
Fernandez-Ortega JF, Baguley IJ, Gates TA, et al. Catecholamines and paroxysmal sympathetic hyperactivity after traumatic brain injury. *J Neurotrauma.* 2017;34(1):109–114. doi:10.1089/neu.2015.4364

4. Correct Answer: b
While all of the conditions mentioned can be complications of severe TBI, PSH increases risk for development of HO.

Further Reading:
Meyfroidt G, Baguley IJ, Menon DK. Paroxysmal sympathetic hyperactivity: the storm after acute brain injury. *Lancet Neurol.* 2017;16(9):721–729. doi:10.1016/S1474-4422(17)30259-4
Bargellesi S, Cavasin L, Scarponi F, et al. Occurrence and predictive factors of heterotopic ossification in severe acquired brain injured patients during rehabilitation stay: cross-sectional survey. *Clin Rehabil.* 2018;32(2):255–262. doi:10.1177/0269215517723161

5. Correct Answer: a
Based on the Modified Clinical Feature Severity Scale, within the first 5 days post-injury, the only measure predictive of PSH development was elevated temperature.

Further Reading:
Hinson HE, Schreiber MA, Laurie AL, et al. Early fever as a predictor of paroxysmal sympathetic hyperactivity in traumatic brain injury. *J Head Trauma Rehabil.* 2017;32(5):E50–E54. doi:10.1097/HTR.0000000000000271

REFERENCES

The full reference list appears in the digital product found on http://connect.springer-pub.com/content/book/978-0-8261-4768-4/part/part04/chapter/ch49

MOVEMENT DISORDERS

BRUNO S. SUBBARAO AND BLESSEN C. EAPEN

GENERAL PRINCIPLES

Definition

A movement disorder is a neurological phenomenon that affects the ability to generate or control movement. It can occur as a result of traumatic brain injury (TBI) and present in either a transient or persistent, hyper- or hypokinetic, focal or generalized fashion.[1]

Epidemiology

The incidence of movement disorders following severe TBI ranges from 13% to 66%.[2]

In a large study of survivors of severe TBI, posttraumatic movement disorders were reported in 22.6%, and persisted in 12.2%. The most common persisting movement disorder was tremor, followed by dystonia. Generalized cerebral edema on computed tomography (CT) at admission and focal cerebral lesions seen on follow up CT scans were found to have a significant association with the future development of movement disorders.[3]

Movement disorders are less prevalent following mild to moderate TBI. In a survey study of mild to moderate TBI survivors, posttraumatic movement disorders were reported in 10.1%, and persisted in 2.6%.[3]

Classification

Hyperkinetic disorders—characterized by excessive, abnormal involuntary movement

- Tremor
- Dystonia
- Ballism and chorea
- Tics and tourettism
- Myoclonus
- Stereotypy, hyperekplexia, and akathisia

Hypokinetic disorders—characterized by slowness or paucity of movement

- Parkinsonism

The previously listed disorders will each be discussed in more detail in subsequent sections of this chapter.

The full reference list appears in the digital product found on http://connect.springerpub.com/content/book/978-0-8261-4768-4/part/part04/chapter/ch50

Etiology and Pathophysiology

Posttraumatic movement disorders are caused by:

- Primary injury
  - Focal contusions to the basal ganglia and associated pathways as well as cortical regions that modulate basal ganglia function indirectly
  - Diffuse axonal injury preferentially affecting the superior cerebellar peduncles, brainstem, and subcortical regions
  - Hemorrhage and ischemia from arterial injury caused by trauma-associated rotational forces
- Secondary injury
  - Associated hypoxia, hypotension, and cerebral edema
  - Release of toxic cytokines and oxidative stress, resulting in free radical production
  - The restorative process of neuroplasticity including collateral sprouting and changes in neurotransmitter sensitivity[4]

General Guiding Principles for Treatment

- A "start low, go slow" approach is important, as patients with TBI are particularly susceptible to adverse effects from medications.
- Movement disorders cannot be treated in isolation because other sequelae of TBI such as balance or cognitive impairments may be exacerbated by standard treatments.[5] As such, the focus of treatment should be aimed at optimizing function.
- Some posttraumatic movement disorders may resolve spontaneously, so it is important to withdraw medications after several months to determine whether they continue to be necessary. Additionally, it would be prudent to wait up to 1 year before considering higher risk or invasive surgical procedures for treatment, to allow sufficient time for spontaneous resolution.

HYPERKINETIC MOVEMENT DISORDERS

Tremor

Definition

Rhythmic, oscillatory movement due to alternate or synchronous contraction of agonist and antagonist muscles.[6]

Subtypes

- Resting—present when body part is inactive
- Postural—present when maintaining body part in an antigravity position
- Kinetic—present when moving from one position to another
- Intention—only present when nearing goal of movement ("endpoint tremor")

Epidemiology

- 10% to 20% of posttraumatic movement disorders[7]

Risk Factors

- Prolonged coma

Timing

- Often appears in the first weeks after injury when voluntary movement begins to recover, but can develop years after injury.[5]

Clinical Presentation

▪ Posttraumatic tremor typically does not occur in isolation, as its emergence is associated with injury to the deeper regions of the brain responsible for motor control and coordination. Additionally, presentation can be mixed, as the tremor depends on the structural components injured (cerebellum, substantia nigra, etc.).[8] Tremor usually occurs bilaterally, affecting the upper greater rather than lower extremities, and is commonly associated with ataxia of the affected limb.[7,9] Affected limbs are evaluated in different postures, and the frequency and amplitude of tremor are described.

Differential Diagnosis

▪ Seizure; rigors; tremor due to hyperthyroidism, hepatic failure, hypercapnia, or medication side effects (e.g., amiodarone, lithium, valproic acid)

Treatment

▪ Tremors occurring after mild to moderate TBIs typically resolve spontaneously.[10]
▪ Medications—to date, there have been no studies performed to demonstrate efficacy. There are anecdotal reports of treatment with the following medications: primidone, propranolol, benzodiazepines (e.g., clonazepam), antiepileptics (e.g., carbamazepine, leviteracetam, gabapentin), glutethimide, L-tryptophan, anticholinergics, L-dopa/carbidopa, isoniazid, and botulinum toxin injections. In general, use of medications with greater potential for sedative side effects, such as benzodiazepines, should be avoided if possible. Choice of initial therapy can also be guided by tremor phenomenology (e.g., for action and posture tremor consider an antiepileptic or anticholinergic; for resting tremor consider L-dopa/carbidopa).
▪ Physical modalities—light weights on affected limb to dampen tremor.
▪ Surgery—consider at least 1 year after onset of tremor if not adequately responsive to conservative measures:
  ● Deep brain stimulation (DBS): surgical method of choice to treat disabling posttraumatic tremors, but less effective for treatment of posttraumatic tremor compared to essential tremor or Parkinson's tremor.[3,11] No consensus exists for the best anatomical location for stimulation.
  ● Stereotactic surgery (e.g., radiofrequency lesioning or g-knife thalamotomy): In one study, radiofrequency lesioning in the ventrolateral thalamus demonstrated tremor improvement in 88% of patients. However, there was an increase in dysarthria and/or gait disturbance in up to 90% of patients immediately postoperatively and in 63% persistently.[7]

Prognosis

▪ Posttraumatic tremor may decrease spontaneously within 1 year after onset.[2] However, for the majority, this tremor remains a persistent problem.[9]

Dystonia

Definition

Involuntary, simultaneous sustained—but not fixed—contraction of opposing muscles resulting in repetitive twisting movements or abnormal postures that are usually exacerbated or elicited by voluntary activity.

Subtypes

▪ Focal, segmental, generalized, and hemidystonia[12]

Epidemiology

▪ 4.8% to 16% of posttraumatic movement disorders; occurs more commonly in men.[6] Hemidystonia is the most common subtype.

Risk Factors

■ Younger age at time of trauma (first two decades of life) and severe TBI.[13] Frequently preceded by, or associated with, ipsilateral hemiparesis.[9]

Timing

■ Onset is likely to be delayed (1 month to 9 years), with mean latency of 20 months.[12] Initially, there is slow progression with spread over months to years followed by eventual stabilization.

Clinical Presentation

■ May occur at rest but usually exacerbated by voluntary movement. Characterized by twisting movements or involuntary postures. Evaluate for abnormal posture exacerbated by limb activation. Examples include torticollis (cervical dystonia), dystonia of the eyelids known as blepharospasm, and writer's cramp.

Differential Diagnosis

■ Rule out other possible causes of abnormal posturing such as muscle, joint, or bone injuries, ocular or vestibular abnormalities that could lead to head or trunk tilt, and toxic or metabolic conditions (e.g., Wilson's disease).[5]

Treatment

■ Acquired dystonias have various causes. Thus, identifying any treatable underlying comorbid conditions is recommended at the onset.
■ Physical modalities: range of motion to prevent contractures
■ Medications[5]—variably effective:
  ● Anticholinergics (e.g., trihexyphenidyl)—major side effect is sedation; better tolerated in the pediatric population
    ■ Tetrabenazine—major side effects include sedation, parkinsonism, and depression
  ● Neuroleptics—often effective but may interfere with neuroplasticity and functional recovery in TBI patients; carries long-term risk of tardive dyskinesias
    ■ Antiepileptics (e.g., gabapentin, carbamazepine)—can be tried, but not usually effective
  ● Benzodiazepines—ineffective as a sole agent but may be useful as adjuvant; major side effect is sedation and may interfere with neuroplasticity and functional recovery
    ■ Botulinum toxin injections— is the treatment of choice for many focal dystonias[14]
    ■ Oral baclofen—major side effect is sedation
    ■ L-Dopa/carbidopa—may be effective in patients with dopa-responsive dystonia
■ Surgery
  ● Intrathecal baclofen pump—recommended for generalized dystonia associated with significant spasticity, but not usually beneficial for isolated dystonia. Response to oral baclofen does not necessarily predict response to intrathecal baclofen
  ● Functional stereotactic surgery—less effective for secondary dystonia (e.g., due to TBI) than for primary dystonia
  ● Deep brain stimulation—for generalized, focal, segmental, and hemidystonia. Long-term efficacy data are limited
  ● Pallidal radiofrequency lesioning (pallidotomy)—improvement may take several months to occur postoperatively

Prognosis

■ Spontaneous remission is unlikely

Chorea, Ballism, and Athetosis

Definitions

- *Chorea*: rapid unpredictable, flowing dance-like movements. Chorea occurs predominantly in the distal limbs. There have been rare case reports of a possible association with epidural and subdural hematomas.
- *Ballism*: repetitive, but variable, high-amplitude purposeless movement that often is characterized by jerking or flinging of an extremity. Ballism occurs predominantly in the proximal limbs.
- *Athetosis*: slower writhing movement of the proximal limbs, often described as "snake-like."

Timing

Latency of weeks to months after injury.

Treatment

Similar to dystonia except for the following:

- *Chorea*: consider amantadine. Deep brain stimulation and botulinum toxin injections are not recommended.
- *Hemiballism*: responsive to intrathecal baclofen in a single case report.[15]

Tics and Tourettism

Definition

Tics are semivoluntary repetitive, nonrhythmic, sudden movements or vocalizations, often with an associated premonitory urge to make a movement or sound. Examples include blinking, jerking of body parts, grunting, or clearing of the throat. Over time, tics can increase in complexity and involve multiple sequential movements and/or vocalizations.[16] Tourettism is a set of symptoms that are virtually identical to Tourette's syndrome, such as motor tics and vocalizations, but the cause is different, such as TBI. Older age of onset and a clear history of onset after TBI help to distinguish tourettism from idiopathic Tourette's syndrome.[3]

Epidemiology

- 0.9% of posttraumatic movement disorders.[6] In one case series describing six patients, all were male with a mean age of 28 years, had suffered a mild to moderate TBI, and had experienced pain in the affected body part prior to the development of a tic.[10]

Clinical Presentation

- Simple tics can present as sudden repetitive movements involving a limited number of muscles groups, such as eye blinking or head jerking. Complex tics often present as patterned movements involving several muscle groups, such as flapping of the upper extremities or hopping. One of the hallmarks of tics is that they can be suppressed briefly. However, a premonitory urge will usually result in expression of a tic, which then briefly relieves this urge.

Differential Diagnosis

- Rule out idiopathic tic disorder such as Tourette's syndrome as well as other differential diagnoses including complex partial seizures, frontal lobe syndrome with frontal release signs, sleep-related movement disorders, and neurological effects of illicit drugs such as cocaine.

Treatment

- Tics can resolve spontaneously within 6 months of initial onset.[16]

- Psychoeducation should be provided to all patients and families. Behavioral therapy can be considered as well.[17]
- Medications
  - Neuroleptics (e.g., pimozide)—one of the most effective agents and the only medication class FDA approved for the treatment of tics.[17] However, they are relatively contraindicated in TBI due to risk of interference with neuroplasticity and functional recovery. Use is also associated with long-term risk of tardive dyskinesia.
  - Clonidine—potential side effects include sedation and orthostatic hypotension.
  - Clonazepam—major side effect is sedation and may interfere with neuroplasticity and functional recovery.
  - Selective serotonin reuptake inhibitors (SSRIs)—generally well tolerated. However, use with caution as the administration of two or more serotonergic drugs or an overdose of one agent may cause serotonin syndrome, a potentially life-threatening disorder.
  - Low-dose dopamine agonists (e.g., pramipexole)—may be effective, particularly if symptoms are associated with restless legs syndrome, and may also offer a secondary cognitive benefit in TBI.
  - Botulinum toxin injections—may possibly be effective for focal motor tics.[18]

Myoclonus

Definition
Sudden, brief, shock-like arrhythmic involuntary movement resulting from paroxysmal aberrant depolarization of individual or small groups of cortical or subcortical motor neurons. Any disease process that causes cortical irritability can produce myoclonus and once the cortical irritability resolves, over weeks to months, myoclonus can also subside.[5]

Epidemiology
- Accounts for 0.5% of posttraumatic movement disorders.[6]

Subtypes
- Focal, multifocal, and generalized.[5]

Clinical Presentation
- Myoclonus, particularly following hypoxemic-ischemic encephalopathy, is often stimulus induced (e.g., provoked by sudden loud noise). Look for segmental versus generalized presentation.
- Positive myoclonus occurs with active muscle contraction, whereas negative myoclonus occurs when muscles are inhibited. Electromyography (EMG) can help differentiate negative myoclonus from other conditions.[8]

Differential Diagnosis
- Consider metabolic causes such as renal or hepatic failure or electrolyte shifts during hemodialysis, as well as medication side effects (propofol, antiepileptics, and serotonergic medications such as trazodone, buspirone, SSRIs) and toxins such as lithium or bismuth. Obtaining a brain magnetic resonance imaging (MRI) study and/or performing lumbar puncture can help assess for new central nervous system (CNS) lesion or infection. An electroencephalogram (EEG) can help rule out myoclonic seizures.[5]

Treatment
- Medications such as valproic acid, clonazepam, levetiracetam, and tryptophan may be trialed for generalized myoclonus, although there is no evidence in the literature regarding their efficacy in the treatment of this condition.

Stereotypy, Hyperekplexia, and Akathisia

Definitions

- *Stereotypy*: involuntary, patterned movement (e.g., self-caressing); 0.9% of posttraumatic movement disorders.[6]
- *Hyperekplexia*: exaggerated startle response; 0.5% of posttraumatic movement disorders.[6]
- *Akathisia*: inner sense of restlessness; 0.9% of posttraumatic movement disorders.

Treatment

- These disorders are very difficult to treat. May respond to amantadine or propranolol.

HYPOKINETIC MOVEMENT DISORDERS

Parkinsonism

Definition

A neurological disorder characterized by four cardinal features: bradykinesia, rigidity, resting tremor, and postural instability. Posttraumatic parkinsonism is likely due to injury to the substantia nigra.

Epidemiology

- 0.9% of posttraumatic movement disorders.[6]
- Studies have found that those with idiopathic Parkinson's disease also have a higher frequency of remote TBI.[5]
- In general, posttraumatic parkinsonism is thought to be due to multiple, repeated closed head injuries as opposed to a single TBI.[3] A case control study in 93 twin pairs did demonstrate, however, that a TBI with loss of consciousness or amnesia significantly increased the risk of development of Parkinson's disease.[19] Notably, the frequency of posttraumatic parkinsonism in boxers ranges from 20% to 50%, and severity correlates with the number of bouts and length of boxing career.[20]

Clinical Presentation

- Tremor—4 to 7 Hz, more distal than proximal, often asymmetric initially, worsened by distraction techniques and walking.
- Rigidity—described as stiffness and an inability to relax the muscles, such that the resistance feels like a "lead-pipe." Cogwheeling may also be present if tremor is superimposed on the rigidity. Rigidity can be asymmetric.
- Bradykinesia—decreased movement velocity. Best indicator of disease severity.
- Postural instability—refers to imbalance and loss of the righting reflex. It is the least specific feature of the four.[8]

Differential Diagnosis

- Idiopathic Parkinson's disease
- Drug-induced parkinsonism
- Normal pressure hydrocephalus
- Polyarthropathy
- Depression

Timing

- Onset is typically within months after injury. In boxers, onset may occur years after ending their careers.[21] TBI can also exacerbate Parkinsonian features transiently in those with Parkinson's disease without increasing/accelerating disability.[11]

Treatment

■ Onset/progression of Parkinsonism within days or weeks after injury should prompt diagnostic imaging, as the cause may be an intracranial bleed, and drainage may fully resolve symptoms.[22]

■ Medications are similar to those used for idiopathic Parkinson's disease, with dopaminergic medications including carbidopa–levodopa and dopamine agonists being the mainstay for treatment. However, patients with posttraumatic parkinsonism have a less predictable response to these medications compared to patients with idiopathic Parkinson's disease.[3]

KEY POINTS

■ Movement disorders are more common in severe TBI compared to mild or moderate injury. The most common persisting movement disorder in this population is tremor, followed by dystonia.

■ Posttraumatic movement disorders can be broadly classified into hyperkinetic disorders (e.g., tremor, dystonia, ballism and chorea, tics and tourettism, myoclonus, stereotypy, hyperekplexia, and akathisia) or hypokinetic disorders (e.g., parkinsonism).

■ Guiding principles for treatment should include a "start low, go slow" approach, avoidance of medication associated with the potential to impair neuroplasticity or impede functional recovery, and focus on optimizing overall function.

STUDY QUESTIONS

1. A 50-year-old man is 6 months post severe TBI due to a motor vehicle collision. He now has a resting tremor. On physical examination, the patient is very slow on alternating tasks such as finger tapping. You also note mild rigidity in ranging his upper extremities. What medication is most likely to help this patient?
   a. Carbidopa/levodopa
   b. Clonazepam
   c. Levetiracetam
   d. Propranolol

2. An 18-year-old man was hit by a motor vehicle while he was on his bicycle. He suffered a severe TBI and developed left-sided hemiparesis. He presents to the clinic 5 years later complaining of twisting movements in his left limbs that are worsened with activity. What condition is this patient most likely suffering from?
   a. Tremors
   b. Myoclonus
   c. Dystonia
   d. Parkinsonism

3. A 36-year-old man fell off a 6-foot ladder onto a concrete driveway and suffered a severe TBI. After several months, he noted a twisting motion in his head and neck and was later diagnosed with posttraumatic torticollis. Which of the following is the best option for management of his condition?
   a. Botulinum toxin injection

    b. Oral baclofen
    c. Intrathecal baclofen
    d. Functional stereotactic surgery

4. A 64-year-old man suffered a severe TBI over two decades ago. He subsequently developed parkinsonism. Which of the following is true in regard to posttraumatic parkinsonism?
   a. Progression of parkinsonian findings within days or weeks after injury should prompt diagnostic imaging
   b. Use of carbidopa–levodopa in posttraumatic parkinsonism results in a more predictable favorable response than in idiopathic parkinsonism
   c. Posttraumatic parkinsonism encompasses 9% of all posttraumatic movement disorders
   d. Use of serotonergic medications is the mainstay treatment for posttraumatic parkinsonism

5. A 31-year-old man was involved in a high-speed motor vehicle collision. He suffered a severe TBI and underwent acute rehabilitation for 2 months. He presents to the clinic now 3 months later reporting head jerks. He is able to prevent them momentarily, but the urge becomes too great with time. Which is true about the medication class most effective in the treatment of this condition?
   a. It works by inhibiting the reuptake of serotonin and norepinephrine
   b. It can be injected locally into affected muscles
   c. There are no absolute or relative contraindications to use of this class of agents in TBI
   d. It carries a long-term risk of tardive dyskinesia

ADDITIONAL READING

Dystonia Medical Research Foundation: https://dystonia-foundation.org/wp-content/uploads/2018/12/DMRF_Traumatic_Brain_Injury_and_Dystonia.pdf

Krauss JK. Movement disorders secondary to craniocerebral trauma. In: Grafman J, Salazar AM, eds. *Handbook Clinical Neurology*. 3rd series. Elsevier; 2015; Vol. 128:475–496. doi:10.1016/B978-0-444-63521-1.00030-3

Krauss JK, Jankovic J. Head injury and posttraumatic movement disorders. *Neurosurgery*. 2002;50(5):927–939; discussion 939–940. doi:10.1227/00006123-200205000-00003

Krauss JK, Trankle R, Kopp KH. Posttraumatic movement disorders after moderate or mild head injury. *Mov Disord*. 1997;12(3):428–431. doi:10.1002/mds.870120326

Krauss JK, Trankle R, Kopp KH. Post-traumatic movement disorders in survivors of severe head injury. *Neurology*. 1996;47(6):1488–1492. doi:10.1212/WNL.47.6.1488

ANSWERS TO STUDY QUESTIONS

1. Correct Answer: a
   This patient is suffering from posttraumatic parkinsonism and may benefit from utilizing dopaminergic agents such as carbidopa/levodopa.

   Further Reading:
   O'Suilleabhain P, Dewey RB, Jr. Movement disorders after head injury: diagnosis and management. *J Head Trauma Rehabil*. 2004;19(4):305–313. doi:10.1097/00001199-200407000-00005

2. **Correct Answer: c**
Dystonia is an involuntary, simultaneous sustained—but not fixed—contraction of opposing muscles resulting in repetitive twisting movements or abnormal postures that are usually exacerbated or elicited by voluntary activity. Hemidystonia is the most common subtype, and a risk factor for presentation is younger age at time of injury.

Further Reading:
Krauss JK, Mohadjer M, Braus DF, et al. Dystonia following head trauma: a report of nine patients and review of the literature. *Mov Disord.* 1992;7(3):263–272. doi:10.1002/mds.870070313

3. **Correct Answer: a**
Botulinum toxin is the treatment of choice for many focal dystonias, including posttraumatic torticollis. Because of the focal nature of the condition, injection with botulinum toxin would be preferred over oral or intrathecal baclofen.

Further Reading:
Kemp S, Kim SDH, Cordato DJ et al. (2012). Delayed-onset focal dystonia of the leg secondary to traumatic brain injury. *J Clin Neurosci.* 19:916–917. doi:10.1016/j.jocn.2011.08.025

4. **Correct Answer: a**
Progression of Parkinson's within days or weeks after injury should prompt diagnostic imaging, as onset in this timeframe may be due to an evolving hematoma. Drainage of the hematoma will most likely spur resolution of symptoms. Treatment responsiveness to carbidopa-levodopa is less predictable in posttraumatic parkinsonism, even though dopaminergic medications are the mainstay treatment. Posttraumatic parkinsonism accounts for 0.9% of posttraumatic movement disorders.

Further Reading:
O'Suilleabhain P, Dewey RB, Jr. Movement disorders after head injury: diagnosis and management. *J Head Trauma Rehabil.* 2004;19(4):305–313. doi:10.1097/00001199-200407000-00005

5. **Correct Answer: d**
Neuroleptics, such as pimozide, are the most effective class in treating a tic disorder. These medications typically block dopamine receptors in the dopaminergic pathways of the brain. They are relatively contraindicated in TBI as they may impair neuroplasticity. Additionally, they do carry a long-term risk of tardive dyskinesia.

Further Reading:
Jimenez-Shahed J. Medical and Surgical Treatments of Tourette Syndrome. *Neurol Clin.* 2020;38(2):349–366. doi:10.1016/j.ncl.2020.01.006

REFERENCES

The full reference list appears in the digital product found on http://connect.springer-pub.com/content/book/978-0-8261-4768-4/part/part04/chapter/ch50

SPASTICITY IN TRAUMATIC BRAIN INJURY

BONNY S. WONG, MARY ALEXIS IACCARINO, AND ROSS ZAFONTE

BACKGROUND

Definition

Spasticity is a velocity-dependent, muscular resistance to passive joint range of motion (ROM) often manifested in patients with upper motor neuron syndrome.[1,2]

Epidemiology

The prevalence of spasticity in traumatic brain injury (TBI) is 18% to 75%.[3-5] Increased severity of TBI escalates the likelihood of spasticity occurring. Development of spasticity is more likely in patients who have experienced prolonged loss of consciousness and is negatively associated with functional independence 1-year post injury.[5,6]

Pathophysiology

Spasticity refers to increased muscular tone due to disruption of inhibitory modulation of descending alpha motor neurons. It results from aberrant neuronal pathway input from gamma afferent motor neurons: reticulospinal and vestibulospinal input combined with exacerbations from irritant noxious stimuli.[7] Spasticity may be aggravated by urinary tract infections, decubitus ulcers, hydrocephalus, fractures, ingrown toenails, heterotopic ossification, kinked and dislodged urinary catheters, restrictive clothing, stool impaction, nephrolithiasis, or sources of physiologic or emotional stress.[2,8]

ASSESSMENT

Clinical Manifestations

The sequelae of spasticity are grossly classified into beneficial and deleterious effects. The beneficial aspects of spasticity are the inadvertent functional and medical advantages conferred by the presence of increased tone: (a) facilitation of ambulation, standing, and transfers; (b) maintenance of muscle bulk; (c) promotion of venous return; (d) reduction of deep vein thrombosis risk; (e) lessening of orthostatic hypotension; (f) prevention of osteoporosis; and (g) decrement of pressure ulcer formation. Conversely, the deleterious sequelae of spasticity include (a) pain, (b) immobility, (c) contractures, (d) skin breakdown, (e) increased energy expenditure, (f) muscle spasm, (g) fracture, (h) tendon injury, (i) increased risk of heterotopic ossification, (j) joint subluxation or dislocation, (k) insomnia, and (l) interference with nursing care and hygiene.[1,2,7-9]

The full reference list appears in the digital product found on http://connect.springerpub.com/content/book/978-0-8261-4768-4/part/part04/chapter/ch51

Physical Examination

Spasticity is elicited by performing passive motion across an affected joint: this motion induces an involuntary velocity-dependent activation of the stretch response. Occasionally, one may also see other corroborating signs such as the Westphal phenomenon, which is a passively activated stretched muscle response in its shortened state. Passive stretch may also trigger spasms, or involuntary contractions, of agonist–antagonist groups, neighboring limb, girdle, and/or trunk muscles.[9]

Assessment Scales

One of the first clinical scales employed to evaluate spasticity is the Ashworth Scale, developed in 1964 and modified by Bohannon and Smith in 1967.[9]

The Modified Ashworth Scale (MAS) is characterized as follows:
- 0: no increase in muscle tone with ROM
- 1: slight increase in muscle tone with or without a catch and release at the end of ROM
- 1+: slight increase in muscle tone, manifested by a catch, followed by slight resistance through the remainder (less than half) of ROM
- 2: more marked increase in muscle tone through most of ROM, but affected part(s) easily moved
- 3: considerable increase in muscle tone, passive movement difficult
- 4: affected part(s) rigid in flexion or extension

MAS has been shown to have good intra-rater and inter-rater reliability in the hands of trained medical professionals.[10,11,12] However, it is frequently criticized for its limited precision in detecting subtle effects of antispasmodic medications. A more practical assessment technique is to quantify the specific condition being treated; for example, pain, function, ambulation distance, gait analysis, or performance tests of the involved extremity.[9,10]

The Tardieu Scale is an alternative to the MAS. The Modified Tardieu Scale (MTS) is characterized as follows:

Quality of muscle reaction:
- 0: no resistance throughout the course of the passive movement
- 1: slight resistance throughout the course of passive movement, with no clear catch at precise angle
- 2: clear catch at precise angle, interrupting the passive movement, followed by release
- 3: fatigable clonus (less than 10 seconds when maintaining pressure) occurring at precise angle
- 4: infatigable clonus (greater than 10 seconds when maintaining pressure) occurring at precise angle

Velocity to stretch:
- $V1$: as slow as possible (used to measure passive ROM)
- $V2$: speed of limb segment falling under gravity
- $V3$: as fast as possible

Joint angle:
- R1: the angle in which a catch or clonus is found during a quick stretch (V3)
- R2: angle of full ROM taken at a very slow speed (V1)

Spasticity angle or dynamic tone component of the muscle: R1 subtracted from R2

Proponents of this scale find that it better captures dynamic spasticity. While studies assessing the reliability of the MTS have largely been mixed in various populations,[13] one study of adults with severe brain injury and impaired consciousness demonstrated significantly higher test-retest and interrater reliability compared to the MAS.[14]

TREATMENT

Considerations

There are multiple indications for the treatment of spasticity after TBI[8]:

- Pain management: Painful spasticity is common in TBI. For patients that cannot effectively communicate, painful spasticity may manifest as agitation, restlessness, sleep disturbance, and/or autonomic dysfunction (sweating, hypertension, tachycardia).
- Patient care needs: Adequate spasticity control can reduce caregiver burden and allow for ease of nursing care, personal hygiene, dressing, and positioning to help prevent contractures and deformities. Spasticity reduction may prevent pressure ulcer formation or act as an adjunctive treatment for healing a pressure ulcer.
- Patient independence: Treatment of spasticity can enhance functional mobility in performing activities of daily living (ADLs), transfers and ambulation, reducing energy expenditure and the need for assistive devices and physical support from another person.

Goal

Spasticity abolishment is often undesirable, as spasticity occasionally facilitates function. Therefore, the goal of treatment should be directed at the minimization of spasticity only as it relates to functional or symptomatic impairment. One should begin treatment by removing noxious stimuli or triggers, followed by minimally invasive interventions.

There are few studies that evaluate treatment of spasticity specific to the TBI population. Most of the evidence is gleaned from the spinal cord injury and stroke literature. However, with thoughtful consideration of the symptoms and side effects most common to TBI patients, the following treatments can be safely applied using a multi-modal, synergistic approach.

Nonpharmacological Management

Positioning

The first step in managing spasticity is the maintenance of neutral joint positioning. This may be implemented by piloting each limb through its full ROM, multiple times a day, and stretching shortened muscle groups. The maintenance of position may be further augmented with casting and splinting, which provide a prolonged period of stretch. Although there is insufficient evidence to support the benefit of manual stretching, prolonged stretching through casting has been shown to increase joint ROM and reduce spasticity.[15,16] Casting should be performed by an experienced physician or physiotherapist with frequent monitoring for adverse effects, including pain, skin breakdown, neurovascular compromise, and fracture.

Physiotherapy and Modalities

Physiotherapy techniques (such as the Bobath and Brunnstrom programs) and modalities (such as cryotherapy) have been documented to be effective in spasticity management. In particular, a 15- to 20-minute application of cryotherapy to spastic muscles has been shown to enact a 35° improvement in ROM.[8] Transcutaneous electrical stimulation has been shown to improve spasticity when compared to placebo and in conjunction with standard physical therapy.[17,18] Local heat, ultrasound, electromyographic biofeedback, vibration, and feedback of tonic stretch reflex are used clinically, although evidence for their use is limited.[8] All modalities should be used with caution, as TBI patients may have insensate dermatomes and/or impaired communication, which may limit the patient's ability to detect/communicate adverse effects of treatment.

Pharmacological Management

Oral medications are frequently employed in the management of spasticity.[19] Common side effects such as sedation and drowsiness may worsen cognitive function, however, limiting their use in the brain injury population. Therefore, consideration of side-effect profiles is the largest determinant of selection of an antispasmodic agent. Concomitant use of oral medication for secondary indications such as pain, mood, sleep, or paroxysmal sympathetic hyperactivity should be considered as well. Initiate any new medication slowly, followed by gentle dose escalation. Though often prescribed, the evidence for the efficacy of oral antispasmodics has not been well substantiated.[7,9] A description of commonly used antispasmodics follows.

Baclofen

This is the most frequently utilized oral antispasmodic agent.[7] It is an inhibitory GABA-B receptor agonist, which inhibits the release of excitatory neurotransmitters at the junction of the presynaptic nerve and muscle.

- Dosing: start with 5 mg two to three times a day and increase dose by 5 mg every 3 to 5 days. Max dose: 80 mg/day.
- Side effects: sedation, hallucinations, convulsions, rigidity, lowered seizure threshold, and severe withdrawal syndrome.[7,9]
- Considerations: in widespread use despite paucity of evidence of efficacy.[9]

Tizanidine

This is an alpha-2 adrenergic receptor agonist that targets supraspinal and spinal receptors.[7,17]

- Dosing: start with 2 to 4 mg/day and increase to 8 mg three times a day; max dose: 36 mg/day.
- Side effects: mirrors baclofen in most of its side effects, with sedation and asthenia being its most common dose-limiting adverse effects.[7] Weakness is less frequently reported in comparison to baclofen and diazepam.[20]
- Considerations: studies have failed to demonstrate functional improvement.[20] Recommend slow up-titration and monitoring for hypotension as a result of inhibition of central sympathetic outflow.

Diazepam

This agent stimulates GABA-A neurotransmission resulting in presynaptic inhibition of stretch reflexes.[20]

- Dosing: start with 2 mg twice a day; max dose: 60 mg/day.
- Side effects: delayed cognition, sedation, drowsiness, memory and attention impairment, tolerance, dependence, weakness, and motor incoordination.[20]
- Considerations: this agent has a long half-life of approximately 30 hours; exacerbation of cognitive impairment and potential impediment of neurorecovery limit the usefulness of diazepam for the TBI population.

Dantrolene

This is unique as an antispasmodic agent because it is peripherally acting. It inhibits calcium ion release from the muscular sarcoplasmic reticulum.[7] While this avoids the cognitive adverse effects of antispasmodics, dantrolene will weaken affected and unaffected muscles alike.

- Dosing: start with 25 mg/day; max dose 400 mg/day.
- Side effects: gastrointestinal intolerance, sedation, and hepatotoxicity. Monitoring of liver function tests is required with use of this agent especially in those at higher risk for dantrolene-associated hepatotoxicity: females, patients over age 30, prior history of liver dysfunction, on longer duration and higher doses of dantrolene, or concomitant use of other potentially hepatotoxic medications.[7,20,21]
- Efficacy in spasticity reduction has been proven in placebo studies, but data supporting functional improvement are lacking.[20]

Other less commonly used antispasmodic agents (e.g., clonazepam, ketazolam, tetrazepam, progabide, gabapentin, piracetam, clonidine, pregabalin, and glycine)[2,7,19,20] are beyond the scope of this chapter. Please see the noted references for a more detailed discussion of these agents.

Interventional Approaches

Botulinum Toxin Injection

Botulinum toxin (BoNT) injection is a common intervention for focal spasticity and is a Level A recommendation (American Academy of Neurology classification) for treatment of upper and lower limb spasticity.[22,23] BoNT is produced by the *Clostridium botulinum* bacterium and acts at the neuromuscular junction to inhibit acetylcholine release.[2,8,9,24] Of the seven antigenically distinct serotypes of BoNT, only serotypes A and B are available for commercial use.[8] Both serotypes have demonstrated efficacy for spasticity.[24–26] In the United States, there are four commercially available toxins that are distinctly different in formulation, purification, and dosing: onabotulinumtoxinA (Botox™), abobotulinumtoxinA (Dysport™), incobotulinumtoxinA (Xeomin™), and rimabotulinumtoxinB (Myobloc™). OnabotulinumtoxinA and abobotulinumtoxinA are Food and Drug Administration (FDA)-approved for the management of upper and lower limb spasticity in adults, while incobotulinumtoxinA is FDA-approved for only upper limb spasticity in adults. An advantage of BoNT compared with oral medications is its lack of systemic effects. Application requires identification of the muscle of interest, followed by injection of the toxin solution. Studies have consistently demonstrated that instrumented guidance via electromyography (EMG), electrical stimulation or ultrasound, is superior to anatomic localization through muscle palpation.[27] The onset of action of BoNT is observed in 1 to 3 days with maximum effect in a few weeks and a duration of effect of 1 to 6 months.[2,8] Repeat injections should not be more frequent than every 3 months because frequent exposure may lead to diminished effect from antibody-mediated resistance.[8,9] A recent systematic review found a 1% prevalence of neutralizing antibodies when BoNT was used for limb spasticity.[28] Neutralizing antibodies were more likely to be found in those on longer duration of therapy, higher doses, and shorter intervals between injections. Immunogenicity and the relationship between neutralizing antibodies and secondary non-response to BoNT is still a controversial topic.[28]

The benefits of BoNT effect may be enhanced by physiotherapy, splinting, casting, or electrical stimulation.[9,29,30] Adverse effects include localized reaction, bleeding, infection, nerve trauma, unintentional weakening of the targeted or surrounding muscles, and cervical dysphagia (rarely associated with cervical injection).[2,8] Additional considerations include cost, insurance approval, transient nature of effect, and need for repeated injections.[2,7-9]

Nerve Block

Nerve blocks eliminate neurological input responsible for the spastic activity.[8] Temporary blocks using short-acting local anesthetics such as bupivacaine or lidocaine can be useful for diagnostic purposes, e.g., to identify the role of spasticity versus contracture. For therapeutic treatment of spasticity, nerve or motor point blocks using lytic agents such as phenol (5%–7%) or alcohol (35%–60%) can be effective.[2,8,9] Nerves are identified using a variable intensity stimulator.[8,9] The duration of effect of temporary blocks is 1 to 6 hours while sustained blocks are effective for 3 to 9 months.[8] Adverse effects include weakness, sensitivity, injection site pain, phlebitis, central nervous system or cardiovascular compromise (rarely), phenol nerve fibrosis (which potentially adulterates anatomy for repeat injections), and dysesthesias.[2,8] Dysesthesias may exacerbate spasticity; therefore, mixed sensorimotor nerves are avoided while motor-only nerve branches are targeted.[9] When comparing phenol neurolysis to BoNT injection for spasticity management, advantages of phenol neurolysis include lower cost, faster onset of action, potentially longer duration of benefit, and safety to perform repeat injections at shorter intervals. However, technical difficulties and concerns of safety profiles with phenol neurolysis must be considered.[31]

Intrathecal Baclofen Pump

Intrathecal baclofen (ITB) delivery is an effective technique for managing generalized or regional spasticity. It should be carefully considered in those recalcitrant to an oral regimen or when adverse effects make use of oral agents untenable.[32] Therapeutic effects can be achieved with much smaller doses of baclofen delivered intrathecally rather than orally, thus reducing the central side effects associated with oral baclofen use. As with all spasticity interventions, it is important to establish ITB therapy goals prior to pump implantation. A 50-mcg test dose is typically administered via lumbar puncture or temporary catheter in adults.[8,33] Patients unresponsive to the standard trial dose may require 75-mcg or 100-mcg bolus.[33] If the trial is successful and the patient and caregiver are agreeable, a pump is subcutaneously implanted.[34] Potentially life-threatening adverse events associated with ITP pump use include complications associated with baclofen withdrawal (increase in tone, pruritus, irritability, altered mental status, hypotension, hyperthermia, rhabdomyolysis, seizure, coma, death) or overdose (nausea, vomiting, dizziness, hypotonia, altered mental status, decreased respiratory drive, death).[2,7-9,35] These may be related to pump-related malfunction, programming error, or catheter-related issues such as breakage, migration, or kinking.[35] It is important for patients and caregivers to be educated on signs and symptoms of baclofen withdrawal and overdose, stay compliant with refill appointments, and plan ahead for pump replacement (average pump battery life is 7 years) and revision surgeries when necessary.

Surgical Treatment

Permanent orthopedic and neurosurgical procedures are usually the last resort in tone management.[8] They include neurotomy, rhizotomy, dorsal root entry zone–otomy (DREZ-otomy), cordotomy, neurectomy, split tibialis transfer (SPLATT) procedure, tendon lengthening, and muscle tenotomies and transposition.[2,8,9]

KEY POINTS

- Spasticity is a velocity-dependent resistance to passive muscle stretch, which can occur as a sequela of TBI.
- Diagnosis of spasticity is made by clinical examination and is often graded using the MAS or a description of the motion limitation and its functional impact.
- The goal of treating spasticity is to improve patient quality of life, including reducing pain, improving caregiver ease, and hygiene management, and maximizing independence and functional mobility.
- A multimodal therapeutic approach is most beneficial and can include physical therapeutic modalities, pharmacotherapy, local neurotoxin injections, intrathecal baclofen pump therapy and surgical interventions.

STUDY QUESTIONS

1. A 60-year-old woman with history of cirrhosis is in inpatient rehabilitation after sustaining a severe TBI due to a motor vehicle collision. She has significant spasticity and episodes of paroxysmal sympathetic hyperactivity. If you were to start an oral medication to target both increased tone and dysautonomia, which medication might you be cautious about starting?
   a. Baclofen
   b. Tizanidine
   c. Dantrolene
   d. Gabapentin

2. A 35-year-old man who is currently in an unresponsive wakefulness state after a TBI presents to your clinic with significant bilateral ankle plantar flexor and invertor spasticity. He underwent BoNT injections to his upper extremities 4 weeks ago. Next, you consider performing tibial nerve phenol injections. In comparison to BoNT injections, which of the following is TRUE regarding phenol neurolysis:
   a. Slower onset of action
   b. Risk of dysesthesias
   c. Shorter duration of benefit
   d. More expensive

3. A 40-year-old woman with generalized spasticity presents to your clinic 1 year after a TBI. Her spasticity is significantly limiting her transfers and mobility. You perform BoNT

injections every 90 days in her lower extremities, but she is unable to tolerate oral baclofen given the cognitive side effects. You would like to consider ITB therapy and you schedule her for a trial. What is the starting baclofen test dose?

   a. 25 mcg
   b. 50 mcg
   c. 75 mcg
   d. 100 mcg

4. When evaluating a patient's elbow flexion spasticity in clinic, you are able to passively extend the elbow through its full range of motion without too much difficulty but notice significant tone throughout. What Modified Ashworth Scale does this correlate to?

   a. MAS 1
   b. MAS 1+
   c. MAS 2
   d. MAS 3
   e. MAS 4

5. What is the mechanism of action of baclofen?

   a. Alpha-2 adrenergic agonist
   b. Facilities GABA's effect on GABA-A receptors
   c. Blocks presynaptic release of acetylcholine at the neuromuscular junction
   d. GABA agonist at GABA-B receptors

ADDITIONAL READING

Brashear A. *Spasticity: Diagnosis and Management, 2nd ed.* Demos Medical Publishing; 2016.

Esquenazi A, Albanese A, Chancellor M, et al. Evidence-based review and assessment of botulinum neurotoxin for the treatment of adult spasticity in the upper motor neuron syndrome. *Toxicon.* 2013;67:115–128. doi:10.1016/j.toxicon.2012.11.025

Simpson DM, Hallet M, Ashman EJ, et al. Practice guideline update summary: botulinum neurotoxin for the treatment of blepharospasm, cervical dystonia, adult spasticity, and headache. *Am Acad Neurol.* 2016;86:1818–1826. doi:10.1212/WNL.0000000000002560

Boster AL, Adair RL, Gooch JL, et al. Best practices for intrathecal baclofen therapy: dosing and long-term management. *Neuromodulation.* 2016;19:623–631. doi:10.1111/ner.12388

Saulino M, Anderson DJ, Doble J, et al. Best practices for intrathecal baclofen therapy: troubleshooting. *Neuromodulation.* 2016;19:632–641. doi:10.1111/ner.12447

ANSWERS TO STUDY QUESTIONS

1. Correct Answer: c

   Although dantrolene may not affect cognition as much as other anti-spasmodic medications due to its peripheral mechanism of action, adverse effects include hepatotoxicity—especially in higher risk patients: females, older age, history of liver dysfunction. If starting dantrolene, it is important to monitor liver function tests regularly especially after dose adjustments.

   Further Reading:
   Utili R, Boitnott J, Zimmerman H. Dantrolene-associated hepatic injury. *Gastroenterology.* 1977;72:610–616. doi:10.1016/S0016-5085(77)80141-8

2. Correct Answer: b
   Phenol is cheaper, has a faster onset of action, and potentially longer duration of benefit compared to BoNT. Possible adverse effects include dysesthesias, particularly when injecting mixed sensory/motor nerves. The incidence of dysesthetic pain is variable in the literature (0%–32%). The onset dysesthesias is seen a few days to 2 weeks after the procedure and typically lasts several weeks (ranges from a few days to even up to a year). Treatment includes repeating the block and/or symptomatic management.

   Further Reading:
   Horn LJ, Singh G, Dabrowski ER. Chemoneurolysis with phenol and alcohol: a "dying art" that merits revival. In: Brashear A, Elovic E. *Spasticity Diagnosis and Management*. 2nd ed. Demos Medical Publishing; 2016:111–127. doi:10.1891/9781617052422.0010

3. Correct Answer: b
   The standard baclofen test dose is a 50-mcg bolus in adults. Spasticity assessments should be done at least twice within 4 hours after the trial. Patients should be closely monitored for adverse events (spinal headaches, nausea/vomiting, sedation, hypotension, seizures, urinary retention, and respiratory depression).

   Further Reading:
   Boster AL, Bennett SE, Bilsky GS et al. Best practices for intrathecal baclofen therapy: screening test. *Neuromodulation*. 2016;19:616–622. doi:10.1111/ner.12437

4. Correct Answer: c
   Marked increase in muscle tone throughout most of the range of motion with ability to move the affected part easily correlates to a MAS of 2.

   Further Reading:
   Brashear A, Zafonte R, Corcoran M, et al. Inter- and intrarater reliability of the Ashworth Scale and the Disability Assessment Scale in patients with upper limb poststroke spasticity. *Arch Phys Med Rehabil*. 2002;83(10):1349–1354. doi:10.1053/apmr.2002.35474

5. Correct Answer: d
   Baclofen acts as a GABA agonist at presynaptic and postsynaptic GABA-B receptors. Both clonidine and tizanidine are central acting alpha-2 adrenergic agonists. BoNT affects the SNARE complex in the presynaptic terminal and prevents the exocytosis of ACh-containing vesicles into the neuromuscular junction. Diazepam stimulates GABA-A neurotransmission.

   Further Reading:
   Zafonte R, Co S, Srikrishana A. Spasticity in traumatic brain injury. In: Brashear A, Elovic E, eds. *Spasticity: Diagnosis and Management*. Demos Medical Publishing; 2011:371–386.

REFERENCES

The full reference list appears in the digital product found on http://connect.springer-pub.com/content/book/978-0-8261-4768-4/part/part04/chapter/ch51

SCREENING FOR EMOTIONAL DISTRESS AFTER TRAUMATIC BRAIN INJURY

ANGELLE M. SANDER

GENERAL BACKGROUND

- Emotional distress, including depression and/or anxiety, is present in a substantial number of persons with mild to severe traumatic brain injury (TBI).[1-4] Information on epidemiology, classification, etiology, and pathophysiology of mood disorders following TBI can be found in Chapter 53. This chapter will focus on screening for mood disorders in persons with moderate to severe TBI.
- Mood disorders are often underdiagnosed and undertreated in persons with TBI, due to their overlap with the cognitive and behavioral symptoms of TBI.[5]
- Use of rating scales to screen for emotional distress in medical settings has been recommended to avoid undertreating, but also to prevent overdiagnosis that can lead to unnecessary medication use.[6]
- Accurate use of screening in medical settings serving persons with TBI requires understanding of the potential for under- or over-diagnosing emotional distress in a population with cognitive and behavioral impairments.

TERMINOLOGY WITH RESPECT TO SCREENING FOR EMOTIONAL DISTRESS VERSUS DIAGNOSIS OF MOOD DISORDERS

- **Screening**—assessment of symptoms in order to guide treatment and/or detect potential for mood disorder; often uses cut-off scores to indicate how consistent symptom presence and severity is with diagnostic criteria for mood disorders; does not enable diagnosis, but indicates the need for more comprehensive assessment that can result in diagnosis
- **Diagnosis**—assessment aimed at establishing the presence or absence of disease; is the result of multiple inputs, including review of records, formal psychiatric or psychological assessments, clinical interview, proxy interview, and so on; established using formal diagnostic criteria, such as the *Diagnostic and Statistical Manual of Mental Disorders* (*DSM*)
- **Sensitivity**—ability of a measure to correctly detect presence of depression or anxiety; typically determined by comparison with a gold standard, such as confirmed diagnosis of depression or anxiety, often via a structured diagnostic interview[7]
- **Specificity**—ability of a measure to correctly identify the absence of depression or anxiety; that is, not falsely identifying someone as having depression or anxiety when they do not

---

The full reference list appears in the digital product found on http://connect.springerpub.com/content/book/978-0-8261-4768-4/part/part04/chapter/ch52

- **Positive predictive value**—probability that a person meeting the cut-off for depression or anxiety on a screening measure actually has the disorder[7]
- **Negative predictive value**—probability that a person who does not meet the cut-off for depression or anxiety on a screening measure does not have the disorder

DIAGNOSTIC TOOLS: STRUCTURED INTERVIEWS

- The gold standard for diagnosis of emotional distress is to use formal diagnostic criteria, such as the *DSM*, currently in its fifth edition,[8] or the World Health Organization's (WHO) International Classification of Diseases (ICD).[9]
- Several structured interviews exist to assist with determining whether a person's symptoms meet the diagnostic criteria for specific psychiatric disorders, such as Major Depressive Disorder or Generalized Anxiety Disorder. The most commonly used diagnostic interviews in persons with TBI are the Structured Clinical Interview for DSM Disorders (SCID),[10] the MINI-International Neuropsychiatric Interview (MINI),[11] and the Schedules Clinical Assessment in Neuropsychiatry (SCAN).[12] The SCID is based on the diagnostic criteria of the *DSM*, while the MINI and SCAN are based on a combination of *DSM* criteria and those of the ICD.
- Advantages—use interviewing to assess frequency and severity of symptoms required to meet diagnostic criteria; allows for probing to obtain exact information necessary, including fluctuation of symptoms over time; map directly on to diagnostic criteria.
- Disadvantages—long and requires expert staff to administer; can be impacted by cognitive deficits in person with injury, including impaired awareness and impaired memory.
- Diagnostic interviews that probe for information over a shorter time-frame, like the past 2 weeks, tend to yield higher estimates than those probing for information over longer periods (past 2 weeks to a month), perhaps due to impaired recall across longer time periods.[3]

USE OF SELF-REPORT QUESTIONNAIRES TO SCREEN FOR EMOTIONAL DISTRESS

- Advantages—quick to administer; many can be given by phone or mailed to patients ahead of time; can be used as a basis of referral for more comprehensive assessment and diagnosis via structured diagnostic interviews; can detect subclinical emotional distress associated with TBI that may not require medication but could still respond to counseling, support groups, and so on.
- Disadvantages—cannot be used to diagnose; varying rates of specificity, sensitivity, and positive and negative predictive values for detecting presence of mood disorders, such as depression or anxiety.
- The most commonly used self-report measures of depression and evidence for their usefulness in screening for depression in persons with TBI are described in Table 52.1. All of these measures have adequate internal reliability and good concurrent validity, as indicated by acceptable correlations with other measures of symptom severity. They differ with respect to their sensitivity, specificity, and positive and negative predictive values with respect to distinguishing persons with TBI who do or do not meet diagnostic criteria for depression or anxiety.

TABLE 52.1 Characteristics of Commonly Used Screening Measures for Emotional Distress in Persons With Traumatic Brain Injury

Measure	No. of Items	Time Interval Assessed	Comparison Standard	Recommended Cut-Off Score	Specificity	Sensitivity	Positive Predictive Value	Negative Predictive Value	Conclusions
Depression									
PHQ-9[13,14]	9	Past 2 weeks	SCID-IV;[15] clinical diagnosis of Major Depressive Disorder[16]	At least five symptoms rated as present for at least several days, with at least one being anhedonia or sad mood	0.89;[14] 0.60[16]	0.93;[14] 0.92[16]	63%	99%	The PHQ-9, administered in person or by phone, is a valid and reliable method for screening for depression in persons with TBI who are oriented.
Hospital Anxiety and Depression Scale-Depression (HADS-D)[17,18]	7	Past week	SCID-IV	7–8	0.92	0.62	81%	82%	Good method of assessing symptoms over past week, but not a means for clinical diagnosis of depression.
Beck Depression Inventory-II (BDI-II)[19,20]	21	Past 2 weeks	SCID-IV	≥19 for mild TBI; ≥35 for moderate to severe TBI ≥6 for mild TBI; ≥23 for moderate to severe TBI	0.79 0.59	0.87 0.10	Not calculated	Not calculated	BDI-II is a useful screening tool to identify people who require more comprehensive assessment/ diagnostic interviewing.

Measure	Items	Time frame	Reliability/Validity	Comments
Brief Symptom Inventory (BSI)[21,22]	53	Past week	Not reported	Persons with TBI showed elevations on 7 of 9 subscales, with the most frequent elevations being on scales with symptoms that overlap physical and cognitive symptoms of TBI (Obsessive-Compulsive and Somatization). Global severity index appears to be valid as an overall indicator of emotional distress, but further evidence is needed for meaning of elevations on individual subscales—they may not be used diagnostically.
BSI-18 [23,24]	18	Past week	Not reported	BSI-18 Global severity index has good reliability and concurrent validity for assessing depressive symptoms following TBI. Impact of physical TBI-related symptoms on individual subscale scores has yet to be determined.

(continued)

TABLE 52.1 Characteristics of Commonly Used Screening Measures for Emotional Distress in Persons With Traumatic Brain Injury (*continued*)

Measure	No. of Items	Time Interval Assessed	Comparison Standard	Recommended Cut-Off Score	Specificity	Sensitivity	Positive Predictive Value	Negative Predictive Value	Conclusions
Center for Epidemiologic Studies-Depression Scale (CES-D)[25–27]	20	Past week	Not reported						Factor structure inconsistent across studies, with one study, conducted with primarily mild TBI, finding one main factor, replicating the original factor structure of the CES-D with normal.[26] The other study, conducted with moderate to severe TBI, found four factors.[25]
Symptom Checklist-20 (SCL-20)[28,29]	20	Past week	Not reported						SCL-20 required some modifications due to 6 items showing unacceptably low correlations with the overall measure and to not enough items assessing the lower end of the depression severity continuum.

Hamilton Depression Rating Scale (HAM-D)[30,31]	17	Past week	SCID-IV	7	0.78	0.93	Not calculated	Not calculated	HAM-D is a useful screening tool for depression in persons with TBI, but requires modification due to several items showing unacceptably low correlations with the overall measure and to not enough items assessing the lower end of the depression severity continuum.
Anxiety									
Hospital Anxiety and Depression Scale-Anxiety (HADS-A)[17,18]	7	Past week	SCID-IV	7/8	0.69	0.75	57%	83%	Caution is recommended when using the anxiety scale.

- The PHQ-9[14] has the most empirical support in terms of sensitivity for major depressive disorder as determined by structured diagnostic interviews.[32,33] The PHQ-9 items map directly on to *DSM* diagnostic criteria and do not assess any symptoms that are not included in those criteria. People who endorse five or more of the nine symptoms as occurring on more than half of the days, with both items 1 and 2 (sad mood and anhedonia) endorsed, are considered likely to have Major Depressive Disorder. The PHQ-8 omits the ninth PHQ-9 item that inquires about suicidal ideation. This version is used primarily in research, when procedures to follow up on suicidal ideation are not possible, but omission of the suicide item is not recommended for clinical purposes. PHQ-9 scores can be used to identify severity of depressive symptoms in the following manner: 5 (mild); 10 (moderate); 15 (moderately severe); and 20 (severe).
- The PHQ-2 assesses the two cardinal symptoms of depression: anhedonia and sad mood. The PHQ-2 has shown good specificity and sensitivity in large samples of primary care patients[32] and older adults.[34] A comparison of PHQ-9 and PHQ-2 in persons with TBI showed that PHQ-2 scores ≥2 had a sensitivity of .90 for predicting persons with PHQ-9 scores ≥10, and thus could be used in lieu of PHQ-9 scores following TBI.[35] PHQ-2 scores ≥2 also showed .95 specificity for classification of persons who endorsed active or passive suicidal ideation on the PHQ-9. Thus a score of ≥2 on the PHQ-2 should trigger questions about suicidal Ideation.
- Investigation of anxiety following TBI is in its infancy. Widely used measures of anxiety include the GAD-7[36] and the Beck Anxiety Inventory,[37] but the sensitivity and specificity of these measures have not been investigated in persons with TBI. As shown in Table 52.1, caution is recommended when using the anxiety scale of the Hospital Anxiety and Depression Scale, as it has shown low specificity in persons with TBI.
- Posttraumatic Stress Disorder (PTSD) occurs in approximately 11% of civilians with TBI[38] and in 12% to 30% of military veterans with TBI.[39,40] The Posttraumatic Checklist (PCL) is a screening tool that can be used to assess symptoms that map on to *DSM-5* criteria for PTSD.[41]
- Patient Health Questionnaire Anxiety and Depression Scale (PHQ-ADS)—this scale combines the PHQ-9 and the GAD-7.[42] This measure has been shown to comprise a general distress factor, with two subfactors of the PHQ-9 and GAD-7. In a recent study with a large sample of persons with TBI at 6 months post-injury, factor analysis of the PHQ-ADS showed a general mood factor that accounted for most of the variance in item responses, with two subfactors of depression and anxiety that each accounted for less variance. The general factor had a higher sensitivity rate for classifying moderate to severe PTSD than did the PHQ-9 or GAD-7 individually (95% sensitivity based on PHQ-ADS cut-off score of 20).[43] Thus, the PHQ-ADS can be used to detect depression and/or anxiety in persons with TBI, in lieu of administering the PHQ-9 and GAD-7; however, definitive diagnosis requires detailed clinical interview and medical record review, as with any self-report measure.

CAVEATS AND SPECIAL ISSUES WHEN SCREENING FOR EMOTIONAL DISTRESS IN PERSONS WITH TRAUMATIC BRAIN INJURY

- The evidence supports counting all symptoms endorsed by persons with TBI toward a diagnosis of depression, rather than attempting to subtract symptoms that overlap with sequelae of TBI.[44] Standard diagnostic criteria for depression and anxiety should be applied to persons with TBI.[2]

- Self-report can be impacted by impaired awareness, which is common among persons with TBI, particularly during the early stages of recovery.[45] Therefore, these measures should be used with caution during inpatient rehabilitation. A score below the cut-off during inpatient rehabilitation should be followed up with another screening following discharge, as emotional distress may increase as persons with TBI become more aware of injury-related impairments and associated life changes.
- Impaired memory can impact recall of symptoms, particularly when the time interval assessed is longer (e.g., past 2 weeks to a month versus past week).[3]
- Impaired attention can result in patients with TBI having difficulty holding the response options in their minds when questionnaires are being administered verbally. Providing them with written response options, perhaps on laminated cards, can help to compensate for attention problems.
- Higher rates of emotional distress have been found when a self-report measure is mailed to persons with TBI to complete at home versus when it is completed over the phone.[3] This may reflect a social desirability effect, or the patient being reluctant to admit verbally to symptoms.

KEY POINTS

- Self-report questionnaires are screening tools; they cannot be used to diagnose depression or anxiety.
- Patients who meet the cut-offs for emotional distress on these questionnaires should be referred for definitive diagnosis and potential treatment.
- Physical and cognitive symptoms associated with TBI should not be ignored as potential symptoms of depression or anxiety.
- Structured diagnostic interviews are the gold standard against which self-report measures are compared; however, the presence of emotional distress that does not meet diagnostic criteria still warrants attention, as supportive counseling/psychotherapy may be beneficial.
- The impact of cognitive deficits, such as impaired awareness, attention, and memory, must be considered when using self-report measures of emotional distress.

STUDY QUESTIONS

1. Which of the following refers to the ability of a screening measure to reduce false positives, or to correctly identify the absence of a mood disorder?
   a. Positive predictive value
   b. Negative predictive value
   c. Sensitivity
   d. Specificity

The contents of this publication were developed under grants from the National Institute on Disability, Independent Living, and Rehabilitation Research (grant numbers 90DPTB0016 and 90DP0028). NIDILRR is a Center within the Administration for Community Living (ACL), Department of Health and Human Services (HHS). The contents of this publication do not necessarily represent the policy of NIDILRR, ACL, HHS, and you should not assume endorsement by the Federal Government.

2. Which is not an advantage of most self-report questionnaires to screen for emotional distress in persons with TBI?
   a. Quick to administer
   b. Map easily on to clinical diagnostic criteria
   c. Can indicate even mild symptoms that may not meet diagnostic criteria, but may still benefit from treatment
   d. Can be mailed out or administered by phone to save time in the office

3. Which of the following is the most accurate statement about use of the Patient Health Questionnaire (PHQ) as a screening measure in persons with TBI?
   a. Administering the full PHQ-9 is the best way to identify persons with depression who need treatment
   b. Administering the PHQ-2 is just as good as the PHQ-9 in terms of sensitivity and does not really have a disadvantage
   c. Administering the PHQ-2 has similar sensitivity to the PHQ-9 and can save time, but clinicians should follow up with a question about suicidal ideation if the score is ≥2
   d. The PHQ-8, which does not include a question on suicidal ideation, is best in an outpatient setting when clinicians do not have the time to follow up on patients who have suicidal ideation

4. Which of the following statements best describes best practice when interpreting scores on a self-report questionnaire of depression in a person with TBI?
   a. Symptoms that overlap depression and TBI-related cognitive impairment, such as decreased concentration and low initiation, should be factored out when interpreting scores
   b. All symptoms endorsed by persons with TBI should be counted toward a diagnosis of depression
   c. All symptoms endorsed by the person with TBI should be counted toward a diagnosis of depression, except those that are clearly TBI-related, such as difficulty making decisions and difficulty concentrating
   d. Responses to a self-report questionnaire should not be considered when deciding whether to treat depression in persons with TBI

5. Which of the following is true about the impact of TBI-related cognitive impairment on response to self-report screening measures for depression?
   a. Impaired self-awareness can impact responses, particularly during the acute phases of recovery
   b. Most self-report questionnaires of depression are not impacted by memory because they only ask people to reflect on symptoms over a short time period
   c. Most self-report measures cannot be administered to people with attention difficulties
   d. Visuospatial difficulties preclude administration of most self-report measures of depression in persons with TBI, as most require a written response

ADDITIONAL READING

Agency for Healthcare Research and Quality. Comparative effectiveness review no. 25. Traumatic brain injury and depression: Executive Summary. 2011;6–7. https://effectivehealthcare.ahrq.gov/sites/default/files/related_files/depression-brain-injury_executive.pdf

Hart T, Rabinowitz A, Fann JR. Mood and anxiety disorders. In: Silver JM, McAllister TW, Arciniegas DB, eds. *Textbook of Traumatic Brain Injury*. American Psychiatric Association; 2019:331–346.

Osborn AJ, Mathias JL, Fairweather-Schmidt AK. Depression following adult, non-penetrating traumatic brain injury: a meta-analysis examining methodological variables and sample characteristics. *Neurosci Behav Rev*. 2014;47:1–15. doi:10.1016/j.neubiorev.2014.07.007

Osborn AJ, Mathias JL, Fairweather-Schmidt AK. Prevalence of anxiety following adult traumatic brain injury: a meta-analysis comparing measures, samples, and postinjury intervals. *Neuropsychology*. 2016;30:247–261. doi:10.1037/neu0000221

Zaninotto AL, Vicentini JE, Fregni F, et al. Updates and current perspectives of psychiatric assessments after traumatic brain injury: A systematic review. *Front Psychiatry*. 2016;7:95. doi:10.3389/fpsyt.2016.00095

ANSWERS TO STUDY QUESTIONS

1. Correct Answer: d
   Specificity is the ability of a measure to correctly identify the absence of depression or anxiety; that is, not falsely identifying someone as having depression or anxiety when they do (not making a false positive). Sensitivity is the ability of a measure to correctly detect the presence of depression or anxiety (not making a false negative).

   Further Reading:
   Anderson JE, Michalak EE, Lam RW. Depression in primary care: tools for screening, diagnosis, and measuring response to treatment. *BCMJ*. 2002;8:415–419.

2. Correct Answer: c
   Self-report questionnaires are quick to administer and can be mailed out ahead of an appointment, or administered by phone, to follow up on during an appointment. Most screening measures of emotional distress do not map directly on to diagnostic criteria (PHQ-9 is the exception).

   Further Reading:
   Osborn AJ, Mathias JL, Fairweather-Schmidt AK. Depression following adult, non-penetrating traumatic brain injury: a meta-analysis examining methodological variables and sample characteristics. *Neurosci Biobehav Rev*. 2014;47:1–15. doi:10.1016/j.neubiorev.2014.07.007

3. Correct Answer: c
   The PHQ-2 has similar specificity to the PHQ-9, but it does not assess suicidal ideation, so anyone who scores ≥2 should be probed for suicidal ideation. The PHQ-2, with the suicide question added as needed, can save time over administration of the PHQ-9.

   Further Reading:
   Li C, Friedman B, Conwell Y, Fiscella K. Validity of the patient health questionnaire-2 (PHQ-2) in identifying major depression in older people. *J Am Geriatr Soc*. 2007;55(4):596–602. doi:10.1111/j.1532-5415.2007.01103.x

4. Correct Answer: b
   Research has indicated that all symptoms endorsed by persons with TBI should be counted when determining whether to treat for depression, rather than attempting to subtract symptoms that may overlap with the sequelae of TBI.

Further Reading:
Teymoori A, Gorbunova A, Haghish FE, et al. CENTER-TBI Investigators and participants, Steinbuchel NV. Factorial structure and validity of depression (PHQ-9) and anxiety (GAD-7) scales after traumatic brain injury. *Journal of Clinical Medicine* 2020;9:873–894. doi:10.3390/jcm9030873

5. Correct Answer: a
Self-report can be impacted by impaired awareness, which is common in persons with TBI, especially during the early stages of recovery.[44] Impaired memory can impact recall of symptoms, particularly when the time interval assessed is longer, and many self-report measures ask about symptoms over the past 2 weeks or month.[3] There are ways to compensate for the impact of attentional and visuo-spatial difficulties, such as providing written response options for those with attention problems and reading the questions to those with visuo-spatial impairment.

Further Reading:
Cook KF, Bombardier CH, Bamer AM, et al. Do somatic and cognitive symptoms of traumatic brain injury confound depression screening? *Arch Phys Med Rehabil.* 2011;92(5):818–823. doi:10.1016/j.apmr.2010.12.008
Osborn AJ, Mathias JL, Fairweather-Schmidt AK. Depression following adult, non-penetrating traumatic brain injury: a meta-analysis examining methodological variables and sample characteristics. *Neurosci Biobehav Rev.* 2014;47:1–15. doi:10.1016/j.neubiorev.2014.07.007

REFERENCES

The full reference list appears in the digital product found on http://connect.springer-pub.com/content/book/978-0-8261-4768-4/part/part04/chapter/ch52

SLEEP DISTURBANCES

FELISE S. ZOLLMAN AND ERIC B. LARSON

BACKGROUND

What Is a Sleep Disturbance?

- Dyssomnias—disorders that result in insomnia (e.g., sleep apnea)
- Parasomnias—disorders of arousal or sleep stage transition (e.g., nightmares, sleep-walking)
- Sleep disorders caused by medical or psychiatric illness (e.g., traumatic brain injury [TBI], stroke, depression, chronic pain)

The focus of this chapter is on the most common type of post-TBI sleep disturbance—insomnia. Another common problem often associated with sleep disturbances, fatigue, is addressed in Chapter 13. Although some authors have proposed an association between TBI and other sleep disorders such as sleep apnea, periodic limb movements, and narcolepsy, it is not clear to what extent these conditions may have been present prior to (and perhaps even contributed to the occurrence of) TBI.[1] Detailed discussion of these conditions is beyond the scope of this chapter.

Sleep Architecture

- Five stages—stages I to IV and rapid eye movement (REM) sleep.
- Non-REM sleep—stages I to IV. Stage I is lightest; Stage IV is deep sleep.
- REM sleep—approximately 20% to 25% of total sleep time. During REM sleep, the brain exhibits heightened activity. This is associated with dreaming and with actively maintaining an atonic state, which is mediated by signaling between the pons and the medulla.

Neurophysiology of Sleep and Wakefulness

- Sleep and wakefulness are regulated by interaction between the ventrolateral preoptic (VLPO) nucleus of the hypothalamus and arousal centers in the hypothalamus and brainstem.
- Melatonin-producing cells in the suprachiasmatic nucleus (SCN) of the hypothalamus induce sleep and regulate circadian rhythms.
- Serotonin and norepinephrine pathways promote wakefulness and are thought to play a role in regulating the stages of non-REM sleep.
- Acetylcholine helps maintain arousal and plays a role in REM sleep.

The full reference list appears in the digital product found on http://connect.springerpub.com/content/book/978-0-8261-4768-4/part/part04/chapter/ch53

Neuropharmacology and Sleep

- Stimulants (e.g., catecholaminergic medications like methylphenidate) increase wakefulness and decrease REM sleep.
- Caffeine shortens REM latency and decreases non-REM sleep time.
- Antihistamines (e.g., diphenhydramine) increase non-REM sleep via blocking a descending activating histaminergic pathway from the hypothalamus to the tegmentum.
- GABA-ergic drugs (e.g., benzodiazepines) decrease time to sleep onset and increase total sleep time, but this is at the expense of deep (Stages III and IV) sleep and perhaps also REM sleep.
- Melatonin agonists (e.g., ramelteon) decrease sleep onset latency and regulate circadian rhythms.

INSOMNIA

Definition

Insomnia can be clinically defined as the occurrence of trouble sleeping characterized by difficulty falling asleep (i.e., requiring more than 30 minutes to get to sleep), and/or difficulty maintaining sleep (i.e., more than 30 minutes of nocturnal awakening), which occurs at least three nights per week, and results in impairment in daytime functioning.[2]

Epidemiology

The widely accepted prevalence figure for insomnia in the general population is 30%.

Diagnosis[2]

- Subjective means include self-report and clinician rating scales such as the Insomnia Severity Index, the Epworth Sleepiness Scale, or the Pittsburgh Sleep Quality Index.
- Objective means of quantifying sleep or insomnia include sleep logs (for inpatients), actigraphy, and polysomnography (PSG).
  - Sleep log—typically completed by a nurse on an inpatient unit. Patient is briefly observed on an hourly basis and notation of sleep versus wake status is noted for each hour. *Drawback*—report is typically based on observations of 5 minutes or less per hour. Such a limited sample can result in inaccurate data.
  - Actigraphy—uses a small motion-sensing device; activity level is sampled every tenth of a second and aggregated at a constant interval, referred to as an epoch. A computerized algorithm translates these data into a representation of time awake versus asleep. *Drawback*—accurate measurement requires (a) that the device be worn continuously during the period of interest and (b) that the individual have little or no motor impairment, the presence of which can compromise accurate reading of movement as a surrogate for awake time.
  - PSG—gold standard for measurement of sleep. PSG monitors many body functions through electroencephalogram (EEG), electro-oculogram (EOG), electromyogram (EMG), and electrocardiogram (ECG) during sleep. *Drawback*—because of the complexity of the equipment required, PSG is costly, labor intensive, and not convenient for routine use.

INSOMNIA AND TRAUMATIC BRAIN INJURY

- Insomnia may occur immediately following injury and may continue for several years thereafter.
- Incidence is reported to range from 36% to 81%.[3-7] The wide variability is in part due to variability in operational definitions of insomnia and due to challenges in accurately applying assessment technology. A recent meta-analysis of 21 studies using both objective and self-report measures estimated the prevalence of insomnia in TBI at 50%.[8]

Mechanism

- Acutely, insomnia results from diffuse disruption of cerebral functioning because of both direct physical damage to deep brain structures (including the hypothalamus and/or brainstem) and because of secondary neuropathological events, which may cause damage because of cerebral pathways essential for the maintenance of normal sleep architecture.
- In moderate to severe TBI, these acute processes result in severe fragmentation of the rest-activity cycle, which is worse with greater injury severity. An earlier return to consolidated rest-activity cycle is associated with a shorter duration of posttraumatic amnesia and lower disability at discharge.[9]
- Melatonin deficiency also appears to play a role, having been demonstrated in TBI patients in the intensive care unit (ICU) setting.[10] This observation raises the prospect that use of a melatonin agonist may be of specific benefit in this population.
- Chronically, behavioral and affective factors also come into play.

Clinical Presentation

TBI patients present with a variety of symptoms, which may be a direct result of their injuries or may be secondary to insomnia, including[5,11]:

- Fatigue
- Irritability
- Cognitive deficits
- Pain

The significant overlap between symptoms that may be due to TBI and those which may be due to insomnia makes the accurate diagnosis of insomnia in the setting of TBI challenging.

MANAGEMENT OF INSOMNIA IN TRAUMATIC BRAIN INJURY

Behavioral and Environmental Interventions

Sleep hygiene practices and environmental modifications that encourage sleep should be implemented early in the course of treatment:

- Time of awakening—Waking up at the same time each morning regardless of the time one goes to sleep helps maintain consistent circadian rhythms.
- Caffeine, alcohol, or nicotine use—Each of these substances interferes with normal sleep architecture and should be avoided. For regular caffeine users, recommend cutting back on daily intake and not having any caffeine past noontime.

■ Environmental factors—Advise turning off lights and minimizing noise or other distractors (e.g., late night activity in an inpatient unit, a TV left on overnight).
■ Regular exercise—Exercise may benefit sleep via anxiolytic and antidepressant effects, circadian phase-shifting effects, and elevating levels of adenosine.[12]

Stimulus control, reducing practices that condition a patient to associate the bed with wakefulness, should also be encouraged early in treatment:

■ Limit time in bed for waking daytime activities—As much as possible, when patients are active and awake (e.g., watching TV), they should be out of bed.
■ Limit time in bed at night when unable to sleep—If it is safe to do so, patients who cannot sleep within 15 minutes of bedtime should be encouraged to get out of bed and find another place to engage in relaxing activities (e.g., reading) until they become drowsy.

Pharmacological Treatment Options[13]

■ Melatonin agonists (e.g., ramelteon)—decrease sleep latency and modestly improve total sleep time. Ramelteon should be a first-line consideration in TBI because of its excellent side effect profile.
■ Benzodiazepines—mainstay treatment for insomnia in the general population. Approved for short-term use—not as a chronic treatment intervention. Benzodiazepines bind nonselectively to the GABA(A) receptor subtype, potentiating the inhibitory effect of GABA in the central nervous system (CNS). In those with TBI, benzodiazepine use is associated with contemporaneous impairment in cognitive function as well as impaired CNS recovery due to inhibition of neural plasticity. In the general population, chronic use has resulted in impairment in memory and learning—likely at least in part due to interfering with long-term potentiation—even after months of abstinence. For these reasons, the use of benzodiazepines in those with TBI is discouraged.
■ Atypical GABA agonists (e.g., zolpidem)—selective for the GABA(A) receptor 1 subtype. Generally have fewer cognitive side effects and shorter half-life than benzodiazepines; however, studies in normals have shown that this class of agent impairs short-term memory and psychomotor speed immediately after administration and in some cases for as long as 24 hours afterward. There are limited data available to assess the effect of these agents in those with neurological impairment; however, given the demonstrated adverse effects in normals, and the likelihood that these effects would be magnified in those with TBI, these agents should be used with caution in the TBI population.
■ Antidepressants:
   • Those with significant anticholinergic side effects (e.g., amitriptyline) are generally to be avoided in patients with TBI because of the risk of exacerbating cognitive impairment, daytime "hangover" effect, orthostatic hypotension, and urinary retention.
   • Selective serotonin reuptake inhibitors may be effective if insomnia is felt to be primarily due to depression.
   • Trazodone is a triazolopyridine derivative that is approved by the Food and Drug Administration as an antidepressant but that is also used off-label for treatment of insomnia. It is frequently used to treat insomnia in those with TBI, although no studies have been conducted to assess the effect of this agent on cognition in this population. A recent retrospective study of other patients with neurological impairment (Alzheimer's disease) showed that, in doses from 50 to 125 mg (25th–75th percentile of dosing range), trazadone was associated with reduced sleep disturbance and slower cognitive decline, possibly secondary to improved slow wave

sleep.[14] Trazodone is typically used in a dosage range from 50 to 200 mg nightly. Some studies of general populations have suggested that doses of 100 mg or more may result in modest cognitive impairment.

- Antihistamines (e.g., diphenhydramine)—generally not used in those with TBI because anticholinergic effects can cause CNS impairment, urinary retention, and orthostatic dizziness.[7]
- Herbal supplements, including melatonin and valerian root can be considered:
  - The usual over-the-counter melatonin formulation comes in a 3-mg tablet, although at least one study has shown that one-tenth that dose, or 0.3 mg, may be optimally effective.[15] Higher doses may be associated with some degree of hypothermia, although the clinical implication of this is uncertain.
  - Data supporting the efficacy of valerian root have been inconsistent[16]; however, it generally has a favorable side effect profile and so may be an appropriate consideration in some cases.

Complementary and Alternative Medicine Options

A study addressing the use of acupuncture to treat insomnia in patients with TBI suggests that this modality is well tolerated, may have equal efficacy to medication use without introducing untoward CNS side effects, and may result in improvement in mood and cognitive function.[18] This may be a promising area for continued future exploration.

OUTCOME

Individualized treatment of sleep–wake disorders in chronic TBI (including education regarding sleep hygiene, pharmacological interventions, and apnea treatment), was shown to result in significant improvements in sustained and divided attention, working memory, speed of language processing, and mood.[17]

KEY POINTS

- Behavioral and environmental interventions should be first-line treatment options for insomnia following TBI.
- Melatonin agonists are a reasonable first-line pharmacological treatment option, given their favorable side effect profile.
- Benzodiazepines, other GABA agonists, and antihistamines should be used with caution, if at all, in the TBI population.

STUDY QUESTIONS

1. Objective means of quantifying sleep include all of the following except:
   a. Sleep log
   b. Pittsburgh Sleep Quality Index
   c. Actigraphy
   d. Polysomnogram

2. Sleep and wakefulness are regulated by interactions between arousal centers in the hypothalamus and brainstem and which of the following:
   a. Somatosensory cortex
   b. Medial geniculate nucleus
   c. Dorsolateral prefrontal cortex
   d. Ventrolateral preoptic nucleus of the hypothalamus

3. An earlier return to consolidated rest-activity cycle is associated with:
   a. Longer duration of PTA and lower disability at discharge
   b. Shorter duration of PTA and lower disability at discharge
   c. Longer duration of PTA and higher disability at discharge
   d. Shorter duration of PTA and higher disability at discharge

4. In people with TBI, benzodiazepine use is associated with:
   a. Contemporaneous cognitive impairment and poor long-term outcome
   b. Contemporaneous cognitive enhancement but later inhibition of neural plasticity
   c. Contemporaneous cognitive enhancement and improved long-term outcome
   d. Contemporaneous cognitive impairment but eventual CNS recovery

5. Which of the following is a triazolopyridine derivative used as an off-label treatment of insomnia for people with TBI?
   a. Zolpidem
   b. Ramelteon
   c. Trazodone
   d. Melatonin

ADDITIONAL READING

https://craighospital.org/uploads/Educational-PDFs/Model-Systems/334.Model-System-TBI-and-Sleep.pdf

Barshikar S, Bell KR. Sleep disturbance after TBI. *Curr Neurol Neurosci Rep.* 2017;17(11):87. doi:10.1007/s11910-017-0792-4

Grima NA, Ponsford JL, Pase MP. Sleep complications following traumatic brain injury. *Curr Opin Pulm Med.* 2017;23(6):493–499. doi:10.1097/MCP.0000000000000429

Larson EB, Zollman FS. The effect of sleep medications on cognitive recovery from traumatic brain injury. *J Head Trauma Rehabil.* 2010;25(1):61–67. doi:10.1097/HTR.0b013e3181c1d1e1

Sandsmark DK, Elliott JE, Lim MM. Sleep-wake disturbances after traumatic brain injury: synthesis of human and animal studies. *Sleep.* 2017;40(5):zsx044 doi:10.1093/sleep/zsx044

ANSWERS TO STUDY QUESTIONS

1. Correct Answer: b
   The Pittsburgh Sleep Quality Index is a self-report measure, not an objective measure.

   Further Reading:
   Buysse DJ, Reynolds CF 3rd, Monk TH, et al. The Pittsburgh Sleep Quality Index: a new instrument for psychiatric practice and research. *Psychiatry Res.* 1989;28(2):193–213. doi:10.1016/0165-1781(89)90047-4

2. Correct Answer: d
Sleep and wakefulness are regulated by interaction between the ventrolateral preoptic (VLPO) nucleus of the hypothalamus and arousal centers in the hypothalamus and brainstem.

Further Reading:
Saper C, Scammell T, & Lu J. Hypothalamic regulation of sleep and circadian rhythms. *Nature* 2005 Oct 27;437(7063):1257–63. doi:10.1038/nature04284

3. Correct Answer: b
Actigraphy showed that 16 patients with acute moderate/severe TBI had an altered rest-activity cycle, probably reflecting severe fragmentation of sleep and wake episodes, which globally improved over time. It was concluded a faster return to rest-activity cycle consolidation may predict enhanced brain recovery

Further Reading:
Duclos C, Dumont M, Blais H, et al. Rest-activity cycle disturbances in the acute phase of moderate to severe traumatic brain injury. *Neurorehabil Neural Repair*. 2013:28(5):472–482. doi:10.1177/1545968313517756

4. Correct Answer: a
In those with TBI, benzodiazepine use is associated with contemporaneous impairment in cognitive function as well as impaired CNS recovery due to inhibition of neural plasticity.

Further Reading:
Rao V, Rollings P. Sleep disturbances following traumatic brain injury. *Curr Treat Options Neurol*. 2002;4:77–78. doi:10.1007/s11940-002-0006-4

5. Correct Answer: c
Trazodone is FDA-approved as an antidepressant, but has been used successfully as a treatment for insomnia. Its use is advocated by some due to a more favorable side effect profile, particularly with respect to cognition.

Further Reading:
Yi XY, Ni SF, Ghadami MR, et al. Trazodone for the treatment of insomnia: a meta-analysis of randomized placebo-controlled trials. *Sleep Med*. 2018;45:25–32 doi:10.1016/j.sleep.2018.01.010

REFERENCES

The full reference list appears in the digital product found on http://connect.springer-pub.com/content/book/978-0-8261-4768-4/part/part04/chapter/ch53

54 CHRONIC NEUROPSYCHIATRIC SEQUELAE I: MOOD DISORDERS

HAZEM SHAHIN AND RICARDO E. JORGE

GENERAL PRINCIPLES

Background

Mood disorders occur in the context of profound changes in cognitive and emotional processing following traumatic brain injury (TBI). Studies have described the detrimental effect of traumatic prefrontal injury on patients' performance in social cognition as well as in the identification and modulation of emotions.[1] These changes may result in poorly integrated self-representations and dysfunctional interpersonal relationships, increasing patients' vulnerability to develop affective disorders.

Epidemiology

Neuropsychiatric illness is a highly prevalent complication of TBI, with a published incidence of 49% following moderate to severe TBI and 34% following mild TBI.[2] Major depressive disorders are the most common diagnosis. Prospective studies with predominantly mild TBI (MTBI) samples report fairly consistent prevalence rates, ranging from 17.0% to 23.1% at 3 months, 18.5% to 23.2% at 6 months, and 13.9% to 18.6% at 12 months post injury.[3] Approximately half of moderate to severe TBI patients will develop depression during the first year after a TBI,[4-6] with a lifetime prevalence of 26% to 64% compared to 17% in the general population.[7] Up to 9% of TBI patients may develop mood disorders within the bipolar spectrum.[8] However, the lifetime risk of bipolar disorder is similar to the general population.[9]

Classification

Following the *Diagnostic and Statistical Manual of Mental Disorders* (DSM-5) diagnostic nomenclature, mood disorders associated with TBI are categorized as *mood disorder due to* Another Medical Condition with subtypes of (a) *with major depressive-like episode* (if the full criteria for a major depressive episode are met) or (b) *with depressive features* (prominent depressed mood but full criteria for a major depressive episode are not met); and (c) *with mixed features* (e.g., significant irritability, pressured speech and formal thought disorder). *Bipolar and related disorders due to TBI* are subdivided in: (a) *with manic or hypomanic like episode*; (b) *with manic features*; and (c) *with mixed features.*

Pathophysiology

The changes in neuronal circuitry seen in TBI may constitute the neurological substrate of cognitive and behavioral deficits that are frequently seen following injury. Mood disorders

---

The full reference list appears in the digital product found on http://connect.springerpub.com/content/book/978-0-8261-4768-4/part/part04/chapter/ch54

may result from deactivation of the lateral and dorsal frontal cortex and increased activation in the ventral limbic and para-limbic structures including the pre-limbic cortex and the amygdala.[10,11] High levels of amygdala activation may be associated with an increased prevalence of anxiety symptoms and negative affect. Moreover, faulty prefrontal modulation of medial limbic structures could explain the impulsive and aggressive behavior frequently observed in these patients.[12] Overall, injury severity, type, or mechanism of injury does not predict the likelihood of development of mood disorders in the aftermath of TBI.[13]

ASSESSMENT

Risk Factors

- Genetic polymorphisms modulating central dopaminergic pathways can affect prefrontal function following TBI.[14,15] However, an association between 5-HTT serotonin transport receptor gene polymorphisms and depression following TBI has not been shown.[16].
- Personal history of mood and anxiety disorders, and previous poor social functioning are associated with the occurrence of major depression in the aftermath of TBI.[4,17]
- A history of alcohol misuse increases the risk of developing a mood disorder during the first year following TBI. It is plausible that alcohol toxicity and TBI interact to produce more severe structural brain damage and more profound changes in the ascending aminergic pathways that modulate reward, mood, and executive function.[18]

Clinical Presentation and Symptoms

Mood disorders due to TBI are frequently associated with other behavioral disorders. For instance, anxiety disorders coexist with depressive disorders in up to two thirds of cases.[12] In addition, clinically significant aggression and alcohol misuse coexist in approximately half of the patients who develop a mood disorder following TBI.[18,19]

(Note that screening tools commonly used for assessment of emotional distress post-TBI will not be addressed here; they are reviewed in Chapter 53. For additional information on diagnostic criteria for TBI-related mood disorders, refer to the *DSM-5*.)

Differential Diagnosis

- The differential diagnosis of *Post-TBI Major Depression* includes adjustment disorder with depressed and/or anxious mood, acute stress disorder, posttraumatic stress disorder (PTSD), apathy, and emotional lability or pathological laughter and crying (PLC).
  - Patients with adjustment disorders develop short-lived and relatively mild emotional disturbances within 3 months of a stressful life event. Although they may present with depressive symptoms, they do not meet *DSM-5* criteria for major depression.
  - PTSD is characterized by symptoms of re-experiencing the trauma ranging from transient flashbacks to severe dissociative states, as well as avoidant behavior, hypervigilance, emotional blunting, and social withdrawal.[13] There is a significant degree of overlap between PTSD and mood disorders. For instance, the majority of veterans from the recent military operations in Iraq and Afghanistan who developed combat related PTSD had a coexistent mood disorder.[20] (See also Chapter 19.)
  - PLC is characterized by the presence of sudden and uncontrollable affective outbursts (e.g., crying or laughing), which may be congruent or incongruent with the

patient's mood. These emotional displays are recognized by the patient as being excessive to the underlying mood and can occur spontaneously or may be triggered by minor stimuli. This condition lacks the pervasive alteration of mood, as well as the specific vegetative symptoms associated with a major depressive episode.

- Apathetic syndromes—A recent study of TBI patients referred to a neuropsychiatric clinic because of behavioral disturbance showed that 71% were apathetic. 85% of these apathetic patients were also depressed.[21] Apathy is frequently associated with psychomotor retardation and emotional blunting.

A diagnosis of *Mood Disorder With Manic or Mixed Features* can be made when symptoms of mania or hypomania are also present but do not predominate in the clinical picture. It should not be made if the mood disturbance occurs only during the course of agitation or delirium. The latter is characterized by sudden onset, fluctuating level of consciousness, disorientation, and prominent attention deficits.

The differential diagnosis of *Bipolar Spectrum Related Disorders* includes the following:

- *Substance-Induced Mood Disorder*—This may occur as a result of intoxication or withdrawal from drugs. It is usually identified by a careful clinical interview and/or toxicological screening.
- *Psychosis Associated With Epilepsy*—This may be observed in patients with epileptic foci located in limbic or paralimbic cortices. Psychotic episodes may be temporally linked to seizures or may have a more prolonged interictal course. In the latter case, the clinical picture is characterized by the presence of partial and/or complex–partial seizures, and of a schizoaffective syndrome. Electroencephalography (EEG) and functional neuroimaging studies (e.g., SPECT and PET) will usually define ictal and interictal disturbances.
- *Personality Change Due to TBI*—This may include mood instability, disinhibited behavior, and hypersexuality. These patients lack, however, the pervasive alteration of mood that characterizes secondary manic syndromes.

TREATMENT

Guiding Principles

Patients with brain injury are more sensitive to the side effects of medications, especially psychotropic drugs. Doses of psychotropic drugs must be prudently increased, minimizing side effects (i.e., start low, go slow). However, the patient must receive an adequate therapeutic trial with regard to dosage and duration of treatment. Brain-injured patients must be frequently reassessed to determine changes in treatment schedules. Special care must be taken in monitoring drug interactions. Finally, if there is evidence of a partial response to a specific medication, augmentation therapy may be warranted, depending upon the augmenting drug's mechanism of action and potential side effects.[22]

Treatment of mood disorders occurring after TBI involves different pharmacological and nonpharmacological strategies. Unfortunately, there is a lack of evidence-based scientific foundation to provide a solid basis for neuropsychiatric treatment. Selection among competing antidepressants is usually guided by their side effect profiles. Mild anticholinergic activity, minimal lowering of seizure threshold, and low sedative effects are the most important factors to be considered in the choice of an antidepressant drug in this population.

Specific Pharmacological Recommendations for Treating Depression (See Also Chapter 37)

- Tricyclic antidepressants (TCAs):
  - Desipramine may be effective for treating depression in patients with severe TBI.[23]
  - TCAs with significant anticholinergic effects (e.g., amitriptyline) should be avoided.
- Selective serotonin reuptake inhibitors:
  - Sertraline—A small study in patients with MTBI showed statistically significant improvement in psychological distress, anger, and aggression as well as in the severity of postconcussive symptoms.[24] Sertraline may also lead to a beneficial effect on cognitive functioning via improvement in mood state.[25] That said, a more recent and larger randomized clinical trial from the same group of investigators found that sertraline was not superior to placebo for post-TBI depression.[26]
  - Citalopram—An open-label study suggested that citalopram may be effective in treating major depression occurring in the setting of TBI.[27] There have not been randomized controlled trials of citalopram for this indication.

Specific Pharmacological Recommendations for Treating Manic Syndromes

There have been no systematic studies of the treatment of manic syndromes in TBI.[13] Lithium, carbamazepine, and valproate therapies have been reported to be efficacious in individual cases.[27] It has been proposed that both lithium and valproate have neuroprotective properties, which would certainly constitute an important therapeutic effect among brain-injured populations.[28] However, data from the only controlled trial of valproate in TBI fail to identify a beneficial effect on cognitive or functional outcomes.[29] The role of other anticonvulsants such as lamotrigine or topiramate as mood stabilizers has not been rigorously assessed in TBI populations. An isolated case report showed adequate control of problematic behaviors with lamotrigine.[30] In addition, there have been brief reports that suggest a beneficial effect of quetiapine on aggression and mania following TBI.[31,32]

Nonpharmacological Interventions

- There is consensus that psychosocial support, reassurance, counseling, and TBI education for patients and their caregivers should be part of the treatment plan, even if delivered through the telephone or Internet.[8,13,33] Cognitive behavioral therapy (CBT) and supportive psychotherapy (SPT) are the most commonly used modalities for tackling anxiety, depression, agitation, and other problematic behavior, and they have a long-lasting treatment effect.[34]
- Electroconvulsive therapy (ECT) can be used with certain precautions in depressive and manic patients with symptoms refractory to pharmacological treatment.[8] A pilot study of the safety, tolerability, and efficacy of repetitive transcranial magnetic stimulation (rTMS) for post-TBI depression, found rTMS to be safe and well tolerated and to have some utility in improving cognitive function, but did not find a therapeutic effect for post-TBI depression.[35] Similarly, transcranial direct current stimulation (tDCS) showed improvement in apathy scores, but no relevant changes were detected in the severity of depressive symptoms.[36] Further research in these relatively new therapeutic modalities is needed.

Prevention Strategies

Given the high prevalence of depressive disorders during the first year after TBI, depression is an ideal target for selective prevention efforts. Initial data are promising, however further research in this area is required.

A randomized clinical trial looked at the efficacy of sertraline as a preventive treatment. A total of 94 hospitalized subjects with TBI of varying severity and who were initially non-depressed were randomized to receive a daily dose of 100 mg of sertraline or placebo during a 6-month period. Intention to treat analysis demonstrated that, at completion of the protocol, subjects receiving placebo were almost 4 times more likely to develop depression than subjects treated with sertraline [HR = 3.6, 95% CI = 1.1, 16.2]. The pharmacological intervention was well tolerated and there were no clinically relevant differences in the frequency of adverse events between the groups of subjects receiving sertraline or placebo. Subjects receiving sertraline were more likely to experience diarrhea or dry mouth than subjects who received placebo, however. This suggests that selective pharmacological prevention is a viable alternative to reduce the burden of depression among this group of patients.[37]

KEY POINTS

- Mood disorders are very common after TBI and usually occur in the context of multiple cognitive and behavioral changes.
- Patients with pre-injury mood and anxiety disorders, poor social functioning, or with pre or post-injury substance misuse are more prone to mood disorders.
- Pharmacotherapy should be prescribed with caution because of risk of severe adverse effects and/or drug interactions.
- SSRIs are considered agents of first choice to treat post-TBI depression.
- Nonpharmacological interventions to support patients and caregivers are important to address coping with injury, rehabilitation expectations, behavioral/personality changes, social and community reintegration.

STUDY QUESTIONS

1. What is the estimated prevalence of depressive disorders during the first year following moderate to severe TBI?
   a. 10%
   b. 50%
   c. 25%
   d. 75%

2. Which of the following is NOT a risk factor for development of a mood disorder in the aftermath of TBI?
   a. Poor social support
   b. History of alcohol misuse
   c. Genetic polymorphism in the serotonin transporter gene (SLC6A4)
   d. Level of disability

3. Which of the following statements is TRUE when considering the differential diagnosis of post-TBI major depression?

a. Patients with adjustment disorders develop short-lived, emotional disturbances within 6 months of a stressful life event

b. Pathological Laughing and Crying (PLC) is characterized by the presence of sudden and uncontrollable affective outbursts (e.g., crying or laughing), that are always incongruent with the patient's mood

c. Apathy is frequently associated with depression, psychomotor retardation, and emotional blunting

d. The overlap between PTSD and mood disorders is rarely encountered

4. Which of the following statements is TRUE regarding pharmacological treatment of depression in patients with TBI?

   a. All tricyclic antidepressants (TCAs) are effective treatments, regardless of TBI severity, and have negligible side effects

   b. Citalopram was never studied as possible treatment for depression in the setting of TBI

   c. Sertraline is poorly tolerated by TBI patients, producing multiple and occasionally severe side effects.

   d. Sertraline has been shown to be a promising effective agent in preventing the onset of depressive disorders during the first year following TBI.

5. Which of the following statements is TRUE about pharmacological recommendations for treating manic syndromes?

   a. There have been no systematic studies of the treatment of manic syndromes in TBI

   b. The role of anticonvulsants such as lamotrigine or topiramate as mood stabilizers has been rigorously assessed in TBI populations.

   c. There is no beneficial effect of antipsychotics such as quetiapine on aggression and mania following TBI

   d. The use of lithium, carbamazepine, and valproate is not recommended in these cases

ADDITIONAL READING

TBI and depression: https://effectivehealthcare.ahrq.gov/sites/default/files/pdf/depression-brain-injury_research.pdf

Emotional effects of brain injury: https://www.headway.org.uk/about-brain-injury/individuals/effects-of-brain-injury/emotional-effects

Wortzel HS, Arciniegas DB. The *DSM-5* approach to the evaluation of traumatic brain injury and its neuropsychiatric sequelae. *NeuroRehabilitation*. 2014;34(4):613–623. doi:10.3233/NRE-141086

Ashman TA, Spielman LA, Hibbard MR, et al. Psychiatric challenges in the first 6 years after traumatic brain injury: cross-sequential analyses of Axis I disorders. *Arch Phys Med Rehabil*. 2004;85(4 Suppl 2):S36–S42. doi:10.1016/j.apmr.2003.08.117

Gibson R, Purdy SC. Mental health disorders after traumatic brain injury in a New Zealand caseload. *Brain Inj*. 2015;29(3):306–312. doi:10.3109/02699052.2014.896471

ANSWERS TO STUDY QUESTIONS

1. Correct Answer: b
   Approximately half of moderate to severe TBI patients will develop depression during the first year after a TBI.

Further Reading:
Bombardier CH, Fann JR, Temkin NR, et al. Rates of major depressive disorder and clinical outcomes following traumatic brain injury. *JAMA.* 2010;303(19):1938–1945. doi:10.1001/jama.2010.599
Hibbard MR, Uysal S, Kepler K, et al. Axis I psychopathology in individuals with traumatic brain injury. *J Head Trauma Rehabil.* 1998;13(4):24–39. doi:10.1097/00001199-199808000-00003, doi:10.1097/00001199-199808000-00005
Seel RT, Kreutzer JS, Rosenthal M, et al. Depression after traumatic brain injury: a National Institute on Disability and Rehabilitation Research model systems multicenter investigation. *Arch Phys Med Rehabil.* 2003;84(2):177–184. doi:10.1053/apmr.2003.50106

2. Correct Answer: c
Genetic polymorphisms modulating central dopaminergic pathways can affect prefrontal function following TBI.[14,15] However, an association between 5-HTT serotonin transport receptor gene polymorphisms and depression following TBI has not been shown.

Further Reading:
Lipsky RH, Sparling MB, Ryan LM, et al. Association of COMT Val158Met genotype with executive functioning following traumatic brain injury. *J Neuropsychiatry Clin Neurosci.* 2005;17(4):465–471. doi:10.1176/jnp.17.4.465
McAllister TW, Flashman LA, Harker Rhodes C, et al. Single nucleotide polymorphisms in ANKK1 and the dopamine D2 receptor gene affect cognitive outcome shortly after traumatic brain injury: a replication and extension study. *Brain Injury.* 2008;22(9):705–714. doi:10.1080/02699050802263019
Chan F, Lanctôt KL, Feinstein A, et al. The serotonin transporter polymorphisms and major depression following traumatic brain injury. *Brain Inj.* 2008;22(6):471–479. doi:10.1080/02699050802084886

3. Correct Answer: c
A recent study of TBI patients referred to a neuropsychiatric clinic because of behavioral disturbance showed that 71% were apathetic; 85% of these apathetic patients were also depressed. Apathy is frequently associated with psychomotor retardation and emotional blunting.

Further Reading:
Tateno A, Jorge RE, Robinson RG. Clinical correlates of aggressive behavior after traumatic brain injury. *J Neuropsychiatry Clin Neurosci.* 2003;15(2):155–160. doi:10.1176/jnp.15.2.155

4. Correct Answer: d
Sertraline 100 mg per day may be effective in preventing development of depression post TBI.

Further Reading:
Jorge RE, Acion L, Burin DI, Robinson RG. Sertraline for preventing mood disorders following traumatic brain injury a randomized clinical trial. *JAMA Psychiatry.* 2016;73(10):1041–1047. doi:10.1001/jamapsychiatry.2016.2189

5. Correct Answer: a
There have been no systematic studies of the treatment of manic syndromes in TBI. Lithium, carbamazepine, and valproate have been reported to be efficacious in individual cases. In addition, there have been brief reports that suggest a beneficial effect of quetiapine on aggression and mania following TBI.

Further Reading:

Jorge RE. Mood disorders. *Handb Clin Neurol.* 2015;128:613–631. doi:10.1016/B978-0-444-63521-1.00038-8

Warden DL, Gordon B, McAllister TW, et al. Guidelines for the pharmacologic treatment of neurobehavioral sequelae of traumatic brain injury. *J Neurotrauma.* 2006;23(10):1468–1501. doi: 10.1089/neu.2006.23.1468

Kim E, Bijlani M. A pilot study of quetiapine treatment of aggression due to traumatic brain injury. *J Neuropsychiatry Clin Neurosci.* 2006;18(4):547–549. doi:10.1176/jnp.2006.18.4.547

Oster TJ, Anderson CA, Filley CM, et al. Quetiapine for mania due to traumatic brain injury. *CNS Spectr.* 2007;12(10):764–769. doi:10.1017/S1092852900015455

REFERENCES

The full reference list appears in the digital product found on http://connect.springer-pub.com/content/book/978-0-8261-4768-4/part/part04/chapter/ch54

CHRONIC NEUROPSYCHIATRIC SEQUELAE II: BEHAVIORAL DISTURBANCES

JASON KRELLMAN AND THEODORE TSAOUSIDES

INTRODUCTION

Acute behavioral manifestations of moderate to severe traumatic brain injury (TBI) are common, occurring in varying degrees of severity in up to 96% of patients.[1] These acute symptoms include agitation, disinhibition, emotional lability, apathy, and/or aggression, and are typically managed pharmacologically, with anticholinergics or dopaminergic antagonists, and behaviorally, with environmental modification such as minimization of agitating stimuli. Individuals with lesions in the prefrontal (e.g., orbitofrontal) cortex or temporal lobe, either mesial (e.g., amygdala) or neocortical (e.g., temporal pole), are particularly vulnerable to behavioral sequelae. Behavioral disruption is thought to be due to loss of tonic balance between those neural regions that underlie the expression of affect, impulses, and drives and those regions that inhibit or otherwise modulate that expression based on the environmental context.

Behavioral sequelae of TBI can persist beyond the immediate post-injury period and become chronic in those with lesions in the aforementioned regions. Individuals with premorbid histories of impulsive or aggressive behavior, such as may be seen in the setting of substance abuse, violence, and/or criminality, are also at higher risk.[1] Therefore, the presence of behavioral symptoms is likely multifactorial, reflecting both the characteristics of the brain injury and the individual's preinjury temperament and personality. Regardless of etiology, chronic behavioral symptoms often result in significantly poorer outcomes, including response to rehabilitation, employment potential, psychosocial functioning, and community reintegration.

The long-term behavioral consequences of TBI can be classified into three broad categories: those arising from executive dysfunction, emotion dysregulation, and anosognosia. Though overlapping to some degree, certain behavioral presentations are more common within each category.

EXECUTIVE DYSFUNCTION

Executive functions are a set of complex and hierarchically nested cognitive functions critical for goal-directed behavior.[2] Executive deficits are associated with frontal lobe pathology, but the sheer number of functions classified under the executive umbrella as well as the high degree of interconnectivity between the frontal lobe and other neural regions means that more posterior neuropathology can also manifest in executive deficits. Patients with lesions of the frontal lobes or within more diffuse frontal systems show impairments

---

The full reference list appears in the digital product found on http://connect.springerpub.com/content/book/978-0-8261-4768-4/part/part04/chapter/ch55

in anticipation, planning, execution, and/or self-regulation. Deficits in executive functioning are among the most disabling consequences of TBI and affect critical long-term outcomes such as return to work, community integration, and social autonomy.

The anatomical and functional complexity of the frontal lobes means that damage to this region can result in a broad range of behavioral symptoms that interfere with emotional, social, and vocational functioning. Three different syndromes have been identified in the literature based on the anatomical features of the injury.[3]

- Abulic syndrome
  - Associated with damage to the medial frontal cortex, abulic syndrome results in an amotivational state characterized by motoric, cognitive, emotional, affective, and motivational apathy. Patients with abulia appear lethargic and unmotivated. They lack initiation, exhibit diminished interest in people and events, respond more slowly to stimuli, have reduced ideational fluency, and are emotionally flat. Very often, patients suffering from abulia are misdiagnosed with depression. Indeed, these individuals appear depressed, but they do not meet criteria for a depression spectrum diagnosis etiologically or symptomatically. This condition has been identified in the literature as pseudo-depression.[2-4]
- Dysexecutive syndrome
  - Damage to the dorsolateral prefrontal cortex is associated with a dysexecutive syndrome characterized by impairment in different aspects of goal-directed behavior. Goal-directed behavior comprises volition, planning, implementation, monitoring, and adjusting behavior.[4] Patients with dysexecutive problems present with significant deficits in planning and organization, monitoring, and set-shifting. Behaviorally, they appear distractible, disorganized, and inefficient. They have difficulty suppressing habitual responses, are unable to develop and employ effective strategies, and tend to perseverate.[2-4]
- Disinhibition syndrome
  - Damage to the orbitofrontal cortex can result in a range of emotional and behavioral disturbances. These include interpersonal disinhibition, poor social judgment, and impulsive decision-making. Affected individuals often exhibit utilization behavior, that is, appropriate but impulsive use of objects in view, in an inappropriate setting or context (e.g., a patient may see the clinician's sunglasses on the desk, during a session, pick them up, and wear them). They can also have difficulty appreciating the impact of their behavior on others, lack empathy and perspective taking, and disregard social conventions. They can appear childish and selfish, and they can engage in aggressive and/or abusive behavior. They may depend on cueing from others and broader environmental supports to assist in exhibiting socially appropriate behavior. Their inability to inhibit behavior and anticipate or appreciate the consequences can result in violating rules, breaking the law, and committing minor crimes. This syndrome has been referred to as pseudo-psychopathy in the literature.[2-4]

Treatment

A meta-analysis of studies examining the efficacy of interventions for post-TBI executive dysfunction concluded that the use of metacognitive strategies results in improvements in goal management,[5] planning and organization,[6] and problem solving,[7,8] with favorable results extending to personally relevant functional activities.[9] Metacognitive strategies involve using and internalizing step-by-step procedures to enhance awareness and self-regulation.[10] Interventions for executive functioning are administered individually, in groups or a combination of individual and group treatment.[9,10] Interventions for executive dysfunction have also been embedded in comprehensive-holistic day treatment programs (CDHPs) with improvements in problem solving.[11,12]

EMOTION DYSREGULATION

Emotion regulation is described as a set of heterogeneous processes involved in monitoring, evaluating, and modifying emotional responses.[13] Individuals with brain injuries can have difficulty modulating emotions and modulating behavioral responses according to the social or broader environmental context, which increases the negative impact of already impaired cognition on psychosocial functioning.[14] Emotion dysregulation may also contribute to higher rates of depression, anxiety, and other types of psychopathology compared to the general population.[15]

Emotion regulation deficits have been linked to disruptions in neuropsychological processes involving the frontal and temporal lobes, including the anterior cingulate and amygdala. Three behavioral types of emotion dysregulation have been observed as a function of lesion location.[16]

- Impaired appraisal of emotional valence
  - Individuals with TBI may lose the ability to appraise the emotional valence (attractiveness or aversiveness) of a stimulus. These individuals have difficulty distinguishing between reward and punishment and sustaining their motivation accordingly. They are unable to avoid situations that elicit undesirable emotions and to select situations that elicit desirable emotions. As a result, they show poor judgment and they appear to gravitate toward situations that eventually negatively impact both their mood and the outcomes of their choices and behavior, resulting in frustration or confusion.[16]
- Impaired modulation of emotional response
  - Individuals with TBI can have difficulty appropriately modulating the intensity of their emotional responses. Their ability both to inhibit as well as amplify emotions is impaired. They appear to be experiencing a type of emotional perseveration. Due to the prolonged latency of and delayed recovery from intense emotions, emotionally laden events have a more profound effect on their moods, and they generate more exaggerated behaviors. Difficulty modulating emotion dynamics leads to rage, explosive temper, aggression, hostility, irritability, and anxiety. Conversely, this difficulty can manifest as placidity, passivity, apathy, depression, and blunted affect due to diminished ability to alter low-intensity emotional states.[16]
- Impaired production of facial expression of emotions
  - Individuals with TBI can present with pseudobulbar affect (PBA), pathological crying or laughing following the presentation of a stimulus, which is not commensurate to the internal subjective experience of the individual. PBA is a motor disorder attributable to pathological disinhibition of motor pathways involved in emotional expression and must be distinguished from a mood disorder for proper management.[17] As a result of PBA, individuals with TBI may often laugh or cry inappropriately in social situations, with little ability to consciously control their reactions. In addition, individuals with these types of emotion regulation deficits have difficulty producing facial expressions conforming to social norms in the absence of an emotional experience (e.g., remaining somber at a funeral or smiling when greeting a familiar person).

Treatment

Emotion dysregulation is a significant obstacle to long-term community integration. However, few interventions have included emotion regulation as a direct target of treatment, and findings on efficacy are mixed. Interventions reported in the literature include behavioral, psychoeducational, and pharmacological approaches, targeting a variety of aspects of emotion dysregulation (e.g., anger, agitation, irritability, depression, PBA).

A behavioral intervention targeting emotion regulation directly as a group intervention has shown significant improvements in emotion self-regulation.[18] Other behavioral interventions include embedding training in emotion regulation in comprehensive day treatment programs[11,12] as a component for improving executive dysfunction. Psychoeducational interventions based on principles of cognitive behavioral therapy (CBT) have also been developed, with promising findings.[19]

Pharmacological interventions including the use of methylphenidate for combative behavior; propranolol, methylphenidate, valproic acid, and olanzapine for agitation, amantadine hydrochloride for irritability; and dextromorphan/quinidine for PBA[20,21,22] have also been effective in reducing manifestations of specific dysregulated behaviors, but as mentioned, the treatment target of these interventions is too narrow in scope to encompass the self-regulatory aspect of emotion awareness and management.

ANOSOGNOSIA

Anosognosia is a failure to recognize frank impairments and their functional consequences and is often comorbid with emotional indifference or "anosodiaphoria." Anosognosia is more commonly observed in individuals with nondominant hemisphere injury, but a definitive neuropathological substrate has not yet been identified.[23] The term generally connotes neurologically based lack of awareness and/or indifference, but psychogenic denial and/or characterologic lack of insight can contribute to the clinical presentation. Therefore, both neurological and psychological contributors to impaired awareness of deficits should be assessed clinically. Not surprisingly, these presentations are associated with reduced response to rehabilitation interventions, treatment noncompliance, and poorer functional outcomes. On a positive note, awareness of deficits generally seems to improve as time since injury increases among individuals with TBI, likely reflecting neurological recovery, more practical experience with functional deficits, and/or the benefit of rehabilitation intervention to improve awareness.

Treatment

Treatment of anosognosia is comprised primarily of CBT interventions and includes education about TBI symptoms and functional deficits; review of discrepancies between self- and other-ratings of functioning; recording and review of patient failures or errors in everyday life by patient, caregivers, and/or therapists; group therapy interventions that emphasize supportive identification of deficits and constructive criticism from peers; and "predict-perform" exercises, wherein an individual's expectation for their performance on a therapist-provided task is compared to their actual performance.[24] Despite the number of available interventions and sizeable portion of patients who improve, lack of awareness of neurological deficits remains among the most challenging post-injury deficits for both patients and clinicians. However, thoughtfully selected neuropsychological interventions delivered in a flexible therapeutic style that emphasizes collaborative problem solving rather than motivation through confrontation can raise an individual's awareness of deficits, thereby increasing their safety and functional ability.

KEY POINTS

- Behavioral sequelae of TBI that persist beyond the immediate post-injury period, may become chronic, and can result in significantly poorer long-term outcomes.
- Long-term behavioral consequences of TBI can be classified into three broad categories: those arising from executive dysfunction, emotion dysregulation, and anosognosia.
- Interventions using metacognitive strategies have been effectively implemented to improve executive dysfunction.
- Behavioral, psychoeducational, and pharmacological interventions have been used in the treatment of aspects of post-TBI emotion dysregulation, with mixed results.
- Psychoeducation and CBT interventions are most commonly used to increase awareness of deficits following TBI.

STUDY QUESTIONS

1. What is the prevalence and clinical relevance of post-TBI behavioral disorders?
   a. 24%
   b. 52%
   c. 74%
   d. 96%

2. Which of the following is not a commonly identified post-TBI behavioral disorder?
   a. Executive dysfunction
   b. Prosopagnosia
   c. Emotion dysregulation
   d. Anosognosia

3. Lesions to which neural regions are associated with anosognosia?
   a. Damage to white matter tracts that interconnect different cortical regions
   b. Damage to subcortical motor pathways
   c. Damage to the frontal or parietal cortex
   d. Damage to the cerebellum

4. Treatment to improve emotion regulation post-TBI includes:
   a. Behavioral interventions
   b. Pharmacological interventions
   c. Psychoeducational interventions
   d. All of the above

5. The clinical presentation of anosognosia, the impaired awareness of deficits, may be further complicated by:
   a. Neuropathy
   b. Psychological factors
   c. Spasmodic dysphonia
   d. Pseudobulbar affect

ADDITIONAL READING

Brain Injury Association of America webpage about pseudobulbar affect: https://www.biausa.org/wp-content/uploads/PBA-Facts-2018.pdf

Ochsner KN, Gross JJ. The neural architecture of emotion regulation. In: Gross J, ed. *Handbook of Emotion Regulation*. The Guilford Press; 2007.

Cicerone KD, Goldin Y, Ganci K, et al. Evidence-based cognitive rehabilitation: systematic review of the literature from 2009 through 2014. *Arch Phys Med Rehabil*. 2019;100(8):1515–1533. doi:10.1016/j.apmr.2019.02.011

Williamson D, Frenette AJ, Burry LD, et al. Pharmacological interventions for agitated behaviours in patients with traumatic brain injury: a systematic review. *BMJ Open*. 2019;9(7):e029604. doi:10.1136/bmjopen-2019-029604

Cantor J, Ashman T, Dams O'Connor K, et al. Evaluation of the short-term executive plus intervention for executive dysfunction after traumatic brain injury: a randomized clinical trial with minimization. *Arch Phys Med Rehabil*. 2014;95:1–9. doi:10.1016/j.apmr.2013.08.005

ANSWERS TO STUDY QUESTIONS

1. Correct Answer: d

Estimates of prevalence in acutely injured individuals are as high as 96%, and these disorders can significantly limit response to rehabilitation, treatment compliance, re-employment, and community reintegration.

Further Reading:
Kim E. Agitation, aggression, and disinhibition syndromes after traumatic brain injury. *NeuroRehabilitation*. 2002;17:297–310. doi:10.3233/NRE-2002-17404

2. Correct Answer: b

While prosopagnosia may occur in a subset of individuals with lesions to the fusiform face area, it is not considered a common behavioral sequelae of TBI. Conversely, executive dysfunction (an impairment in one or more of the interrelated set of cognitive functions required for goal-directed behavior, such as planning, inhibition, social awareness, and behavioral selection based on situational factors), emotion dysregulation (an impairment in recognizing, experiencing, and/or expressing emotions, often resulting in significantly attenuated or exaggerated emotional responses and emotion-driven behaviors in response to legitimate triggers), and anosognosia (a neurologically-based lack of awareness of injury-related cognitive, emotional, physical, and/or behavioral changes that result in inappropriate emotional responses and behaviors) are commonly reported behavioral impairments post TBI.

Further Reading:
Kim E. Agitation, aggression, and disinhibition syndromes after traumatic brain injury. *NeuroRehabilitation*. 2002;17:297–310. doi:10.3233/NRE-2002-17404

Stuss D. Traumatic brain injury: relation to executive dysfunction and the frontal lobes. *Curr Opin Neurol*. 2011;24:584–589. doi:10.1097/WCO.0b013e32834c7eb9

Cummings JL, Miller BL. Conceptual and clinical aspects of the frontal lobes. In: Miller LB, Cummings JL, eds. *The Human Frontal Lobes: Functions and Disorders*. The Guilford Press; 2007.

3. Correct Answer: c

Anosognosia results from damage to frontal or parietal cortical areas, usually in the non-dominant hemisphere. Damage to white matter tracts is associated with executive dysfunction, damage to subcortical motor pathways has been linked to pseudobulbar affect, and damage to the cerebellum results in poor motor control and balance deficits.

Further Reading:

Zappala G, Thiebaut de Schotten M, Eslinger PJ. Traumatic brain injury and the frontal lobes: what can we gain from diffusion tensor imaging? *Cortex*. 2012;48(2):156–165. doi:10.1016/j.cortex.2011.06.020

4. Correct Answer: d

All three types of interventions provide an empirical basis that supports their use in post-TBI rehabilitation for the treatment of discrete behavioral problems (e.g., anger, agitation, depression). However, only one, behavioral intervention, has focused on emotion regulation as a broad target, showing promising results.

Further reading:

Tsaousides T, Spielman L, Kajankova M, et al. Improving emotion regulation following web-based group intervention for individuals with traumatic brain injury. *J Head Trauma Rehabil*. 2017;32(5):354–365. doi:10.1097/HTR.0000000000000345

5. Correct Answer: b

Psychogenic denial, characterological lack of insight, general mental health, and level adjustment to disability are additional factors that could complicate the clinical presentation of anosognosia for diagnostic and treatment purposes.

Further reading:

Stuss D. Traumatic brain injury: relation to executive dysfunction and the frontal lobes. *Curr Opin Neurol*. 2011;24:584–589. doi:10.1097/WCO.0b013e32834c7eb9doi:10.1097/WCO.0b013e32834c7eb9

Zappala G, Thiebaut de Schotten M, Eslinger PJ. Traumatic brain injury and the frontal lobes: what can we gain from diffusion tensor imaging? *Cortex*. 2012;48(2):156–165. doi:10.1016/j.cortex.2011.06.020

Cummings JL, Miller BL. Conceptual and clinical aspects of the frontal lobes. In: Miller LB, Cummings JL, eds. *The Human Frontal Lobes: Functions and Disorders*. The Guilford Press; 2007.

REFERENCES

The full reference list appears in the digital product found on http://connect.springer-pub.com/content/book/978-0-8261-4768-4/part/part04/chapter/ch55

CUMULATIVE EFFECTS OF REPEATED MILD TRAUMATIC BRAIN INJURY AND CHRONIC TRAUMATIC ENCEPHALOPATHY

PHILIP H. MONTENIGRO AND ROBERT C. CANTU

INTRODUCTION

In recent years there has been increasing attention to and controversy over the potential long-term cumulative effects of exposure to multiple concussions (MC) and repetitive head impacts (RHI). Today, the evidence linking cumulative exposure to MC and RHI to long-term cognitive, mood, and behavioral impairment, structural and functional changes on neuroimaging, as well as biological markers of neuronal injury, blood–brain barrier dysfunction, neuroinflammation, and the neurodegenerative disorder known as Chronic Traumatic Encephalopathy (CTE), is unequivocal.[1-23] MC and RHI occur in a variety of contexts but are most commonly observed in contact and collision-style sports. Given the number of persons involved in these sports, the public health implications may be considerable. The objective of this chapter is to summarize what is currently known about the consequences of long-term exposure to RHI and MC, with special emphasis on CTE.

PATHOPHYSIOLOGY

When a concussion is experienced, there is injury to the blood–brain barrier[12] and activation of the brain's inflammatory response.[14-16] This response causes a disrupted neuronal metabolic cascade characterized by an imbalance of ions across the cellular membrane, mitochondrial dysfunction, increased excitatory amino acids, dysregulation of neurotransmitter synthesis, and free radical production.[11,19] Ultimately, this metabolic cascade makes neurons more vulnerable to secondary ischemic injury.[1,11,19] Cumulative neuronal injury is evidenced through blood and cerebrospinal fluid biomarkers (i.e., tau, neurofilament light, amyloid-beta [Ab], and sTREM2[5,13,15,22]); however, additional research is needed to establish clinical utility.

   Even in the absence of a concussion there is a net cumulative effect of exposure to subconcussive RHI on structural and functional brain neuroimaging,[3,10] biomarkers of neuronal–axonal injury,[15,22] blood–brain barrier dysfunction,[12] neuroinflammation,[15,16] and CTE neurodegenerative pathology.[20,23] Genetics is also felt to play a role in modifying the pathophysiological cascade. One study found the ApoE4 allele in combination with MC is more likely to result in dementia.[24] Though studies in the literature are conflicting, two noted a significantly higher frequency of ApoE4 homozygotes among CTE cases.[25,26]

The full reference list appears in the digital product found on http://connect.springerpub.com/content/book/978-0-8261-4768-4/part/part04/chapter/ch56

Neuropathology of Chronic Traumatic Encephalopathy

While CTE is associated with exposure to MC and RHI, not everyone exposed to brain trauma develops CTE, suggesting its development is influenced by other factors as well (e.g., genotype, comorbidities). Since not everyone exposed to MC and RHI necessarily develops CTE, the minimum amount of exposure required for development is not yet known. Like other neurodegenerative disorders, the diagnosis can only be confirmed postmortem. In 2015, the National Institute of Neurological Disorders and Stroke (NINDS) and National Institute of Biomedical Imaging and Bioengineering (NIBIB) developed consensus-based diagnostic criteria for CTE.*

■ The pathognomonic lesion, which must be present for the diagnosis of CTE, consists of immunoreactive hyperphosphorylated tau (p-tau) aggregates in neurons, astrocytes, and cell processes around small vessels in a patchy multifocal distribution at the depths of the cortical sulci. This pattern of neuropathological changes is unique to CTE and is specifically distinct from all other neurodegenerative tauopathies.[27,28]
■ Supportive, but not in of themselves, diagnostic neuropathological features of CTE include
  ● p-tau preferentially affecting superficial cortical layers II–III (in contrast to layers III–V in Alzheimer's Disease [AD])
  ● p-tau preferentially affecting CA2 and CA4 of the hippocampus (in contrast to CA1 in AD)
  ● p-tau distributed throughout the subcortical nuclei (amygdala, thalamus, etc.)
  ● p-tau in thorny astrocytes in the subpial and periventricular areas
  ● p-tau aggregates in large grainlike, dotlike, threadlike structures (e.g., p-tau in neurites)
  ● non-tau–related macroscopic features (e.g., dilated third ventricle, cavum septum)
  ● TAR DNA-binding protein of approximately 43 kd (TDP-43) immunoreactive aggregates within neurons and dotlike structures in the hippocampus, anterior medical temporal cortex, and amygdala[28]
■ The consensus neuropathological diagnostic criteria for CTE demonstrate good inter-rater reliability (75%–78%).[28,29]
■ AD is a frequent comorbidity with CTE (CTE-AD); however, Ab plaques and Ab1–40 aggregation in CTE-AD cases are significantly increased in the sulcus compared to the gyral crest,[25] which is consistent with a biomechanical etiology.[19]
■ Efforts to refine and advance the pathological criteria for CTE are ongoing. As the neuropathology of CTE becomes better defined, the critical next step will be to diagnose CTE during life.

CLINICAL PRESENTATION

Since a definitive diagnosis of CTE cannot be made during life, the incidence and prevalence of CTE remain unknown. Identifying the clinical features associated with CTE and developing valid clinical criteria and biomarkers to diagnose CTE during life is of critical importance.

---

*Editor's note: See also TBI/CTE Research Group (2021). The Second NINDS/NIBIB Consensus Meeting to Define Neuropathological Criteria for the Diagnosis of Chronic Traumatic Encephalopathy. *Journal of Neuropathology and Experimental Neurology*, 80(3), 210-219. This publication, which came out after this chapter was produced, provides results of the second consensus conference, with updated discussion of ongoing pathological instigation and characterization of CTE.

Cases of confirmed CTE with no comorbid disease, referred to here as primary CTE (pCTE), are an important initial reference point. Retrospective structured interviews with informants (e.g., family, primary care physician) of pCTE cases[26,27] have led to a preliminary clinical depiction of CTE. The core characteristic symptoms of CTE typically arise in one of three clinical domains: cognition, behavior, and mood.[26] Additionally, a subset of cases manifest *concomitant* motor impairments at various points in the disease course[19]:

- *Cognitive*: decrease in memory, executive function, attention, learning, and dementia
- *Mood*: depression, anxiety, apathy, irritability, hopelessness, and possibly suicidality
- *Behavioral*: having a "short fuse," explosiveness, violence, impulsiveness, and aggression
- *Motor*: parkinsonism, ataxia, and dysarthria

The overall clinical picture of CTE can be characterized into phenotypes as follows:

- A behavioral phenotype with an earlier age of symptom onset
- A cognitive phenotype with a latent symptom onset
- A mixed behavioral/mood and cognitive onset phenotype

A percentage of cases from all three symptom-onset phenotypes progress to dementia.[19,21] Of all published cases in the literature thus far, 68% have had a progressive clinical course.[30]

Clinical Diagnostics

- In 2014, preliminary clinical diagnostic criteria for CTE were proposed, primarily for use in a research context[30] (Table 56.1). This set of proposed criteria utilizes diagnostic modifiers "possible" and "probable" to designate the clinical likelihood that the clinical diagnosis represents underlying CTE (Table 56.1.C).
- To be diagnosed with "possible/probable CTE" one must first meet diagnostic criteria for the clinical syndrome associated with MC and RHI, designated traumatic encephalopathy syndrome (TES; Table 56.1.A).[30]
- The criteria require two steps to make a clinical diagnosis, first diagnose TES and then determine the likelihood of underlying CTE pathology. (The designation TES was not intended to be specific for CTE but rather encompasses a broader spectrum of likely outcomes associated with MC and RHI exposure.)
- To make a *"possible* CTE-TES" diagnosis there must be evidence of a progressive clinical course.
- To make a *"probable* CTE-TES" diagnosis requires at least one positive potential biomarker for CTE (Table 56.1.C).
- A *probable* CTE-TES diagnosis cannot be made when a case meets criteria for TES and for another disorder; however, *possible* CTE-TES can.
- As previously mentioned, comorbidity is common among neurodegenerative disease, including CTE, and the criteria allow one to consider the likelihood that TES is due to concomitant underlying etiologies. When there is strong suspicion of comorbid disorders it is recommended that each be labeled as potentially being either primary, secondary, or mixed.[30]
- Preliminary results from a validation study identified a sensitivity of 0.95, specificity 0.44, and diagnostic accuracy of 0.84 for *possible* CTE-TES.[31]
- It is important to emphasize that these criteria are primarily of value in a research context. They have not been validated for clinical use. Additional research is needed to evaluate potential CTE biomarkers to make the diagnosis of *probable* CTE-TES. It is likely that inclusion of biomarkers will further improve specificity.

TABLE 56.1 Proposed Research Criteria for Diagnosis of Traumatic Encephalopathy Syndrome (TES) and Likelihood of Underlying Chronic Traumatic Encephalopathy (CTE) Pathology

A. General criteria for TES (all four criteria must be met for TES diagnosis)
1. History of MC/RHI (at least 1 of the 3 must be present)
a. At least 4 concussions or mild TBIs
b. At least 2 moderate/severe TBIs
c. Subconcussive trauma (as defined by at least 1 of the following types of exposure)
   i. At least 6 years of organized contact sports
   ii. Military service with combat exposure
   iii. Other significant RHI (e.g., domestic abuse)
2. Core clinical features (at least 1 of the 3 domains must be present)*
*Cognitive***: significant impairment in memory, orientation, language, attention, executive function, or visuospatial function
Behavioral: described as explosive, short fuse, out of control, physically, and/or verbally violent. Or intermittent explosive disorder
Mood: feeling overly sad, depressed, or hopeless, or diagnosis of major depressive disorder or persistent depressive disorder
3. Supportive features (at least 2 must be present)
Documented decline (at least 1 year), delayed symptom onset after exposure, impulsivity, anxiety, apathy, paranoia, suicidality, headache, and motor impairment
4. Clinical features must be present for a minimum of 12 months

B. Proposed criteria for TES diagnostic subtypes and modifiers
Diagnostic subtypes (select only 1 of 4)

1. Cognitive	Cognitive core features are present without behavioral or mood core features and without functional impairment
2. Behavioral/Mood	Behavioral and/or mood core features are present without cognitive core features
3. Mixed	Both cognitive and behavioral/mood core features are present, but without functional impairment
4. Dementia	Cognitive core features and functional impairment are present
The above subtypes may occur with the following motor features:	Dysarthria, dysgraphia, bradykinesia, tremor, rigidity, gait change, falls, and/or other features of parkinsonism

Clinical course modifier (select only one designation)

Stable	History or tests indicate little if any change
Progressive	Clear indication of progression over 2 years
Unknown/inconsistent	Unknown or inconsistent information

C. Proposed CTE likelihood criteria

Probable CTE-TES (all of the following):	Progressive course
	Another neurological disorder cannot better account for the clinical presentation and/or biomarkers.

(continued)

TABLE 56.1 **Proposed Research Criteria for Diagnosis of Traumatic Encephalopathy Syndrome (TES) and Likelihood of Underlying CTE Pathology (*continued*)**

At least one positive potential biomarker must be present:	Positive PET tau imaging
	Negative PET amyloid imaging
	Elevated CSF p-tau/tau ratio
	Normal amyloid-beta CSF levels
	Cavum septum pellucidum on an imaging study
	Cortical thinning or atrophy on an imaging study
	If PET tau imaging was performed, it must be positive
Possible CTE-TES	Does not meet criteria for probable CTE
	Progressive course
	If PET tau imaging was performed, it must be positive
Unlikely CTE-TES	Does not meet criteria for probable or possible CTE-TES

*The core diagnostic clinical symptoms were selected for inclusion in the diagnostic criteria if and only if that symptom appeared in 70% or more of neuropathologically confirmed CTE cases reviewed.[30]

**By augmenting the criteria core features to require the presence of cognitive symptoms the diagnostic specificity markedly increases.[32]

CSF, cerebrospinal fluid; CTE, chronic traumatic encephalopathy; MC, multiple concussions; RHI, repetitive head impacts; TBI, traumatic brain injury; TES, traumatic encephalopathy syndrome.

Source: Montenigro PH, Baugh CM, Daneshvar DH, et al. Clinical subtypes of chronic traumatic encephalopathy: literature review and proposed research diagnostic criteria for traumatic encephalopathy syndrome. *Alzheimers Res Ther*. 2014;6:1–17.

Neuroimaging

The long-term effects of exposure to MC and RHI have also been demonstrated through various imaging studies.

- Imaging abnormalities have been shown to occur after a single season of contact–collision sport exposure.[3,6–12]
- Changes are seen in the corpus callosum, external capsule, inferior fronto-occipital fasciculus, ventricular system, and cavum septum pellucidum.[18,19]
- Even after the resolution of symptoms, ultrastructural and functional brain alterations may be seen via both anatomic and functional neuroimaging studies (see also Chapter 12).[18,19,24]

CLINICAL CONSEQUENCES

In the acute setting, those who experience a concussion while still symptomatic from a previous concussion are at a higher risk for developing postconcussion syndrome (PCS) or second impact syndrome (SIS).[19] (See also Chapters 11, 15, and 16.)

Cumulative exposure: Until recently, there had not been a metric to accurately estimate cumulative exposure to subconcussive RHI. To address this need, the Cumulative Head

Impact Index (CHII) was developed.[1] The CHII takes into account the total number of years played at each level (e.g., Pee-Wee, High-School, Division-1), positions played (e.g., first position as quarterback), and head impact frequencies derived from reported helmet acceler-ometer data. A threshold dose–response relationship between the CHII and risk for later-life cognitive clinical sequelae was developed using an objective neuropsychological measure of cognition and validated self-report measures of behavior and mood (Figure 56.1A–F).

Former NFL players' CHII was associated with:

■ The burden of white-matter abnormalities identified on magnetic resonance imaging (MRI)[4]

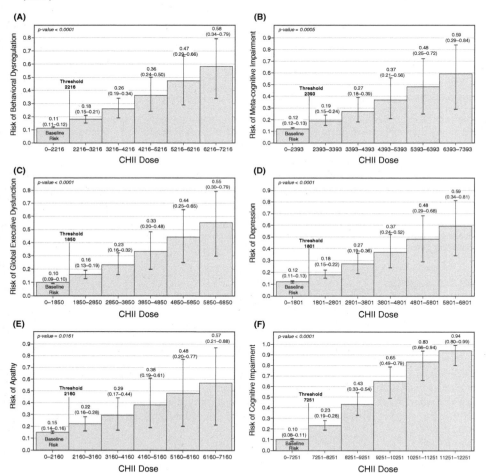

FIGURE 56.1 **Threshold dose–response relationship between the CHII and clinical impairment.**

A linear dose–response relationship between Cumulative Head Impact Index (CHII) exposure and later-life clinically significant behavioral dysregulation (A), executive dysfunction (B, C), depression (D), apathy (E), and cognitive impairment (F).

Source: From Montenigro P, Alosco M, Martin B, et al. Cumulative head impact exposure predicts later-life depression, apathy, executive dysfunction, and cognitive impairment in former high school and college football players. *J Neurotrauma.* 2017;34(2):328–340. doi:10.1089/neu.2016.4413

- Structural volumetric measures of the brain on MRI[5]
- Parietal white-matter creatine on MRI spectroscopy[7]
- Plasma total tau[22]
- Cerebrospinal fluid tau, Ab, and sTREM2 (i.e., measure of neuroinflammation)[15]
- Risk of premature death[21]

The long-term consequences of MC among living contact–collision sport athletes have been well documented.

- Athletes who participate in contact and collision-style sports have an increased likelihood of developing cognitive impairment, depression, emotional instability, executive dysfunction, memory impairment, and neurodegeneration later in life.[1,2,5,9,17,18]
- Functional impairment or dementia is five times more likely to develop in retired contact–collision sport athletes after the age of 50.[14] The delayed onset of symptoms may be explained by an underlying mechanism that permits normal function (e.g., cognitive reserve)[33] until a critical threshold of damage has accumulated or until underlying pathology has progressed.[19]

GAPS IN KNOWLEDGE AND FUTURE DIRECTIONS

Although a great deal of progress has been made in the study of long-term consequences of MC and RHI exposure and CTE, critical questions and gaps in knowledge remain.

- It is not yet known why some develop latent impairments and/or CTE following exposure to MC/RHI while others with similar exposure histories do not.
- A lot of progress has been made in evaluating the association between MC/RHI exposure in living athletes with clinical impairments and/or biomarkers. Studies are needed to assess the clinical utility of these findings for the individual. Predictive models cannot determine an individual's personal risk.

KEY POINTS

- RHI, even in the absence of concussion, have potential long-term serious consequences. New methods to estimate lifetime exposure have demonstrated a threshold dose–response relationship with cognitive, behavioral, and mood impairments, as well as strong predictive associations with in vivo biomarkers.
- CTE is an increasingly well-defined neurodegenerative disease associated with exposure to MC and RHI.
- Clinical diagnostic criteria for CTE have been proposed and preliminary studies of validity are ongoing. Early reports indicate the criteria for *possible* CTE-TES has good sensitivity and diagnostic accuracy, but needs improvement in specificity.
- Potential biomarkers for CTE have been studied in living individuals with high exposure to MC and RHI. Studies associating these biomarkers with postmortem CTE pathology are needed.

STUDY QUESTIONS

1. A seasoned semiprofessional baseball player reports having had a total of two concussions during his playing career. His wife confirms his report as do medical records from his primary care physician. He asks about the likelihood that he will develop neurological problems. What is the most appropriate response?
   a. Reassure him that he is not at risk for long-term clinical outcomes.
   b. Inquire about his plans going forward for involvement in baseball.
   c. Inquire more broadly about his history of involvement in sports or other head injury exposures.
   d. Caution him that he is at risk for long-term clinical sequelae due to his head injury history.

2. A patient comes to your office and asks you to evaluate him for CTE. The most appropriate next step is:
   a. Measure CSF p-tau and Ab.
   b. Apply CTE-TES clinical criteria.
   c. Obtain Ab and tau PET scans.
   d. Undertake a comprehensive history and physical.

3. Involvement in what sport is thought to carry the greatest risk of CTE?
   a. Rugby
   b. Baseball
   c. Football
   d. Basketball

4. The greatest risk factor for developing neurodegeneration later in life as identified in postmortem case reports appears to be:
   a. ApoE4 homozygote genotype
   b. Male gender
   c. Years playing contact sports
   d. Race or ethnicity

5. What does not correlate with risk of CTE?
   a. Cumulative head impact exposure
   b. Years playing contact sports
   c. Sports played
   d. Number of concussions

ADDITIONAL READING

https://concussionfoundation.org/CTE-resources

CTE multicenter clinical research project: www.diagnosecte.com

Budson AE, McKee AC, Cantu RC, Stern RA. *Chronic Traumatic Encephalopathy: Proceedings of the Boston University Alzheimer s Disease Center Conference.* Elsevier Health Sciences; 2017.

McKee A, Alvarez V, Bieniek K, et al. Preliminary results of the NINDS/NIBIB consensus meeting to evaluate pathological criteria for the diagnosis of CTE. *Neurology.* 2015;(P2):178

Montenigro PH, Alosco ML, Martin BM, et al. Cumulative head impact exposure predicts later-life depression, apathy, executive dysfunction, and cognitive impairment in former high school and college football players. *J Neurotrauma*. 2017;34(2):328–340. doi:10.1089/neu.2016.4413

ANSWERS TO STUDY QUESTIONS

1. Correct Answer: c
   Before you can even begin to discuss his risk, you should first determine if he is or was ever involved in any contact–collision sports. These include but are not limited to American-style football, ice-hockey, soccer, boxing, and rugby. While baseball is his current primary sport, he may have participated in contact sports at some point during his lifetime. Recall that current evidence demonstrates a strong dose–response relationship between exposure to repetitive head impacts and risk for later-life cognitive, behavioral, and mood impairment. Answer (a) is a tempting distractor because he has only had two confirmed concussions and evidence associates three or more concussions with risk. Answer (b) is partially correct and is therefore a good answer, but it is not the best answer choice. Although he may only have two concussions, if he has another concussion before retirement his risk will increase. Answer (d) is wrong because you do not have all the information needed to evaluate his history of exposure to MC and RHI.

   Further Reading:
   Montenigro PH, Alosco ML, Martin BM, et al. Cumulative head impact exposure predicts later-life depression, apathy, executive dysfunction, and cognitive impairment in former high school and college football players. *J Neurotrauma*. 2017;34(2):328–340. doi:10.1089/neu.2016.4413
   Seichepine DR, Stamm JM, Daneshvar DH, et al. Profile of self-reported problems with executive functioning in college and professional football players. *J Neurotrauma*. 2013;(30):1299–1304 doi:10.1089/neu.2012.2690
   Iverson GL, Brooks BL, Lovell MR, Collins MW. No cumulative effects for one or two previous concussions. *Br J Sports Med*. 2006;40(1):72–75. doi:10.1136/bjsm.2005.020651

2. Correct Answer: d
   Answers (a) and (c) are potential biomarkers for CTE that have yet to be validated as diagnostic for CTE in living persons. Answer (b) is incorrect because the proposed clinical criteria are still preliminary and intended for research purposes only at this time. Taking a history and performing physical exam, answer (d), represents the key first step in determining whether the patient has been exposed to MC and/or RHI.

3. Correct Answer: c
   The distinguishing feature between football and all other choices is the frequency of head impacts. Helmet accelerometer studies report heavy head impact burdens at all levels of football.

   Further Reading:
   Montenigro PH, Alosco ML, Martin BM, et al. Cumulative head impact exposure predicts later-life depression, apathy, executive dysfunction, and cognitive impairment in former high school and college football players. *J Neurotrauma*. 2017;34(2):328–340. doi:10.1089/neu.2016.4413

4. Correct Answer: c

Years playing contact–collision sports is a useful proxy for cumulative head impact exposure in postmortem studies. The relationship between race (d) and the ApoE4 genotype remains unclear.

Further Reading:

Mez J, Daneshvar DH, Abdolmohammadi B, et al. Duration of American football play and chronic traumatic encephalopathy. *Ann Neurol.* 2020;87(1):116–131. doi:10.1002/ana.25611

5. Correct answer: d

Number of concussions has not been shown to correlate with the extent of CTE pathology seen in autopsy studies.[27] All other choices are associated with the development of CTE.

Further Reading:

McKee AC, Stern RA, Nowinski CJ, et al. The spectrum of disease in chronic traumatic encephalopathy. *Brain.* 2013;136(1):43–64. doi:10.1093/brain/aws307

REFERENCES

The full reference list appears in the digital product found on http://connect.springer-pub.com/content/book/978-0-8261-4768-4/part/part04/chapter/ch56

57 POSTTRAUMATIC HEADACHE

THOMAS K. WATANABE

GENERAL PRINCIPLES

Definition

According to *International Classification of Headache Disorders*, third edition (*ICHD-3*), headaches (HAs) that develop within 1 week after head trauma (or within 1 week of regaining consciousness or discontinuation of medications that impair the ability to report HA after injury) are referred to as posttraumatic headaches (PTHs). PTHs that last longer than 3 months are referred to as persistent PTH.[1] This definition may not be adequate in describing the incidence and prevalence of PTH (see section titled Natural History).

Epidemiology

- HAs may develop in up to 90% of patients with traumatic brain injury (TBI).[2]
- A systematic review found an aggregate prevalence of 57.8%.[3]
- Risk factors include female gender and pre-injury history of HA.[4]
- In children, pre-injury HA and family history of migraine HA are associated with PTH 3 months after injury.[5]

Natural History

- 28% of those who experienced moderate to severe TBI in a civilian population did not report onset of PTH until more than 3 months post injury.[4]
- Only 27% of returning war veterans who developed HAs after TBI had initial complaints in the first week after injury.[6]
- Overall prevalence of 78% 5 years after moderate to severe TBI.[7]
- Overall incidence of 91% in a civilian mild TBI population over the course of the first year post injury.[8]

Classification

- HAs are often classified based on their clinical features.
- Most studies identify migraine as the most common type of PTH in both mild and moderate to severe TBI civilian populations, with tension-type HA being the next most common type.[7-9] Migraine is also the most common HA type among service members in a large Gulf War study.[10]
- Less common are cervicogenic HA, neuritic pain, musculoskeletal HA, dysautonomic HA, sinus HA, posttraumatic cluster HA, and medication overuse HA.
- PTH may also present as mixed or difficult to classify.
- *ICHD-3* classification (does not differentiate based on clinical features)[1]:

The full reference list appears in the digital product found on http://connect.springerpub.com/content/book/978-0-8261-4768-4/part/part04/chapter/ch57

- HA attributed to trauma or injury to the head and/or neck
  - Acute HA attributed to traumatic injury to the head
    - ☐ Acute HA attributed to moderate or severe traumatic injury to the head
    - ☐ Acute HA attributed to mild traumatic injury to the head
  - Persistent HA attributed to traumatic injury to the head
    - ☐ Persistent HA attributed to moderate or severe traumatic injury to the head
    - ☐ Persistent HA attributed to mild traumatic injury to the head
  - Acute HA attributed to whiplash
  - Persistent HA attributed to whiplash
  - Acute HA attributed to craniotomy
  - Persistent HA attributed to craniotomy

Pathophysiology

Pathophysiology is poorly understood and is likely often multifactorial. There are a number of potential sources of pain after head trauma, including injury to bones, skin, nerves, dura, joints (cervical and mandibular), ligaments, and muscles. Central mechanisms, psychological factors, vascular changes, neuroinflammation, and medications (including those being used to treat HA) may also play roles in generating pain.[11] The development of PTH may be a warning sign of a serious intracranial process (see section titled Diagnosis).

DIAGNOSIS

History

- Quality of pain—COLDER (character, onset, location, duration, exacerbation, relief).
- Ask about severity, frequency, temporal associations, and postural relationships.
- Associated symptoms—nausea, vomiting, dizziness, visual dysfunction, and auras.
- Patients with family history of HA are more likely to develop PTH.[12]

Clinical Presentation (Based on International Headache Society Classification of Headache)

Clinical presentation is often mixed rather than falling into only one of the following categories.

- *Migraine HA*—throbbing, moderate to severe intensity, aggravated by activity, unilateral, lasts 4 to 72 hours, may be associated with nausea or vomiting, photophobia, and/or phonophobia, may have aura. Basilar artery migraines can occur secondary to traction on the vertebral–basilar circulation from acceleration–deceleration injury.
- *Tension-type HA*—moderate diffuse nonpulsating pain in forehead or temples, mild to moderate intensity, usually bilateral, often described as pressure, or bandlike, which is not typically aggravated by activity. For episodic tension-type HA, either photophobia or phonophobia may be seen, but not both, and without nausea or vomiting.
- *Neuritic pain*—sharp, shooting, electric pain. Most commonly originating from greater or lesser occipital nerves, with pain located periocular and radiating from back to front of head.
- *Musculoskeletal HA*—"cap-like" in quality, trigger points may be present. Patient may have history of skull fracture or bruxism.

- *Cervicogenic HA*—typically originates in the cervical or occipital region and radiates rostrally. Often active trigger points can be identified, palpation of which reproduces the pain pattern.
- *Dysautonomic HA*—unilateral episodic throbbing pain associated with autonomic changes.
- *Sinus HA*—localized to the sinuses and associated with sinus tenderness.
- *Temporomandibular joint dysfunction syndrome*—typically located in the temporal region; may be exacerbated by chewing or yawning. Clicking or malocclusion of the jaw may be appreciated.[1]

Ominous Symptoms That May Indicate Intracranial Pathology

- *Increased intracranial pressure (ICP)*—worsening and constant cephalgia, associated nausea and vomiting, decreased arousal. May be secondary to a space-occupying lesion (e.g., bleed), tension pneumocephalus, hydrocephalus, or shunt failure.
- *Low ICP*—HA exacerbation in upright position. Usually secondary to overshunting or CSF leak.
- Acute or delayed vascular dysfunction (see also Chapter 58):
  - *Carotid artery injury*—severe and ipsilateral pain, involving orbital or periorbital regions as well as the neck.
  - *Vertebral artery injury*—severe pain in cervical or ipsilateral occipital regions, ipsilateral facial dysesthesia, vertigo, nausea/vomiting.
  - *Carotid cavernous fistula*—frontal HA, facial pain, chemosis, proptosis, and diplopia.[12]

Physical Examination

- Comparison to baseline (whenever possible) is key.
- *Migraine or tension HA*—likely normal neurological examination, but may have transient neurological changes during initial phase of a migraine attack.
- *Neuritic HA*—palpation of affected nerve may reproduce HA pain.
  - *Greater occipital nerve*—best palpated below base of skull, off midline, pain referred to vertex.
  - *Lesser occipital nerve*—best palpated behind sternocleidomastoid, one third of muscle length from mastoid; pain often radiates to mastoid, ear, and/or lower temple.
- *Sinus HA*—sinuses may be tender with palpation.
- *Musculoskeletal and cervicogenic HA*—identify trigger points that may reproduce pain; palpate paracervical and/or suboccipital muscles or muscles of mastication in temporomandibular joint dysfunction. Pain may also be reproduced with cervical range of motion.[12]

Ominous Examination Findings That May Indicate Intracranial Pathology

- *Increased ICP*—deterioration in mental status, focal neurological deterioration, and papilledema.
- *CSF leak*—clear rhinorrhea, otorrhea that may worsen with Valsalva.
- *Vascular injury*—external evidence of neck trauma, cervical carotid bruit, ocular bruit, sensory changes, visual deficits, and Horner's syndrome.
- *Infection*—fever, nuchal rigidity, purulent drainage from wound or postsurgical site.[12]

Laboratory Studies

- Limited utility—if infection is suspected, CSF may be studied.

Radiographic Assessment

▪ In the absence of signs of increased ICP, new or worsening focal neurological deficits, bruits, or meningeal irritation, cerebral imaging is generally not warranted.

▪ If focal neurological findings are noted, computed tomography (CT) or magnetic resonance imaging (MRI) of the brain should be considered.

▪ *Increased ICP*—CT of brain is imaging of choice because of the ease of obtaining study and will also identify cerebral swelling and pneumocephalus. If situation is not acute, MRI is more sensitive.

▪ *Vascular injury*—MRI or MRA of neck will assess blunt carotid trauma. Ultrasound can also detect vascular lesions and vasospasm but is limited by technique. Angiography may be considered in selected cases (e.g., as a pre-op assessment).

▪ *Infection*—CT or MRI with contrast can identify abscesses.

▪ *Musculoskeletal HA*—consider C-spine plain films (lateral, open-mouth, flexion–extension); C-spine MRI if disc disease is suspected and symptoms are not responsive to conservative measures.

▪ *Sinus HA*—CT can be used to evaluate for sinusitis and anatomic or structural problems.[12]

TREATMENT

Guiding Principles

▪ There is insufficient evidence to support any particular treatment protocol.

▪ Interventions should be based on HA phenotype; migraine HA is the most common type in most TBI populations.

▪ For HAs due to identified intracranial pathology, address the underlying pathology directly.

▪ Evaluate for depression or other psychological factors, including PTSD, which may contribute to HA frequency, persistence, and severity.[13]

▪ Identify and counsel patient on PTH triggers—including, for example, sleep, caffeine, stress, exercise, or diet.[14]

Initial Management

▪ Consider the need for evaluation for acute intracranial pathology.[2]

▪ Categorize HA phenotype.

▪ Consider time-limited use of opioid medications for severe HA (see section titled Pharmacological Treatment for discussion of precautions with use in this patient population).

▪ Consider time-limited use of acetaminophen or nonsteroidal anti-inflammatory medication for mild to moderate HA.

▪ For HAs that meet the criteria for migraine, start with a trial of a triptan, provided there are no contraindications (e.g., complicated migraine, cardiovascular disease).

▪ For HAs that are associated with cervical spine pain, consider a referral to physical therapy that may include gentle cervical range of motion exercises without resistance and modalities to decrease symptoms once structural spine pathology has been ruled out.

▪ Identify and address existing comorbidities that may be contributing to symptoms such as sleep dysfunction, stress/anxiety, visual problems, and inadequately treated pre-existing HA disorder.

Ongoing Care

- Reconsider the need to evaluate for intracranial pathology.[2]
- (Re)categorize HA phenotype.
- For HAs that meet criteria for migraine/probable migraine, assess efficacy and frequency of use of abortive medication; consider trial of different type if not efficacious (including a different triptan if one has been trialed previously). If the patient is experiencing more than three migraine HAs per month, initiate trial of preventive migraine HA medication.
- For any HA type, if there is evidence of muscle tension or cervicogenic component, initiate physical therapy including cervical flexibility, strengthening and endurance exercises, manual therapy, neuromuscular re-education, home exercises, and aerobic conditioning.
- Consider behavioral therapy interventions.

Nonpharmacological Treatment

- Cognitive behavioral therapy, relaxation, education, and biofeedback have shown favorable results in uncontrolled studies.[2]
- Physical therapy may be useful if the PTH is caused by musculoskeletal or biomechanical dysfunction.[2] Myofascial pain can be addressed with trigger point injections.[14]
- Neuritic pain may respond to local anesthetic block of the affected nerve, most commonly the greater occipital nerve.[15]
- Acupuncture has been shown to be effective as both an abortive and a prophylactic management approach for migraine HAs and for tension HA in the general HA population.[16,17]

Pharmacological Treatment

Abortive Agents

- Nonsteroidal anti-inflammatory drugs (NSAIDs)—can be effective for musculoskeletal HA, migraine HA, and tension HA.[14,18-21]
- Muscle relaxants—use not supported; may worsen concomitant cognitive deficits.
- Acetaminophen—effective for musculoskeletal and tension HA.
- Opioids—consider time-limited use for severe, functionally disabling pain, with caution due to high-abuse potential and risk of sedation/cognitive impairment.
- Vasoactive medications—serotonin receptor agonists (triptans) and ergotamine derivatives are first line for migraine HA pain, provided that no cerebrovascular or cardiovascular contraindications are present. A positive response to these medications also helps confirm the diagnosis of migraine HA.

Prophylactic Agents

- β-Blockers (propranolol, metoprolol)—primary choice for migraine prophylaxis in patients who do not have cognitive impairment due to TBI. Exercise caution in the setting of cognitive impairment.
- Calcium channel blockers (verapamil)—most evidence for efficacy pertains to cluster HA.
- Antidepressants—tricyclic antidepressants (nortriptyline, amitriptyline) and selective serotonin reuptake inhibitors (venlafaxine) are frequently used for migraine prophylaxis.
- Anticonvulsants (valproate, topiramate) also may be beneficial in migraine prophylaxis.

Other Agents
- Pulsed corticosteroids—may abort an attack of intractable migraine.
- Inhalation of 100% oxygen for cluster HA (not a typical posttraumatic HA presentation).
- Antiemetics—can be considered for patients with severe nausea who cannot ingest other medications.
- Botulinum toxin—FDA approval for chronic migraine; some lower-quality evidence for use in tension-type and cervicogenic HA has also been published.[22,23]
- Calcitonin gene-related peptide receptor (CGRP) antagonists—FDA approved for migraine prophylaxis (CGRP monoclonal antibodies) and for abortive treatment (CGRP antagonists).

Outcome Measures
- Use of a HA log is recommended to accurately assess frequency and severity of HAs and to determine treatment efficacy.
- Quality of life measures, for example, Migraine Disability Assessment (MIDAS) and HA Impact Test (HIT-6), are also useful tools to evaluate impact of HA on activity and participation and to help determine the need for alterations in the treatment plan.[24]

Treatment Controversies
- There may be an inverse correlation between TBI severity and the presence of PTH.[25]
- Many patients with PTH have pending litigation; there is a possibility that secondary gain may interfere with response to treatment.[26]
- Inadequacy of current ICHD criteria, including rigidity of definition of PTH (development within 1 week of trauma) and lack of differentiation of HA type.[1]

Additional Considerations

Posttraumatic Headache and Sport-Related Concussion
- HA is the most common symptom after sport-related concussion, with rates as high as 92% being reported.[27]
- HAs can also be a manifestation of physical exertion in the absence of head trauma, making the diagnosis of persistent postconcussive symptoms on the basis of exertional PTH problematic.[28] Additionally, there is increasing awareness of the role of autonomic dysfunction as a cause of persisting HA symptoms after, and possibly triggered by, head trauma.[29]
- One needs to consider other conditions that may provoke or exacerbate HAs in athletes, including dehydration, sleep disruption, stress, and overuse of analgesic medications.
- Postconcussion migraine HA has been shown to be associated with a more protracted recovery from concussion in young athletes.[30,31]
- Management of sport-related concussion HA does not differ significantly from the aforementioned recommendations regarding PTH in general.

Pediatric Posttraumatic Headache Management
- Age less than 18 and posttraumatic migraine HA may independently and to some degree additively predict slower recovery after concussion.[32]
- Pre-existing migraine is a risk factor for prolonged recovery (return to school and sports).[33]
- Treatment generally follows recommendations for treating primary HA disorders in children; note that only a few triptans are FDA approved for pediatric use (almotriptan, rizatriptan, and sumatriptan/naproxen sodium).

KEY POINTS

- PTH is an important complication of TBI, with an incidence up to 90%.
- It is recommended that initial treatment strategies be derived from determination of HA phenotype (e.g., migraine, tension type, neuritic).
- The most common type of PTH is migraine or probable migraine HA.
- PTH may have a mixed phenotype and may be exacerbated by other injury-related factors (e.g., sleep dysfunction, mood disorder, visual deficits, intracranial pathology).

STUDY QUESTIONS

1. The most common type of PTH is:
   a. Tension
   b. Migraine
   c. Neuralgic
   d. Cluster

2. According to *ICHD-3* criteria, to meet the definition of PTHs, the HAs must arise within what time period after injury (assuming that the patient is conscious and able to report the HA)?
   a. 1 day
   b. 7 days
   c. 14 days
   d. 30 days

3. A mild to moderate intensity, bilateral HA described as band-like is most consistent with what type of HA?
   a. Tension
   b. Neuralgic
   c. Migraine
   d. Dysautonomic

4. What type of postconcussion HA is associated with a more protracted recovery from concussion in young athletes?
   a. Tension
   b. Cervicogenic
   c. Migraine
   d. Cluster

5. Botulinum toxin has FDA approval for which type of HA?
   a. Tension
   b. Chronic migraine
   c. Cluster
   d. Neuralgic

ADDITIONAL READING

International Headache Society website: https://journals.sagepub.com/doi/full/10.1177/03331024177 38202

Lucas S, Hoffman JM, Bell KR, Dikmen S. A prospective study of prevalence and characterization of headache following mild traumatic brain injury. *Cephalgia.* 2014;34:93–102. doi:10.1177/0333102413499645

Lucas S, Hoffman JM, Bell KR, et al. Characterization of headache after traumatic brain injury. *Cephalgia.* 2012;32;600–606. doi:10.1177/0333102412445224

Marmura MJ, Silberstein SD, Schwedt TJ. The acute treatment of migraine in adults: The American Headache Society evidence assessment of migraine pharmacotherapies. *Headache.* 2015;55:3–20. doi:10.1111/head.12499

Watanabe TK, Bell KR, Walker WC, Schomer K. Systematic review of interventions for post-traumatic headaches. *PM&R.* 2012;4(2):129–140. doi:10.1016/j.pmrj.2011.06.003

ANSWERS TO STUDY QUESTIONS

1. Correct Answer: b

The most common type of PTH is migraine. This is true for both mild and moderate to severe HAs.

Further Reading:

Stacey A, Lucas S, Dikmen S, et al. Natural history of headache five years after traumatic brain injury. *J Neurotrauma* 2017;34(8):1558–1564. doi:10.1089/neu.2016.4721

Lucas S, Hoffman JM, Bell KR, Dikmen S. A prospective study of prevalence and characterization of headache following mild traumatic brain injury. *Cephalgia.* 2014;34(2):93–102. doi:10.1177/0333102413499645

2. Correct Answer: b

This definition is somewhat problematic because studies have reported an onset of HAs attributable to a TBI several weeks or longer after the incident.

Further Reading:

Headache Classification Committee of the International Headache Society. The International Classification of Headache Disorders. 3rd ed. *Cephalalgia.* 2018;38(1):1–211. doi:10.1177/0333102417738202

3. Correct Answer: c

Tension HAs are typically bilateral and mild to moderate in intensity. Neuralgic HAs are usually described as sharp, shooting, or electrical. Migraine HAs are throbbing, unilateral, moderate to severe, and often accompanied by nausea and photophobia. Dysautonomic HAs are often episodic with evidence of autonomic changes.

Further Reading:

Lucas S, Hoffman JM, Bell KR et al. Characterization of headache after traumatic brain injury. *Cephalgia* 2014;34(2):93–102. doi:10.1177/0333102413499645

4. Correct Answer: c

Posttraumatic migraine HA has been found to be associated with prolonged recovery in youths following concussion.

Further Reading:
Kontos AP, Elbin RJ, Sufrinko A, et al. Recovery following sport-related concussion: integrating pre- and postinjury factors into multidisciplinary care. *J Head Trauma Rehabil* 2019; 34(6): 394–401. doi:10.1097/HTR.0000000000000536

5. Correct Answer: b
Chronic migraine (HAs on 15 or more days per month) is the only HA type for which high-quality evidence has been published showing demonstrable efficacy.

Further Reading:
Simpson DM, Hallett M, Ashman EJ, et al. Practice guideline update summary: botulinum neurotoxin for the treatment of blepharospasm, cervical dystonia, adult spasticity, and headache: report of the Guideline Development Subcommittee of the American Academy of Neurology. *Neurology.* 2016;86(19):1818–1826. doi:10.1212/WNL.0000000000002560
Escher CM, Paracka L, Dressler D, Kollewe K. Botulinum toxin in the management of chronic migraine: clinical evidence and experience. *Ther Adv Neurol Disord.* 2017;10(2):127–135. doi:10.1177/1756285616677005

REFERENCES

The full reference list appears in the digital product found on http://connect.springer-pub.com/content/book/978-0-8261-4768-4/part/part04/chapter/ch57

NEUROVASCULAR COMPLICATIONS AFTER NONPENETRATING BRAIN INJURY

SUNIL KOTHARI AND BEI ZHANG

INTRODUCTION

Blunt cerebrovascular injury (BCVI) is a nonpenetrating traumatic injury to the vertebral and/or carotid arteries. Although relatively uncommon, BCVI after traumatic brain injury (TBI) can have devastating consequences. The most common manifestation of BCVI, especially in extracranial arteries, is arterial dissection. Two forms of BCVI that can occur intracranially are aneurysms and fistulas, especially carotid-cavernous fistulas (CCFs).

- Recognizing BCVI after TBI is complicated by several factors:
  - Patients may be asymptomatic or may have nonspecific symptoms.
  - Symptoms may be delayed in their presentation, sometimes for weeks to months.
  - Symptoms (e.g., headache) may mistakenly be attributed to the TBI itself, rather than to a BCVI.
  - Although uncommon, patients with mild TBI can develop BCVI.
- Clinicians need to maintain a high index of suspicion in order to expediently identify these conditions.

BLUNT CEREBROVASCULAR INJURY

Description

- Can present in up to 9% of patients with severe TBI.[1,2]
- Of patients with BCVI, 10% to 40% may develop stroke, which commonly occurs within the first 72 hours of injury.[2–4]
- Can occur intracranially or extracranially, either in the internal carotid artery or in the vertebral artery; occur extracranially more commonly than intracranially.
  - Carotid artery injuries significantly outnumber vertebral artery injuries.[5]
  - Can be bilateral 30% to 40% of the time.[6]
  - Usually, there is no external evidence of trauma over the affected vessel.
  - The Denver Scale, or the Biffl Scale, is a widely used classification scheme based on imaging findings.[3,7]
- Grade I: luminal irregularity or dissection with <25% luminal narrowing
- Grade II: dissection or intramural hematoma with ≥25% luminal narrowing
- Grade III: traumatic aneurysms
- Grade IV: vessel occlusion
- Grade V: vessel transection

The full reference list appears in the digital product found on http://connect.springerpub.com/content/book/978-0-8261-4768-4/part/part04/chapter/ch58

▪ Screening criteria have been proposed in asymptomatic patients. Although the specific criteria vary, most recommend screening, via imaging, all patients with significant TBI, especially if high-velocity and/or accompanied by other traumatic injuries.[4,8–10]

▪ An example of a screening algorithm can be found online.[11]

TRAUMATIC ARTERIAL DISSECTION

▪ Traumatic arterial dissection may occur either within the connective tissue and vasa vasorum of the media or, more commonly, within the intima.[12] Involvement of the media or adventitia can result in aneurysms, pseudoaneurysms, or fistulae.

▪ Can occur as a result of stretch injury or direct trauma, resulting in a tear in the wall of an artery (dissection), which allows intrusion of blood within the layers of the arterial wall.

▪ Intimal disruption can lead to thrombus formation, which can result in vascular obstruction in situ and/or result in distal embolization. Expansion of the subintimal blood causes luminal narrowing, sometimes resulting in obstruction.

Clinical Presentation

▪ Symptoms may be a result of local effects or due to ischemia.

▪ Often, but not always, local symptoms precede the development of ischemia. Therefore, early recognition of local symptoms and timely intervention may reduce the risk of the development of ischemia.

Extracranial Carotid Artery Dissection

Local Symptoms

▪ Headache and neck pain are usually the most prominent symptoms.[12] The pain is typically ipsilateral, sharp or constant, and affects the jaw and face or frontoparietal area.

▪ Patients may report pulsatile tinnitus or a subjective bruit.

▪ A partial Horner's syndrome (miosis and ptosis) can be seen on the ipsilateral side as a result of involvement of the sympathetic fibers that travel along the internal carotid artery.

▪ Ipsilateral cranial nerve palsies can also be seen. The lower cranial nerves are more often involved, with taste disturbance and tongue weakness being the most common manifestations.[12]

Ischemic Symptoms

▪ Ischemic symptoms (cerebral or retinal) are common in carotid dissections, occurring in the majority of patients[13] and resulting in either transient ischemic attacks or infarctions.

▪ Ischemic symptoms usually follow local symptoms by hours or days.

▪ Specific symptoms are referable to the vascular territories of the involved vessel and can include visual loss (e.g., amaurosis fugax), aphasia, hemiparesis, and so on.

Extracranial Vertebral Artery Dissection

Local Symptoms

▪ Neck pain, often severe, is the most prominent local symptom. The pain is primarily located in the ipsilateral occipitocervical region.

Ischemic Symptoms

- Ischemic symptoms may not occur if there is adequate collateral circulation.
- When ischemic symptoms occur, symptoms usually reflect involvement of brainstem or cerebellar structures and can include ataxia, vertigo, dysarthria, and diplopia.

Intracranial Dissection

- Ischemic symptoms, not local symptoms, are usually the first manifestation. Ischemic symptoms tend to be more severe than in extracranial dissection.
- Intracranial dissections are much more likely to rupture, resulting in subarachnoid hemorrhage.[12]

Imaging

- Although digital subtraction angiography (DSA) remains the gold standard, noninvasive options, especially computed tomography angiography (CTA), are frequently used for screening.[1,8,10,14]

Treatment

- Treatment is broadly divided into medical and interventional.
- Treatment is geared toward prevention of extension of the dissection and/or vessel occlusion/cerebral ischemia.
- Medical treatment consists of either antiplatelet therapy or anticoagulation. Although anticoagulation has generally been viewed as the primary therapeutic approach, recent studies found that there is currently not enough evidence to definitively recommend one modality over another.[3,15] Early and uninterrupted antithrombotic treatment is often helpful in preventing ischemic stroke.[10,16] However, the bleeding risk needs to be carefully weighed against the protective effects in the setting of polytrauma.[3]
- Interventional treatment includes surgery, stenting, or balloon occlusion.
- Choice of treatment depends on many factors including the patient's symptoms, time course of symptom progression, nature of lesion, etiology of ischemia (e.g., embolic vs. vessel occlusion), patient's overall neurological status, contraindications to certain treatments (e.g., anticoagulation), and availability of newer interventional modalities.
- Most patients will require follow-up imaging to monitor status of the BCVI, especially if being treated medically.[10]

CAROTID-CAVERNOUS FISTULA

Description

- Although fistulas can occur in any artery after dissection or occlusion, the most common posttraumatic fistula occurs between the internal carotid artery and the cavernous sinus.[13]
- The cavernous sinuses contain a number of venous channels. They are located on either side of the sella turcica and posterior to the orbits.
- A number of important structures pass through the cavernous sinus, including the internal carotid artery and cranial nerves (CN) III, IV, V, and VI.
- Although there are several different types of CCFs, by far the most common after trauma is one in which a fistula develops directly between the internal carotid artery and the cavernous sinus. These traumatic CCFs are known as Barrow type A CCF or

direct CCF.[17] Traumatic CCFs represent high-flow shunts because there is shunting of blood between a high-flow arterial system and a low-flow venous system. The high-flow shunt created by the CCF increases venous resistance, which impedes the venous drainage into the cavernous sinus.

- Although traumatic CCFs can develop at the time of or shortly after the initial injury, they can also develop much later, when an initially injured internal carotid artery finally erodes or ruptures into the cavernous sinus.
- Bilateral traumatic CCFs have been reported.[18]

Clinical Presentation

- The symptoms of traumatic CCFs are a result of vascular congestion in the regions that are normally drained by the cavernous sinus.
- Orbital and periorbital manifestations are the most common and include ipsilateral chemosis, scleral injection, proptosis (sometimes pulsatile), and pain.
- An orbital or facial bruit may be auscultated.[19,20]
- Extraocular palsy (especially of CN VI) and diminished visual acuity can also occur.
- Increased intraocular pressure (because of impaired aqueous humor drainage through the canals of Schlemm) may result in glaucoma and loss of vision (ischemic optic neuropathy).[19]
- In addition to orbital and ophthalmic symptoms, patients may complain of headache, epistaxis, upper facial numbness, and tinnitus (often described as buzzing or "swishing").[18]
- The possibility of significant or even complete visual loss (from retinal hypoxia and/or ischemic optic neuropathy) warrants early detection and management of a traumatic CCF.[18] Other serious complications include cerebral ischemia (because of "vascular steal") and hemorrhage, both subarachnoid and parenchymal.

Imaging

The gold standard modality is four-vessel DSA. However, CTA and MR angiography (MRA) are often used as first-line noninvasive imaging modalities to evaluate CCFs.[21]

Treatment

- Traumatic CCFs are most often treated with endovascular techniques.[13,18] These include the use of balloons, liquid embolic agents, and coils to achieve occlusion or embolization.[22]
- Direct surgical repair may be indicated in some cases.[13]
- Although closure of the fistula usually results in resolution of most symptoms, visual function may not return because of permanent injury to the optic nerve.[20]

TRAUMATIC INTRACRANIAL ANEURYSM

Description

- Traumatic intracranial aneurysms (TICAs), although rare, are associated with significant morbidity and mortality rates of 50% after rupture.[23]
- Although more often associated with severe TBI, they can occur after even mild head trauma.[23]
- Traumatic aneurysms can be classified by both histological type and location.

- Histologically, TICAs fall into one of three main categories:
  - True aneurysms involve disruption of the intima and media with preservation of the adventitia, which forms the aneurysm wall.
  - In false aneurysms (or pseudoaneurysms), all three layers (intima, media, and adventitia) are disrupted and the extravasated blood is contained only by arachnoid, brain parenchyma, or the hematoma itself.
  - Mixed aneurysms represent false aneurysms that are formed after the contained rupture of a true aneurysm.
- TICAs are also classified by their anatomic location. In particular, they can be distinguished by whether they arise proximal or distal to the circle of Willis.
  - Aneurysms that arise proximal to the circle of Willis can involve the carotid artery (either the supraclinoid or the intraclinoid segment) or the vertebrobasilar arteries.
  - Aneurysms that arise distal to the circle of Willis involve cortical or subcortical arteries (or their branches).

Clinical Presentation

- The clinical presentation depends on whether the aneurysm has ruptured or not. Unfortunately, most aneurysms are asymptomatic until rupture, thereby minimizing the possibility of early detection.
- Patients with supraclinoid carotid artery aneurysms can present with headache, memory disturbance, and visual changes before rupture. Patients with unruptured infraclinoid carotid artery aneurysms can present with cranial nerve deficits, diabetes insipidus, recurrent epistaxis, or symptoms of a CCF.[23,24]
- Most traumatic aneurysms present after rupturing, resulting in subdural, subarachnoid, or intraparenchymal hemorrhages. Symptoms of a ruptured aneurysm typically include decreased level of consciousness, focal neurological deficit, and/or seizure.
- The average time from initial trauma to aneurysmal hemorrhage is approximately 21 days, although rupture can be delayed for months or even years.[23]

Imaging

- Because TICAs are rare, routine screening is not recommended.[25]
- Unruptured aneurysms are difficult to detect with routine, noncontrast computed tomography (CT) or magnetic resonance imaging (MRI) scans. CTA or MRA may be considered, especially given the cost and risk of complications associated with DSA, the diagnostic gold standard.[23]
- After rupture, CT or MRI will demonstrate intracranial hemorrhage. DSA should be performed as soon as possible in order to identify the underlying lesion.

Treatment

- The goal of treatment is to exclude the aneurysm from the circulation by surgical or endovascular methods.
- Endovascular procedures are more difficult with traumatic aneurysms because of the lack of an aneurysmal neck, the extent of the arterial wall involved, the fragile nature of these aneurysms, and the lack of a defined wall in cases of pseudoaneurysm. Despite this, endovascular techniques utilizing balloons, flow diversion, or embolization with detachable coils have been used with some success.[23,26]
- Surgical clipping has advantages in that it allows for removal of the hematoma, provides definitive isolation of the aneurysm, and allows for the reconstruction of the parent artery, if needed.[23] Otherwise, trapping, excision, and wrapping of the aneurysm may be viable options.[27]

▧ Ultimately, considerations such as aneurysm structure, location, clinical status of the patient, and availability of appropriately skilled personnel will dictate the optimal treatment method.

KEY POINTS

▧ Although uncommon, BCVI after TBI can have devastating consequences.
▧ Most often seen after TBI are arterial dissections, CCFs, and TICAs.
▧ Clinicians should familiarize themselves with the clinical presentations of these complications and maintain a high index of suspicion in order to expediently identify these conditions.

STUDY QUESTIONS

1. What is the most common manifestation of BCVI?
   a. CCF
   b. Arterial dissection
   c. TICA
   d. Arterial transection

2. Which of the following is true about BCVI after TBI?
   a. Vertebral artery injuries outnumber carotid artery injuries
   b. There is usually evidence of trauma over the affected vessel
   c. Symptoms may mimic those related to the TBI itself
   d. Patients with mild TBI are not at risk for development of BCVI

3. On the Denver Scale, a dissection or an intramural hematoma with ≥25% luminal narrowing indicates:
   a. Grade I
   b. Grade II
   c. Grade III
   d. Grade IV
   e. Grade V

4. Which of the following symptoms is unlikely to be caused by extracranial carotid artery dissection?
   a. Horner's syndrome
   b. Taste disturbance and tongue weakness
   c. Aphasia and hemiparesis
   d. Dysarthria and diplopia
   e. Amaurosis fugax

5. Which of the following is true about TICAs?
   a. Although TICAs are rare, routine screening is recommended
   b. In true aneurysms, all three layers (intima, media, and adventitia) are disrupted
   c. Most aneurysms are usually asymptomatic until rupture
   d. The average time from initial trauma to aneurysmal hemorrhage is around 7 days

The authors would like to recognize and thank Ana Durand-Sanchez, MD, and Michael Green, MD, for their contributions to previous versions of this chapter.

ADDITIONAL READING

Anatomy of the cavernous sinus: https://radiopaedia.org/articles/cavernous-sinus?lang=us

Plitt A, Kafka B, Rickert K. Blunt cervical vascular injury. In: Madden C, Jallo J, eds. *Neurotrauma*. Oxford University Press; 2020:121–128. doi:10.1093/med/9780190936259.003.0014

Kafka B, Plitt A, Rickert K. Blunt intracranial cerebrovascular injury. In: Madden C, Jallo J, eds. *Neurotrauma*. Oxford University Press; 2020:129–136. doi:10.1093/med/9780190936259.003.0015

Esnault P, Cardinale M, Boret H, et al. Blunt cerebrovascular injuries in severe traumatic brain injury: incidence, risk factors, and evolution. *J Neurosurg*. 2017;127(1):16–22. doi:10.3171/2016.4.JNS152600

Brommeland T, Helseth E, Aarhus M, et al. Best practice guidelines for blunt cerebrovascular injury (BCVI). *Scand J Trauma Resusc Emerg Med*. 2018;26(1):90. doi:10.1186/s13049-018-0559-1

Kim DY, Biffl W, Bokhari F, et al. Evaluation and management of blunt cerebrovascular injury: a practice management guideline from the Eastern Association for the Surgery of Trauma. *J Trauma Acute Care Surg*. 2020; 88(6):875–887. doi:10.1097/TA.0000000000002668

ANSWERS TO STUDY QUESTIONS

1. Correct Answer: b

High-energy, nonpenetrating trauma can result in a disruption in one or more layers of the cervical carotid or vertebral artery wall (dissection). The most common manifestation of BCVI, especially in extracranial arteries, is arterial dissection. CCF and TICA are uncommon.

Further Reading:

Harrigan M. Ischemic stroke due to blunt traumatic cerebrovascular injury. *Stroke*. 2020;51(1):353–360. doi:10.1161/STROKEAHA.119.026810.

2. Correct Answer: c

Carotid artery injuries significantly outnumber vertebral artery injuries. Usually, there is no external evidence of trauma over the affected vessel. Although uncommon, patients with mild TBI can still develop BCVI.

Further Reading:

Thanvi B, Munshi SK, Dawson SL, Robinson TG. Carotid and vertebral artery dissection syndromes. *Postgrad Med J*. 2005; 81(956):383–388. doi:10.1136/pgmj.2003.016774.

3. Correct Answer: b

Grade II is defined as dissection or intramural hematoma with ≥25% luminal narrowing.

Further Reading:

Biffl WL, Moore EE, Offner PJ, et al. Blunt carotid arterial injuries: implications of a new grading scale. *J Trauma*. 1999; 47(5):845–853. doi:10.1097/00005373-199911000-00004.

4. Correct Answer: d

Dysarthria and diplopia occur in extracranial vertebral artery dissection.

Further Reading:

Thanvi B, Munshi SK, Dawson SL, Robinson TG. Carotid and vertebral artery dissection syndromes. *Postgrad Med J*. 2005; 81(956):383–388. doi:10.1136/pgmj.2003.016774.

5. Correct Answer: c

Because TICAs are rare, routine screening is not recommended. In false (pseudo) aneurysms, all three layers (intima, media, and adventitia) are disrupted. The average time from initial trauma to aneurysmal hemorrhage is around 21 days.

Further Reading:

Larson PS, Reisner A, Morassutti DJ, et al. Traumatic intracranial aneurysms. *Neurosurg Focus*. 2000; 8(1):e4. doi:10.3171/foc.2000.8.1.1829.

Zangbar B, Wynne J, Joseph B, et al. Traumatic intracranial aneurysm in blunt trauma. *Brain Inj*. 2015; 29(5):601–606. doi:10.3109/02699052.2015.1004559.

REFERENCES

The full reference list appears in the digital product found on http://connect.springerpub.com/content/book/978-0-8261-4768-4/part/part04/chapter/ch58

V

SPECIAL CONSIDERATIONS AND TRAUMATIC BRAIN INJURY RESOURCES

PEDIATRIC CONSIDERATIONS IN TRAUMATIC BRAIN INJURY CARE

SHARIEF TARAMAN, RACHEL PEARSON, AND JONATHAN ROMAIN

GENERAL PRINCIPLES

Definitions

Pediatric traumatic brain injury (TBI) is injury to the brain from a biomechanical etiology occurring in patients under 18 years of age, including inflicted abusive head trauma and sport-related concussions, but excluding obstetrical complications.

Pediatric concussion, a form of mild TBI (MTBI), is a traumatically induced disturbance of neurological function and mental state, occurring with or without loss of consciousness; this generally occurs without evidence of gross structural pathology on acute neuroimaging with functional disturbances resolving over time.[1]

Epidemiology

TBI is a leading cause of morbidity/mortality among pediatric patients, and it is responsible for the majority of trauma-related hospitalizations and deaths in the pediatric population. While children are generally viewed as having better outcomes than adults, TBI sustained at a young age (less than 4 years old) typically results in worse long-term prognosis.[2,3]

MTBI accounts for approximately 80% of pediatric TBI; a significant proportion of this is secondary to recreation and sport-related injuries.[2] It is estimated that 1.6 to 3.8 million sport-related concussions occur in the United States per year in all ages.[2] Among high school athletes, 5% to 6% of all injuries involve the head.[4] Youth athletes represent the largest at-risk population for sport-related concussion, with an estimated 135,000 high school athletes sustaining concussions/MTBIs annually.[5] After a single concussion, the risk of sustaining another concussion during the same season increases threefold.[6]

Classification

Uses modified pediatric Glasgow Coma Scale (GCS)[7]:

- Mild: GCS 13 to 15, includes concussion, constitutes 75% to 85% of all head injuries
- Complicated mild: GCS 13 to 15 with evidence of intracranial pathology (contusions, hemorrhage, axonal injury, etc.)
- Moderate: GCS 9 to 12
- Severe: GCS 3 to 8 after initial resuscitation

The full reference list appears in the digital product found on http://connect.springerpub.com/content/book/978-0-8261-4768-4/part/part05/chapter/ch59

- Limitations in pediatrics: difficult to assess verbal score in preverbal infants and older children with language/developmental delays; pediatric GCS may be used for children under 2 years old.

Pathophysiology

Specific pediatric implications:

- Concussion/MTBI—often recurrent in child and adolescent contact sports. Multiple potential physiological injury mechanisms may occur following concussive impact. These include spreading neuronal depression/migraine, seizure activity, changes in cerebral blood flow, perturbations of brain metabolism, altered neuronal activation, neurotransmitter disruption, and/or axonal dysfunction, blood–brain barrier disruption, and/or activation of inflammatory pathways.
- Contusion—less common in infants/toddlers than in adolescents or adults.
- Diffuse cerebral edema—more common in infants/toddlers than in adolescents or adults.
- Diffuse axonal/shearing injury—frontal white matter networks (controlling attention, executive function, and emotion) are not fully mature until the early 20s. In infants, unmyelinated white matter may be particularly vulnerable.
- Hypoxia-ischemia—particularly associated with abusive head trauma, especially infants.
- Penetrating injuries—rare in pediatrics.
- Seizures—more common in infants and younger children than adolescents/adults.
- Skull fractures—slightly more common in younger children.

Mechanism

The most common mechanisms of pediatric TBI vary by age group:

- Infants: inflicted abusive head trauma (due to shaking and/or impact; may be recurrent or have delayed presentation, often with concurrent hypoxic-ischemic injury) and falls
- Toddlers: falls
- Children/adolescents: motor vehicle accidents and sport-related concussions

PEDIATRIC CONCUSSION AND MILD TRAUMATIC BRAIN INJURY—ASSESSMENT

Signs and Symptoms

Usually self-limited, with the majority (70%–85%) resolving within 21 days. In general, however, adolescents and patients with certain pre-existing conditions have longer recovery periods.[8,9]

- *Acute symptoms and signs:* essentially mirror those seen in adults. Subjective symptoms are more challenging to assess in young children, and the practitioner should take care to avoid suggestibility that can bias symptom reporting. Common, freely available tools such as the Sport Concussion Assessment Tool — 5th edition (SCAT5) and Child

SCAT5 are used to quantify symptoms using a Likert scale; however, formal validation in pediatric patients, especially under age 5 years, is still lacking.[10]

- *Risk factors for prolonged symptoms*: Persistent postconcussion symptoms, commonly defined as symptoms lasting for more than 3 months from time of injury, occurs in 13% to 30% of pediatric patients.[11] Risk factors for prolonged recovery include history of a prior concussion with prolonged recovery, adolescent age, certain pre-existing comorbidities (migraine, attention-deficit/hyperactivity disorder [ADHD], learning disability, or psychiatric diagnosis), lower socioeconomic status, and family history of migraine, psychiatric disorder, or learning disability.[12]

Physical Exam

- General physical exam should include a thorough neck exam to assess range of motion, discomfort with any particular movements, and/or tenderness to palpation.
- Neurological exam with emphasis on mental status (helpful to use Standardized Assessment of Concussion from SCAT5 or Child SCAT5), vestibular-ocular motor screening (VOMS), and balance testing.
- Ancillary testing that may be helpful includes the Balance Error Scoring System (BESS) or modified BESS, King Devick, and/or reaction time.

Diagnostic Testing

- Neuroimaging is typically not indicated for MTBI. Validated neuroimaging rules, such as the Pediatric Head Injury/Trauma Algorithm (PECARN), should be employed in acute care settings.[13]
- Serum biomarkers are not validated for clinical use in pediatric MTBI.[1]
- Neuropsychological testing may aid in the management of concussion, especially in situations of unreliability of patient self-report.[14] Results from neuropsychological testing should be interpreted in the context of other variables, including academic history, mental health history, and effort to task, as these factors can influence test performance; it should never be used as a stand-alone diagnostic tool or to make definitive return-to-play recommendations.

PEDIATRIC CONCUSSION AND MILD TRAUMATIC BRAIN INJURY—MANAGEMENT

Guiding Principles

Specific pediatric-focused recommendations have been published by the American Academy of Neurology (2013), the American Academy of Pediatrics (2018), and the Ontario Neurotrauma Foundation (2019).[15–17] Pediatric considerations are also mentioned in the Consensus Statement on Concussion in Sport (2016).[18] In addition, the Centers for Disease Control and Prevention has published the HEADS UP to Youth Sports Initiative to provide concussion education to athletes, coaches, and parents.[19]

Management of Sport-Related Concussion

Issues unique to pediatric concussion include:

- *School:* May require adjustments for cognitive, behavioral, and/or fine motor deficits.[20–22]

- Initial support: Alert school personnel to injury, reintegrate into school progressively with goal of preventing prolonged absence from school, provide extra assistance, adjust educational curricula as needed, and provide time and resources to facilitate completion of makeup work.[23]
- General school-based support: Monitor student carefully for a period following recovery. Watch for subtle cognitive or behavioral problems.
- Specific classroom-based support: Delay or provide additional time for tests, offer flexibility for assignment due dates, provide preferential seating to allow for closer monitoring and less distraction, provide examples of completed work, allow rest breaks or partial days as needed.

■ ***Return to play***: Concerns guiding return-to-play recommendations include mitigating risk of Second Impact Syndrome (SIS), repeat injury, and/or worsened symptoms after repeated concussions. Additionally, concerns exist that multiple concussions may lead to persistent postconcussive symptoms, chronic neurocognitive impairment, or chronic traumatic encephalopathy; however, a causal connection remains unclear and further studies are needed to better understand the relationship between repetitive head trauma and chronic neurocognitive sequeulae.[24,25]

PEDIATRIC MODERATE TO SEVERE TRAUMATIC BRAIN INJURY

Note: Initial management MUST start concurrently with initial assessment.

History

- Risk factors for worse outcome: Developmental delay/learning disabilities, comorbid medical conditions (coagulopathy, epilepsy, psychiatric disorder), low-socioeconomic status, prior TBI.
- Symptoms of TBI in children are similar to those seen in adults, with the exception that subjective symptoms (pain, dizziness, etc.) may be challenging to assess in preverbal or developmentally delayed individuals. Parental assessment of whether the child is different from baseline is helpful.

Physical Examination

The following exam considerations are unique to the pediatric population:

- General physical exam for other signs of trauma:
  - External signs of head injury—assess for bulging fontanelle.
  - Other physical exam findings—retinal hemorrhages, burns, multiple old scars/bruises/fractures—may indicate abuse-related injury.
  - Neurological exam findings—assess age-specific reflexes.

Laboratory Studies

CBC, chemistry panel, toxicology screen (particularly for adolescents)

Radiographic Assessment

- A skeletal survey may be indicated to rule out inflicted trauma.
- Validated neuroimaging rules, such as PECARN, should be employed in acute care settings.[13] Imaging indications are otherwise similar to those used for adults.

Neurodiagnostic Studies

Continuous video electroencephalography (cvEEG) is helpful in identifying subtle/subclinical seizures, which may occur in roughly 15% of children with moderate to severe TBI.[26]

MODERATE TO SEVERE PEDIATRIC TRAUMATIC BRAIN INJURY—MANAGEMENT

Guiding Principles

See Guidelines for the Management of Pediatric Severe Traumatic Brain Injury, third edition.[3]

Initial Management

- ABCs (airway, breathing, circulation, etc.)
- Assess GCS score: if 3 to 14, obtain head computed tomography (CT). Consider insertion of intracranial pressure (ICP) monitor if GCS <8 or if any evidence of herniation, hydrocephalus, or intraventricular hemorrhage; maintain cerebral perfusion pressure.
- Stepwise approach to treating elevated ICP.
- If diffuse swelling on CT: consider decompression via craniectomy with duraplasty.
- If active ictal focus on EEG: consider high-dose barbiturates or other anticonvulsants.
- Prophylactic moderate (32°C to 33°C) hypothermia, while not recommended, may be used for ICP control in some instances.

Supportive Care

- Acute seizure prophylaxis may be warranted (first 7 days post-injury only) but its role is unproven in children. Prophylactic use of antiseizure medications has not been shown to decrease long-term risk of posttraumatic epilepsy.
- Nutrition: early caloric supplementation greater than 130% to 160% of resting metabolic requirements.
- General care: oral hygiene, skin care/decubitus ulcer prevention, corneal protection, bowel/bladder regimen.
- Institute early intervention with physical therapy, occupational therapy, and speech therapy.

Treatment Controversies

- Many sedatives and anticonvulsants show developmental toxicity in animal models (exceptions: topiramate, levetiracetam), and therefore use, if necessitated, should be undertaken with caution.[27]

KEY POINTS

- Outcomes after TBI are generally viewed as better in children than adults; however, TBI sustained in younger age groups (less than 4 years) actually results in worse long-term prognosis.
- Patients may require accommodations for cognitive, behavioral, and/or fine motor deficits, specifically with respect to schooling.
- cvEEG is helpful in identifying subtle/subclinical seizures, which may occur in roughly 15% of children with moderate to severe TBI.

STUDY QUESTIONS

1. Which of the following factors are associated with prolonged recovery time after pediatric concussion?
   a. History of migraine
   b. History of ADHD
   c. History of depression
   d. Prior concussion with prolonged recovery
   e. All of the above

2. Which of the following is more commonly seen after TBI in infants and young children than in adolescents and adults?
   a. Posttraumatic headache
   b. Mood disturbance
   c. Seizures
   d. Elevated ICP.

3. A 14-year-old male presents to the emergency department after sustaining a head injury while skateboarding without a helmet and falling. There was no loss of consciousness; however, the patient does not recall walking home after his injury. His parents brought him to the emergency department where he is alert and oriented. His exam is notable for clear fluid drainage from his nose and hemotympanum on the left side. What is the appropriate next step in management for this patient?
   a. Stat magnetic resonance imaging (MRI) brain
   b. Stat head CT
   c. Observe overnight (without imaging)
   d. Discharge from the emergency department

4. Which of the following tools is most helpful in the routine assessment of acute pediatric concussion?
   a. MRI brain
   b. Serum biomarker panel
   c. SCAT5 or the Child SCAT
   d. BESS

5. Which of the following may affect results on neuropsychological testing after concussion?
   a. Sleep disturbance
   b. History of learning disability
   c. History of ADHD
   d. Posttraumatic headache
   e. All of the above

ADDITIONAL READING

CDC concussion website: http://www.cdc.gov/concussion/HeadsUp/youth.html

Swaiman KF, Ashwal S, Ferriero DM. *Pediatric Neurology: Principles and Practice.* 6th ed. Elsevier; 2017 (Part XII). doi:10.1016/j.pediatrneurol.2017.01.021

Kochanek PM, Tasker RC, Carney N, et al. Guidelines for the management of pediatric severe traumatic brain injury, 3rd ed. Update of the Brain Trauma Foundation guidelines. *Pediatr Crit Care Med.* 2019;20:S1–S82. https://pubmed.ncbi.nlm.nih.gov/30829890

McCrory P, Meeuwisse W, Dvorak J, et al. Consensus statement on concussion in sport—the 5th International Conference on Concussion in Sport held in Berlin, October 2016. *Br J Sports Med.* 2017;51(11):838–847. doi:10.1136/bjsports-2017-097699

ANSWERS TO STUDY QUESTIONS

1. Correct Answer: e

Risk factors for prolonged recovery and persistent post-concussive symptoms include personal or family history of migraine, ADHD, learning disability, mood disorder, anxiety, sleep disturbance, female sex, adolescent age group, and lower socioeconomic status.

Further Readings:

Halstead ME, Walter KD, Moffatt K. Sport-related concussion in children and adolescents. *Pediatrics.* 2018;142(6). doi:10.1542/peds.2018-3074

Barlow KM. Postconcussion syndrome: a review. *J Child Neurol.* 2016;31(1):57–67. doi:10.1177/0883073814543305

2. Correct Answer: c

Infants and young children are more likely to have posttraumatic seizures than adolescents and adults. Infants are less likely to have elevated ICP due to open fontanels and sutures.

Further Reading:

Arndt DH, Goodkin HP, Giza CC. Early posttraumatic seizures in the pediatric population. *J Child Neurol.* 2016;31(1):46–56. doi:10.1177/0883073814562249

3. Correct Answer: b

According to PECARN criteria, patients with GCS <14, altered mental status, or signs of basilar skull fracture should have further evaluation with a head CT. Head CT versus observation is appropriate for patients with severe mechanism of injury, severe headache, recurrent vomiting, or loss of consciousness >5 seconds. This patient has cerebrospinal fluid (CSF) rhinorrhea and hemotympanum, concerning for basilar skull fracture.

Further Reading:

Kuppermann N, Holmes JF, Dayan PS, et al. Identification of children at very low risk of clinically important brain injuries after head trauma: a prospective cohort study. *Lancet.* 2009;374(9696):1160–1170. doi:10.1016/S0140-6736(09)61558-0

4. Correct Answer: c

The SCAT5 and Child SCAT are validated tools that evaluate postconcussive symptoms and neurological functioning. While balance tests have been shown to be useful in older adolescents with sport-related concussion, symptom scales and cognitive tests are generally helpful in assessing recovery and predicting outcomes. Structural abnormalities are not typically seen on neuroimaging in concussion, and imaging is typically not indicated. No serum biomarkers have been validated in pediatric concussion.

Further Reading:
Lumba-Brown A, Yeates KO, Sarmiento K, et al. Centers for Disease Control and Prevention guideline on the diagnosis and management of mild traumatic brain injury among children. *JAMA Pediatr.* 2018;172(11):e182853. doi:10.1001/jamapediatrics.2018.2853

5. Correct Answer: e
Persistent cognitive difficulties in the context of more minor injury, such as concussion, raise suspicion for external variables, including pre-existing ADHD, learning disability, and developmental delay. Additionally, pain, insomnia, depressed mood, anxiety, acute stress reactions, and posttraumatic stress disorder can develop as a result of TBI, and these too can affect test performance.

Further Reading:
Corwin DJ, Zonfrillo MR, Master CL, et al. Characteristics of prolonged concussion recovery in a pediatric subspecialty referral population. *J Pediatr.* 2014;165(6):1207–1215. doi:10.1016/j.jpeds.2014.08.034

REFERENCES

The full reference list appears in the digital product found on http://connect.springer-pub.com/content/book/978-0-8261-4768-4/part/part05/chapter/ch59

SPECIAL CONSIDERATIONS IN CARING FOR THE WORKERS' COMPENSATION PATIENT

FELISE S. ZOLLMAN

BACKGROUND

The need for a no-fault workers' compensation (WC) system came into being in the context of the emergence of modern industrial society. In the United States, the first state-specific WC legislation was enacted in Maryland in 1902,[1] followed by Congress' 1906 Employers' Liability Act.[2] This legislation shifted the traditional view that employees accepted the risk associated with the work they did, and could only sue if they could prove gross negligence on the part of the employer, to the notion that employers bore responsibility for providing a safe work environment. The first federal WC system in the United States was enacted in 1908 in the form of the Federal Employer Liability Act, which covered railway workers. The first state WC system was established in Wisconsin in 1911. The last state to put such a system in place was Mississippi, in 1948.[1,2]

The core concept of WC is that it is a no-fault compensation system in which the employee is entitled to collect a percentage of lost wages and have medical and rehabilitation care paid for by the employer or the employers' agent or insurer. In return, the employee may not sue the employer because of the injury.

WORKERS' COMPENSATION AND TRAUMATIC BRAIN INJURY

Much of the available data on the incidence, prevalence, and costs associated with traumatic brain injury (TBI) in the context of the WC system comes from a few select states such as Washington, because these states have created a single large State Fund, which covers the vast majority of workers in the state, and therefore have access to a large centralized database containing injury and claim-related information. A handful of large employers may opt out and serve as their own insurers, and these workers are not reflected in published data. Federal employees covered under federal WC programs are also not included.

Epidemiology

Studies have reported that work-related TBIs (wrTBIs) account for between 5% and 14% of all TBIs.[3] The average annual incidence of wrTBI is approximately 10 per 100,000 full-time equivalent (FTE) employees.[4] The top three causes of wrTBI are falls, motor vehicle accidents, and being struck by objects.[4] A recent study reviewed the number of lost time wrTBIs per FTE position in the state of Ohio.[5] The three top-ranked causes of injury in this study (based on time lost from work claims, not medical claims) were falls to a lower level,

The full reference list appears in the digital product found on http://connect.springerpub.com/content/book/978-0-8261-4768-4/part/part05/chapter/ch60

being struck by an object/equipment, and motor vehicle collisions. The industries with the most lost time from work per FTE were trucking and construction.[5]

The gender differential for occupational injuries is greater than it is in the civilian sector in general: Various studies have suggested a ratio of men to women affected by wrTBI ranging from 2:1 to 10:1.[4,6,7] One Canadian mild TBI (MTBI) study, however, did find a higher *prevalence* of MTBI claims among female employees versus males (although the incidence was 2:1 male:female). The authors postulated that the reversal in gender ratio for prevalence of MTBI might be due to an observed longer duration of claims remaining open for female workers with MTBI.[7] The highest incidence of wrTBI for women was in education and healthcare, and for men, manufacturing, transportation, and construction.[8] The annual case fatality rate for wrTBI is reported by various authors to be between 6.7% and 8%.[6,9]

A study from Washington State published in 2006 reported an annual claim cost per TBI of $25,400. Medical costs were $12,600, time lost was $3,200, and disabled pension benefits were $4,000. Median claim cost was $61,000. This study concluded that the highest risk/most costly industries included logging, construction, janitorial services, and roofing.[6]

Information gleaned from studies such as those described earlier can be helpful in suggesting which industries see the greatest number of days of lost work due to TBI and which causes of TBI may be of most concern for a given industry, leading to a framework for developing industry-specific injury prevention programs.

MANAGEMENT OF WORK-RELATED TRAUMATIC BRAIN INJURY

Personnel

- In addition to the usual clinical care personnel, injured workers are usually followed by a medical case manager (MCM), typically an RN by training. The role of this individual is to direct and move the case forward through the medical or rehabilitation care process and see the case to closure. MCMs are guided by the Code of Professional Conduct for Case Managers (see Additional Reading section).
- WC carriers will typically identify a primary treating physician (PTP) for an injured worker. This physician is the individual who is primarily responsible for managing the treatment of the injured worker. Some states set forth detailed guidelines for PTPs, including case coordination and reporting duties. The American College of Occupational and Environmental Medicine's (ACOEM) treatment guidelines are also a widely recognized tool for steering care for this population (see Additional Reading section).
- WC carriers will also typically assign an adjustor to each case, whose responsibility it is to manage the financial aspect of a claim. The adjustor will typically work in conjunction with the MCM on behalf of the insurance company in monitoring claims-related costs.

Management Approach

Typical injury cases would be expected to progress through a sequence of stages, from acute care to medical rehabilitation to vocational rehabilitation (VR). A study by Wrona revealed, however, that only 48% of TBI survivors seen for acute medical management (identified based on hospital discharge records) progressed to medical rehabilitation; 46% were referred for VR. Sixty-five percent of those referred for VR did ultimately return to the work force. The author hypothesized that the reason a minority of cases were referred for medical rehabilitation was because "most cases do not occur in the area served by clinical model treatment programs and do not follow the clinical trajectory of short intensive initial inpatient care, followed closely by intensive rehabilitation and referral for return to work."[10]

KEY POINTS

■ The WC system was developed to provide a no-fault means of providing injured workers with injury-related care and some measure of compensation for lost wages while shielding employers from accident-related litigation.

■ The top three causes of wrTBI are falls, motor vehicle collisions, and being struck by an object.

■ MCMs typically shepherd cases through the continuum of medical and rehabilitation care, to the point of case closure. Adjustors monitor claims and costs.

■ The majority of injured workers who go through VR do return to the workforce in some capacity.

STUDY QUESTIONS

1. The three most common causes of TBI resulting in lost days of work include all of the following except:
   a. Motor vehicle collisions
   b. Falls on same level
   c. Falls to a lower level
   d. Being struck in the head

2. The following statements about MCMs are all true except
   a. MCMs are typically RNs
   b. MCMs manage an injured worker's case from care needs to claims review
   c. MCMs are involved with a work-related injury case from initial assignment post-injury through rehabilitation/VR needs
   d. The Code of Professional Conduct for Case Managers guides professional practice for MCMs

3. WC coverage is designed to meet all of the following needs except:
   a. Provide a vehicle through which an employee may recover damages through the courts
   b. Compensate an employee who is injured on the job
   c. Cover costs of healthcare associated with work-related injury
   d. Provide oversight of care needs via an MCM

4. Which of the following statements regarding the epidemiology of wrTBI is correct?
   a. wrTBIs account for between 5% and 14% of all TBIs
   b. The gender differential for occupational injuries is the same as is seen in civilian TBI
   c. The highest incidence of wrTBI for women is seen in education and healthcare positions
   d. The highest incidence of wrTBI for men is seen in manufacturing, transportation, and construction

ADDITIONAL READING

Case Manager Code of Conduct: https://ccmcertification.org/sites/default/files/docs/2018/ccmc-18-code-of-conduct_1.pdf

American College of Occupational and Environmental Medicine's (ACOEM) treatment guidelines: https://www.dir.ca.gov/dwc/MTUS/MTUS-Guidelines.html

Rondinelli, R. *Guidelines to the Evaluation of Permanent Impairment*. 6th ed. American Medical Association; 2007.

Wrona RM. Disability and return to work outcomes after traumatic brain injury: results from the Washington state industrial insurance fund. *Disabil Rehabil*. 2010;32(8):650–655. doi:10.3109/09638280903186327

ANSWERS TO STUDY QUESTIONS

1. Correct Answer: b
The three most common causes of TBI resulting in time lost from work include falls to a lower level, blows to the head from objects/equipment, and motor vehicle collisions.

Further Reading:
Konda S, Al-Tarawneh IS, Reichard AA, et al. Workers' compensation claims for traumatic brain injuries among private employers—Ohio, 2001–2011. *Am J Ind Med*. 2020;63:156–169 doi:10.1002/ajim.23073

2. Correct Answer: b
Adjustors handle the financial aspect of an injured worker's case, not MCMs.

Further Reading:
Case Manager Code of Conduct: https://ccmcertification.org/sites/default/files/docs/2018/ccmc-18-code-of-conduct_1.pdf

3. Correct Answer: a
WC is a no-fault system. The employee is entitled to a portion of wages and medical/rehabilitation care. In return, the injured worker may not sue the employer because of the injury.

Further Reading:
Guyton GP. A brief history of workers' compensation. *Iowa Orthop J*. 1999;19:106–110.

4. Correct Answer: b
The gender differential is greater for wrTBI than for civilian TBI, with a larger proportion of wrTBI occurring in men.

Further Reading:
Chang VC, Ruseckaite R, Collie A, Colantonio A. Examining the epidemiology of work-related traumatic brain injury through a sex/gender lens: analysis of workers' compensation claims. *Occup Environ Med*. 2014;71:695–703. doi:10.1136/oemed-2014-102097

REFERENCES

The full reference list appears in the digital product found on http://connect.springer-pub.com/content/book/978-0-8261-4768-4/part/part05/chapter/ch60

DEVELOPING A LIFE CARE PLAN

ROGER O. WEED AND DEBRA E. BERENS

BACKGROUND

- Definition: "A life care plan is a dynamic document based upon published standards of practice, comprehensive assessment, data analysis and research, which provides an organized concise plan for current and future needs with associated costs, for individuals who have experienced catastrophic injury or have chronic health care needs."[1]
- Use: Identification of lifelong anticipated care for patients/clients who will not fully recover (i.e., have a permanent disability).
- Historical relevance: The term "life care plan" was introduced into the legal literature in 1981 and came to be recognized as a valuable tool within the rehabilitation profession that identifies and projects the effects of catastrophic injury on an individual's future.[1,2]
- Includes expected short- and long-term or lifelong needs and costs of medical care; residential placement (facility and in-home); transportation; home/architectural modifications; medical and nonmedical supplies, equipment, and adaptive devices; physical, occupational, speech, recreational, and other therapies; medications; and other needs as related to, or a result of, the traumatic brain injury (TBI).[1]
- Routine healthcare needs/costs typically are not included in most jurisdictions, as the need or service would have occurred independent of the brain injury. Similarly, pre-existing conditions typically are not included unless the brain injury exacerbated the condition or had another concomitant effect.
- Quality of life considerations may be relevant for the life care planning for many individuals with TBI.[3]

DIAGNOSIS: FOR WHOM IS A LIFE CARE PLAN APPROPRIATE?

- Life care plans for individuals with TBI may be generated for the following situations[2,4–9,10]:
  - Hospital or rehabilitation facility discharge planning
  - Medical-legal cases (e.g., personal injury litigation, medical malpractice litigation, federal litigation, contract law/wrongful adoption)
  - Adoption of special needs children
  - Care planning for older adults
  - Workers' compensation claims
  - FELA (Federal Employees Liability Act) claims
  - Managed care health plans and insurance reserve-setting
  - Trust-funded care for people with disabilities (includes special needs trusts and family-funded trusts)

The full reference list appears in the digital product found on http://connect.springerpub.com/content/book/978-0-8261-4768-4/part/part05/chapter/ch61

- Medicare set-asides
- Vaccine injury fund cases
- Family consulting for lifetime care needs
- Wounded warriors or veterans with injuries

MANAGEMENT: HOW IS A LIFE CARE PLAN GENERATED?

Elements of the Life Care Plan (see also Figure 61.1)[1,10]

These include the following:

- Projected evaluations: nonphysician or allied health evaluations that will occur on a periodic basis. For example, evaluations for physical therapy (PT), occupational therapy (OT), speech-language pathology (SLP), cognitive therapy, dietary/nutrition, therapeutic recreation, music therapy, audiology, vision screening, and/or swallow studies.
- Projected therapeutic modalities: ongoing or episodic treatment generated from the aforementioned evaluations as well as case management, behavior management, individual/family counseling, and/or other recommended therapeutic modalities.
- Diagnostic testing/educational assessments, for example, neuropsychological, psychological, vocational evaluations, and, for children, neurodevelopmental and/or psychoeducational testing.
- Wheelchair needs, accessories, and maintenance: type and configuration of recommended wheelchairs, specialty cushions and covers, carry bags, gloves, and yearly maintenance/service requirements as well as estimated replacements throughout lifetime.
- Aids for independent function (includes assistive technology and adapted devices).
- Orthotics and prosthetics.
- Home furnishing and accessories.
- Drug and supply needs: prescribed and over-the-counter drugs, and supplies including incontinence, feeding, tracheostomy, wound care, and so on.
- Home care/facility care: living in the least restrictive setting is preferred. However, home care may not be the most cost-effective alternative or the most medically appropriate for the client depending on their needs and brain injury sequelae.
  - For clients recommended to live at home, the level of in-home care is identified (e.g., skill level of providers, hours per day the providers are needed, shift care vs. hourly care vs. live-in care).
  - Facility care may be most appropriate for those who have no capability of living at home or whose needs exceed capabilities available in a home environment.
  - There may also be need for specialty programs such as yearly summer camps, brain injury clubhouses, or other productive activity for adults and children.[11]
- Future medical care—routine: typically provided by a physiatrist or neurologist with expertise in brain injury.
- Transportation: adapted driving evaluation and training if the client has potential to drive, vehicle modifications, wheelchair modifications, private driver, or public transportation.
- Health and strength maintenance (a.k.a. recreation and leisure time activities): home exercise program, adapted sports or recreation activities, and gym or health club membership as an avenue for structured exercise and socialization or community integration.

✓ **Projected evaluations**: Have you planned for different types of nonphysician **evaluations** (e.g., physical therapy, speech therapy, recreational therapy, occupational therapy, music therapy, dietary assessment, audiology, vision screening, swallow studies)?

✓ **Projected therapeutic modalities**: What therapies will be needed (based on the evaluations given previously)? Will a case manager help control costs and reduce complications? Is a behavior management or rehab psychologist, pastoral counseling, or family education appropriate?

✓ **Diagnostic testing/educational assessment**: What testing is necessary and at what ages? Vocational evaluation? Neuropsychological? Educational levels? Educational consultant to maximize IDEA?

✓ **Wheelchair needs**: What types and configuration of wheelchairs will the client require—power? Shower? Manual? Specialty? Ventilator? Reclining? Quad pegs? Recreational?

✓ **Wheelchair accessories and maintenance**: Has each chair been listed separately for maintenance and accessories (bags, cushions, trays, etc.)? Have you considered the client's activity level?

✓ **Aids for independent functioning**: What can this individual use to help themselves? Environmental controls? Adaptive aids? Omni-reachers?

✓ **Orthotics/prosthetics**: Will the client need braces? Have you planned for replacement and maintenance?

✓ **Home furnishings and accessories**: Will the client need a specialty bed? Portable ramps? Hoyer or other lift?

✓ **Drug/supply needs**: Have prescription and nonprescription drugs been listed, including size, quantity, and rate at which to be consumed? All supplies such as bladder and bowel program and skin care?

✓ **Home care/facility care**: Is it possible for the client to live at home? How about specialty programs such as yearly camps? What level of care will they require?

✓ **Future medical care—routine**: Is there a need for an annual evaluation? Which medical specialties? Orthopedics? Urology? Internist? Vision? Dental? Lab?

✓ **Transportation**: Are hand controls sufficient or is a specialty van needed? Can local transportation companies be used?

✓ **Health and strength maintenance**: What specialty recreation is needed? Blow darts? Adapted games? Row cycle? Annual dues for specialty magazines? (Specialty wheelchairs should be placed on wheelchair page.)

✓ **Architectural renovations**: Have you considered ramps, hallways, kitchen, fire protection, alternative heating/cooling, floor coverings, bath, attendant room, equipment storage, and so on?

✓ **Future medical care/surgical intervention or aggressive treatment**: Are there plans for aggressive treatment or additional surgeries such as reconstruction?

✓ **Orthopedic equipment needs**: Are walkers, standing tables, tilt tables, body support equipment needed?

✓ **Vocational/educational plan**: What are the costs of vocational counseling, job coaching, tuition, fees, books, supplies, technology, and so on?

✓ **Potential complications**: Have you included a list of potential complications which can occur, such as skin breakdown, infections, psychological trauma, contractures, and so on? (Usually "possible" rather than "probable")

FIGURE 61.1   Life care plan checklist.

Source: Original copyright by Roger O. Weed, Ph.D., 1989, with revisions. Weed R, Berens D. Life care planning after TBI: clinical and forensic issues. In: Zasler N, Katz D, Zafonte R, eds. *Brain injury medicine.* 2nd ed. Demos Medical Publishing; 2012:1437–1453.

- Architectural renovations: typically included for clients who are to be cared for at home.
  - For the military, the Veterans Administration has established certain allowances that are re-evaluated each year. See www.benefits.va.gov/homeloans/adaptedhousing. asp for current allowances.
- Potential complications: conditions for which the client with TBI is at higher risk. Included for information only, as no frequency or duration of complications are typically predictable. Costs of complications generally are not included unless they are "expected" and can be quantified, in which case the expected complication would be listed in the life care plan with the other expected recommendations, and associated cost of the expected complication included.
- Future medical care/surgical intervention or aggressive treatment. Examples include orthopedic or plastic surgery, or admission to address serious behavioral sequelae of TBI.
- Equipment needs/durable medical equipment.
- Vocational/educational plan.

Life Care Plan Authors

- Qualified life care planning authors can be certified by one of three organizations (see Additional Reading).
- Authors of a life care plan may come from a variety of professional settings including rehabilitation consultants, nurses, physicians, and others (see the following).
- Qualified life care planners follow a standard of practice prescribed by their respective organizations.

Life Care Planning Team Members

These include the following:

- *Client or evaluee* (i.e., the person with the disability)[12]: Assuming that the client/evaluee is accessible (i.e., legally permitted) and capable of appropriate interaction, interview them, preferably in-person in their home environment. If not possible, one alternative is to have a videotaped "day in the life" of the client. It is recommended that the client interview take place in the client's residence (home or facility) for (a) client convenience, (b) the opportunity to assess potential home modification needs, and (c) observing medications, equipment, and supplies.
- *Family members/caregivers*
- *Physiatrist or neurologist:*
  - Often designated the team leader.
  - Can assist in establishing medical foundation for a life care plan.[1,13,14]
  - The physician evaluation should include functional limitations, expected future medical treatment including referral to other specialties, review of medications, supplies, and/or durable medical equipment and related topics.
- *Neuropsychologist:* will establish cognitive, affective, behavioral, social, and functional capabilities as well as identify current and future needs, including aging-related needs.
- *Occupational therapist:* addresses seating and positioning needs (may also be done by physical therapist), activities of daily living training, adaptive aids, safety in the residence, and other vocationally related issues.
- *Speech-language pathologist* (may also be called *communication disorders specialist or speech therapist*): identifies speech and language abilities as well as augmentative communication needs for clients with severe communication disorders; cognitive remediation needs, swallowing techniques and feeding/PEG tubes and supplies, and assistive technology recommendations.

- *Physical therapist:* reviews durable medical equipment needs including mobility devices such as wheelchair design and specifications. If appropriate, may conduct a functional capacity evaluation (may also be performed by the occupational therapist).
- *Educational consultant:* identifies needed educational programs/services. Under the federal Individuals with Disabilities Education Act (IDEA), the public school system is responsible for providing specialized services to *eligible* school-age children with disabilities up to the age of 22. Each state also offers early intervention programs for children with brain injury from birth to age 3.
- *Case manager:* coordinates care, liaises with treatment providers, equipment acquisition, and problem-solving support.
- *Vocational evaluator* (if client has work potential): Identifies client's vocational capabilities.[6]
- *Rehabilitation counselor* (a.k.a. vocational *rehabilitation counselor*): assists in coordinating a job and/or labor market analysis. Provides vocational guidance and counseling including job-seeking skills training, job development, selective job placement, supported employment, and/or postplacement services, and may serve as a job coach and/or provide work adjustment training. A rehabilitation counselor with at least a master's degree who holds the national CRC (certified rehabilitation counselor) credential is recommended. (See also Chapter 70 for a more detailed discussion of return-to-work after brain injury.)
- *Economist:* if litigation-related (forensic), calculates the cost of "damages" over the client's lifetime as related to the brain injury. The economist will rely on the base costs of the items and services recommended in the life care plan to project the cost of care throughout the client's life expectancy.[15] Table 61.1 shows an example entry from a life care plan that provides relevant information for the economist to calculate appropriate cost projections. In order for an economist to project the cost of care, certain details must be included in the life care plan, including the expected type and amount of treatment or service, date to start treatment, date to stop treatment, and base cost of treatment (in today's dollars). For products such as durable medical equipment and supplies, include specifications, date to purchase, expected costs, and replacement schedules. It is strongly recommended that the life care planner defer to an economist or other trained and qualified professional to determine the "bottom line" or total lifetime cost of the life care plan, unless (a) they have specific training in this specialized area or (b) they are in a position to apply special rules pertaining to economic projections (e.g., the Alaska Rule) that eliminate complex formulas.

TABLE 61.1 EXAMPLE: Relevant Life Care Plan Information for Economist

Example of Minimum Information Needed for an Economist to Project Costs
Neuropsychiatric evaluation performed in 6/2020 at a cost of $750 (includes complete evaluation with report and recommendations).
Expect counseling to start in 7/2020, frequency one time per week, for 1-hour session each, for 26 weeks at a cost of $150 per hour from PhD-level brain injury counselor or psychologist.
Expect group counseling beginning 1/2021, frequency one time per week for 12 months then one time every 2 weeks for 12 months at a cost of $60 per session.
Expect medical follow-up four times per year until 1/2022 by psychiatrist at a cost of $95 each visit (med check visit only).
Expect medication as prescribed: Prozac, one 20 mg/day, from 7/2020 to 1/2021 at cost of $371–$383 for 30 pills. (Note: Generic fluoxetine is available for $4 for a 30-day supply at many of the large retail pharmacies.)

General Life Care Planning Procedures and Additional Considerations

Client-Specific Considerations

■ Request and review all medical records and (if available for forensic cases) deposition transcripts of the client and family/caregivers, as well as healthcare professionals regarding the client's brain injury.[1] May also be appropriate to request pre-injury records and/or records regarding pre-existing or comorbid conditions to determine the client's overall general health condition. For children or college-age adults, review of pre-injury and post-injury school records is also appropriate.

■ Conduct an in-person interview, if possible, with the client and/or reliable family member/caregiver, preferably in their home/residential environment. While there is no established standard for life care planners using telehealth procedures to conduct client/evaluee interviews, exigent circumstances (e.g., the COVID-19 pandemic of 2020–2021) may at times warrant such practices. The life care planner is responsible for knowing the laws, ethical codes, and standards and scope of practice for their professional discipline in this regard.

■ Begin identifying long-term and lifelong care issues and options, including considerations for aging.[16]

■ Define the foundation for each recommendation, consistent with appropriate and reasonable care.

■ Ensure familiarity with the client's particular situation and the literature with regard to probable needs as related to the TBI. Are the clinicians' recommendations reasonable and consistent with the accepted standard of care?[16]

■ Once an adequate foundation is established for the future care needs and recommendations, an initial life care plan is developed. The process of developing a life care plan also includes an investigation into resources, availability of services in the client's geographic area, and cost research.

■ The life care plan is then typically presented to, and reviewed by, the client/family (if clinically appropriate and, if in forensic settings, permissible) and, at times, the treatment team. An alternative is to have the physician or healthcare provider(s) who participated in development of the plan review and sign off or endorse their medically based recommendations.

■ Pediatric life care plans require special attention and expertise. For example, the life care planner must consider the stages of child development, availability of school-based services provided under the federal IDEA, likely functional potential as the child reaches adulthood, as well as aging issues over the child's lifetime.

Medicolegal Considerations

■ Some states require that the calculation of life care plans consider collateral financial sources. The life care plan expert must thoroughly understand jurisdictional requirements.[17,18]

■ Life care planners must exercise caution when including household services. For example, payment of loss of income may include compensation for services normally purchased, leading to "double dipping" as per rules within various jurisdictions.[19]

Best Practices

■ Consensus and Majority Statements that summarize best practices in life care planning were developed by the community of life care planners during the biennial Life Care Planning Summits, held initially in 2000 and occurring approximately every other year with the most recent Summit as of this publication held in 2017. Familiarity with current best practices is essential for life care planners.[20,21]

> **KEY POINTS**
>
> ▪ The life care plan encompasses a comprehensive lifelong expectation of medical *and* nonmedical needs for the client/evaluee, including expected cost of the needs as related to TBI.
> ▪ The life care planner must be qualified to author the plan.
> ▪ The life care planner relies on a variety of other qualified specialties, the patient/client/evaluee and their family/caregivers, and relevant medical records and other related documents to accumulate data needed so that the comprehensive life care plan outlines the totality of the client's needs and costs associated with a TBI.
> ▪ When preparing a litigation-related life care plan, rules for what are allowable damages vary from jurisdiction to jurisdiction and state to state and the life care planner must fully understand the nuances of each prior to preparation of the life care plan.

STUDY QUESTIONS

The reference for all questions is *Life Care Planning and Case Management Handbook* (Weed & Berens, 2019); see the reference list located in the Additional Reading section.

1. Life care planning in forensic settings means:
   a. Working with an attorney to set up guardianship
   b. Presenting a life care plan in personal injury litigation
   c. Authoring a life care plan for a family trust
   d. Writing a life care plan for wounded warriors

2. Life care plans are designed for:
   a. People with catastrophic injuries
   b. People with complex healthcare needs
   c. People who are represented by an attorney
   d. People with catastrophic injuries and/or complex healthcare needs

3. Regarding qualified life care planners, which is most true?
   a. Qualified life care planners follow life care planning standards of practice
   b. One problem with finding a qualified life care planner is there are no standards of practice against which to measure the person's performance
   c. Unless life care planners are certified, they will not be allowed to testify in the courtroom
   d. Only nurses with a BA or above are qualified to be a life care planner

4. Regarding life care planning, which is most true?
   a. The life care plan is designed to only identify medically related needs
   b. A life care plan is not relevant to workers compensation cases
   c. Life care plans can be a useful tool for identifying current and future medical and nonmedical needs
   d. Only physicians are qualified to write life care plans

5. Regarding life care planning, which is most true?
   a. The life care plan lists expected needs but not prices
   b. A significant purpose of the life care plan is to identify lifelong care needs and their costs
   c. Qualified life care planners are required to have continuing education in economic projection
   d. Once a life care plan is submitted, no revisions are allowed

ADDITIONAL READING

American Association of Nurse Life Care Planners: http://www.aanlcp.org

The International Academy of Life Care Planners peer-reviewed standards of practice (3rd revision, 2015): http://www.rehabpro.org/sections/ialcp/focus/standards/ialcp-standards-of-practice

Physician life care planning certification: https://www.physicianlcp.com/

Weed R, Berens D. eds. *Life Care Planning and Case Management Handbook.* 4th ed. Routledge; 2019. doi:10.4324/9781315157283

Summary guide for people who are beginning life care planners. In: Weed R, Owen T. *Life Care Planning: A Step-by-Step Guide.* 2nd ed. E & F Vocational Services; 2018.

Neulicht A, Berens D. PEEDS-RAPEL: a case conceptualization model for evaluating pediatric cases with acquired brain injury. *NeuroRehabilitation.* 2015;36:275–287. doi:10.3233/NRE-151216

ANSWERS TO STUDY QUESTIONS

1. Correct Answer: b
Forensic means litigation related.

2. Correct Answer: d
As noted in the accepted definition, life care plans are appropriate for people with serious or catastrophic injuries as well as people with complex healthcare needs. Typically, the person is expected to need lifelong care.

3. Correct Answer: a
Although people who are not certified may author plans, the official position by the International Academy of Life Care Planners is that people need to follow the standards of practice in order to meet the accepted methodology threshold.

4. Correct Answer: c
As noted in several areas of the chapter, "medical" needs comprise only a part of the formula. For brain injuries, it is common that "medical" needs is only one component of the lifelong needs identified in the life care plan document.

5. Correct Answer: b
There is no requirement that life care planning authors have education in economics other than the basic criteria needed by someone who is qualified to project the costs into the future then reduce to present value. Table 61.1 in the chapter offers an example. A life care plan is a dynamic document and can be updated as needed.
The reference for all questions is Weed R. *Life care planning: past, present and future.* In: Weed R, Berens D, eds. *Life Care Planning and Case Management Handbook.* 4th ed. Routledge, 2019.

REFERENCES

The full reference list appears in the digital product found on http://connect.springer-pub.com/content/book/978-0-8261-4768-4/part/part05/chapter/ch61

TRAUMATIC BRAIN INJURY IN A FORENSIC CONTEXT

JERRY J. SWEET, KRISTEN M. KLIPFEL, AND
LAURA M. BENSON

INTRODUCTION

Clinical referrals leading to psychometric evaluation of well-documented or suspected traumatic brain injury (TBI) have become common within many healthcare disciplines, such as neurology, neurosurgery, and neuropsychology. Increasingly common are contacts from lawyers regarding former or current patients who suffered a TBI due to the actions of others, such as in a motor vehicle accident, and who have ongoing injury-related complaints. In modern society, such individuals frequently end up in litigation. All healthcare professionals whose work includes frequent contact with injured individuals need to know about forensic aspects of clinical practice.

ESTABLISHED RESEARCH OUTCOMES

- Approximately 2.87 million TBI-related emergency department visits occur annually in the United States, including over 837,000 TBIs among children. Of these individuals, approximately 75% are diagnosed as concussion or some form of mild TBI (MTBI).[1] A similar pattern is observed among civil litigants, with the vast majority presenting for forensic evaluation having sustained an MTBI.[2]
- *MTBI:* Cognitive deficits, when present, are typically experienced during the first 2 weeks after sustaining an MTBI. While experts do not completely agree as to when deficits resolve, sequelae are usually time limited, with resolution expected by 3 months post injury.[3,4] Somatic, cognitive, and/or emotional symptoms persisting beyond this point are often related to other factors associated with the TBI such as pain, fatigue, baseline characteristics, or unrealistic appraisal of pre-injury condition, rather than having a neurological basis. The presence of litigation has also been associated with persistence of symptom complaints.[2,5]
- Many individuals return to work within 2 to 3 weeks, with over 90% doing so within 2 months post-MTBI; a small subset continue to experience persisting difficulties beyond this time frame. Predictors of delayed return-to-work or unemployment following MTBI include lower level of education, nausea or vomiting on hospital admission, extracranial injuries, a high level of pain early after the injury, and limited job independence and decision-making latitude.[6] Additionally, individuals with complicated MTBIs (i.e., trauma-related intracranial abnormalities on neuroimaging) may take longer to return to work.[7]

The full reference list appears in the digital product found on http://connect.springerpub.com/ content/book/978-0-8261-4768-4/part/part05/chapter/ch62

■ *Moderate to severe TBI:* Recovery from moderate to severe TBI largely varies with severity of injury (e.g., penetrating vs. nonpenetrating injury). However, in general, the majority of cognitive recovery occurs within the first 5 months post-injury, with improvement reaching a plateau between 1 and 2 years post injury. With severe injury, the risk of significant residual problems is high, as only about one in four severe TBI survivors has disability-free recovery on categorical outcome measures like the Disability Rating Scale.[8] Additionally, ability to effectively exhibit social communication skills, including spoken language comprehension, verbal reasoning, social inference, reading, and politeness in social discourse, has been linked to successful employment outcomes following a moderate or severe TBI.[9]

CONSIDERATION OF DOSE–RESPONSE

■ In general, a dose–response relationship is expected with regard to TBI severity and subsequent cognitive and functional changes. Moderate to severe TBI is associated with an increased risk of persistent and meaningful impairments, as well as functional limitations. In contrast, MTBI has not been found to produce severe cognitive impairments.[10] Following MTBI, very severe complaints are viewed as unexpected and may be associated with invalid cognitive testing.[11]

■ Within a forensic context, empirical dose–response relationships may be violated, with a subset of litigants reporting excessive cognitive impairments and functional limitations that are discrepant with the severity of TBI sustained. Commonly seen in personal injury cases, those with mild uncomplicated TBI may be reporting cognitive impairments known only to occur with moderate to severe TBI.[10] Although some litigants may genuinely perceive themselves as impaired, some will be reporting symptoms disingenuously related to secondary gain.

SHORTCOMINGS IN METHODOLOGICAL RESEARCH

■ In 2014, only 34% of eligible studies met criteria for International Collaboration of Mild Traumatic Brain Injury Prognosis (ICMTBIP) inclusion. Even though research on MTBI has greatly expanded in recent years, the quality of research continues to be lacking, as evidenced by poorly designed studies, many unanswered clinical and research questions, and a lack of uniformity in the definitions used to describe MTBI. Clinicians, therefore, may draw erroneous conclusions based on inaccurate definitions and faulty methodologies.[12]

■ These methodological shortcomings can greatly impact work in the legal realm as well. In fact, certain articles in the literature have come to be relied on solely for the purpose of arguing highly improbable neuropsychological presentations in a litigation environment, typically without referencing meta-analytical studies that contrast these views.[11]

CLINICAL VERSUS FORENSIC CONTEXT

■ Individuals presenting in a routine clinical context (i.e., not involved in current litigation or planning to litigate) are commonly understood to be pursuing services in order to address symptoms for which there is motivation and strong desire to become symptom free.

- A forensic context to evaluation and treatment adds a risk of change in motives, in the direction of documenting problems, with the desired outcome being a favorable decision from the legal system, rather than identifying and receiving clinical care that resolves problems. There is risk that behavior will change independently of actual injury (i.e., a risk of behaviors manifested to effect an outcome other than injury recovery). This is termed risk of *secondary gain* (i.e., the goal is external reward, rather than symptom relief). Related to the risk of invalid presentations on examination, intentional exaggeration or fabrication of symptoms, known as malingering, must be assessed proactively.[2] Empirical research suggests a 30% to 40% risk of spurious symptom reporting or contrived behavior change in TBI forensic contexts, which requires that both symptom reporting and behavior change biases be evaluated.[13] There are additional explanations for symptom exaggeration, which may include litigating patients being influenced by "symptom knowledge" after reading about their conditions or being coached by their attorneys regarding what to say and how to present in a clinical context.
- By far, one of the most common types of forensic proceedings related to TBI is personal injury litigation, wherein healthcare experts are asked to assess damages. The adjudication of disability claims may also focus on effects of TBI.
- During some criminal proceedings, acute or chronic effects of TBI may also become relevant, related to issues of culpability, or to be considered at the time of sentencing as a mitigating circumstance. In such scenarios, care must be taken to rely on objective evidence of impairment or disability because of concern that a motive for secondary gain or an attempt to justify criminal behavior has altered symptom reporting or behavior.

ROLE DISTINCTIONS IN FORENSIC PROCEEDINGS

- Healthcare professionals possess certain areas of specific knowledge that are greater than that of lay persons; thus, the court considers that healthcare professionals are experts in these areas.
- Within litigation, expert status is commonly divided into two categories: (a) *treating* expert (sometimes referred to as a *treater*) and (b) *retained* expert, with the distinction primarily based on the former having had contact with the litigant in the course of providing routine clinical evaluation or treatment, whereas the latter was retained specifically to provide opinions related to the subsequent litigation. Additionally, experts may be narrowly retained as undisclosed consultants for one side or the other. When in this role, they will assist the side that retains them to best understand the complexities of the case, and they may help develop questions that can be asked during legal proceedings. Such undisclosed consultants will neither interview the patient themselves nor testify.
- Treating experts may also be referred to as fact witnesses, as most often the expectation is that opinions offered will be limited to facts known and opinions formed at the time clinical care was delivered. In contrast, retained experts are considered opinion witnesses who are allowed to offer broad-ranging opinions based on all relevant information available, including opinions regarding causation.
- Forensic specialists tend to view the distinction between treating experts and retained experts as relatively immutable; changing roles from being a treating expert to being a retained expert for a particular case is generally considered to be very ill advised and potentially fraught with ethical problems.[14]

DIAGNOSTIC ISSUES RELATED TO FORENSIC TRAUMATIC BRAIN INJURY CASES

- *Self-report reliability*: It is well known that self-report in general can be unreliable with regard to fully or accurately detailing events and functioning, even in individuals who are highly motivated to provide accurate information.[15] Research has demonstrated an even greater degree of unreliability in individuals who provide historical information and descriptions of functioning in a forensic context.[16] Even reporting of facts, such as pre-injury academic attainment[17] and pre-injury psychological status, has been shown to be inaccurately reported more frequently in personal injury litigants.
- *Good-old-days bias/diagnosis threat/misattribution*: Separate research findings have demonstrated a tendency among litigants and claimants to (a) report pre-injury function as more favorable than it actually had been,[18,19] (b) perform more poorly on cognitive tasks in response to the *suggestion* that a brain injury had occurred,[20] and (c) attribute perceived neuropsychological changes to the wrong factor (e.g., reduced processing speed attributed to traumatic injury, rather than serious depression, pain, and narcotic pain medications).
- *Nonspecificity of mild injury symptoms*: At the mild end of the uncomplicated brain injury severity range, frequently referred to as *concussion*, the absence of objective medical findings is common and often results in a diagnosis of MTBI based solely on historical data. This is problematic, especially when initial diagnosis is made long after the alleged injury, in that symptoms of concussion and MTBI are nonspecific and can be seen in individuals without brain injury who are experiencing depression, anxiety, or chronic pain or have other nonbrain injury problems.[21] Notably, numerous studies have found that pre-existing depression, anxiety, and other psychological and behavioral conditions predict post MTBI.[22–25]

NEUROPSYCHOLOGICAL CONTRIBUTIONS TO TRAUMATIC BRAIN INJURY EVALUATION

- Neuropsychological evaluations quantify neurobehavioral disturbances through use of detailed, standardized measures that allow for the mapping of the possible effects onto the nature of the specific TBI at issue. Through objective assessment, dose–response relationships can be evaluated in terms of whether measured symptoms and performances are credibly related to type and severity of TBI, as well as available injury evidence, such as brain imaging.
- Performance validity and symptom validity measures can identify individuals who are or are not reporting symptoms and performing in a valid, credible manner.
- In combination with other forms of available information, such as neuroimaging and neurological examinations, neuropsychological data can contribute to the overall understanding of a litigant's, claimant's, or defendant's presentation. Objective neuropsychological data are particularly useful with MTBI, which most often does not produce neurological examination or brain imaging abnormalities.

IMPORTANT ISSUES WHEN LAWYERS ARE INVOLVED

- *Bases of opinions*: In routine clinical activities, healthcare professionals have a degree of diagnostic certainty that is most often based on evidence-based practice within their specialties. When informing the legal system of opinions, experts are expected to provide a clear basis for each opinion. In recent years, the U.S. legal system has increasingly expected bases of opinions to be scientific, rather than to simply reflect a judgment based on clinical experience. Effective forensic opinions are based on objective and widely accepted diagnostic criteria that can be identified in the medical literature. Similarly, statements about treatment effectiveness can include personal professional experience, but are most effective when resting on accepted practice guidelines and outcome studies.

- *Strength of opinion threshold*: A common expectation when answering questions posed by lawyers is that the certainty or degree of conviction regarding an expert's opinion is also expressed. The legal system often requires that an opinion be beyond *possible* to *probable* in order to warrant consideration by the court. Unlike clinical opinions, which are often much more stringent, the legal threshold identified as *probable* is simply more likely than not, even if the likelihood is only 51%.

- *Initial injury versus subsequent symptoms and function*: At all injury severity levels, but particularly at the milder end of the continuum, lawyers often seek opinions regarding whether an initial injury occurred and, if it did, the rating of initial injury severity, as well as, separately, whether there are persistent or permanent residual injury effects. When persistent effects are alleged to have taken place because of an initial TBI, an effective opinion would be based on being able to trace those effects backward in time through healthcare record documentation to the time of injury, with no evidence of similar pre-injury problems. Evaluation of pre-injury function is most often reliably based on school, vocational, military, medical, or other records predating the injury, when available. Without such records, limits of opinion certainty should be expressed, particularly in light of the unreliability of self-report in a forensic context.

MEANS OF EXPRESSING FORENSIC OPINIONS

- *Written reports*: Treating experts rely on routine clinical documentation when providing testimony as a treating expert. Retained experts most often construct a specific forensic report that is intended to provide lawyers with a very specific opinion and the basis for each opinion that will be expressed in court. There is no single format for such reports, but most provide a detailed listing of specific sources of information that form the basis of opinions, as well as a detailed narrative that attempts to fully explain opinions. When the report includes information pertaining to the evaluation of a litigant, claimant, or criminal defendant, all relevant information gathered is expected to be identified in the report. Experts viewed as "cherry picking" information will be portrayed as biased.

- *Discovery deposition*: Legal system procedures have been created to facilitate a level playing field by providing all relevant information to all interested parties prior to a trial or an adjudicated outcome. Deponents are under oath to be honest and are expected to speak only when questions elicit a response, and at that time to respond with only information that is responsive to the question posed. Questions may be broad and far reaching, attempting to uncover all the limits of expected expert testimony. Objections by attorneys may occur, with a judge ruling at a later point whether certain questions and certain answers will be allowed at time of trial. Experts should be prepared to provide all relevant opinions at the time of the discovery deposition.

- *Evidence deposition/trial testimony*: If a testifying expert cannot attend trial, a more formal deposition, sometimes videotaped, will be taken and presented at trial. There is an expectation that what an expert said during a discovery deposition will be consistent with later trial testimony. In general, only the introduction of new facts would be expected to alter opinion at trial. Questions raised during evidence depositions and trial testimony often are more focused than the discovery deposition. Attempts will be made by attorneys from both sides to emphasize facts that favor their own perspectives of the case. This often involves attempts to devalue the relevance or competence of the expert and to create an appearance of not being objective, whether accurate or not.

FORCES OPERATING ON EXPERTS/GUIDANCE FOR WORKING WITH ATTORNEYS

- For both treating experts and retained experts, there is a common goal of expressing opinions objectively, rather than advocating for one side's preferred position. That is, though treating experts sometimes assume their roles include advocating for their patients, the legal system expects objectivity that will stand apart from the advocacy positions of the lawyers. Experts are to advocate only for their own opinions, not for the patient or for one side or the other of the case. Unique characteristics of forensic proceedings can make this difficult, requiring special consideration.[26]
- Strong advocacy positions of lawyers can create pressure on an expert to agree with and support one side of the case.[27] For retained experts, recommendations for maintaining objectivity in the face of these pressures include (a) use of the same evaluation procedures and interpretive methods when retained by either side, (b) use of objective decision rules or algorithms when forming opinions, (c) creating consistency between opinions and relevant mainstream empirical research, (d) requesting payment be provided in advance or at the time services are rendered, and not based on any form of contingency plan, (e) not allowing even the appearance of having negotiated opinions with lawyers, (f) proactively considering response bias when evaluating symptom reporting and behavioral presentations of the litigant or defendant, which means gathering corroborative data and performing objective testing, (g) being cognizant of symptom base rates in healthy non-injured individuals when rendering diagnoses, (h) placing only the amount of confidence in collateral information that it deserves, and (i) avoiding exaggerated or dramatic descriptors in reports.[28,29]
- It is statistically unlikely that a retained expert's evaluation of the case would always agree with the retaining attorney's understanding of the case. Therefore, unbiased experts will at times disagree with the retaining attorney's preferred position. Given that an attorney's understanding of an alleged TBI cannot always be correct at the outset, if an expert does not ever give disappointing news to a retaining attorney then it seems very likely that the expert is not offering an objective, independent opinion.

KEY POINTS

- Individuals who have sustained a TBI often end up in personal injury litigation within which healthcare professionals may be needed to provide testimony as treaters or retained experts.
- Understanding TBI outcome and dose–response expectations can provide a solid basis for expert forensic opinions.

- Consideration of objective findings from multiple specialties (e.g., neurology, neuroradiology, neuropsychology) may best inform the legal system.
- Understanding pre-injury function and credibility of post-injury presentation is essential.
- Objectivity can be strained by the forensic context, but must be maintained when providing an expert opinion.

STUDY QUESTIONS

1. Is there a meaningful difference between individuals presenting in a clinical context versus individuals presenting in a legal context following an MTBI?
   a. Yes, individuals presenting in a clinical context seek to address current symptoms with the goal of becoming symptom free, whereas many individuals presenting in a forensic context are not doing so primarily to pursue treatment, but instead seek to receive a favorable decision from the legal system
   b. Yes, individuals presenting in a forensic context routinely seek to address current symptoms with the goal of becoming symptom free, whereas individuals presenting in a clinical context want to receive a favorable decision from the legal system
   c. Yes, individuals presenting in a clinical context seek to address current symptoms and file for disability. Individuals presenting in a forensic context seek to file for disability
   d. There is no meaningful difference between the two groups

2. In the eyes of the U.S. legal system, which statement best describes expectations for a treating expert?
   a. A treating expert is expected to answer questions regarding treatment, as well as offer opinions as to causation, damages, or other forensic matters pertinent to the case
   b. A treating expert is expected to answer only questions regarding treatment
   c. A treating expert can decide on a case-by-case basis which questions can be answered
   d. A treating expert should do whatever the lawyers involved in the case say

3. When the goal of the person being assessed is external reward, rather than symptom relief, there is a context-specific potential for what is referred to as:
   a. Primary gain
   b. Tertiary gain
   c. Secondary gain
   d. Malingering

4. In what type of legal determination is TBI commonly a focus?
   a. Fitness for duty
   b. Personal injury damages
   c. Competency to stand trial
   d. Criminal responsibility

ADDITIONAL READING

Sweet JJ, Klipfel, KM. Forensic primer for the non-forensic neuropsychologist: When clinicians participate in forensic proceedings. In: Schroeder RW, Martin PK, eds. *Validity Assessment in Clinical Neuropsychological Practice*. Guilford; 2021.

Bush S. NAN Policy & Planning Committee. Independent and court-ordered forensic neuropsychological examinations: official statement of the national academy of neuropsychology. *Arch Clin Neuropsychol*. 2005;20(8):997–1007. doi:10.1016/j.acn.2005.06.003

Cheshire WP, Hutchins JC. Professionalism in court: the neurologist as expert witness. *Neurol Clin Pract*. 2014;4(4):335–341. doi:10.1212 /CPJ.0000000000000041

Heilbronner RL, Sweet JJ, Morgan JE, et al. American Academy of Clinical Neuropsychology consensus conference statement on the neuropsychological assessment of effort, response bias, and malingering. *Clin Neuropsychol*. 2009;23(7):1093–1129. doi:10.1080/13854040903155063

Vanderploeg RD, Belanger HG, Kaufmann PM. Nocebo effects and mild traumatic brain injury: legal implications. *Psychol Inj Law*. 2014;7(3):245–254. doi:10.1007/s12207-014-9201-3

Woodcock JH. Medical legal consultation in neurologic practice. *Neurol Clin Pract*. 2014;4(4):329–334. doi:10.1212/01.CPJ.0000437696.56006.94

ANSWERS TO STUDY QUESTIONS

1. Correct Answer: a

Individuals presenting in a routine clinical context pursue services in order to address symptoms for which there is motivation and strong desire to become symptom-free, whereas those presenting in a forensic context are typically motivated to receive a favorable decision from the legal system, rather than identifying and receiving clinical care that resolves problems.

Further Reading:
Sweet JJ, Goldman DJ, Guidotti Breting LM. Traumatic brain injury: guidance in a forensic context from outcome, dose-response, and response bias research. *Behav Sci Law*. 2013;31:756–778. doi:10.1002/bsl.2088

2. Correct Answer: b

Treating experts may also be referred to as fact witnesses, as most often the expectation is that opinions offered will be limited to facts known and opinions formed at the time clinical care was delivered. In contrast, retained experts are considered opinion witnesses, who are allowed to offer broad-ranging opinions based on all relevant information available including opinions regarding causation.

Further Reading:
Boone KB. *Clinical Practice of Forensic Neuropsychology: An Evidence-Based Approach*. The Guildford Press; 2013.

3. Correct Answer: c

Secondary gain occurs when the goal is external reward, rather than the ostensible overt reason for seeking medical care, that is, symptom relief.

Further Reading:
Sherman EMS, Slick DJ, Iverson GL. Multidimensional malingering criteria for neuropsychological assessment: a 20-year update of the malingered neuropsychological dysfunction criteria. *Arch Clin Neuropsych*. 2020;00:1–30. doi:10.1093/arclin/acaa019

4. Correct Answer: b

As a majority of TBIs involve injury scenarios associated with falls, motor vehicle accidents, being struck by or against an object, and assault, it is not uncommon for the injured party to become involved in the legal system, seeking personal injury damages.

Further Reading:

Sweet JJ, Goldman DJ, Guidotti Breting LM. Traumatic brain injury: guidance in a forensic context from outcome, dose-response, and response bias research. *Behav Sci Law*. 2013;31:756–778. doi:10.1002/bsl.2088

REFERENCES

The full reference list appears in the digital product found on http://connect.springer-pub.com/content/book/978-0-8261-4768-4/part/part05/chapter/ch62

ALCOHOL MISUSE AND TRAUMATIC BRAIN INJURY

RANDI DUBIEL AND JOHN D. CORRIGAN

GENERAL PRINCIPLES

Note that this chapter addresses alcohol but not illicit drugs or misuse of prescription drugs except as a complicating factor. (See Chapter 64 for more information on these topics.)

Definitions

Alcohol Use Disorders in the ICD-10

- *Dependence (ICD-10).*[1] Three or more of the following occurring together for at least 1 month; or if less than 1 month, occurring together repeatedly within a 12-month period[1]:
  - Need for significantly increased amounts of alcohol to achieve intoxication or desired effect; or markedly diminished effect with continued use of the same amount of alcohol
  - Physiological symptoms characteristic of the withdrawal syndrome for alcohol; or use of alcohol (or closely related substance) to relieve or avoid withdrawal symptoms
  - Difficulties controlling drinking (where, when, or amounts consumed)
  - Alternative pleasures or interests reduced or neglected in order to accommodate drinking or its effects
  - Persisting with drinking despite clear evidence and knowledge of harmful physical or psychological consequences
  - Strong desire or sense of compulsion to drink alcohol
- *Abuse/harmful use (ICD-10).*[1] Clear evidence that alcohol use contributed to physical or psychological harm, which may lead to disability/adverse consequences (pattern of use has persisted 1 month or occurred repeatedly over a 12-month period)

Alcohol Use Disorder DSM-5

The fifth edition of the *Diagnostic and Statistical Manual of Mental Disorders* (DSM-5) merges alcohol abuse and alcohol dependence into a single category, Alcohol Use Disorder (AUD).

- AUD is characterized by an inability to stop or control alcohol use despite adverse physical or social consequences. The occurrence of at least two of the 11 symptoms listed in Table 63.1 in a 12-month period suggests a problematic pattern indicative of AUD.[2]
- Severity of AUD determined by number of symptoms:
  - Mild = two to three symptoms
  - Moderate = four to five symptoms
  - Severe = six or more symptoms

The full reference list appears in the digital product found on http://connect.springerpub.com/content/book/978-0-8261-4768-4/part/part05/chapter/ch63

TABLE 63.1   **The 11 Symptoms of Alcohol Use Disorder in the *DSM-5***

1. Drinking more than intended
2. Attempts to cut down are unsuccessful
3. A majority of time is spent drinking or recovering from its effects
4. Experiences strong cravings to use alcohol (new in the *DSM-5*)
5. Alcohol use interferes with obligations at work, school, or home
6. Drinks despite social or interpersonal consequences of alcohol use
7. Alcohol use replaces other vocational or avocational activities
8. Drinks in situations that create a risk for physical harm
9. Drinks despite awareness of physical or psychological harm to oneself
10. Has developed a tolerance for the effects of alcohol
11. Experiences withdrawal or takes alcohol or other substances to avoid withdrawal symptoms

Source: Adapted from American Psychiatric Association. *Diagnostic and Statistical Manual of Mental Disorders.* 5th ed. Author; 2013. doi:10.1176/appi.books.9780890425596

AUD DSM-5 Versus ICD-10

- Classifications highly convergent for both absence of AUD and presence of most severe AUD[3]
- Divergence between systems:
  - *DSM-5* "mild" use disorder primarily split between "no diagnosis" and "misuse"
  - *DSM-5* "moderate" use disorder primarily categorized as "dependence" and to a lesser degree "misuse"
- ICD-10 does not include the following *DSM-5* indicators:
  - Taking larger amounts of the substance over time
  - Significant amount of time spent obtaining, using, or recovering from use
  - Failure to fulfill role obligations at home, work, and/or school
  - Interpersonal conflict attributed to use
  - Use in dangerous situations

Recommended Maximum Consumption Versus Alcohol Misuse[4]

- Men:
  - ≤65 years old—no more than four drinks in a sitting or 14 drinks in a week.
  - >65 years old—no more than three drinks in a sitting or seven drinks in a week.
- Women—no more than three drinks in a sitting or seven drinks in a week.
- Less use may be considered misuse in the presence of medication interactions or contraindicated medical conditions.
- Binge drinking—four or more drinks for women and five or more drinks for men within around 2 hours.
- Low risk use—use that does not meet criteria for misuse.
- Abstinence—no use of alcohol.
- There is no expert consensus whether a traumatic brain injury (TBI) is a contraindicated medical condition; however, many clinicians have concluded that abstinence from alcohol is the only safe recommendation that can be made following TBI.

Epidemiology

- Among those hospitalized due to TBI, approximately half will engage in binge drinking 1 year after injury.[5]
- In the United States, for those greater than 15 years old who are treated in acute rehabilitation for a primary diagnosis of TBI, approximately 23% have problem alcohol use prior to injury.[6]

■ In the United States, among those greater than 15 years old who are treated in acute rehabilitation for a primary diagnosis of TBI who are alive 5 years later, 14% report problem alcohol use.[7]

■ Substances most likely misused follow national trends, but alcohol is the most available, most used, and most misused.[8]

■ The greater one's intoxication at time of injury the more likely the injury will include a TBI.[9]

■ The strongest predictor of post-injury AUD is drinking before injury. Individuals with a history of AUD prior to injury are as much as 10 times more likely to exhibit problematic alcohol use post-injury, when compared to those without such history.[10]

■ Early childhood TBI may predispose to adolescent and early adulthood substance misuse.[11]

DIAGNOSIS

Screening

■ Clinical interview
  ● Determine levels of use and consequences.
  ● To promote transparency, a supportive and nonjudgmental presentation is essential.
  ● Open-ended questions normally elicit more information than multiple, yes/no, or short response questions.

■ Structured screening instruments (for brief descriptions, content, and cut-off scores see the American College of Surgeons Committee on Trauma Alcohol Screening and Brief Intervention Quick Guide: www.facs.org/trauma/publications/sbirtguide.pdf).[12]
  ● AUDIT: ten items, requiring 2 to 3 minutes of administration; extensive validation; sensitive to entire spectrum of drinking problems.[13]
  ● AUDIT-C: three items, requiring 1 minute. Scores range from 0 to 12; maximum score is 12; greater than three identifies 86% of men who report problem drinking; greater than two identifies 84% of women.[14]
  ● Binge drinking question: single item inquiring when last time the individual had five or more drinks in a single occasion. If in last month, considered positive. Allows conclusion that misuse or worse is present.[4]
  ● CRAFFT: six items, designed for screening in adolescents by asking about risky use situations but not actual questions about consumption.[15]
  ● S2BI: one item (second item if first response positive) to quickly screen adolescents. Initial question asks if the individual used alcohol, tobacco, or marijuana in the past year. Can be self-administered.[16]

■ Laboratory studies
  ● Blood alcohol content at time of injury:
    ■ Indicates intoxication at time of injury but not history of misuse.
    ■ High values (e.g., 80 mg/dL exceeds the legal limit for operating a motor vehicle in all 50 states) are a basis for assuming at least misuse.
    ■ Very elevated values may suggest tolerance for alcohol associated with dependence.
    ■ To estimate level at the time of injury, add 15 mg/dL for each hour from injury to blood draw.[12]
  ● Indices of impaired liver functioning are only sensitive to chronic use.

TREATMENT

In a rehabilitation setting, recommended interventions are education, screening, brief intervention, and referral for treatment, as indicated.[17]

- Education
  - It is recommended that all patients in rehabilitation for TBI receive education about the negative consequences of alcohol use.[17,18]
    - Even if there was no premorbid misuse, an individual should know that their acute recovery, if not lifetime health, will be more vulnerable to alcohol use than people who have not had serious TBIs.[18]
    - Patient and family defensiveness can be minimized by emphasizing that alcohol use education is relevant to everyone who has had a TBI.
  - Content recommendations have been published (see Table 63.2).[18,19]
- Brief intervention
  - Standard structure (National Institute of Alcoholism and Alcohol Abuse Pocket Guide [see References])
    Screening:
    - Distinguish among abstainers, low-risk use, at-risk use, and substance use disorder.
    Intervention:
    - If low risk, advise not to increase.
    - If at-risk, advise and assist depending on readiness to change.
    - If substance use disorder, advise, refer, and/or treat.

TABLE 63.2   Eight Educational Messages Presented in a *User's Manual for Faster, More Reliable Operation of a Brain After Injury*

1. People who use alcohol or other drugs after they have a brain injury don't recover as much
2. Brain injuries cause problems in balance, walking, or talking that get worse when a person uses alcohol or other drugs
3. People who have had a brain injury often say or do things without thinking first, a problem that is made worse by using alcohol and other drugs
4. Brain injuries cause problems with thinking, like concentration or memory, and using alcohol or other drugs makes these problems worse
5. After brain injury, alcohol and other drugs have a more powerful effect
6. People who have had a brain injury are more likely to have times that they feel low or depressed, and drinking alcohol and getting high on other drugs makes this worse
7. After a brain injury, drinking alcohol or using other drugs can cause a seizure
8. People who drink alcohol or use other drugs after a brain injury are more likely to have another brain injury

Source: Adapted from Ohio Valley Center for Brain Injury Prevention and Rehabilitation. *Substance Use and Abuse After Brain Injury: A Programmer's Guide*. Ohio State University; 2001.

  - "FLO" method[20]
    FLO components:
    - *Feedback on screening results:* Share results nonjudgmentally and ask for their reactions.
    - *Look for any change talk:* Explore importance they place on changing, confidence that they can, and pros and cons. Reinforce comments in the direction of change.

- *Options explored:* elicit what they see as options, seek permission to offer advice, close on good terms.

Tips:

- Use Motivational Interviewing technique (see *Center for Substance Abuse Treatment training manual*[20]).
- When in doubt, use reflection.
- Don't argue—keep fishing for positive change talk.

◼ Referral for treatment[18]

- Locate appropriate referral source in the person's home community.
- Discuss referral with the person and obtain release for referral and follow-up.
- Contact referral source, verify cultural relevance, and make referral.
- Facilitate patient's contact with the referral source to make an appointment.
- Forward information including biographical data and plans for discharge.
- Identify possible barriers to referral, such as transportation, scheduling, or family compliance, and address, prior to initial appointment.
- Follow up with referral source after initial appointment to confirm attendance. If patient did not attend determine how to facilitate participation.

KEY POINTS

◼ Medical professionals caring for persons with TBI should be competent in screening for alcohol use and conducting brief intervention and/or referral as indicated.

◼ Both ICD-10 and *DSM-5* offer criteria for diagnosing alcohol-related conditions; the key distinctions between the two were reviewed herein.

◼ There is no expert consensus on whether brain injury is a medical condition that contraindicates any alcohol use nor do guidelines for maximum consumption in adults after TBI exist—clinical judgment must be used.

STUDY QUESTIONS

1. Persons intoxicated at the time of sustaining a TBI are more likely to be:
   a. Older in age
   b. Younger in age
   c. Have no prior history of substance misuse
   d. None of the above

2. The U.S. Dietary Guidelines for Americans defines high-risk drinking for men under 65 years of age as the consumption of:
   a. Four or more drinks on any day
   b. Five or more drinks on any day
   c. Eight or more drinks per week
   d. Twenty or more drinks per week

3. What is the dietary guideline for maximum consumption of alcohol in adults with TBI?
   a. Less than two drinks per day
   b. Less than two drinks per week

    c. Drinking alcohol is safe following TBI

    d. There are no clear consensus guidelines on a safe amount of alcohol after TBI

4. When referring individuals with TBI for AUD treatment, it is important to:

    a. Identify possible barriers to referral, including transportation and cultural preferences

    b. Discuss the referral with the accepting provider

    c. Establish follow-up communication with either the patient or treating provider to ensure that initial planned contact actually occurred

    d. All the above

5. What is the greatest predictor for individuals having AUD following TBI?

    a. Age at time of injury

    b. Being female

    c. Having prior history of alcohol misuse

    d. Severity of TBI

ADDITIONAL READING

American College of Surgeons Committee on Trauma Alcohol Screening and Brief Intervention Quick Guide www.facs.org/trauma/publications/sbirtguide.pdf

NIAAA Pocket Guide for Alcohol Screening and Brief Intervention https://pubs.niaaa.nih.gov/publications/Practitioner/pocketguide/pocket_guide.htm

Corrigan JD. Substance abuse as a mediating factor in outcome from traumatic brain injury. *Arch Phys Med Rehabil.* 1995;76(4):302–309. doi:10.1016/S0003-9993(95)80654-7

Ohio valley center for brain injury prevention and rehabilitation. *Substance Use and Abuse After Brain Injury: A Programmer's Guide.* Ohio State University; 2001. www.ohiovalley.org

Ohio valley center for brain injury prevention and rehabilitation. *User's Manual for Faster More Reliable Operation of a Brain After Injury.* Ohio State University; 2004. www.ohiovalley.org

ANSWERS TO STUDY QUESTIONS

1. Correct Answer: b

Persons intoxicated at the time of TBI are more likely to be young and have prior histories of misuse.

Further Reading:

Parry-Jones BL, Vaughan FL, Miles Cox W. Traumatic brain injury and substance misuse: a systemic review of prevalence and outcomes research (1994-2004). *Neuropsychol Rehabil.* 2006:16(5):537–560 doi:10.1080/09602010500231875

2. Correct Answer: b

High-risk drinking is the consumption of five or more drinks on any day or 15 or more drinks per week for men under the age of 65. High-risk drinking for women and men over the age of 65 is the consumption of four or more drinks on any day or eight or more drinks per week. Moderate drinking is the consumption of up to one drink per day for women of legal drinking age and up to two drinks per day for men of legal drinking age.

Further Reading:
www.niaaa.nih.gov/alcohol-health/overview-alcohol-consumption/moderate
-binge-drinking

3. Correct Answer: d
   Although there are dietary guidelines for a "safe" amount of alcohol intake for the general population of healthy adults, risk factors associated with brain injury (such as heightened seizure risk) make it difficult to identify a level of consumption, other than abstinence, that is certain to not be detrimental.

   Further Reading:
   Corrigan J, Mysiw J. Substance misuse among persons with traumatic brain injury. In: Zafonte R, Katz D, Zasler N, eds. *Brain Injury Medicine: Principles and Practice, 2nd ed.* *Demos Medical Publishing*; 2013:1315–1328. doi: 10.1891/9781617050572.0079

4. Correct Answer: d
   Patients identified at greatest risk for or diagnosed as having AUD after TBI need special attention, including appropriate referral for treatment. Providers should have a method for making referrals acceptable, accessible, and useful to improve compliance. Community providers are most effective when they are adequately prepared for the patient and their needs. Ideally, follow-up should occur to ensure referral was completed as planned and if not, help should be provided in order to trouble shoot and establish a treatment plan.

   Further Reading:
   Corrigan J, Mysiw J. Substance misuse among persons with traumatic brain injury. In: Zafonte R, Katz D, Zasler N, eds. *Brain Injury Medicine: Principles and Practice, 2nd ed.* Demos Medical Publishing; 2013:1315–1328. doi:10.1891/9781617050572.0079

5. Correct Answer: c
   The strongest predictor of post-injury AUD is drinking before injury. Individuals with a history of AUD prior to injury are as much as 10 times more likely to have problematic alcohol use post-injury, when compared to those without such history.

   Further Reading:
   McKinlay A, Grace R, Horwood J, et al. Adolescent psychiatric symptoms following preschool childhood mild traumatic brain injury: evidence from a birth cohort. *J Head trauma Rehabil.* 2009;24(3):221–227. doi:10.1097/HTR.0b013e3181a40590

REFERENCES

The full reference list appears in the digital product found on http://connect.springer-pub.com/content/book/978-0-8261-4768-4/part/part05/chapter/ch63

64 SUBSTANCE ABUSE AND TRAUMATIC BRAIN INJURY

RANDI DUBIEL AND JOSHUA M. MASINO

GENERAL PRINCIPLES

This chapter addresses use of substances other than alcohol. While literature regarding alcohol use and traumatic brain injury (TBI) is robust, the literature that addresses other substances, including illicit drugs or misuse of prescription drugs, is generally less expansive.

Definitions

Substance Misuse and Substance Use Disorder

- *Intoxication:* reversible syndrome resulting from use of a specific substance.[1]
- *Misuse:* use of a substance in a way that is unhealthy/risky in greater amounts, more often, or longer than recommended, or use not directed by a prescriber, excluding abuse or dependence, in the past year.[1]
- Substance Use Disorders (SUDs) are manifested by at least two symptoms during a 12-month period (see Table 64.1)[2] and represent a maladaptive pattern of substance use, leading to clinically significant impairment or distress.[1]
- SUD in the *DSM-5* combines the *DSM-IV* categories of substance abuse and substance dependence into a single disorder, measured on a continuum from mild (two to three symptoms), moderate (four or five symptoms), to severe (six or more symptoms).[1]
- In the *DSM-5*, each specific substance is addressed as a separate use disorder (including alcohol, caffeine, cannabis, hallucinogens, inhalants, opioids, sedatives, hypnotics or anxiolytics, stimulants, tobacco, or other) but nearly all substances are diagnosed based on the same predominant criteria.
- *Withdrawal:* cluster of symptoms that occur reliably, has a clear onset closely following cessation of the substance abused, and create clinically significant consequences when they occur.

Epidemiology

- Approximately 20.3 million people ≥12 years old (one in seven) in the United States are estimated to have SUD, which is similar to the number of people with diabetes and more than 1.5 times the annual prevalence of all cancers.[3]
- In 2018, over 53 million people ≥12 years old in the United States reported use of illicit drugs (including marijuana, heroin, cocaine, methamphetamines, hallucinogens, inhalants) or misuse of prescription drugs in the previous year. Just over 25% of persons meeting criteria for SUD accessed treatment for medical problems associated with illicit drug use or to reduce/stop illicit drug use, including prescription misuse.[4]

The full reference list appears in the digital product found on http://connect.springerpub.com/content/book/978-0-8261-4768-4/part/part05/chapter/ch64

TABLE 64.1   Symptoms of Substance Use Disorder in the *DSM-5*

- The substance is taken more or longer than intended
- Attempts to cut down use are unsuccessful or a continued desire to quit is present
- A majority of time is spent using the substance or recovering from its effects
- Strong cravings to use the substance (new in the *DSM-5*)
- Substance use interferes with obligations at work, school, or home
- Uses substance despite social or interpersonal consequences of its use
- Use of the substance replaces other vocational or avocational activities
- Substance use in situations that create a risk for physical harm
- Uses substance despite awareness of physical or psychological harm to oneself
- Has developed a tolerance for the effects of the substance
- Experiences withdrawal or takes other substances to avoid withdrawal symptoms

Source: From the American Psychiatric Association. *Diagnostic and Statistical Manual of Mental Disorders* (5th ed.). Author; 2013; Black DW, Grant JE. *DSM-5® Guidebook: The Essential Companion to the Diagnostic and Statistical Manual of Mental Disorders*. 5th ed. American Psychiatric Association Publishing; 2014.

- Substance use and intoxication are established risk factors for TBI.[5]
- SUD is the third most frequent neuropsychiatric diagnosis among individuals with TBI.[6]
- TBI has been found to be common among individuals who are seeking treatment for substance use, with up to two thirds of people in rehab for either TBI or SUD having a history of both TBI and SUD.[7]
- Experiencing early-life TBI has been implicated in problematic substance use during adolescence.[8,9] Relative to adolescents without a TBI, those who self-reported history of TBI had odds 2 times greater for binge drinking, 2.5 times greater for daily cigarette smoking, 2.9 times greater for nonmedical use of prescriptions drugs, and 2.7 times greater for consuming an illegal drug in the past 12 months.[10]
- Individuals with pre-injury history of SUD, a diagnosis of depression since TBI, being male, younger age, and non-married status have been found to be at higher risk for post-injury substance misuse.[11]
- Data from the 2012–2013 National Epidemiologic Survey on Alcohol and Related Conditions revealed that a past-year TBI was significantly associated with past-year SUD.[12]
- In a Canadian study using the Canadian Community Health Survey, individuals with TBI had significantly increased odds of past-year illicit drug use compared to a non-injured control group.[13]
- While substance use is often decreased in the months following TBI it has been found that drug use often returns to premorbid use levels by 1 year post TBI.[14]

Pathophysiology

- Extensive study on how TBI affects addiction vulnerability is lacking.
- Impact of TBI can damage the frontal lobes, ventral medial prefrontal cortex, and orbital frontal cortex. This can disrupt mesolimbic dopaminergic neurocircuits and result in a stunted reward system[15] and reduced impulse control, both of which may influence the self-regulation of substance use.
- Given that substance use can lead to increased dopamine (DA) transmission, it has been suggested that DA depletion or malfunction after TBI contributes to compulsive and addictive behaviors such as those seen with substance misuse.[16]

- Disinhibition, impaired executive functioning, and impulsivity as a result of TBI could additionally contribute to an individual's risk taking, which has been shown to have a strong association to substance misuse.[17]
- Impaired cognitive function after TBI may result in unintentional misuse of medication(s) and possibly lead to consuming more than prescribed.
- SUD has also been considered as a coping mechanism for physical, psychological, and psychosocial stressors of disability rendered by TBI.[18]

Substances

Use at Time of Injury Resulting in TBI[19]:

- 23.7% positive for cannabis
- 13.2% positive for cocaine
- 8.8% positive for amphetamine
- 37.7% for one or more illicit drugs

Cannabis

- In 2018, approximately 4.4 million people ≥12 years old in the United States had a marijuana use disorder in the past year.[3]
- Marijuana impairs short-term memory and judgment and distorts perception; therefore its use in persons with TBI can be problematic, theoretically exacerbating impairments that may already exist as a result of brain injury.
- In a U.K. longitudinal birth cohort, sustaining childhood TBI (ages 1–11 years) correlated with problematic cannabis use, while sustaining adolescent TBI (ages 12–16 years) correlated with problematic cannabis and alcohol use, when compared to age-matched individuals with isolated orthopedic injuries.[20]
- In an observational study in Colorado, 74% of adults with TBI reported cannabis use pre-injury with 45% reporting use after their injury. Individuals cited reasons for use as recreational, reducing stress/anxiety, and to facilitate sleep.[21]

Cocaine

- In 2018, an estimated 5.5 million people ≥12 years old in the United States had past-year use of cocaine, inclusive of over 800,000 users of crack.[3] There are no available estimates for how commonly such substances are used in persons with TBI.
- Acts by blocking the reuptake of DA, norepinephrine, and serotonin via binding to pre-synaptic transporters thereby amplifying the natural effect of these substances on the post-synaptic neuron. Chronic cocaine exposure in animals has been found to diminish functioning of the orbitofrontal cortex leading to a negative impact on decision-making and self-awareness.[22]
- There is a paucity of research exploring the consequences of coexisting TBI and cocaine use.

Amphetamines

- Of the U.S. population, 1.9% or 5.1 million people ≥12 years old misused prescription stimulants in the past year.[3] Currently, there are no published estimates for how commonly amphetamines are misused/abused in persons with TBI.
- Amphetamines are similar in structure to DA, can increase presynaptic release, and reduce reuptake of DA as well as provoke excitability of dopaminergic neurons.
- Methamphetamine is a synthetic drug chemically similar to amphetamine that exerts a preferential neurotoxic effect on the frontostriatal systems,[23] impacting emotional and neurocognitive regulation. Use has been associated with reduced hippocampal volume, damage to the prefrontal cortex and limbic systems, as well as impaired DA transmission.

■ When presenting with TBI, individuals testing positive on urine toxicology for methamphetamines were more likely to have had a violent mechanism of injury compared to those negative for methamphetamines.[22]

Opiates

■ Opiate Use Disorder (OUD) has been identified as an epidemic in the United States, with over 10.3 million people in the United States reporting opiate misuse and an estimated 2 million people ≥12 years old having OUD. However, little remains known about the prevalence of opiate misuse or abuse among people with TBI.[3]

■ Opiate prescribing is common in individuals with TBI due to coexistence of acute and chronic pain.[24] A multicenter study found that over 70% of people discharged from acute inpatient rehabilitation for TBI were prescribed opiates.[25]

■ Studies using the National Survey of Drug Use and Health (NSDUH) data have revealed that individuals with disability, not specific to TBI, were more likely to misuse prescription pain medicine than those without disabilities.[26]

■ Clinicians should use caution when considering prescribing opiates for pain. Clinical guidelines for management of opioid therapy and mild TBI, developed by the Veterans Administration/Department of Defense (VA/DoD), recommend against prescribing opiates to individuals with history of TBI.[27]

DIAGNOSIS

In order to minimize the negative consequences of SUD, it is critical to identify individuals with TBI who are at risk for substance use post-injury through formal clinical screening. Although surveys reveal that rehabilitation staff perceive 22% of patients to have substance misuse problems, structured clinical screening suggests the actual rate is two to three times higher. This highlights the importance of active screening for SUD in all patients with TBI.

■ Clinical interview
  ● Determine levels of use pre- and post-TBI via screening (discussed later).
    ▪ All patients with TBI should be asked about use. If the patient is unable to provide an accurate history, then family or care partners should aid in estimating pre-injury use.
  ● Establish rapport.
■ Physical exam
  ● While acute withdrawal from substances is not commonly encountered during an inpatient rehabilitation setting, there may be an occasion where a patient presents for rehabilitation early after injury and displays symptoms/signs that are consistent with withdrawal. Such symptoms/signs include tachycardia, dilated pupils, elevated blood pressure, diaphoresis, delusions, and paranoia; these symptoms may mimic symptoms often encountered after TBI. The symptoms/signs of drug withdrawal and the length of withdrawal vary depending on the substance and duration of misuse. This underscores the importance of recognizing substance use at the time of injury and pre-TBI and establishing the time line from last use so that withdrawal can be accurately considered in the differential diagnosis.
■ Screening measures

While there are a number of screening questionnaires available, consideration of social desirability, patient demographics, and administrative burden must be considered when selecting a particular questionnaire.

- CAGE-AID (adapted to include drugs): screening tool adapted from the CAGE alcohol assessment tool to include questions about drug use.[28]
  - CAGE is an acronym for four questions:
    - ☐ Cut down—Have you ever felt the need to cut down on your drinking or drug use?
    - ☐ Annoyed—Have people annoyed you by criticizing your drinking or drug use?
    - ☐ Guilty—Have you ever felt guilty about your drinking or drug use?
    - ☐ Eye opener—Have you ever felt you needed a drink or used drugs first thing in the morning to steady your nerves ("eye opener") or to ease the effect of a hangover?
  - Answering "yes" to one item or more indicates a possible SUD.
  - Sensitivity and specificity in TBI population are more reliable than longer measures, such as the Michigan Alcohol Screening Test (MAST) and Substance Abuse Subtle Screening Inventory—third edition (SASSI-3).
- Alcohol, Smoking, and Substance Involvement Screening Test (ASSIST).[29]
  - Developed by the World Health Organization
  - Version 3.1 includes different languages.
  - Allows for screening for multiple potential substances of abuse with one tool.
- SASSI-3
  - Constructed using both direct and subtle items, intending to ask items that appear unrelated to substance use in hopes of reducing defensive behavior or denial of use.[30]
  - Better choice for illicit drugs than CAGE-AID.
  - Ages 18 and up.
  - Found to have 95% sensitivity in TBI.[31]
- Laboratory studies
  - Biological screening tests, such as blood or urine samples, provide information on current consumption, but are not sufficient to establish substance use history or the presence of SUD.

TREATMENT

Given the unique needs of individuals with TBI and co-occurring SUD, there are special considerations for treating SUDs in the TBI population. During rehabilitation, interventions should focus on education, brief intervention if screening is positive for SUD, and, if indicated, referral for further treatment.

- Education
  - Education regarding SUD and its negative effects on TBI recovery and outcomes should be provided to all patients receiving rehabilitation for TBI.[32]
  - General consensus supports treatment via a combination of education and an integrated multidisciplinary team approach. Treatments focusing on (a) education regarding both conditions and their resulting symptoms, (b) implementation of coping strategies to minimize symptoms of both conditions, and (c) teaching the consequences of risky behavior may be most successful.[33]
  - There is some evidence that education is most effective for patients who have experienced negative consequences of substance misuse or can link their injury to substance misuse, therefore using these experiences as teachable moments is advantageous.

■ Brief intervention
  ● Screening, Brief Intervention (SBI)—standard of care for trauma patients for screening, required by the American College of Surgeons since 2007.
    ▪ Consists of screening for substance misuse, feedback/education regarding risks of use, and brief motivational interview.
    ▪ Shown to reduce alcohol consumption and reduction in trauma recidivism.[34]
  ● Screening, Brief Intervention, and Referral to Treatment (SBIRT).[35]
  ● Also designed to reduce substance use and prevent its negative consequences, such as trauma recidivism with added referral for treatment for more severe substance misuse.
    ▪ Involves systematic screening for substance use, followed by application of a brief motivational intervention (BMI) in patients that test positive. The BMI includes exploring motivation for substance use, reviewing consequences of use, weighing the pros and cons of use, negotiating terms of consumption, and allowing the patient to summarize with their own conclusions and questions.
    ▪ Has been shown to increase the belief that alcohol use will have negative effects, including increasing cognitive and physical impairments, in persons with more severe TBI which could influence future use.[36]
■ Counseling
  ● Commonly employed components of treatment for SUD may not be effective in individuals with TBI due to challenges such as impaired cognition and/or behavior, reduced insight, and restricted access to transportation.
  ● Misinterpretation of TBI-related cognitive and behavioral impairments as willful resistance to treatment or low motivation can undermine treatment relationships; thus knowing that a dual diagnosis of TBI and SUD exists is paramount.
  ● Consideration needs to be given to the structure, location, length, and frequency of treatment sessions, and treatments should be tailored to an individual's needs based on their TBI-related impairments.
  ● Motivational Interviewing (MI) has been shown to be beneficial and is generally supported[37,38] in patients with TBI. MI takes into account the many factors that influence a person's motivations to use substances based on the expected positive and negative consequences of using the substance. The goals of MI are to increase a person's motivation and commitment for change.
■ Medications
  ● While pharmacological interventions for opiate dependence are approved and available,[39] the efficacy of such interventions has not been thoroughly studied in those with co-occurring TBI. Medications are most effective when used in a structured treatment program which includes medication administration monitoring, urine toxicology screening, medical, psychological, and vocational services.
■ Referral for treatment
  ● Taking an active role in referral to community resources for those with identified SUD is imperative.
  ● Efforts should focus on (a) locating appropriate referral source in a patient's home community, (b) discussing the referral with the patient and obtain release for referral and follow-up, (c) connecting with the referral source to verify appropriate relevance, (d) facilitating making the appointment, (e) forwarding patient information and discharge plans, (f) identifying possible barriers to accessing the appointment and assisting with problem-solving, and (g) following up with referral source to confirm the appointment occurred.[42]

KEY POINTS

- All patients with TBI should be screened for pre-existing substance use and SUD, as well as advised that substance use following TBI creates greater risk for consequences affecting brain function and functional outcomes.
- Research has identified a link between TBI and increased vulnerability to alcohol and illicit drug use, with similar expectations in OUD.
- Abstinence or a reduction in substance use is common immediately following TBI for a variety of reasons (reduced access, mobility impairments, close supervision), thus continued follow-up is paramount to capture those who relapse or begin substance misuse later in recovery.
- More data are needed to establish efficacy of treatment for illicit drug use and prescription drug misuse in survivors of TBI.

STUDY QUESTIONS

1. What is *most* true regarding substance use following TBI?
   a. Return to pre-injury use is common immediately following TBI
   b. Individuals with TBI rarely return to substance use once they are 1 year or more post TBI
   c. Return to pre-injury use is common by 1 year after TBI
   d. Long-term substance abuse is rarely a problem after TBI

2. Which is *not* a risk factor for development of SUD after TBI?
   a. Prior use of a substance
   b. The stress and anxiety induced by a prolonged recovery after TBI
   c. Age older than 65 years
   d. Early age occurrence of TBI

3. Who should be provided education about substance use after TBI?
   a. Only patients at risk to develop substance misuse
   b. All patients with TBI
   c. Family members of those surviving TBI
   d. Only those with moderate to severe TBI
   e. b and c

4. Regarding treatment of co-occurring SUD and TBI, it is helpful to:
   a. Employ traditional methods of treatment
   b. Avoid peer-based support
   c. Provide MI techniques alongside skill-based interventions
   d. Establish longer and more frequent treatment sessions

ADDITIONAL READING

Substance Abuse and Mental Health Services Administration (SAMHSA) https://www.samhsa.gov/find-help/disorders

CDC drug surveillance publication https://www.cdc.gov/drugoverdose/pdf/pubs/2018-cdc-drug-surveillance-report.pdf

Parry-Jones B, Vaughan F, Miles Cox W. Traumatic brain injury and substance misuse: a systematic review of prevalence and outcomes research (1994–2004). *Neuropsychological Rehabil.* 2006;16(5):537–560. doi:10.1080/09602010500231875

McHugo GJ. The prevalence of traumatic brain injury among people with co-occurring mental health and substance use disorders. *J Head Trauma Rehabil.* 2017;32(3):E65. doi:10.1097/HTR.0000000000000249

Babor TF, McRee BG, Kassebaum PA, et al. Screening, Brief Intervention, and Referral to Treatment (SBIRT): toward a public health approach to the management of substance abuse. *Subst Abus.* 2007:28(3):7–30. doi:10.1300/J465v28n03_03

ANSWERS TO STUDY QUESTIONS

1. Correct Answer: c

There is usually a decrease in alcohol and other drug use with higher rates of abstinence observed immediately following TBI. However, return to substance use has been found to be common and occurs at pre-injury use amounts (or more) by 1 year after TBI.

Further Reading:

Ponsford J, Whelan-Goodinson R, Bahar-Fuchs A. Alcohol and drug use following traumatic brain injury: a prospective study. *Brain Inj.* 2007;21(13–14):1385–1392. doi:10.1080/02699050701796960

2. Correct Answer: c

A population-based study found that those with a pre-injury history of SUD, a diagnosis of depression since TBI, being male, younger age, and non-married status were more at risk for post-injury substance misuse.

Further Reading:

Horner MD, Ferguson PL, Selassie AW, et al. Patterns of alcohol use 1 year after traumatic brain injury: a population-based, epidemiological study. *J Int Neuropsychol Soc.* 2005;11(3):322–330.

3. Correct Answer: e

All patients and their family members should be provided education about substance use and the associated risks following TBI. This should occur early in the recovery process. Screening for substance use prior to and after TBI are important for identifying those at risk and appropriately directing treatment interventions.

Further Reading:

Corrigan JD, Mysiw WJ. Substance abuse among persons with TBI. In: Zasler ND, Katz DI, Zafonte RD, Arciniegas DB, Bullock MR, Kreutzer JS (eds). *Brain Injury Medicine: Principles and Practice,* 2nd Edn. Demos Medical Publishing. 2012: 1315–1328.

4. Correct Answer: c

General consensus for treatment of SUD in TBI supports a combination of education and an integrated multidisciplinary approach. Structure of treatment needs to be flexible and may need to be altered in duration and frequency based on individual needs. Peer support has been found to be well received by persons with TBI and can be of benefit. Motivational counseling may help limit substance use while also having a beneficial impact on other aspects of behaviors in those with TBI seeking substance abuse treatment.

Further Reading:

Bombardier CH, Rimmele CT. Motivational interviewing to prevent alcohol abuse after traumatic brain injury: a case series. *Rehabilitation Psychology*. 1999;44(1):52.

Cox WM, et al. Outcomes of systematic motivational counseling for substance use following traumatic brain injury. *Journal of Addictive Diseases*. 2003;22(1):93–110.

REFERENCES

The full reference list appears in the digital product found on http://connect.springer-pub.com/content/book/978-0-8261-4768-4/part/part05/chapter/ch64

ETHICAL CONSIDERATIONS

TERESA A. SAVAGE AND DEBJANI MUKHERJEE

OVERVIEW

■ Ethics is a group of principles that help people determine what are right or wrong actions in the context of a given situation.

■ Various theories and frameworks can be used to analyze ethical considerations, including a focus on principles, relationships, virtues, consequences, rules, or processes.

■ Traumatic brain injury (TBI) can pose unprecedented ethical dilemmas about what it means to live a good life. There are webs of lives affected by one injury.[1]

■ Core principles of biomedical ethics[2] include:
- *Beneficence*: providing benefit and balancing risks to bring forth the best results
- *Respect for autonomy*: fostering self-determination and respecting individual differences
- *Nonmaleficence*: doing no harm
- *Justice*: upholding concepts of fairness and equity

■ An ethics of care (or care ethics) focuses on relationships, interdependencies, vulnerabilities, and context. After a TBI, each one of these aspects may be altered as a direct result of brain injury.[3]

■ Clinical ethics involves analyzing and resolving practical ethical issues, drawing on an analysis of medical indications, patient preferences, quality of life (QOL), and contextual factors.[4]

■ Ethical issues may arise when there are competing interests or values, or disagreements about the "right" or "wrong" way to approach a problem; terms such as moral dilemma, moral uncertainty, and moral distress describe the tension between the perceived course of right action and constraints.[5]

■ Ethical considerations in TBI range from withdrawal of life support decisions in severe TBI to the ability of a participant with a mild TBI to consent to a low-risk research project. There are numerous frameworks and philosophies that can be used to analyze ethical issues in TBI. The nature of the injury, striking at the core of the sense of self and personhood, can lead to philosophical and practical ethical considerations. The list of factors to consider is presented as a starting point to understanding the complexities involved. It is organized according to time post-injury, and within each time frame, some examples of issues across the continuum of brain injury are highlighted.

PARTIAL LIST OF ETHICAL ISSUES IN TRAUMATIC BRAIN INJURY

In the Acute Phase

■ The acute phase is marked by uncertainty, fluctuating prognoses, and time-sensitive medical decisions. For more severe injuries, surrogates are typically making decisions

---

The full reference list appears in the digital product found on http://connect.springerpub.com/content/book/978-0-8261-4768-4/part/part05/chapter/ch65

for the person who sustained the TBI; the surrogate uses substituted judgment, which means making the decision that the surrogate believes the patient would make, if capable.

- *With mild TBI (MTBI)*, there may be pressure to clear the patient to return to work, or the athlete to return to play. Deficits in cognitive functioning that may not be apparent may put the patient at risk for greater injury, especially should they return to the activity that caused the injury, for example, contact sports. Physicians may feel pressure to release the patient prematurely or, in the setting of injury-related litigation, to verify the presence of impairments that are not objectively noted.[6]
- With more serious injury, there may be discussions about potential withdrawal or withholding of life support; prognostic information is critical for the surrogate decision maker who must understand the various degrees of uncertainty in predicting eventual functional outcome. Palliative care consultation may be useful when discussing goals of care and the possibility of withdrawal of treatment. In this context, a new subspecialty of neuropalliative care is emerging.[7]
- *Allocation decisions pertaining to use of scarce life support* resource (ventilators, ICU admission) may arise during a pandemic or other disaster.
- *Pervasive nihilism* may factor in when a patient's condition is viewed as hopeless: "marginalized and sequestered from the evolving fruits of neuroscience."[8]
- *Diagnostic and prognostic uncertainties* can come into play. Prediction of unlikelihood of survival or high likelihood of unacceptable QOL if the patient survives may lead to a self-fulfilling prophecy. Prediction of mortality or high morbidity influences the decision to withdraw treatment; outcome data which factors into decision-making may be communicated or received in skewed fashion.[9]
- Requests from families for *novel diagnostic and therapeutic interventions* are not unusual; through the Internet, families learn of possible interventions being studied and may desire these for the patient, but the intervention is only available through participation in research, and efficacy has not been established. Guidelines for communication with a surrogate that can aid in these discussions have been published.[10]
- *Honoring advance directives* is a challenge if faced with a discrepancy between the advance directive instructions and the surrogate's request. For example, a surrogate may request continued aggressive treatment in conflict with the expressed wishes of the patient to discontinue unwanted treatment, or vice versa.[11]
- *A decision to have a guardian appointed* can be burdensome for families without financial means to afford the guardianship process. This can result in lack of adequate surrogate/advocacy support for the brain injury survivor.
- *Decisions for the unbefriended, incapacitated patient* who lacks a surrogate decision-maker may require institutional policies for surrogate decision making.[12]

In the Inpatient Rehabilitation Phase

- The inpatient rehabilitation phase often involves initial adjustment to impairments, waxing and waning decisional capacity, respect for emerging abilities, greater involvement of surrogates as caregivers, and limited discharge options.
- In MTBI (e.g., when seen as a comorbid presentation alongside spinal cord injury), patients may not appreciate any cognitive deficits, and so may decline rehabilitation therapies and/or reassessment. There may be issues with the employer or family if the patient's behavior or cognitive abilities have changed.
- *Consideration of pre-injury and post-injury interests and "selves"* may arise, often because persons with TBI may have personality changes and will no longer seem like the same person to family and friends, which makes surrogate decision-making more challenging.

- *The reverberating impact of the injury on the family system* is apparent as the patient's role in the family may change drastically if the patient is no longer able to return to work or fulfill roles as a spouse, parent, or child.
- *Assessment of decision-making capacity* (see also Chapter 42).
- *Decisional capacity versus performative capacity* (see also Chapter 42).
- *QOL judgments by persons other than the injured patient* is deferred to the surrogate if the patient is unable to make such decisions during their inpatient rehabilitation stay. The surrogate decision-maker may hold the view that the QOL would be unacceptable to the patient, so requests a "Do Not Resuscitate" order be placed and/or tube feedings be discontinued.
- *Identifying surrogate decision-makers*, in the absence of a durable power of attorney for healthcare, or state statute, may be difficult, particularly when more than one family member may lay claim to the role (e.g., an unmarried adult with more than one adult child).
- *Assent versus consent* in medical decision-making means that patients may be unable to give consent, but can give assent (an affirmative agreement) for treatment or participation in research. Generally, assent should be sought if the patient is able do so.
- Patients may have *emerging capacities* and when capable, decision-making should revert back to the patient.
- *Infantilization of adults with TBI* should be avoided. Although the patient may only be able to understand gestures or two-word phrases, the patient should not be treated as though they are a child.
- *Use of behavioral restraints* should be a last resort. Most facilities have explicit policies and procedures for use of chemical or physical restraints when the patient poses a risk of harm to self or others.
- *Access to and timing of inpatient rehabilitation* is critical in order to maximize benefit of intense rehabilitation; some patients who may not be able to benefit from rehabilitation in the early post-injury phase may benefit later in their recovery process. Navigating the admission process and coverage issues so as to secure therapy at the optimal time may be complicated.
- *Safe discharge options* may be a source of disagreement. Some patients may not recognize their deficits or may disagree with the rehabilitation team that their discharge arrangements put them at risk of harm; discharge can be especially challenging if the patient desires to return home, yet lacks support from family or friends or the financial resources to hire assistance in order to live at home.[13]
- *Allocation of resources* may depend on where a patient lives, how persistent and resourceful family can be to find services, and whether equipment, supplies, and services are deemed medically necessary.

In Post-Discharge Recovery

- After people with TBI are discharged from inpatient rehabilitation, ethical issues revolve around capacity, self-determination, access to healthcare, as well as return to employment and community activities.
- *Access to healthcare and social services* often depends on geographic location and family support; patients may have barriers in accessing specialty care in their community, and social services, such as transportation, personal assistants, vocational rehabilitation, and mental health services, may also not be readily available.
- *Accountability* for the patient's behavior and decisions *may be* challenging. At what point in the recovery process should patients be held accountable for their decisions and actions?

- *Anosognosia* or impaired self-awareness can be present; some patients lack insight into the deficits caused by their brain injury; this can result in denial of the need for therapy or use of assistive devices.[14]
- *Participation in research* may be a consideration, particularly if the research holds the possibility of direct benefit in balance with potential risks. If there is no possibility of benefit to the patient, but there may be knowledge to be gained for future patients, should the surrogate give consent for a patient who is still lacking the capacity to make this decision for themselves?[10,15]
- Undiagnosed and untreated *psychiatric sequelae of TBI* may appear; mental health services in the community for patients with TBI are often difficult to find; insurance may cover therapy for the patient only and not for any family therapy.
- TBI can impact social and *emotional functioning*, including sexual behaviors. Ethical tensions include protecting vulnerable persons versus facilitating independence.
- *Role of spirituality* in adjustment to TBI can be quite variable; some patients may find comfort in their faith, while other patients may struggle in understanding why they experienced misfortune.
- *Biases and stigma* may be associated with cognitive disability; integrating back into the patient's former community may be challenging when friends and coworkers do not understand the changes in the patient; patients may experience discrimination faced by many people with cognitive, intellectual, or mental health disabilities.

Broader Social Issues

- *Public health advocacy* issues such as gun control, helmet laws, fall prevention for the older adults, services for returning veterans with TBIs, concussion protocols, and responsibility in professional sports should be considered, and are addressed by various relevant professional healthcare societies.
- Many people with TBI belong to *marginalized communities* and are impacted by structural racism and poverty.
- *Reintegration* into the community can be challenging; the patient may first require the services of a long-term care facility or other structured support setting.
- *Return to work* in the same job is often the goal of both the patient and family members, though cognitive, behavioral, and/or physical limitations may result in the need to consider a lower status, lower paying position.

QUALITY OF LIFE

QOL is hard to define and measure.[16] Healthcare providers often rate QOL lower than do individuals living with a disability.[17] Notions of a "good" life change over time and with new life experiences. The best interest standard is often used to discuss QOL, but factors such as the severity of the injury, access to services, premorbid personality characteristics, and social support can complicate the notion of what is in the patient's best interest. Family members and surrogate decision makers are dealing with their own emotional reactions and fears and may not make decisions based on a "substituted judgment"[2] or what the patients themselves would want. Understanding the values, preferences, hopes, and life satisfaction of persons with TBI is important in exploring ethical issues.

SENSE OF SELF AND PERSONHOOD

TBI raises dilemmas about a sense of self and personhood. Are individuals fundamentally changed if their personalities, memories, or functional capacities are altered? The definition of personhood is distinct from personality, and various legal, theological, and philosophical theories define the concept in specific ways.[18] Vegetative states, minimally conscious states, and other disorders of consciousness raise critical issues about how we define the self in relation to QOL, prognosis, and time post injury. As a person with TBI adjusts and recovers, they may have emerging capacities and start a process of redefining themselves, especially in relation to others.

MISDIAGNOSIS

Misdiagnosis of vegetative state and minimally conscious state is common; as many as 30% to 40% of patients diagnosed in vegetative state retain some consciousness.[19] Inappropriate management, including pain management, can occur when patients are misdiagnosed. Unfortunately, premature withdrawal of life-sustaining treatment occurs in a high percentage of patients, often within 72 hours of injury.[19]

ISSUES TO CONSIDER BASED ON BIOETHICAL PRINCIPLES

- Beneficence:
  - Best interest of the patient.
  - Who defines best interest?
  - Benefits and burdens of each treatment.
  - Use of evidence-based guidelines in shared medical decision making.
  - Clear communication of information.
  - Integration into least restrictive environment.
- Respect for patient autonomy/self-determination:
  - What is the patient's current decision-making capacity?
  - Do they have an advance directive?
  - Have they identified a surrogate decision maker?
  - Has the patient made their preferences known? When?
  - Has the TBI fundamentally changed the patient's sense of self?
  - Should the advance directive be honored if the patient is improving and may regain capacity, but the surrogate wants to stop treatment?
- Nonmaleficence:
  - Refers to harms of action as well as harms of inaction.
  - If the patient does not fully understand what is being considered, are they being harmed?
- Justice:
  - Discrimination on the part of healthcare providers and society at large because of diagnosis (e.g., assuming the person lacks capacity).

- Allocation of resources: medical, social, and financial.
- Public health's precautionary principle: in the absence of scientific evidence of harm, preventive measures should be taken.

APPROACH TO CLINICAL ETHICAL ANALYSES

- Identify the moral dilemma, moral uncertainty, or moral distress.
- Determine the facts of the case:
  - Medical: diagnosis, prognosis, deficits, risks, benefits of treatment, and goals of treatment.
  - Social: family support, living situation, social support, occupation, goals, and experiences with the healthcare system, health literacy.
  - Spiritual and cultural: belief systems, values, and religious practices that may influence treatment decisions.
- List the stakeholders and the nature of their interests (e.g., patient, family, healthcare providers, facility, payers, community members, and others).
- Name the problem/dilemma(s):
  - Values in conflict.
  - Communication difficulties.
  - Applicable laws and/or institutional policies.
  - Violations of codes of ethics.
  - Limited resources.
- Gather additional information:
  - Are there any perspectives missing?
  - Where are you getting your facts? Who is telling the story?
  - To what degree does prognostic certainty factor in?
- Consider the alternatives:
  - List arguments for and against each alternative.
  - Eliminate options that are "out of bounds" (illegal, unethical, against policy).
  - Examine how each remaining alternative may affect the patient and other interested parties.
  - Are the choices consistent with the patient's moral, religious, or social beliefs? With the family's beliefs? With the team members' beliefs?
  - How far does the patient's autonomy extend if they make a decision that is contingent upon the surrogate's cooperation?
  - Who ultimately makes the decision/takes action?
- Implementation and follow-up:
  - Develop a plan.
  - Determine the extent of agreement on a course of action consistent with the patient's wishes and acceptability to the family and healthcare team.
  - Decide who should be informed.
  - Accept informed refusal from a patient with decisional capacity or from the surrogate.
  - Reflect on the case: What went right? What went wrong? What would you do differently in the future?

KEY POINTS

- TBI can pose unprecedented ethical dilemmas and bring up age-old debates about QOL and personhood.
- Diagnostic errors are common in disorders of consciousness. This can result in withdrawal of life-sustaining treatment based on incorrect prognostic considerations.
- Ethical issues vary temporally, based on time since injury, as well as based on the severity of the brain injury.

STUDY QUESTIONS

1. When the physician's personal perspective regarding the likelihood of a patient's bad outcome, such as death or severe cognitive and physical disability after TBI, leads to withdrawal of life support, it is referred to as:
   a. Playing the odds
   b. Destiny
   c. Self-fulfilling prophecy
   d. Accepting mortality over morbidity

2. An ethics of care, in contrast to focusing solely on ethical principles for ethical analysis and decision-making, focuses on:
   a. The nursing care a patient receives
   b. The context and web of relationships affected by a patient's situation
   c. The physician's Hippocratic Oath and Code of Ethics
   d. The family who will care for the patient after discharge

3. After discharge from rehabilitation, patients may still experience anosognosia, which leads to:
   a. Denial of deficits and inability to see the need for therapy or use of assistive devices
   b. The need for surgical intervention
   c. Sexual promiscuity or impotence
   d. Seizures

4. One of the ethical issues facing physicians who treat patients with concussion is:
   a. The patient's insistence on extensive testing
   b. The patient's request for analgesia
   c. The patient's refusal to be hospitalized
   d. The patent's desire to return to the activity that caused the brain injury

5. In surrogate decision-making, surrogates are often asked to make a substituted judgment. This means:
   a. They should ask someone else what they would do in the same situation
   b. They should consider what the patient would want in the same situation
   c. They should consider what would be best for the patient
   d. They should make their decision based on financial means

ADDITIONAL READING

Hastings Center Briefing on Brain Injury: Neuroscience and neuroethics: https://www.thehastingscenter.org/briefingbook/the-vegetative-and-minimally-conscious-states

Armstrong MJ. Developing the disorders of consciousness guideline and challenges of integrating shared decision-making into clinical practice. *J Head Trauma Rehabil*, 2019;34(3):199–204. doi:10.1097/HTR.0000000000000496

Fins JJ. *Rights come to mind: Brain injury, ethics, and the struggle for consciousness.* Cambridge University Press, 2015. doi:10.1017/CBO9781139051279

Honeybul S, Gillett GR, Ho KM, et al. Long-term survival with unfavorable outcome: a qualitative and ethical analysis. *J Med Ethics*. 2015;41:963–969. doi:10.1136/medethics-2013101960

Sequeira AL-S, Lewis A. Ethical and legal considerations in the management of an unbefriended patient in a vegetative state. *Neurocrit Care*. 2017;27:173–179. doi:10.1007/s12028-017-0405-8

Tarsney P S, Sandel E, Doyle CK, et al. Putting the pieces together: Advance directives in the rehabilitation setting. *PMR*. 2020;12:73–81. doi:10.1002/pmrj.12295

Seminars in Neurology, 2018;Vol 38:Issue 5:2018: Entire issue is devoted to ethics in neurology

ANSWERS TO STUDY QUESTIONS

1. Correct Answer: c
   Withdrawing treatment allows the patient to die, which fulfills the prophecy that the patient will have a bad outcome.
   "Neurologists and intensivists are acutely aware that, despite interventions, patients with neurologic pathology may ultimately end up with a functional status that would not be acceptable to them which some would consider a fate worse than death. These concerns can lead to the infamous *self-fulfilling prophecy*, where our expectations for a bad outcome reduce our investment and actions, and therefore the poor outcome is likely to occur. We may not even be conscious that our expectation for recovery affects the speed with which we work, the staff we assign to a patient's care, and the medical interventions we offer."

   Further Reading:
   Septien S, Rubin MA. Disorders of consciousness: ethical issues of diagnosis, treatment, and prognostication. *Semin Neurol*. 2018;38(5):548–554. doi: 10.1055/s-0038-1667384

2. Correct Answer: b
   The ethics of care, while also considering ethical principles, focuses on the web of relationships in the patient's life, the concepts of interdependence and vulnerabilities, and the context in which healthcare decisions are being made.
   "an ethics of care...centers on responsiveness in an interconnected network of needs, care and prevention of harm."

   Further reading:
   Beauchamp TL, Childress JF. *Principles of Biomedical Ethics*. 6th ed. Oxford University Press; 2009:36.

3. Correct Answer: a
   Anosognosia is the inability to recognize deficits caused by the brain injury.
   "Persistent impairments in self-awareness appear to relate to a variety of cognitive and behavioral problems. They are also linked to poor decision making and may limit a person's engagement in rehabilitation activities that potentially could be helpful to them."

Further reading:
Prigatano GP. *The Study of Anosognosia*. Oxford University Press; 2010:3.

4. Correct Answer: d
   Although patients may experience symptoms of concussion, they may want to return to the activity where they sustained the brain injury, such as dangerous work on their job, contact sports, or dangerous leisure activity. Physicians may feel pressure from the patient or other parties to allow the patient to return to the activity or return to work, against the physician's better judgment.
   Further Reading:
   Donnelley SD, Kirschner KL, eds. *Mapping the Moral Landscape: Families and Persons With Traumatic Brain Injury: The Hypothetical Case of Jeff*. Brain Injury Association; 2003.

5. Correct Answer: b
   Substituted judgment means that the surrogate uses the knowledge about the patient's wishes and makes the decision that the patient would make, if capable. The best interests standard is used when the patient's wishes are unknown.

   Further Reading:
   Beauchamp TL, Childress JF. *Principles of Biomedical Ethics*. 6th ed. Oxford University Press; 2009:139–140.

REFERENCES

The full reference list appears in the digital product found on http://connect.springer-pub.com/content/book/978-0-8261-4768-4/part/part05/chapter/ch65

SPECIAL CONSIDERATIONS FOR MILITARY PERSONNEL: UNIQUE ASPECTS OF BLAST INJURY

HUNAID HASAN AND MICHAEL S. JAFFEE

OVERVIEW

There has been increased attention and awareness regarding concussions and traumatic brain injury (TBI) and their associated comorbidities in our military service members and veterans. TBI is referred to as a "signature injury of the war."[1] The increase in the use of high explosive devices that produce a shock wave can result in blast-induced neurotrauma (BINT) in personnel exposed to the blast wave.[2] Moreover, a significant proportion of combat BINTs have more than one mechanism of injury. In addition to the blast component, the combination of acceleration–deceleration impacts or fragment injuries are referred to as "blast plus" injuries.[3]

Unfortunately, modern military equipment proves to be not fully effective in TBI prevention.[4,5] A variety of programs to enhance detection and to better standardize quality of care in a multidisciplinary fashion have emerged from this recognition. Although BINTs are an important component of combat injury, not all military injuries have a blast component. The discussion that follows applies to servicemembers with combat-related concussions and TBIs.

DEFINITION

To standardize definitions and terminology, the Department of Defense (DoD) uses the following definition and classification system for mild TBI (MTBI; concussion) and moderate to severe TBI.

A traumatically induced structural injury or physiological disruption of brain function, as a result of an external force, that is indicated by new onset or worsening of at least one of the following clinical signs immediately following the event:

- *Any alteration in mental status (e.g., confusion, disorientation, slowed thinking, etc.).*
- *Any loss of memory for events immediately before or after the injury.*
- *Any period of loss of or a decreased level of consciousness, observed or self-reported.*

External forces may include any of the following events: the head being struck by an object, the head striking an object, the brain undergoing an acceleration/deceleration movement without direct external trauma to the head, or forces generated from events such as a blast or explosion, including penetrating injuries.

The full reference list appears in the digital product found on http://connect.springerpub.com/content/book/978-0-8261-4768-4/part/part05/chapter/ch66

The DoD definition is consistent with the definitions used by the Centers for Disease Control and Prevention (CDC), the American Congress of Rehabilitation Medicine (ACRM), and World Health Organization (WHO).

Of note, loss of consciousness (LOC) is not required for a diagnosis, and the presence of symptoms alone without a known injury does not qualify for a diagnosis. The designation "complicated MTBI" or clinical presentation of MTBI but with abnormal imaging is not part of the DoD system of definition. The classification of mild, moderate, and severe are summarized in the following table.

Mild	Moderate	Severe
Normal imaging	Normal or abnormal imaging	Abnormal imaging
Loss of consciousness (LOC): 0–30 min	LOC >30 min <24 hr	LOC >24 hr
Alteration of consciousness (AOC): up to 24 hr	AOC >24 hr	
Posttraumatic amnesia (PTA): 0–1 d	PTA >1 d and <7 d	PTA >7 d

EPIDEMIOLOGY

- Attacks with high explosives are responsible for about 60% of combat-related deaths.[2]
- From 2000 through the third quarter of 2019, a total of 413,858 cases of TBI have been identified.[6]
- Annual incidence has changed based on circumstances and these trends can be observed at this site: https://dvbic.dcoe.mil/dod-worldwide-numbers-tbi
- Systematic TBI screening programs began in 2007, increasing the yield.
- The largest annual incidence of TBI was in 2011 with 32,834 cases identified.
- The vast majority (82.4%) of cases identified are MTBI (i.e., concussion).

MECHANISMS OF INJURY

- The majority of DoD concussions and TBIs occur in a nondeployed setting and include training accidents, athletic concussions, and motor vehicle crashes (MVCs).
- Combat injuries may include blast as a component of injury.
- Blast injuries often have an additional mechanism such as rollover or impact (i.e., more than a single mechanism, or "blast plus").[3]

BLAST WAVE PHYSICS

Explosive blasts produce transient pressure waves, which can reach the speed of sound.[7] This is characterized by an initial high-pressure wave followed by a protracted low-pressure wave. This has been well studied and known to affect fluid- and air-filled structures (e.g., eyes, ears, lungs, and gastrointestinal tract). Blast waves also may include heat and electromagnetic waves, which can further disrupt the metabolic process and injure tissue.

MECHANISMS OF TRAUMATIC BRAIN INJURY WITH BLAST COMPONENT

Blast waves can cause TBI by several different commonly accepted mechanisms.[8–17] Primary, secondary, and quaternary mechanisms are generally considered unique to blast injury. The tertiary mechanism is similar to traditional closed head injuries.

- *Primary injury* represents the transduction of the blast wave itself, which can disrupt tissues. Understanding of the direct effect upon the brain is incomplete. It is unclear if the direct effect of the blast wave differs from more traditional causes of TBI in pathophysiology, neurological damage, or recovery patterns.[18] The three prevailing theories developed from animal models include:
  - Transduction of blast wave through skull causing biochemical dysfunction.
  - Vascular congestion from thorax injury causing transient pressure oscillations in the brain.[19]
  - Retrograde cerebrospinal fluid pressure from compression in the spinal column causing increased pressure in the cranial cavity.
- *Secondary injury* signifies the damage caused by objects traveling at high rates of speed and striking the victim. TBI can be caused by:
  - Penetrating head injury due to shrapnel or other foreign bodies.
  - Traditional closed head injury patterns with focal contusions and diffuse axonal injury due to rapid acceleration and deceleration.
- *Tertiary injuries* occur when the individual is thrown from high rates of speed and strike stationary objects. TBI is caused by traditional closed head injury mechanics such as rapid acceleration and deceleration in multiple planes.
- *Quaternary injuries* represent effects from thermal and inhalation injuries. Brain injury is thought to be caused by hypoxic or toxic effects upon cerebral tissue.

PATHOPHYSIOLOGY OF BLAST INJURIES

There is evidence through in vitro and animal studies that blast-induced shock waves cause blood–brain barrier (BBB) disruption and associated vascular events.

BBB disruption seems to be the major primary injury leading to neuroinflammation and neurodegeneration post-exposure to blast shock waves.[20]

- Lower-intensity blast shock waves cause oxidative stress and matrix metalloproteinase activation in brain capillaries leading to disruption of the BBB and formation of vascular edema, apoptosis of endothelial cells, and infiltration of leukocytes and macrophages.[20]
- Higher-intensity blast shock waves cause acute rupture of cerebral blood vessels leading to immediate increased oxidative stress and inflammation.[21,22]
- Absence of spontaneous repair of the BBB in days to weeks post-injury leads to a leaky BBB which causes worsening of the neuronal dysfunction, neuroinflammation, and neurodegeneration.[20]

Implications of early pressure surges through the arterial and venous vasculature systems after BINT, concurrent with the spread of shock waves in the body, are as follows.[23]

- Early pressure changes increase in platelet-activating factors induced by neutrophil activation and endothelial cell mediators/modulators leading to early and cyclic opening of the BBB.[4,24–26]

- Hydrodynamic pulse radiates through the vasculature away from the origin. Radiation of the pulse is less resistive in the brain as the brain vasculature has no valves.[27]
- There are temporal differences between the vascular and parenchymal responses to pressure transients. Significant pressure transients in the parenchyma and ventricle lead to tissue deformation and disrupt normal vasoactive function.[23,28-34] Resulting neurological deficits may include memory deficits and other cognitive problems, sleep disorder, and mood issues such as anxiety and depression, based on brain regions involved.[20]

POSTMORTEM FINDINGS

- Neuroanatomical pattern of *astrogliosis* post-exposure to high explosives
  - Brains of deceased servicemembers showed reactive astrocytosis in those that died shortly after a blast injury and severe astroglial scarring in those with chronic history of blast TBIs in the distribution as stated below[2]:
    - Subpial glial plate
    - Penetrating cortical blood vessels
    - Gray–white matter junction
    - Structures lining the ventricles
  - Reactive astrocytes are seen within hours post-injury and undergo cytoplasmic enlargement, nuclear displacement, and increase in glial fibrillary acidic protein (GFAP) expression.[2]
  - They further extend processes, intertwine and consolidate to form an astroglial scar within the same distribution, which is suggestive of a temporal and topographic link to the blast injury.[2]

SYMPTOMATOLOGY

- Blast syndrome soldiers report being stunned and losing consciousness post blast.[35]
- About 65% of blast injury victims experience headaches, tinnitus, deafness, dizziness, cognitive deficits such as memory problems, apathy, and musculoskeletal issues such as back pain.[35]
- BINT patients have been shown to be more sensitive to sudden loud noises and experience emotional and physical exhaustion.[35]
- Recent research has shown prolonged symptoms following BINT often have a psychological component as part of the symptom profile. The psychological component can amplify or exacerbate some of the other physical and cognitive symptoms.[36,37]

COMORBIDITIES AND COMPLICATIONS

- Psychological[38,39]
  Patients with a TBI sustained in combat have an increased risk for having psychological symptoms, including posttraumatic stress. Data show that up to 40% to 45% of combat injuries may have this comorbidity.[40]

- Polytrauma
  Dual sensory impairment with involvement of both visual and auditory function in association with an MTBI can occur, due to both peripheral and central etiologies.
  - More than 60% of veterans of Operation Iraqi Freedom with histories of blast-related MTBI were found to have some degree of sensorineural hearing loss.[41]
  - The presence of central auditory processing impairments appears to be common in soldiers with blast exposure, although the underlying cause is unknown.
  - Research on veterans with blast-related and other forms of TBI found that, in patients with moderate or severe TBI, 38.2% experienced an associated ocular injury. Reduced visual acuity was found in 16.7%, whereas 32.2% had visual field defects.[42]
  - Special expertise in auditory and visual rehabilitation is necessary for the complete rehabilitation approach to blast-injured military personnel.[19]
- Vascular complications[43]
  - Vascular lesions can occur due to exposure to shock waves. After moderate to severe blast injuries there is an increased risk of cerebrovascular injuries and complications, such as traumatic aneurysm, dissections, and vascular fistulae.[22]
  - In those with traumatic aneurysms, almost half develop vasospasm.[43] (See also Chapter 58.)

SCREENING IN A DEPLOYED SETTING

(Identifies those who are experiencing symptoms possibly related to TBI; does not qualify as an official diagnosis).

In 2016, collaboration between the medical corps and the Joint Chiefs of Staff led to new policy for the DoD, summarized in DTM (Directive-Type Memorandum) 09-033. Rather than relying on a service member to self-report symptoms, any and all service members involved in certain situations at risk for concussion are to undergo a screening evaluation and a mandatory 24-hour rest period.

These situations include:

- *Everyone* involved in a vehicle associated with a blast event, collision, or rollover
- Presence within 50 m of a blast (inside or outside)
- A *direct blow* to the head or witnessed *LOC*
- Exposure to *more than one blast event* (the service member's commander shall direct a medical evaluation).

When administered:

Screening occurs in the following settings:
- Post-injury in field (incident-based)—relies on an instrument known as the Military Acute Concussion Evaluation (MACE-2). MACE-2 is not used to make a diagnosis but as a screening tool to identify those who need further evaluation.
  - Similar to the Sport Concussion Assessment Tool (SCAT5) but the history and questions are directed at military injury.
  - In addition to the concussion history questions, there are three parts of assessment ("CNS"):
    - Cognitive screen (uses the Standardized Assessment of Concussion [SAC])
    - Neurological exam (brief and standardized)
    - Symptoms

■ At a Level IV hospital (after a service member is medically evacuated from a war zone), MACE-2 is used to determine if a concussion may be part of polytrauma pattern of injury.

SCREENING UPON RETURN FROM DEPLOYMENT

■ Post-Deployment Health Assessment—included with overall medical post-deployment screening upon return home from deployment—questions based on the Brief TBI Screen instrument (subjective incident and symptom questions) https://dvbic.dcoe.mil/sites/default/files/3-Question-Screening-Tool.pdf
  • Expanded to four questions to include acute symptoms and current symptoms
■ Entry to Veterans Administration (VA) care system—questions based on the four-question adaptation of the Brief TBI Screen instrument.

TREATMENT

Development of guidelines for military TBI was difficult due to individualized variation of mechanisms and severity of each trauma.[43] Approach to therapy has shifted to being more symptom based. BINT concussions are associated with greater psychopathology than concussions that are not blast related.[44] Neuropsychological testing is imperative in differentiating neurological from psychological contributions in those with persistent cognitive deficits.[45]

Acute In-Theater Management

■ Main objective: Safety—identify those who are experiencing TBI-related symptoms and prevent exposure to a recurrent injury until fully recovered.
■ There are training and practice guidelines for each echelon of care.
■ Each of the guidelines includes an assessment for red flags that would be a potential sign of need for a higher level of care.

Levels of care (highest level of care is highest number) in deployed area:

■ Level I: Battalion Aid Station—Medic/Corpsman—MACE-2
■ Level II: Concussion Care Center—physician and occupational therapy tech—cognitive testing
  • Concussion Care Centers have been established in theater with 2-week programs to manage those who may take longer to recover with expectation of recovery and return-to-duty.
■ Level III: Field Hospital—specialty care—neuroimaging

Evacuation

For patients with any significant injury to any part of the body that will lead to impairment, including moderate to severe TBI, evacuation is done by plane to a Level IV hospital facility (Landstuhl, Germany, for Iraq and Afghanistan) for further stabilization before transport to a U.S. Military Hospital.

DoD: Military Treatment Facilities

- Defense and Veterans Brain Injury Center (DVBIC)
  - Network of 14 military treatment facilities and four VA polytrauma facilities specializing in TBI care
- National Intrepid Center of Excellence (NICOE)—located on campus of Walter Reed National Medical Center
  - Provides comprehensive assessments for servicemembers with dual diagnoses and/or prolonged recovery periods
  - Network of 10 associated Intrepid Spirit Centers (seven of which are co-located with DVBIC sites)

VA System of Care—Largest Healthcare System in the United States

- Divided into 23 geographic areas—Veterans Integrated Service Networks (VISNs)
- Polytrauma System of Care
  - Five regional Polytrauma/TBI Rehabilitation Centers—provide acute comprehensive care (Richmond, Palo Alto, Minneapolis, Tampa, San Antonio)
  - 22 Polytrauma Rehabilitation Network Sites—provide post-acute interdisciplinary care
  - 82 Polytrauma Support Clinic Teams—involved in follow-up and management of stable patients
- Systems of care include education of family members and assistance with reintegration into community and education.

Specialized Pharmacotherapy Studied in Military Populations

- *N*-acetylcysteine (NAC): In a randomized, double-blind, placebo study, demonstrated efficacy in decreasing acute postconcussive and neurocognitive symptoms in service personnel in combat zones during the first 7 days post blast-related concussions.[46,47]
- Hyperbaric oxygen: In a randomized, double-blind, placebo study of DoD military injuries, did not show any benefit in patients with postconcussive symptoms both in non-blast- and blast-related concussions.[48]

Management of Return-to-Duty

Guidelines help guide a safe return-to-duty. These include resolution of impairing symptoms both at rest and with exertion and a return to cognitive baseline. If prior concussions have occurred within the previous 12 months, there is a longer required waiting time before being cleared for return-to-duty.

Computer-based cognitive testing is done pre-deployment and repeat testing can be done and compared to baseline as part of a return-to-duty decision-making process, after a service member no longer has impairing symptoms. This testing is not done as either a screen or a diagnostic test; it is used to help inform safe return-to-duty. This is similar to the application of such tests in sport-related concussions.

Differences From Sport-Related Concussion Model

- Combat-sustained blast injuries occur in an emotionally and psychologically complex context. Service members operate at an elevated baseline of attentive hypervigilance for extended periods of time. In addition, combat exposure is associated with significant emotional trauma.
- Global bodily injury from blast dynamics is typically more complex and severe than focal brain injuries caused by sport-related concussion. It is currently unclear whether

the severity and rate of persistent symptoms after concussion due to the blast mechanism itself differ from mechanical-/impact-related concussion.[18] These injuries may represent more than one mechanism ("blast plus") as opposed to a single-mechanism athletic injury.

■ Some lessons learned from the study of sport-related concussion do translate to the combat theater. These include methods for early rapid assessment and consensus guidelines for return-to-duty decisions, similar to those developed for return-to-play decisions in athletes following concussions. Also, cumulative effects of multiple blast exposures may be analogous to cumulative effects of recurrent sport-related concussions.

■ There are significant differences in patterns of comorbid injuries and conditions that occur in military blast injuries from those seen in sport-related concussions. These include comorbid physical trauma such as burns, complex fractures, visual and auditory impairments, and limb loss, as well as comorbid psychological injuries associated with combat exposure.

■ Decisions about return-to-duty must be made with the recognition that residual cognitive or psychomotor impairment can significantly affect the response of the individual to demanding combat-related contingencies, and thus may place other servicemembers' lives at risk.

Available Management Guidelines

Mild Traumatic Brain Injury/Concussion

■ Acute Management—DTM 09-033—June 2010
  ● https://www.documentcloud.org/documents/4411763-2010-Deputy-Secretary-of-Defense-Directive-Type.html
■ Subacute-Chronic Management
  ● See the VA/DoD Guidelines on Management of Concussion/Mild Traumatic Brain Injury 2016: https://www.healthquality.va.gov/guidelines/Rehab/mtbi/mTBICPGFullCPG50821816.pdf

Moderate to Severe Traumatic Brain Injury

■ Guidelines for Management of Severe TBI (2016), Brain Trauma Foundation
  ● https://braintrauma.org/uploads/03/12/Guidelines_for_Management_of_Severe_TBI_4th_Edition.pdf
■ Field Management of Combat Related Head Trauma (2006), focused on military setting
  ● https://www.braintrauma.org/uploads/02/09/btf_field_management_guidelines_2.pdf
  ● Joint Trauma System Guideline for Neurosurgery and Severe Head Injury (2017), DoD Joint Trauma System, guidance for deployed providers
  ● https://jts.amedd.army.mil/assets/docs/cpgs/Neurosurgery_and_Severe_Head_Injury_02_Mar_2017_ID30.pdf

---

KEY POINTS

■ Detection and management of TBI in the military setting continues to evolve. Ongoing research and collaboration with a variety of civilian subject matter experts and centers of excellence allow regular updates in these detection and management programs.

- Screening for TBI and concussions in deployed and combat settings has evolved from subjective symptom-based self-reporting to mandatory incident-based screening.
- Understanding blast effects upon the central nervous system is an evolving science. Both the direct effects of the blast wave upon the brain and the possible sequelae of repeated exposure are currently under investigation.

STUDY QUESTIONS

1. Explosive blast pressure waves possess the following characteristics:
   a. Speed of light; initial high-pressure wave followed by a protracted low-pressure wave
   b. Speed of light; initial low-pressure wave followed by a protracted high-pressure wave
   c. Speed of sound; initial high-pressure wave followed by a protracted low-pressure wave
   d. Speed of sound; initial low-pressure wave followed by a protracted high-pressure wave
   e. Speed of sound; protracted high pressures

2. Reactive astrocytosis and severe astroglial scarring in those deceased with chronic history of blast TBIs was seen in all of the following locations except:
   a. Subpial glial plate
   b. Penetrating cortical blood vessels
   c. Gray–white matter junction
   d. Subcortical white matter tracts
   e. Structures lining the ventricles

3. Which of the following BINT-related postmortem pathological changes are seen:
   a. Meningeal and gray–white matter congested veins
   b. Perineural, capillary, and venular enlargement
   c. Flattened gyri, tentorial grooving, small cerebellar cone
   d. Small cells in the pons and medulla
   e. All of the above

4. What are the implications of early pressure surges through the arterial and venous vasculature systems after BINT?
   a. They cause late pressure changes, decreasing platelet-activating factors
   b. Radiation of the pulse is less resistive in the brain as the brain vasculature has no valves
   c. Mechanisms which underlie the temporal differences between the vascular and parenchymal pressure are well understood and described in the literature
   d. Pressure transients in the parenchyma and ventricle do not lead to tissue deformation and disruption of vasoactive function
   e. Hydrodynamic pulse radiates through the vasculature toward the origin

5. Service members involved in certain situations are at increased risk for concussions and need to undergo a screening evaluation and mandatory 24-hour rest period. This is required in each of the following situations except:
   a. Inside/outside presence within 100 m of a blast
   b. Inside/outside presence within 50 m of a blast
   c. Exposure to more than one blast event
   d. A direct blow to the head or witnessed LOC
   e. Everyone in a vehicle associated with a blast event, collision, or rollover

ADDITIONAL READING

Military Health System Traumatic Brain Injury Center of Excellence: https://health.mil/About-MHS/OASDHA/Defense-Health-Agency/Research-and-Development/Traumatic-Brain-Injury-Center-of-Excellence

VA Polytrauma/TBI System of Care: www.polytrauma.va.gov/understanding-tbi

Hicks RR, Fertig SJ, Desrocher RE, et al. Neurological effects of blast injury. *J Trauma.* 2010;68:1257–1263. doi:10.1097/TA.0b013e3181d8956d

de Lanerolle NC, Hamid H, Kulas J, et al. Concussive brain injury from explosive blast. *Ann Clin Transl Neurol.* 2014;1(9):692–702. doi:10.1002/acn3.98.

Moore DF, Jaffee MS. Special issue: military traumatic brain injury and blast. *Neuro Rehabilitation.* 2010; 26:179–290. doi:10.3233/NRE-2010-0553

Sayer NA, Cifu DX, McNamee S, et al. Rehabilitation needs of combat-injured service members admitted to the VA Polytrauma Rehabilitation Centers: the role of PM&R in the care of wounded warriors. *PMR.* 2009;1(1):23–28. doi:10.1016/j.pmrj.2008.10.003

ANSWERS TO STUDY QUESTIONS

1. Correct Answer: c
Explosive blasts produce transient pressure waves, which can reach the speed of sound. It is characterized by an initial high-pressure wave followed by a protracted low-pressure wave. Answers (a) and (b) describe blast waves traveling at the speed of light which is incorrect. Answer (d) has an initial low-pressure wave followed by a high-pressure wave and the wave pattern is high pressure followed by protracted low pressure. Option (e) describes protracted high-pressure waves which is not accurate given that a protracted low-pressure wave follows an initial high-pressure wave.

Further Reading:
Cullis IG. Blast waves and how they interact with structures. *J R Army Med Corps.* 2001;147(1):16–26. doi:10.1136/jramc-147-01-02

2. Correct Answer: d
Reactive astrocytosis is seen in the subpial glial plate, penetrating cortical blood vessels, gray–white matter junction, and structures lining the ventricles. It is not seen in subcortical white matter tracts.

Further Reading:
Shively SB, Horkayne-Szakaly I, Jones RV, et al. Characterization of interface astroglial scarring in the human brain after blast exposure: a postmortem case series. *Lancet Neurol.* 2016;15:944–953. doi:10.1016/S1474-4422(16)30057-6

3. Correct Answer: e

Postmortem pathological changes related to BINT have been seen in all of the structures in options (a) through (d), so choice (e), all of the above, is correct.

Further Reading:

Mott FW. The microscopic examination of the brains of two men dead of commotio cerebri (shell shock) without visible external injury. *Br. Med. J.* 1917;2(2967):612–615. doi:10.1136/bmj.2.2967.612

Ashcroft PB. Blast injury of the lungs with a curious lesion of the cerebrum. *Lancet.* 1943;241(6234):234–235. doi:10.1016/S0140-6736(00)42226-9

4. Correct Answer: b

As the brain vasculature lacks valves, radiation of the pulse is less resistive. Option (a) is incorrect because early (not late) pressure changes increase (not decrease) platelet-activating factors. Option (c) is incorrect because, at this time, we are not clear of the mechanisms which underlie the temporal differences between the vascular and parenchymal pressure. Option (d) is incorrect because significant pressure transients in the parenchyma and ventricle lead to tissue deformation and disrupt normal vasoactive function. Option (e) is incorrect because hydrodynamic pulse radiates through the vasculature away from (not toward) the origin.

Further Reading:

Bauman RA, Ling G, Tong L, et al. An introductory characterization of a combat-casualty-care relevant swine model of closed head injury resulting from exposure to explosive blast. *J Neurotrauma.* 2009;26(6):841–860. doi:10.1089/neu.2008.0898

Mitchell MJ, Lin KS, King MR. Fluid shear stress increases neutrophil activation via platelet-activating factor. *Biophys J.* 2014;106(10):2243–2253. doi:10.1016/j.bpj.2014.04.001

Lehoux S, Castier Y, Tedgui A. Molecular mechanisms of the vascular responses to hemodynamic forces. *J Intern Med.* 2006;259(4):381–392. doi:10.1111/j.1365-2796.2006.01624.x

Risdall JE, Carter AJ, Kirkman E, et al. Endothelial activation and chemoattractant expression are early processes in isolated blast brain injury. *Neuromolecular Med.* 2014;16(3):606–619. doi:10.1007/s12017-014-8313-y

Simard JM, Pampori A, Keledjian K, et al. Exposure of the thorax to a sublethal blast wave causes a hydrodynamic pulse that leads to perivenular inflammation in the brain. *J Neurotrauma.* 2014;31(14):1292–1304. doi:10.1089/neu.2013.3016

Cernak I, Noble-Haeusslein LJ. Traumatic brain injury: an overview of pathobiology with emphasis on military populations. *J Cereb Blood Flow Metab.* 2010;30(2):255–266. doi:10.1038/jcbfm.2009.203

Cernak I, Wang Z, Jiang J, et al. Ultrastructural and functional characteristics of blast injury-induced neurotrauma. *J Trauma.* 2001;50(4):695–706. doi:10.1097/00005373-200104000-00017

Chavko M, Watanabe T, Adeeb S, et al. Relationship between orientation to a blast and pressure wave propagation inside the rat brain. *J Neurosci Methods.* 2011;195(1):61–66. doi:10.1016/j.jneumeth.2010.11.019

Gupta RK, Przekwas A. Mathematical models of blast induced TBI: current status, challenges, and prospects. *Front Neurol.* 2013;4:59. doi:10.3389/fneur.2013.00059

Chavko M, Koller WA, Prusaczyk WK, Mccarron RM. Measurement of blast wave by a miniature fiber optic pressure transducer in the rat brain. *J Neurosci Methods.* 2007;159(2):277–281. doi:10.1016/j.jneumeth.2006.07.018

Saljo A, Svensson B, Mayorga M, et al. Low levels of blast raises intracranial pressure and impairs cognitive function in rats. *J Neurotrauma.* 2009;26:1345–1352. doi:10.1089/neu.2008.0856

Lu J, Ng KC, Ling G, et al. Effect of blast exposure on the brain structure and cognition in *Macaca fascicularis*. *J Neurotrauma*. 2012;29(7):1434–1454. doi:10.1089/neu.2010.1591

5. Correct Answer: a

Service members involved in the following situations are required to undergo a screening evaluation and mandatory 24-hour rest period: presence within 50 m of a blast, exposure to more than one blast event, a direct blow to the head or witnessed LOC, and everyone involved in a vehicle associated with a blast event, collision, or rollover. Option (a) gives the option of 100 m, when the policy is actually 50 m.

REFERENCES

The full reference list appears in the digital product found on http://connect.springer-pub.com/content/book/978-0-8261-4768-4/part/part05/chapter/ch66

TREATMENT AND REHABILITATION SERVICES FOR MILD TO MODERATE TRAUMATIC BRAIN INJURY IN THE MILITARY

AMY Y. HAO, BLESSEN C. EAPEN, AND AMY O. BOWLES

INTRODUCTION

- Traumatic brain injuries (TBIs) in the military occur before, during, or after operational deployment. Although most TBIs are mild in severity, these injuries can result in serious short-term physical, emotional, and cognitive symptoms, and sometimes result in long-term changes in functioning.
- Advances in battlefield medicine have improved the survival from otherwise life-threatening injuries, which would have been fatal in the past, resulting in an increased survival of service members with TBI.[1]
- Many service members experience a combination of physical injuries, psychological trauma, and mild traumatic brain injury (MTBI). A traumatic stress reaction can occur as a result of the same event, or separate events.
- "Polytrauma clinical triad" of chronic pain, posttraumatic stress disorder (PTSD), and persistent postconcussive symptoms (PPCS) are frequently observed together and 6% to 40% of all veterans screened experience these conditions concurrently.[2,3]
- Service members who are wounded in combat are at an increased risk for chronic pain,[4] depression,[5] and PTSD.[6]

SCOPE OF THE PROBLEM

TBI has become known as the "signature injury" of the wars in Iraq and Afghanistan.[7] During these conflicts, the extensive use of improvised explosive devices (IEDs) has been responsible for up to 50% to 79% of deployment-related TBIs.[8] In 2007, the high incidence of military TBI, coupled with the growing concern of the cumulative effect of multiple concussions, led the Department of Defense (DoD) and Department of Veterans Affairs (VA) to adopt a common definition, screening criteria, and clinical practice guidelines. The VA/DoD classification system for TBI is presented in Table 67.1.

- Postdeployment TBI screening of military personnel returning from Operation Enduring Freedom in Afghanistan (OEF), Operation Iraqi Freedom (OIF), and Operation New Dawn in Iraq (OND) conflicts are positive approximately 20% of the time.[1]

The full reference list appears in the digital product found on http://connect.springerpub.com/content/book/978-0-8261-4768-4/part/part05/chapter/ch67

TABLE 67.1   U.S. DoD/VA Traumatic Brain Injury Classification System

Criteria	Mild	Moderate	Severe
Loss of Consciousness (LOC)	0–30 min	30 min < LOC < 24 hr	≥24 hr
Alteration of Consciousness (AOC)	≤24 hr	If >24 hr, then use other criteria to classify severity	
Posttraumatic Amnesia (PTA)	≤1 day	1 day < PTA < 7 days	≥7 days
Glasgow Coma Scale (GCS) score	13–15	9–12	≤8
Structural Imaging (magnetic resonance imaging [MRI] or computed tomography [CT])	Normal	Normal or abnormal	Normal or abnormal

Source: From The Management of Concussion/MTBI Working Group. *VA/DoD Clinical Practice Guideline for Management of Concussion/Mild Traumatic Brain Injury (MTBI)*. 2009; www.healthquality.va.gov/guidelines/Rehab/mtbi

- It is essential to appreciate that screening positive for TBI on a questionnaire is not definitive evidence that the injury actually occurred. Rather, the gold standard for TBI diagnosis is a thorough clinical evaluation.[7]
- DoD policies direct TBI screening following exposure to a potential injury event and at specified pre-deployment, post-deployment, and periodic health assessments.[10,11] Most concussion patients are managed by a primary care provider, but a comprehensive system of specialty TBI clinics are available to treat those with severe injuries, complex comorbidities, or refractory symptoms.
- Based on DoD surveillance statistics from 2000 to 2019, 82.8% of the 413,858 total traumatic brain injuries diagnosed in the military were categorized as mild, 9.8% moderate, 1.0% severe, 1.3% penetrating and 5.2% not classifiable.[12]
- In the VA, patients who screen positive are sent to a TBI specialty clinic for a comprehensive TBI evaluation (CTBIE) to determine the likelihood of TBI and direct further treatment.

COMORBIDITIES

The evaluation and management of combat-related TBI can be complicated by the presence of other medical and psychiatric factors. These include combat-related injuries such as burns and amputation, as well as various comorbidities such as PTSD, depression and other signs and symptoms which may overlap or interact with those of TBI.

- *PTSD:* Estimates of the prevalence of PTSD among OEF/OIF veterans range from 4% to 17%.[13] In one study, the proportion of veterans who screened positive for TBI and had PTSD was more than double those who had PTSD alone (32% vs. 13%).[14]
  - Screening positive for PTSD is associated with:
    - Number of deployments[15]
    - Deployment-related stressors[16]
    - Greater combat exposure[17]
    - Getting wounded[18]
    - Sustaining an MTBI[8]
    - Greater general medical burden[19]

- Careful diagnostic interviewing by a clinician results in more accurate identification of combat-related PTSD and reduces false-positive diagnoses.[20,21] Depression frequently co-occurs with PTSD in military personnel.[8,21]
- Service members who sustain an MTBI and have high levels of combat stress symptoms have a three to eight times increased likelihood of experiencing postconcussive symptoms, compared to those with low levels of combat stress.[22]

Depression: In post-deployment surveys, 5.7% to 15.7% of service members screen positive for depression,[23,24] although some surveys of those in the VA care system have shown rates of 39% to 48%.[25]

- Similar to screening estimates for MTBI and PTSD, these prevalence estimates decline when screening is followed by interviewing with a clinician.[21]
- There is significant symptom overlap between depression and postconcussion syndrome.[26] Military service members with history of MTBI demonstrate a 34% rate of co-occurring depression diagnoses.[27]
- In those with MTBI, the presence of loss of consciousness (LOC) and/or posttraumatic amnesia (PTA), PTSD, and self-reported cognitive problems were associated with worse depression.[28,29]

Amputation: Between January 2001 and December 2016, 1710 U.S. service members sustained at least one amputation; 73% of these injuries resulted from an IED blast injury and 31% involved amputation of more than one major limb.[30]

- Service members undergoing amputation are at significant risk for depression, anxiety, PTSD, chronic pain, and body image problems.[31]
- Patients who have both a combat-related TBI and amputation utilize more medical and rehabilitative services than those with amputation alone.[32]

Body image: Military personnel who suffer facial disfigurement, complex scars to their limbs or torsos, spinal cord injuries, or amputations frequently deal with psychological problems relating to their body image. Psychological adjustment issues and problems associated with body image can interfere with social and occupational functioning.

- Despite the expectation that the symptom burden increases proportionally with severity of bodily injury, some studies suggest otherwise. In fact, those patients with more extensive bodily injuries report fewer posttraumatic stress and postconcussion symptoms than those who experience minor bodily injuries.[33]

Sensory impairments

- Visual and audiologic symptoms are common following blast-related MTBI. Up to 75% of veterans with a history of MTBI due to blast injury report tinnitus[34] and in a study of visual dysfunction after blast-induced MTBI, 68% of patients reported visual complaints—most commonly photophobia.[35] Symptom-based management with re-evaluation for treatment response and functional improvement is recommended.[9]

Chronic pain: Pain lasting more than 6 months is defined as chronic. Chronic pain is a common problem in veterans,[36] and it is frequently comorbid with TBI.[3,37]

- People who suffer from chronic pain often report subjectively experienced cognitive impairment,[38] and they are likely to report postconcussion-like symptoms in the absence of a past MTBI.[39] Those with chronic pain are also at risk for comorbid depression.

Insomnia: Problems with sleep often occur during deployment,[40] and are commonly reported postdeployment,[41] both in low- and high-combat stress groups.[29] In patients with TBI, and especially those with concurrent TBI and PTSD, insomnia can be especially problematic.[29]

Persistent problems with falling asleep, staying asleep, or waking too early can occur as a primary insomnia condition or be associated with a comorbid condition (e.g.,

PTSD or chronic pain).[42] Sleep problems can be associated with obesity,[43] tinnitus,[44] and perceived impairments with cognition when they become chronic.[34]

- Sleep hygiene counseling and PTSD severity reduction in patients with MTBI has been associated with sustained improvements in headaches, cognitive function, and daytime sleepiness.[45]

■ *Substance misuse, abuse, and dependence:* Substance use is a prevalent issue among service members and veterans. It can co-occur with mental health problems and cause problems with social and occupational functioning.

- In those with concurrent TBI, substance abuse can exacerbate cognitive dysfunction and have an adverse effect on underlying mood disturbances, making an accurate diagnosis more challenging.[46]

■ *Life stress and community re-entry issues:* Some service members struggle with resuming their home and work lives and responsibilities following deployment.[47] These problems can be compounded by the stress of deploying again within a short period. Repeated deployments can contribute to PTSD symptoms[17] as well as substance misuse and mental health problems.

- Veterans with TBI have greater challenges with community reintegration than those without TBI, but this may be influenced by the presence of comorbid depression and/or chronic pain.[48]

■ *Suicidality:* The suicide rate among U.S. military personnel has risen steadily since the initiation of the OEF/OIF conflicts. TBI is thought to be one of the factors contributing to this rising rate.[49]

- History of multiple lifetime TBIs has been associated with increased rate of recent suicidal ideation in Iraq and Afghanistan war-era veterans.[50] OEF/OIF/OND veterans with a history of deployment-related TBI demonstrate a higher risk of suicide attempts as well.[51] A recent study found that a history of TBI was associated with increased suicidal ideation in a population of veterans with depression, but not in the non-depressed sub-sample.[52]

IN-THEATER EVALUATION AND MANAGEMENT

■ Trauma care for military personnel follows five progressive levels, or echelons, which guide both immediate stabilization and appropriate long-term management[53,54] (see Table 67.2).

■ The Military Acute Evaluation (MACE) is used to screen service members with high risk of exposure to blast or TBI, and is most sensitive within 12 hours of injury.[55] It is derived from the Standardized Assessment of Concussion (SAC) and is utilized to preliminarily document neurocognitive deficits as well as screen for red flags.[56] In 2019, the military released an updated version, the MACE-2,[57] which includes a vestibular/ocular-motor assessment piece. These tools can be used in the theater of military operations or at home.

■ As compared to civilian TBI, which is frequently associated with blunt trauma, combat-related TBI is frequently associated with blast injury. Given the higher risk of vascular injury in blast-related severe or penetrating TBI, the use of early decompressive craniectomy,[58] although controversial in civilian trauma cases, as well as aggressive treatment of cerebral vasospasm,[59] has been highlighted in recent military experience.[60] In addition, whereas tension-type headaches are associated with blunt trauma, headaches following blast injury are often more vascular or migrainous in nature.[61]

TABLE 67.2   Military Echelons of Care

Level I: Initial emergency care and evacuation by trained emergency medical technicians (i.e., combat medics, corpsmen, and independent duty medical technicians). Very limited surgical capability.
Level II: Composed entirely of mobile units (e.g., Army forward surgical team). Especially critical in areas where rapid evacuation to Level III is limited. First level at which surgical resuscitation is possible.
Level III: Highest level of medical care available within the combat zone with capability similar to U.S. civilian trauma center (e.g., Army combat support hospital). Generally includes an intensive care unit and medical subspecialty care.
Level IV: First level at which surgical management outside the combat zone can be performed; usually provided by a combat support hospital, fleet hospital, or fixed medical facility depending on situation and evacuation route.
Level V: Final level of care at which definitive stabilization and treatment is performed. Consists of military treatment facilities (MTF) in the United States (e.g., Walter Reed Army Medical Center in Washington, D.C.; National Naval Medical Center in Bethesda, Maryland; Brooke Army Medical Center at Fort Sam Houston in San Antonio, Texas).

Source: From Bagg MR, Covey DC, Powell ET. Levels of medical care in the global war on terrorism. *J Am Acad Orthop Surg.* 2006;14:7–9. doi:10.5435/00124635-200600001-00003

- The immediate effects of blast and explosion exposures can be categorized as follows:
  - Primary blast injuries: caused by over- or under-pressurization shock waves which cause damage to organs at tissue-density interfaces.
  - Secondary blast injuries: result from debris thrown as a result of the explosion or blast which can lead to penetrating injuries or blunt trauma.
  - Tertiary blast injuries: injuries sustained due to the body being thrown against a fixed object, or from structural collapse.
  - Quaternary blast injuries: injuries related to the blast or explosion but not due to primary, secondary or tertiary causes; e.g., burns, inhalation injuries, exacerbation of pre-existing conditions.[62]
- In 2019, the Defense and Veterans Brain Injury Center (DVBIC) released the Concussion Management Tool.[63] This provides an integrated tool for acute evaluation and management of concussion, whether it occurs in combat or at home. It also provides guidance on return to activity.*
- DVBIC has created additional clinical tools for providers, including treatment algorithms and recommendations as well as educational materials for patients (see Additional Reading and References).
- A graduated return to activity process is recommended after acute concussion or MTBI in both deployed and non-deployed settings. There are six stages of activity progressing from rest to unrestricted activity with symptom monitoring throughout.[64]

STATESIDE EVALUATION AND MANAGEMENT

- General and specific principles for managing an uncomplicated MTBI during deployment, as well as providing subsequent treatment and rehabilitation services, are set out

---

* Editor's note: DVBIC is now referred to as the Traumatic Brain Injury Center of Excellence (TBICoE). Some resources have been re-named as a result, though all materials referenced in this chapter are available through this center's website: https://health.mil/About-MHS/OASDHA/Defense-Health-Agency/Research-and-Development/Traumatic-Brain-Injury-Center-of-Excellence

TABLE 67.3   General Principles for Providing Treatment and Rehabilitation Services

Somatic complaints (e.g., headaches, dizziness or coordination problems, vision and hearing changes, sleep disturbance, fatigue)
Assess individual factors and symptom presentation to guide treatment:
• <u>Headache</u>: Single most common symptom. Assessment and management should parallel those for other causes of headache.
• <u>Dizziness and disequilibrium</u>: Treatment interventions based on etiology—peripheral vestibular, central nervous system, psychological, musculoskeletal, or idiopathic.
• <u>Vision</u>: Acute symptoms include light sensitivity, blurry vision, or eye fatigue. Persistence of symptoms may require evaluation by optometry, ophthalmology, neuro-ophthalmology, and/or vision rehabilitation.
• <u>Hearing</u>: Changes in hearing acuity or noise sensitivity typically resolve within a month and permanent impairments in central auditory acuity or processing are rare with MTBI. Audiology evaluation may be indicated for comprehensive hearing assessment.
• <u>Sleep</u>: Comorbidities including sleep apnea, chronic pain, and depression can contribute to sleep disturbance. Nonpharmacological management options include education on sleep hygiene and cognitive behavioral therapy.
• <u>Fatigue</u>: Assess physical activity, cognitive function, and mental health.
Psychiatric signs and symptoms
• Treat according to nature and severity of symptom presentation, including both psychotherapeutic and pharmacological treatment modalities.
Persistent/refractory post-concussive symptoms
• Consideration should be given to other factors, including psychiatric and psychosocial support, and compensatory or litigation issues.

Source: From Management of Concussion-mild Traumatic Brain Injury (MTBI) (2016); https://www.healthquality.va.gov/guidelines/Rehab/mtbi/

by the combined VA/DoD Clinical Practice Guidelines,[9] with salient points outlined in Table 67.3.

■ The primary goal of treatment and rehabilitation in military personnel who have persistent symptoms and comorbidities due to TBI is to reduce symptoms, improve functioning, and in some cases determine eligibility for return to duty.

■ For service members with complex comorbidities, multimodal and interdisciplinary treatment and rehabilitation services are used to address the wide variety of impairments seen in patients with TBI (see Additional Reading and References).

  ● *Medications*
    ▪ Use dual-purpose medications to address commonly concurrent symptoms in TBI patients, such as headaches and mood disturbances, or PTSD and insomnia, to reduce polypharmacy.
    ▪ Give full, therapeutic trials at maximal tolerated doses while monitoring for side effects.
    ▪ Avoid medications that can cause cognitive impairment or that can lower seizure threshold.

  ● *Physical Therapy*
    ▪ Physical therapy interventions can be useful for addressing TBI-related vestibular impairments that can lead to vertigo and imbalance, as well as nonmedication-based treatment for cervicogenic and migraine headaches.[65]

  ● *Occupational Therapy*

- ■ Occupational therapy can target cognitive and memory impairments in MTBI that may hinder community reintegration; this discipline also addresses impairments in activities of daily living (ADLs) and instrumental ADLs in those with moderate to severe TBI.[66]
- ● *Speech and Language Pathology*
  - ■ Craniofacial trauma after blast injury, especially in severe TBI, can result in injuries leading to disorders of swallowing and cognitive-communication impairments, including aphasia and dysarthria.[67]
- ● *Exercise*
  - ■ Exercise has been shown to promote neurogenesis[68,69] and is a good adjuvant treatment for depression and anxiety in people who are slow to recover from an MTBI.[70]
- ● *Psychological and Behavioral Treatment*
  - ■ Psychological care is integral for patients with TBI given the high rate of sleep and mood disturbances; treatment leads to improved functioning with comorbid PTSD[71] and anxiety problems[72] as well as improved sleep and reduced psychological distress.[41]
- ▦ The Polytrauma System of Care, created by the Veterans Health Administration in 2004 to address the growing needs of the OEF/OIF/OND population, serves to provide the aforementioned treatment services.[73,74]
  - ● This system of care is comprised of a well-connected network providing continuum of care, including Polytrauma Support Clinic Teams (PSCT), Polytrauma Network Sites (PNS), Polytrauma Rehabilitation Centers (PRCs), and Polytrauma Transitional Rehabilitation Programs (PTRP).
  - ● PRCs provide acute, comprehensive inpatient rehabilitation, and provide consultations to other VA facilities. PTRPs offer structured residential rehabilitation with a focus on progressive return to independent living. PNS can provide the entry point into the system for veterans who screen positive, and in conjunction with PSCTs, provide continued, specialized outpatient care.[75]
- ▦ The coexistence of chronic pain, PTSD, and PPCS presenting as the polytrauma clinical triad may also be taken into consideration when planning treatment approaches and management, especially in OEF/OIF veterans.[2,3]

KEY POINTS

- ▦ Mild traumatic brain injury (MTBI) has become known as the "signature injury" of the recent wars, including Operation Enduring Freedom in Afghanistan (OEF), Operation Iraqi Freedom (OIF), and Operation New Dawn (OND).[7]
- ▦ The Veterans Healthcare System and Department of Defense have robust TBI screening programs as well as specialty care systems for patients who cannot be successfully managed in primary care.
- ▦ The Defense and Veterans Brain Injury Center (DVBIC) has developed resources to help direct management of combat-related head trauma. The VA/DoD Clinical Practice Guidelines for the Management of Concussion/MTBI are available to help direct stateside management at least 7 days post injury.
- ▦ Unlike in civilian trauma populations, combat-related TBI is commonly due to blast injury.[76] Current evidence does not support changing TBI treatment or prognosis based on mechanism of injury.

STUDY QUESTIONS

1. A 24-year-old U.S. Marine Corps corporal was driving a truck when a vehicle ahead detonated an IED (improvised explosive device). He was thrown from the vehicle and lost consciousness for approximately 1 hour per witness reports. His next memory is of being in the hospital 3 days later. Computed tomography (CT) of the head did not reveal any acute, abnormal intracranial findings. What level of TBI did he incur according to the U.S. DoD/DVA Traumatic Brain Injury Classification system?
   a. No brain injury
   b. Mild
   c. Moderate
   d. Severe

2. All of the following factors are associated with screening positive for PTSD except:
   a. Greater combat exposure
   b. No deployment-related injuries
   c. Sustaining an MTBI
   d. Deployment-related stressors

3. The "polytrauma clinical triad" consists of which of the following diagnoses?
   a. Depression, postconcussive symptoms, insomnia
   b. Generalized anxiety disorder, postconcussive symptoms, chronic pain
   c. PTSD, postconcussive symptoms, chronic pain
   d. Headaches, postconcussive symptoms, PTSD

4. Which of the following headache phenotypes is more common following a blast-related head injury as opposed to a blunt trauma head injury?
   a. Tension-type
   b. Cervicogenic
   c. Migraine
   d. Occipital neuralgia

5. A Navy veteran survives a severe traumatic brain injury resulting from a motor vehicle collision and requires intensive inpatient rehabilitation services. Which center within the Polytrauma System of Care is most appropriate for this veteran?
   a. Polytrauma Network Site (PNS)
   b. Polytrauma Rehabilitation Center (PRC)
   c. Polytrauma Transitional Rehabilitation Program (PTRP)
   d. Polytrauma Support Clinic Team (PSCT)

ADDITIONAL READING

Defense and Veterans Brain Injury Center: Concussion Management Tool. 2019. https://dvbic.dcoe.mil/material/concussion-management-tool

Management of Concussion/MTBI Working Group. *VA/DoD Clinical Practice Guideline for Management of Concussion/Mild Traumatic Brain Injury (mTBI)*. 2016. www.healthquality.va.gov/guidelines/Rehab/mtbi

Eapen BC, Cifu DX. *Polytrauma Rehabilitation. Physical Medicine and Rehabilitation Clinics of North America.* Elsevier. 2019. doi:10.1016/S1047-9651(18)30856-8

Shura RD, Epstein EL, Armistead-Jehle P, et al. (2019). Assessment and treatment of concussion in service members and veterans. In: Eapen B, Cifu D, eds. *Concussion Assessment, Management and Rehabilitation.* Elsevier. doi:10.1016/B978-0-323-65384-8.00013-4

Tapia R, Garg D, Eapen B. Developing a therapeutic approach toward active engagement for veterans with mild traumatic brain injury. *Journal Head Trauma Rehabil.* 2019;34(3):141–149. doi:10.1097/HTR.0000000000000490

Rosenfeld JV, McFarlane AC, Bragge P, et al. Blast-related traumatic brain injury. *Lancet Neurol.* 2013;(12)9:882–893. doi:10.1016/S1474-4422(13)70161-3

ANSWERS TO STUDY QUESTIONS

1. Correct Answer: c

Moderate. He suffered an IED-related brain injury with loss of consciousness greater than 30 minutes but less than 24 hours and PTA greater than 1 day but less than 7 days. This is classified as a moderate TBI.

Further Reading:

Management of Concussion-mild Traumatic Brain Injury (mTBI). 2016. https://www.healthquality.va.gov/guidelines/Rehab/mtbi

2. Correct Answer: b

No deployment related injuries. Factors associated with screening positive for PTSD include: number of deployments, deployment-related stressors, greater combat exposure, getting wounded, sustaining an MTBI and greater general medical burden.

Further Reading:

Stroupe KT, Smith BM, Hogan TP, et al. Healthcare utilization and costs of veterans screened and assessed for traumatic brain injury. *J Rehabil Res Dev.* 2013;50(8):1047–1068. doi:10.1682/JRRD.2012.06.0107

Reger MA, Gahm GA, Swanson RD, et al. Association between number of deployments to Iraq and mental health screening outcomes in U.S. Army soldiers. *J Clin Psychiatry.* 2009;70(9):1266–1272. doi:10.4088/JCP.08m04361

Booth-Kewley S, Larson GE, Highfill-McRoy RM, et al. Correlates of posttraumatic stress disorder symptoms in Marines back from war. *J Trauma Stress.* 2010;23(1):69–77. doi:10.1002/jts.20485

Vasterling JJ, Proctor SP, Friedman MJ, et al. PTSD symptom increases in Iraq-deployed soldiers: comparison with nondeployed soldiers and associations with baseline symptoms, deployment experiences, and postdeployment stress. *J Trauma Stress.* 2010;23(1):41–51. doi:10.1002/jts.20487

Koren D, Norman D, Cohen A, et al. Increased PTSD risk with combat-related injury: a matched comparison study of injured and uninjured soldiers experiencing the same combat events. *Am J Psychiatry.* 2005;162(2):276–282. doi:10.1176/appi.ajp.162.2.276

3. Correct Answer: c

PTSD, postconcussive symptoms, chronic pain. The polytrauma clinical triad consists of chronic pain, PTSD, and persistent postconcussive symptoms. Depression, insomnia, generalized anxiety disorder, and headaches are other common comorbidities in patients with MTBI.

Further Reading:

Lew HL, Cifu DX, Crowder T, Hinds SR. National prevalence of traumatic brain injury, posttraumatic stress disorder, and pain diagnoses in OIF/OEF/OND Veterans from 2009 to 2011. *J Rehabil Res Dev.* 2013;50(9):11–14. doi:10.1682/JRRD.2013.09.0212

Cifu DX, Taylor BC, Carne WF, et al. Traumatic brain injury, posttraumatic stress disorder, and pain diagnoses in OIF/OEF/OND Veterans. *J Rehabil Res Dev*. 2013;50(9):1169–1176. doi:10.1682/JRRD.2013.01.0006

4. Correct Answer: c

Migraine. While blunt trauma head injuries tend to be associated with tension-type headaches, headaches following blast injury are more often migrainous or vascular in nature.

Further Reading:

Defense and Veterans Brain Injury Center: Military acute concussion evaluation 2 (MACE 2). 2018. https://health.mil/About-MHS/OASDHA/Defense-Health-Agency/Research-and -Development/Traumatic-Brain-Injury-Center-of-Excellence/Provider-Resources

5. Correct Answer: b

Polytrauma Rehabilitation Center (PRC). PRCs provide acute, comprehensive inpatient rehabilitation and are the most appropriate settings for veterans who suffer severe TBI requiring intensive, multidisciplinary inpatient rehabilitation.

Further Reading:

Bell JA, Burnett A. Exercise for the primary, secondary and tertiary prevention of low back pain in the workplace: a systematic review. *J Occup Rehabil*. 2009;19(1):8–24. doi:10.1007/s10926-009-9164-5

van Praag H. Neurogenesis and exercise: past and future directions. *Neuromolecular Med*. 2008;10(2):128–140. doi:10.1007/s12017-008-8028-z

REFERENCES

The full reference list appears in the digital product found on http://connect.springer-pub.com/content/book/978-0-8261-4768-4/part/part05/chapter/ch67

MANAGEMENT OF TRAUMATIC BRAIN INJURY IN THE OLDER ADULT

DAVID X. CIFU, BLESSEN C. EAPEN, AND CARLOS A. JARAMILLO

INTRODUCTION

This chapter reviews the general aspects of traumatic brain injury (TBI) rehabilitation of the older adult (aged 65 and older).

Normal age-related changes of the brain include:

- Brain atrophy with deceased brain volume and weight
- Increased bridging vein fragility
- Increased adherence of dura to skull
- Decreased cerebral autoregulation and cerebral perfusion reactivity

These neuroanatomical and neurophysiological changes make the elderly brain susceptible to more severe TBI and its resulting complications.

DEMOGRAPHICS

The U.S. Census Bureau estimates that adults over 65 years of age, who currently make up approximately 12% of the population, will represent nearly 17% of the world's total population, or some 1.6 billion individuals, by 2050, with most of them living in developing countries.[1] In the United States in 2013, more than 1 in 200 Americans aged 65 to 74 years and more than 1 in 50 Americans aged 75 years and older experienced a TBI-related emergency department (ED) visit, hospitalization, or death, and adults aged 75 years or more accounted for 26.5% of all TBI-related deaths and 31.4% of all TBI-related hospitalizations.[2,3]

ETIOLOGY

The most common causes of TBI in older adults, in decreasing frequency, are falls, traffic-related events, including motor vehicle crashes (MVCs) pedestrian struck by vehicle, and assault/violence.[4] Falls, which are typically low-velocity injuries, result in focal brain injuries, most commonly subdural hematomas (SDH) and/or focal cortical contusions. Elders on anticoagulation/antiplatelet agents have a higher likelihood of also having intracerebral hemorrhage. Based on the speed and mechanics of the impact and the presence of safety restraints (e.g., seat belts, air bags), MVCs may result in diffuse axonal injury (DAI),

---

The full reference list appears in the digital product found on http://connect.springerpub.com/content/book/978-0-8261-4768-4/part/part05/chapter/ch68

focal contusions, or SDH. Pedestrian–MVCs frequently occur at crosswalks and in parking lots and these accidents similarly result in DAI, SDH, or focal contusions. Skeletal and visceral injuries are not uncommon in elders involved in MVC or pedestrian–MVCs. Assaults and violent acts, although rare, may result in focal contusions, skull fractures with SDH, epidural hematomas (EDH), and/or intracranial bone or bullet fragments. Age-related physiological changes (e.g., cerebral atrophy) may result in older adults who sustain a TBI of any severity experiencing relatively more severe impairments then might otherwise be expected.

RISK FACTORS

Falls

- *Chronic medical:* central neurological disease (cerebrovascular accident, Parkinson's disease, dementia), peripheral neurological disease (diabetes mellitus, alcohol misuse), visual impairments (glaucoma, cataracts), weakness/pain (musculoskeletal disease, arthritis).
- *Acute medical:* episodic postural hypotension, acute illness, alcohol use, medication effects, polypharmacy.
- *Activity-related:* tripping while walking, descending stairs, climbing ladders, bicycling.
- *Environmental:* poor lighting, nonsecure throw rugs, ill-fitting shoe wear, pets, children.[5]

Traffic-Related Events

Common senescent changes seen in older adults, such as decreased visual acuity, decreased night vision, slowed reaction time, decreased hearing, pain and medication effects, put them at risk for MVCs. In addition to these factors, *the slower walking pace* seen in older adults can predispose older adults to pedestrian–MVCs (e.g., cross walk lights are not timed to older adults). Older drivers have a higher rate of fatality per mile driven compared with those between the ages 30 and 69, with the highest rates among drivers over the age of 85. This appears to be related to age-related susceptibility to serious injury and medical comorbidities, which complicate recovery from injury.[6]

CLINICAL PRESENTATION

Older adults experience a disproportionate incidence of mild TBIs compared to other age groups likely due to greater susceptibility to injury.[7] Elderly individuals are also particularly vulnerable to SDH because bridging veins become more susceptible to shearing forces as the brain naturally atrophies with advancing age.[4] Postconcussive symptoms may worsen pre-existing conditions which are more common in older adults, such as depression, mild cognitive impairment, and mild dementia.

Morbidity

TBI in the older adult often results in a higher morbidity related to concomitant medical problems, for example at least 1 in 10 community dwelling elders 65 years and older have significant cognitive deficits and by age 85 up to 50% have at least mild dementia.[8,9] Clinicians with training and expertise that spans both brain injury and geriatric medicine should be involved from initial hospitalization to assist in minimizing secondary complications such as pressure ulcers, contractures, deep vein thromboembolisms, cardiac deconditioning, aspiration precautions, and bowel and bladder management, in addition to assessing medical comorbidities, such as cardiovascular disease, diabetes, neuromuscular disease, and dementia that may have challenged function before injury.

Common Co-morbid Complications

- Fractures—affect weight-bearing status and need for assistance.
- Cardiopulmonary complications—lower ejection fraction and vital capacity and alterations of cardiac rhythm can affect ability to participate in rehabilitation and live independently.
- Pain—both pre-injury (neuropathic, musculoskeletal, or vascular pain) and post-injury (pain caused by trauma) should be assessed and treated appropriately. As with all individuals, whenever possible manage acute and chronic pain conditions with nonpharmacological modalities (education, exercise, counselling, biofeedback).
- Swallowing—may be compromised from traumatic injury or pre-existing pathology (e.g., cerebrovascular accident, Barrett's esophagus), resulting in need for alternative feeding methods or modified diet.
- Polypharmacy—specific to older adults who may be on multiple preinjury medications and may have difficulty managing medication administration instructions. Care must be taken when choosing medications to adjust for physiological differences in drug metabolism for elderly adults; for example, opioids may easily lead to delirium and nonsteroidal anti-inflammatory drugs (NSAIDs) may further compromise renal function. Side effect profiles should also be considered as central acting medications could exacerbate TBI-related symptoms and increase risk of adverse events such as falls.
- Deep venous thrombosis prophylaxis and treatment—need to consider factors such as optimal timing of initiating prophylaxis, balancing fall risk with optimal treatment approach

TREATMENT

Rehabilitation

The rehabilitation approach to an older adult with TBI requires an understanding of preinjury level of function, medical comorbidities, cognitive impairments, and behavioral issues. In addition to a thorough medical review, a detailed review of the elder's social support network is critical. This is a key factor to help the rehabilitation team set goals that are realistic for the patient's anticipated discharge environment. Specific areas of focus in a rehabilitation program for the older adult are discussed in the following sections.

Medication Management
The majority of the population above 65 years of age takes at least one prescription medication daily, with a majority taking over five medications.[10] Therefore, concern must be given to polypharmacy, which will likely complicate care on discharge and could lead to adverse events and outcomes. This is especially important in elderly patients who may have age-related decline in hepatic and renal drug clearance. Medications may change during the acute and chronic recovery periods. Therefore, educating the patient and caregivers on proper medication timing and dosing is important when

transitioning a patient through the acute phase to rehabilitation, and eventually to discharge from a hospital setting.

Bladder and Bowel Continence

Normal aging may affect bladder function because of prostate hypertrophy, pelvic relaxation (in women), decreased bladder capacity with urinary frequency, and decreased capability to suppress bladder contractions at low volumes, resulting in urinary urgency.[11] TBI can result in urinary incontinence related to an inability to sense bladder fullness, an inability to suppress the pontine micturition center's automatic emptying at key volumes, or increased frequency caused by a urinary tract infection. Assessment of preinjury voiding patterns is helpful in discerning underlying pathology, independent of the effects of TBI. As with the bladder, bowel routines are typically disrupted during hospitalization. In the older adult, disruption of the bowel routine can become a preoccupation unless properly addressed. Assessing preinjury bowel routine is the first step in establishing goals. Continence should be a significant focus of rehabilitation efforts in older adults, because this can determine an individual's independence and level of caregiver burden.

Sensory Health

Vision

Normal aging is associated with changes in visual acuity and refractive power, decrements in extraocular motion, increases in intraocular pressure, decreased tear secretion, and decreased corneal and lens function.[8,9] These conditions could be compounded by additional visual disturbances after head injury and put the patient at increased risk for falls. Identifying visual changes due to TBI as well as pre-existing visual problems is essential to the rehabilitation process.[12]

Hearing

Normal aging is associated with high-frequency hearing loss and signal distortion at higher frequencies, difficulty localizing signals needed for binaural hearing, and difficulty understanding speech in unfavorable listening conditions.[8,11] Traumatic injuries can result in disruption of the ossicular chain, or cranial nerve VIII becoming selectively damaged. Preinjury hearing aids may be less effective, which can hinder the accurate communication needed to help older adults through the rehabilitation process.[12]

Smell

Normal aging is associated with decreased sense of smell and is associated with decreased appetite and poor nutritional intake in the elderly.[8,9] This is important to consider because the olfactory nerve is the most frequently injured cranial nerve after a TBI and further disruption of smell may affect an individual's appetite.[12] Decreased smell may also negatively affect the ability to detect burning objects. Home evaluation should include appropriate placement of smoke detectors.

Taste

Normal aging is accompanied by the loss of lingual papillae, decreased saliva volume, and relative decrement of taste acuity.[8,9] Loss of smell caused by a TBI may further impair the sense of taste, which can result in poor oral intake.[12]

Touch, Vibration, Joint Position Sense

Position sense diminishes with age; this may be accelerated by the presence of peripheral neuropathy, which should be evaluated and treated/managed.[8,9] This is concerning after TBI in the elderly because impaired balance is a common occurrence. Compensation techniques and assistive devices may help an individual adapt to these impairments.[12]

Cognition and Behavior

Dementia affects 3% to 11% of community-dwelling adults above the age of 65, and 20% to 50% of adults above the age of 85.[8,9] Preinjury cognition and behavior need to be assessed in order to set appropriate and realistic rehabilitation goals. Neurostimulants, typically used to address arousal and attention after TBI, should be prescribed with caution in elderly patients because of age-related changes in drug metabolism.[12] Any change in functional status after injury will likely be upsetting to the patient and family, so monitoring for adjustment disorders and related conditions should be routine, with referral provided for counseling services as needed and care used when prescribing CNS acting medications.

Sleep Disturbance

Normalizing the sleep–wake cycle is important after a TBI to optimize recovery.[12] Behavioral and environmental modifications are usually first-line interventions. In considering medication management, note the following considerations specific to older adults: (a) diphenhydramine should not be used owing to the risk for urinary retention and cognitive worsening; (b) benzodiazepines should be avoided due to paradoxical reactions in elderly people; and (c) tricyclic antidepressants can cause postural hypotension and urinary retention, and are poorly tolerated.[8,9]

Sexuality

Sexuality is commonly ignored in older adults, but at any age sexuality gives one a sense of self, and capacity to show love and affection and maintain intimate relationships.[8,9] Normal aging can result in physiologic changes to the vaginal mucosa, erectile function, and orgasmic performance that can be improved with intervention. Sexual desire may change (increase or decrease) after TBI; therefore, it is important to screen for sexual and relationship concerns in older adults and educate patients and families about changes. Age-related, hormonal and cardiovascular factors also play a role in sexual function and clinicians must be aware of potential pharmacological, adaptive, and assistive technology interventions to enhance sexual function, as well as the risks and limitations of these options.[13]

Safety and Home Environment

A home evaluation by the rehabilitation team is important to assess safety risks in the home, to prevent future injury secondary to falls or wandering.[12] Questions should be asked regarding the size of the home, number of floors, flooring type(s), presence of throw rugs, width of doors, and accessibility and usability of bathrooms. Patients should also be asked about who lives in the home with them, including pets, and the proximity of friends and family. Home assessments help with determining functional goals during the rehabilitation process, durable medical equipment needs, and the need for home modifications, which all need to be determined when considering discharge planning.

Substance Abuse

Substance abuse, in particular unhealthy alcohol use, is common among elderly adults[14] and may significantly complicate recovery from a brain injury. In addition, ongoing usage during and after recovery puts the patient at risk for repeated TBI, falls, motor vehicle-related accidents and other adverse events. Screening for substance abuse in older adults is important to improve long-term outcomes and safety, and a tailored treatment program is important if these issues are identified. Family and caregiver education is a key component of treatment. (See also Chapters 63 and 64.)

Community Reintegration

Rehabilitation programs should focus on physical, cognitive, and behavioral deficits after brain injury, while promoting social reintegration and improved quality of life. Community mobility is important and should focus on route finding, negotiating different terrains, and appropriate use of public transportation. Improvements can positively impact the individual's ability to resume leisure activities, increase feelings of independence, and minimize feelings of isolation.

Elder Abuse

Elder abuse, including physical, emotional (e.g., neglect) and financial abuse, has been increasing, especially among those with poor social support.[8,9] When considering and evaluating for abuse after TBI, an understanding of and interactions with the person's social support are important, and providing family education regarding the effects of and limitations after TBI are necessary.[15]

AGING WITH TRAUMATIC BRAIN INJURY

The normal aging process is associated with declines in certain cognitive abilities, such as processing speed and some aspects of memory, language, visuospatial function, and executive function.[8,9] Neuropsychological impairments after a TBI in the older adult often parallel and may aggravate the changes seen with normal aging, with diminished ability to attend, concentrate, and recall, although long-term recall is more often affected due to aging as opposed to TBI. After TBI, a subset of individuals with the $ApoE_4$ allele may have a higher risk of earlier onset Alzheimer's dementia.[15] In addition, repeated TBIs predispose individuals to accelerated degeneration of the brain and associated dementia.[16]

OUTCOMES

Data from the National Institute on Disability, Independent Living and Rehabilitation Research (NIDILRR) TBI Model systems reveal that individuals aged 55 years and older have about a week longer rehabilitation length of stay and marginally higher costs of care, while demonstrating greater disability and a decreased percentage of return to a private residence at discharge than those 50 years of age and younger. Additionally, individuals aged 65 and older generally need a higher degree of supervision for their day-to-day care 1-year post injury.[17]

KEY POINTS

- There is a worldwide increase in the aging population with a concomitant increase in the number of older adults at risk for TBI.
- Falls are the most common cause of TBI in the elderly and fall risk can be stratified and reduced.

- Elderly individuals have slower recovery rates, higher mortality rates, and lower functional status at discharge following moderate to severe TBI.
- Older adults are at increased risk for sustaining SDHs and EDHs.
- Healthcare providers should be cognizant of normal age-related changes that could affect recovery from TBI or be compounded by a brain injury.
- Rehabilitation programs should provide a holistic, patient-centered approach to management of older adults with TBI, with a goal of successful community reintegration to prevent social isolation and improve quality of life.

STUDY QUESTIONS

1. In older adults, the most common cause of TBI is:
   a. Violence/assault
   b. Pedestrian–motor vehicle accidents
   c. Falls
   d. Motor vehicle accidents

2. Common *environmental* causes of falls that can result in TBI in older adults include:
   a. Episodic postural hypotension
   b. Tripping while walking
   c. Poor lighting
   d. Arthritic pain

3. Data from the NIDILRR TBI Model systems reveal that compared to individuals 50 years old and younger, those aged 55 years and older:
   a. Stay about a week longer in inpatient rehabilitation units
   b. Cost considerably more to rehabilitate
   c. Demonstrate similar disability after rehabilitation
   d. Are more likely to return to a private residence after inpatient rehabilitation

4. Which of the following areas of sexual function and sexuality do not commonly diminish with aging:
   a. The ability to maintain intimate relationships
   b. Vaginal mucosa's ability to lubricate
   c. Erectile function
   d. Orgasmic performance

5. Dementia affects approximately what percentage of community-dwelling older adults above 65 years of age?
   a. 5%–10%
   b. 15%–20%
   c. 25%–30%
   d. 35%–40%

ADDITIONAL READING

Older adult fall prevention: https://www.cdc.gov/steadi

Gardner RC, Dams-O'Connor K, Morrissey MR, Manley GT. Geriatric traumatic brain injury: epidemiology, outcomes, knowledge gaps, and future directions. *J Neurotraum.* 2018;35(7):889–906. doi:10.1089/neu.2017.5371

Haller CS, Delhumeau C, De Pretto M, et al. Trajectory of disability and quality-of-life in non-geriatric and geriatric survivors after severe traumatic brain injury. *Brain Inj.* 2017;31(3):319–328. doi:10.1080/02699052.2016.1255777

Papa L, Mendes ME, Braga, CF. Mild traumatic brain injury among the geriatric population. *Curr Tran Geriatr Gerontol Rep.* 2012;1:135–142. doi:10.1007/s13670-012-0019-0

Shimoda K, Maeda T, Tado M, at al. Outcome and surgical management for geriatric traumatic brain injury: analysis of 888 cases registered in the Japan Neurotrauma Data Bank. *World Neurosurg.* 2014;82(6):1300–1306. doi:10.1016/j.wneu.2014.08.014.

ANSWERS TO STUDY QUESTIONS

1. Correct Answer: c
   The most common causes of TBI in older adults, in decreasing order, are falls, traffic-related events, including motor vehicle crashes (MVCs) and pedestrian struck by vehicle, and violence/assault.

   Further Reading:
   Thompson HJ, McCormick WC, Kagan SH. Traumatic brain injury in older adults: epidemiology, outcomes, and future implications. *J Am Geriatr Soc.* 2006;54(10):1590–1595. doi:10.1111/j.1532-5415.2006.00894.x

2. Correct Answer: c
   Common environmental causes of falls in older adults that can result in TBI include poor lighting, nonsecure throw rugs, ill-fitting shoe/shoe wear, pets, and children.

   Further Reading:
   Tinetti ME, Speechley M. Prevention of falls among the elderly. *N Engl J Med.* 1989;320(16):1055–1059. doi:10.1056/NEJM198904203201606

3. Correct Answer: a
   Data from the National Institute on Disability and Rehabilitation Research (NIDILRR) TBI Model systems reveals that individuals aged 55 years and older have about a week longer rehabilitation length of stay and marginally higher costs of care, but demonstrate greater disability and a decreased percentage of return to a private residence at discharge than those 50 years of age and younger.

   Further Reading:
   Frankel JE, Marwitz JH, Cifu DX, et al. A follow-up study of older adults with traumatic brain injury: taking into account decreasing length of stay. *Arch Phys Med Rehabil.* 2006;87(1):57–62. doi:10.1016/j.apmr.2005.07.309

4. Correct Answer: a

At any age sexuality gives one a sense of self, and capacity to show love and affection and maintain intimate relationships. Normal aging can result in physiologic changes to the vaginal mucosa, erectile function, and orgasmic performance.

Further Reading:

Kane RL, Ouslander JG, Abrass IB. *Essentials of Clinical Geriatrics*. 4th ed. McGraw-Hill. 1999:256–291.

5. Correct Answer: a

Dementia affects 3% to 11% of community-dwelling adults above the age of 65, and 20% to 50% of adults above the age of 85.

Further Reading:

Fillit HM, Rockwood K, Young J. *Brocklehurst's Textbook of Geriatric Medicine and Gerontology*. 8th ed. Elsevier; 2016.

REFERENCES

The full reference list appears in the digital product found on http://connect.springer-pub.com/content/book/978-0-8261-4768-4/part/part05/chapter/ch68

COMPLEMENTARY AND ALTERNATIVE MEDICINE IN TRAUMATIC BRAIN INJURY

FELISE S. ZOLLMAN

BACKGROUND

Complementary and alternative medicine (CAM) techniques are widely used for a variety of indications in the United States and throughout the world. Rigorous data demonstrating efficacy in persons with TBI are limited. That said, due to broad acceptance, generally favorable risk/benefit profile, and ability to integrate many CAM practices within a conventional medicine framework, these interventions merit consideration in appropriately selected patients. For example, in the U.S. military, the use of an integrated, conventional plus CAM approach to wellness is broadly accepted.[1]

Definitions

- Complementary and alternative medicine (CAM)—a group of diverse medical and healthcare systems, practices, and products that are not generally considered to be part of conventional medicine.[2]
- Conventional medicine—current accepted Western medical practice.
- Complementary medicine—modalities that complement—but don't replace—conventional medical interventions.
- Alternative medicine—modalities used in lieu of conventional medical interventions.
- Integrative medicine—the combined use of conventional and CAM techniques with a focus on treating the whole person and the use of less invasive treatment approaches where possible/appropriate, with decision-making informed by evidence-based scientific principles.[1]

Partial Listing of Complementary and Alternative Medicine Practices

Homeopathy/naturopathy; herbal medicine; aromatherapy; relaxation techniques (meditation, hypnosis, use of music or humor, guided imagery); biofeedback; energy-based therapies (healing touch, reflexology, Reiki, massage); craniosacral manipulation; electromagnetic therapy (transcranial magnetic stimulation, crystals); music therapy; movement therapies (Alexander, Feldenkrais, Qi Gong, Tai Qi, Yoga); nutraceuticals; hyperbaric oxygen; Chinese medicine/acupuncture. This chapter will focus on those areas for which there is published data addressing use in those with TBI.

The full reference list appears in the digital product found on http://connect.springerpub.com/content/book/978-0-8261-4768-4/part/part05/chapter/ch69

Published Data in Traumatic Brain Injury Exists for the Following:

Meditation (Mindfulness)

Basic principles:

- Mindfulness is a form of meditation, which involves attending to relevant aspects of one's experience in a nonjudgmental manner. The goal of mindfulness is to maintain awareness moment by moment, disengaging oneself from strong attachment to beliefs, thoughts, or emotions, thereby developing a greater sense of emotional balance and well-being.[3]
- Mindfulness in traumatic brain injury (TBI): There is generally a lack of rigorous data demonstrating a clinical benefit with mindfulness interventions in TBI. Published data consist of personal accounts, case series, and a recently published systematic review:
  - Trisha Meili (the "Central Park Jogger") describes learning to "live inside again." In contrast to prevailing medical views, Meili sees lack of memory and insight as an opportunity to develop the ability to focus on the present ("Here it is. . . . This is my situation"), not as an impairment to be overcome.[4]
  - In a pilot intervention study, 10 subjects attended 12 weekly group sessions consisting of meditation, breathing exercises, guided visualization, and group discussion. Outcome: SF-36 (a widely recognized life satisfaction scale in which higher numbers indicate greater satisfaction) increased from 37 to 52.[5] Another study looked at the role of meditation in addressing fatigue post-TBI, and found a beneficial effect.[6]
  - A meta-analysis addressing the use of meditation, mindfulness techniques, and/or yoga for post-TBI symptoms found that, while individual studies were generally of low quality, study subjects experienced significant improvement in quality of life, fatigue, and mood.[7]

Tai Qi/Qi Gong (Also Known as Tai Chi, Chi Gong, Qi Quong)

- Basic principles: Tai Qi, literally meaning "great energy," is both a healing art and martial arts discipline. Qi Gong literally means "energy work." Qi Gong generally involves slower movements, and is considered easier to perform; there is a specific focus on mindfulness and physical health.
- Tai Qi in TBI: While the literature is scant, two case series and two case/control studies showed beneficial effects with respect to motor function[8], mood,[9,10] ability to attend to basic self-care needs,[11] and/or self-esteem.[10]

Music Therapy

- Basic principles: This rehabilitation technique involves using music to facilitate recovery of sensory perception, motor function, cognitive recovery, and emotional responsiveness.
- Music therapy in TBI: The use of music therapy has been shown to improve cognitive function, specifically in the realm of executive function,[12,13] and this improvement correlated with increased cortical volume in the right inferior frontal gyrus by magnetic resonance imaging (MRI).[13]

Acupuncture

Basic principles:

- From a Chinese medicine perspective, the human body is viewed as a microcosmic reflection of the universe. The physician's role is to aid in maintenance of harmonious balance, both internally and in relation to the external environment.
- Vital energy, known as "Qi," flows through channels, or meridians, creating an interwoven network of circulation.
- Meridians are a multilayered, interconnecting network of channels or energy pathways that establish an interface between an individual's internal and external environments.

These energy pathways are named for organs whose realms of influence are expanded from their conventional biomedical physiologies to include functional, energetic, and metaphorical qualities. Pathology involves disharmony/disruption of energy flow.[14] The relationship between these organs and their broader spheres of influence is often represented via a table of correspondences.

- The five phases approach to diagnosis: The dynamic energy balance among pathways/organs can be viewed diagrammatically by arranging five elements, and the organs with which they are associated (Figure 69.1).
- Any of the correspondences (e.g., emotions, organs) from Table 69.1[15] can be overlaid onto this construct to understand the relative influence of one to the other. For example, the emotion of *water* is fear, the emotion of *wood* is anger or irritability, and the emotion of *fire* is joy/mania. The five phases relationship tells us that fear nourishes anger and controls (or mitigates) joy/mania.

Use of acupuncture in TBI:

- TBI from a Chinese medicine perspective: two syndromes are typically recognized: *Qibi* (or blockage of Qi)—presents with an agitated, hyperadrenergic state; *Qituo* (or exhaustion of Qi)—presents with unresponsiveness. Additional factors may include Kidney Yin deficiency and Liver Yin deficiency/Liver Yang excess (capitalized organ names represent both associated characteristic energetic qualities and meridian pathway labels).
- Acupuncture has been reported to be of benefit in TBI with respect to improvement in level of consciousness and extent of injury recovery.[16,17] One study in particular, an interventional controlled study of subjects in coma, compared 17 subjects to 15 historical controls. Diagnoses included TBI and ruptured internal carotid artery. Subjects within 1 week of injury underwent four acupuncture treatments at 12-hour intervals: "A significantly greater number of patients in the acupuncture group (59%) had a

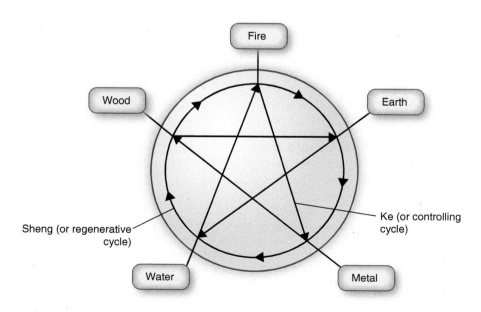

FIGURE 69.1 Five phases relationships.

TABLE 69.1 Table of Correspondences

Element:	Water	Wood	Fire	Earth	Metal
Season	Winter	Spring	Summer	Late summer	Fall
Associated pathogen	Cold	Wind	Heat	Damp	Dryness
Yin organ	Kidney	Liver	Heart and SNS*	Spleen	Lung
Yang organ	Bladder	Gallbladder	Small intestine and PNS†	Stomach	Large intestine
Primary sense organ	Ears	Eyes	Tongue	Mouth	Nose
Body tissue	Bone	Ligaments and tendons	Blood	Muscles	Skin
Emotion	Fear	Anger	Joy/mania	Worry	Grief
Taste	Salty	Sour	Bitter	Sweet	Spicy
Color	Blue	Green	Red	Yellow	White

*Sympathetic nervous system (also known as pericardium or master of the heart).

†Parasympathetic nervous system (also known as triple heater or triple burner).

Source: Adapted from Beinfield H, Korngold, E. *Between Heaven and Earth: A Guide to Chinese Medicine.* Ballantine Books; 1992.

greater than 50% neurological recovery, than the patients in the no acupuncture group (20%) (*p* = .025)." Study conclusion: Early acupuncture intervention may be a reasonable adjunctive treatment for brain-injured patients.[17] Acupuncture has also been shown to be of benefit in treating insomnia post TBI.[18] Finally, a retrospective cohort study suggested that patients with TBI who receive acupuncture had fewer hospitalizations or emergency department visits in the first year after injury.[19]

▪ Acupuncture may also be of value for symptomatic relief of sequelae of TBI, including headache, fatigue, and mood changes.[20] A detailed review of these topics is beyond the scope of this chapter.

ASSESSMENT

▪ Determine candidacy for a particular intervention.
- For meditation/mindfulness: Is the individual able to attend to the mindfulness exercise? Is trying to develop focused attention more likely to increase the patient's frustration level, or is it valuable to them to hone this skill?
- For Tai Qi/Qi Gong: Probably most appropriate for addressing balance/motor deficits, though there is a component of mindfulness about movement that might (theoretically) aid attention as well.
- For music therapy: consider the individual's stage in recovery. Will music be calming, relaxing, stimulating? In the early post-TBI recovery period after severe TBI (i.e. Rancho Level IV), music therapy may be over-stimulating.

- For acupuncture: (a) Will the individual tolerate needle placement? For a Rancho Level IV patient in particular, this may be a challenge. (b) What is the goal of treatment? It is important to identify specific impairments or functional gains which are to be the focus of treatment and monitor progress accordingly.
■ Ensure that appropriately trained/qualified providers are available to provide the service being considered. For example, acupuncturists may be (a) physicians trained in medical acupuncture, (b) licensed acupuncturists (typically trained as Oriental Medical Doctors), and occasionally (c) chiropractors. Physician acupuncturists may be located via the Academy of Medical Acupuncture website (see Additional Reading). Consider the medical complexity of the situation in identifying an appropriate provider: Patients who have significant medical comorbidities (such as someone with a moderate to severe TBI) may be better served by seeing a physician acupuncturist, while someone with residual sequelae of a mild TBI (e.g., headaches, fatigue) may be just as well served by seeing a licensed acupuncturist.

TREATMENT

Meditation/Mindfulness

■ Fundamental principle involves attending to the present and to awareness of self. This process is undertaken in a nonjudgmental fashion, observing our natural tendency for our mind to stray, then returning to self-awareness.[3]
■ This process can be facilitated via breathing exercises, guided imagery, and use of external cues (e.g., meditative object).

Tai Qi/Qi Gong

■ Both disciplines incorporate smooth, balanced movement with mindfulness.
■ Specific "forms" are intended to promote the smooth flow of Qi along certain meridians and/or (particularly with respect to Qi Gong) for the purpose of nourishing certain organs or organ qualities.

Music Therapy

■ Neurologic music therapy (NMT) is a technique that has been developed for the purpose of using music to facilitate sensory, motor, and/or cognitive/emotional recovery after neurological injury or impairment. Specific approach varies based on the target of the intervention. Examples include active engagement in musical activity to facilitate sustained attention, rhythmic movement to augment motor control and recall of music/lyrics to address memory impairment.[12]

Acupuncture

■ The technique involves penetrating the skin with thin, solid, metallic needles that are manipulated by the hands, using a heat source, or by electrical stimulation.[14]
■ Acupuncture needles have unique bioelectrical characteristics:
  - They are typically bimetallic (e.g., stainless steel shaft, copper/silver/bronze alloy handle) and therefore effectively create a battery. One needle inserted causes local agitation. Two or more needles cause a directional current flow. Current flow can be enhanced with the use of heat and electricity.

- Once needles are placed, they may be manipulated in one of the following ways: (a) no manipulation/neutral/dispersion; (b) manual tonification (manipulation); (c) heat; or (d) electrical stimulation, which facilitates the directed flow of Qi (electrons; Figures 69.2–69.4). Low-frequency electrical stimulation results in an endorphin-mediated generalized effect. High-frequency stimulation results in a monoamine-mediated, more rapid onset, segmental response.[14]
- Risks include bleeding/bruising, infection, needle shock/fainting, nerve irritation, and puncture of an organ/vital structure (very rare).
- In general, acupuncture is a very safe and well-tolerated procedure.

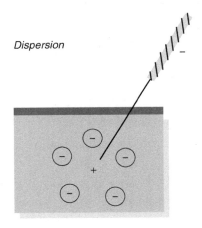

FIGURE 69.2   **Dispersion.**

Source: From Helms JM. *Acupuncture Energetics: A Clinical Approach for Physicians*. Medical Acupuncture Publishers; 1995. Used with permission.

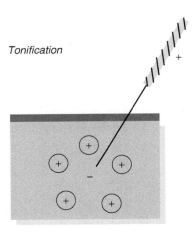

FIGURE 69.3   **Tonification.**

Source: From Helms JM. *Acupuncture Energetics: A Clinical Approach for Physicians*. Medical Acupuncture Publishers; 1995. Used with permission.

Directed electron flow

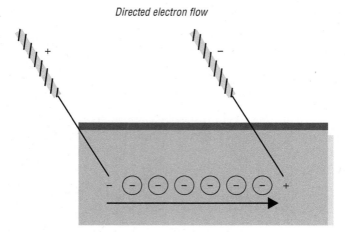

FIGURE 69.4 **Directed flow of Qi facilitated with electrical stimulation.**

Source: From Helms JM. *Acupuncture Energetics: A Clinical Approach for Physicians*. Medical Acupuncture Publishers; 1995. Used with permission.

KEY POINTS

- Published data on the role of CAM practices in TBI are limited.
- Meditation may help with focus on the present, perception of life satisfaction, and fatigue.
- Tai Qi/Qi Gong may benefit motor function, mood, and self-esteem.
- Music therapy may offer some benefit in cognitive recovery, particularly in the realm of executive function.
- Acupuncture has been shown to be of benefit in improving the level of arousal post-TBI and in treating insomnia. It may also be considered for treatment of various sequelae of TBI such as headache, fatigue, and mood changes.

STUDY QUESTIONS

1. Though limited, there is a body of published literature showing benefit with use of acupuncture for some aspects of TBI management. This includes all of the following except:
   a. Level of arousal
   b. Motor control
   c. Insomnia
   d. Headaches

2. Integrative medicine is a term used to describe which of the following:
   a. Use of multiple treatment modalities at the same time
   b. Identifying one provider who coordinates care to ensure a holistic treatment plan
   c. Integrating all rehabilitation team members to develop a unified treatment plan
   d. The combined use of conventional and CAM techniques with a focus on use of less invasive treatment approaches where possible

3. Mindfulness training refers to:
   a. Teaching an individual to be aware of their injury and how to manage it
   b. Teaching an individual to be mindful of the impact of their injury on family and friends
   c. Teaching an individual to focus awareness on the present, moment to moment, in non-judgmental fashion
   d. Improving attention and focus in those with attentional impairment post TBI

4. Music therapy has been shown to benefit which of the following post TBI?
   a. Executive function
   b. Motor control
   c. Speech
   d. Arousal

5. Acupuncture is believed to work via restoring the smooth flow of Qi through what network in the body?
   a. Nervous system
   b. Meridians
   c. Vascular system
   d. Organ channels

ADDITIONAL READING

American Academy of Medical Acupuncture. www.medicalacupuncture.org/

NIH *National Center for Complementary and Integrative Health.* https://www.nccih.nih.gov

Brain Injury Association music therapy information page: https://www.biausa.org/public-affairs/media/neurologic-music-therapy-in-neurorehabilitation

Helms JM. *Acupuncture Energetics: A Clinical Approach for Physicians.* Medical Acupuncture Publishers; 1995.

Ludwig DS, Kabat-Zinn J. Mindfulness in medicine. *JAMA.* 2008;300(11):1350–1352. doi:10.1001/jama.300.11.1350

ANSWERS TO STUDY QUESTIONS

1. Correct Answer: b
   Limited evidence, based on published studies, suggests a role for acupuncture in assisting with all of these aspects of post-TBI clinical management except for motor control.

   Further Reading:
   Frost E. Acupuncture for the comatose patient. *Am J Acupunct.* 1976;4(1):45–48.
   Zollman FS, Larson EB, Wasek-Throm LK, et al. Acupuncture for treatment of insomnia in patients with traumatic brain injury: a pilot intervention study. *J Head Trauma Rehabil.* 2012;27(2):135–142. doi:10.1097/HTR.0b013e3182051397
   https://www.scienceinmedicine.org.au/wp-content/uploads/2018/03/Cochrane-acupuncture-2018.pdf.

2. Correct Answer: d
   Integrative medicine refers to the combined use of conventional and CAM techniques with a focus on treating the whole person and the use of less invasive treatment approaches.

Further Reading:
Madsen C, Vaughan M, Koehlmoos TP. Use of integrative medicine in the U.S. military health aystem. *Evid Based Complement Alternat Med*. 2017;2017:9529257. doi:10.1155/2017/9529257

3. Correct Answer: c
While it is possible to see some improvement in attention with use of CAM modalities such as mindfulness training, the term itself refers to the technique of attending to the present and to awareness of self in non-judgmental fashion.

Further Reading:
Ludwig DS, Kabat-Zinn J. Mindfulness in medicine. *JAMA*. 2008;300(11):1350–1352. doi:10.1001/jama.300.11.1350

4. Correct Answer: a
Music therapy has been shown to benefit executive function post-TBI, and this improvement correlates with increased cortical volume in the right inferior frontal gyrus by MRI.

Further Reading:
Siponkoski ST, Martínez-Molina N, Kuusela L, et al. Music therapy enhances executive functions and prefrontal structural neuroplasticity after traumatic brain injury: evidence from a randomized controlled trial. *J Neurotrauma*. 2020;37(4):618-634. doi:10.1089/neu.2019.6413

5. Correct Answer: b
Meridians are a multilayered, interconnecting network of channels or energy pathways that establish an interface between an individual's internal and external environments. These energy pathways are named for organs whose realms of influence are expanded from their conventional biomedical physiologies to include functional, energetic, and metaphorical qualities. Pathology involves disharmony/disruption of energy flow.

Further Reading:
Helms JM. *Acupuncture Energetics: A Clinical Approach for Physicians*. Medical Acupuncture Publishers; 1995.

REFERENCES

The full reference list appears in the digital product found on http://connect.springer-pub.com/content/book/978-0-8261-4768-4/part/part05/chapter/ch69

RETURN TO WORK FOLLOWING TRAUMATIC BRAIN INJURY

NANCY H. HSU

BACKGROUND

Importance

Traumatic brain injury (TBI) results in cognitive, physical/sensory, neurobehavioral, and psychosocial impairments that present barriers to return to work (RTW).[1-3] At the same time, gainful employment promotes an improved sense of well-being and identity, better health status, greater community involvement, less usage of healthcare services, decreased social isolation, and better quality of life, and reduces potential emotional stressors and substance abuse.[2,4,5] In addition to providing financial support, work has personal therapeutic benefits, including social interaction, providing structure and purpose in life, enhancing perception of quality of life, and positively impacting self-concept. As such, the importance of incorporating successful RTW as part of the TBI rehabilitative goals cannot be overstated.

Incidence

It has been estimated that among survivors of moderate to severe TBI who were employed prior to injury, 40.4% RTW at 1 year and 40.8% at 2 years, with a range reported from 0% to 84% across studies.[6,7] Several factors contribute to the wide range of RTW rates, including varied classification of severity of TBI, differing definitions of RTW, financial incentives that promote or discourage RTW in different countries, and availability of vocational rehabilitation services.[1,2,8,9] RTW rates are higher for individuals with mild TBI (MTBI) of whom more than half RTW by 1 month post-injury, and more than 80% by 6 months.[10]

Durability

A review of U.S. TBI model systems (TBIMS) data collected on patients with moderate to severe TBI who required a course of inpatient rehabilitation post-injury revealed that 34% of survivors were stably employed (i.e., employed at 1-, 2-, and 3- or 4-year follow-up), 27% were unstably employed (employed at one or two of the three follow-up visits), and 39% were unemployed at all three follow-up intervals.[11] On the other hand, data from Australia showed slightly higher levels of employment as well as stability of employment—44% of individuals with moderate to severe TBI were stably employed post-injury at 1, 2, and 3 years, 17% were unstably employed, and the remaining 32% were unemployed for the entire 3-year period.[12] A follow-up TBIMS study that examined long-term employment patterns found that the odds of RTW are highest within the first year post-injury, while the probabilities decline between years 5 and 10.[13] Again, for individuals with MTBI, a considerable majority return to work within 6 months post injury.[10]

The full reference list appears in the digital product found on http://connect.springerpub.com/content/book/978-0-8261-4768-4/part/part05/chapter/ch70

Changes in Occupational Status Post-Return to Work

While RTW rates are relatively low in the setting of moderate to severe TBI, what is often overlooked in the RTW literature is the consistency in occupational status between pre- and post-injury jobs for those who successfully RTW. Consistency rates are higher for those in managerial and professional jobs compared to those in manual labor jobs.[7,12,14,15] Nevertheless, approximately 20% of those who are steadily employed post-injury (i.e., working 3–5 years after the injury) return to jobs for which they are overqualified in terms of education and vocational training requirements.[16] RTW is more positive for those returning to more supportive and nurturing work environments than more competitive and high-risk work environments.[1,17]

Rehabilitation Continuum of Care

The full spectrum of TBI rehabilitative services includes acute inpatient rehabilitation, post-acute rehabilitation, and community re-entry and RTW with assistance as indicated. Vocational support to increase chances of successful RTW may range from instruction on gaining employment to intensive on-the-job training, and outpatient follow-up to help adapt to new challenges and access community resources.[1,18]

Effectiveness

The evidence supporting interventions to improve RTW is weak, consisting mostly of observational and uncontrolled studies.[19–21] A variety of vocational rehabilitation models (e.g., TBI programs with integrated or added vocational components, vocational rehabilitation models adapted for TBI, and case coordination/resource facilitation models) have been shown to increase RTW.[20] Supported employment (discussed in more detail in a following section) is a specific approach that can effectively improve RTW outcomes for individuals with severe TBI.[22] A comprehensive/holistic program features work readiness training and work trials, case coordination, and supported employment.[20,22,23]

Funding Sources for Vocational Interventions

- State vocational rehabilitation agency
- Insurance carrier
- Workers compensation insurance
- Out of pocket

ASSESSMENT

Factors

RTW involves a complex interaction between premorbid characteristics, injury factors, post-injury impairments, and personal and environmental factors, making predicting outcomes only moderately accurate.[8] However, a number of factors have consistently shown to be associated with a reduced chance of RTW (Table 70.1).[5,7,13,14,24,25] Neurobehavioral impairments (e.g., disinhibition, impulsivity, decreased initiation), medical consequences of TBI (e.g., headaches, posttraumatic seizures), and comorbidities (e.g., depression, substance abuse, mood lability) also pose as barriers to RTW.[23]

TABLE 70.1   Risk Factors Associated With Unsuccessful Return to Work Posttraumatic Brain Injury

Age >40 years at time of injury	Lack of knowledge of available work incentives
Unemployed pre-injury	Lack of job placement assistance
Low education level pre-injury	Inability to return to pre-injury job or employer
Unskilled manual laborer pre-injury	Lack of awareness of impairments
Greater number of cognitive deficits	Poor social support network
	Premorbid psychiatric history
Length of inpatient rehabilitation stay	Premorbid alcohol or recreational drug use
Duration of posttraumatic amnesia	Greater level of physical disability
Racial or ethnic minority	Female gender

Evaluation

A thorough physical examination and diagnostic workup including neuroimaging and neuropsychological testing is necessary for accurate diagnosis of the physical, cognitive, neurobehavioral, and emotional sequelae of TBI. If returning to previous work, some type of release to return to duty may be required. Having a member of the team conduct a thorough job analysis can also be very helpful.

Vocational Assessment

- Traditional vocational assessment, that is, a "place once and done" approach, has not been effective for clients with TBI, who often have more significant support needs.[1]
- Functional vocational assessment: This assessment is designed to determine RTW options and support needs. It may involve examining the individual's ability to return to pre-injury employment; a new job that capitalizes on use of the person's residual skills either with pre-injury or new employer; or a different type of job with new employer.[1] Assessment includes interviewing the TBI survivor and/or caregivers as well as a vocational situational assessment in a real (not simulated) work setting.

VOCATIONAL REHABILITATION INTERVENTION

Team Approach

The vocational rehabilitation team may be comprised of a combination of the following: brain injury physician, vocational rehabilitation specialist (including job coach if severe disability), social worker, physical therapist, occupational therapist, vision therapist, speech/language therapist, and neuropsychologist/rehabilitation psychologist. Each discipline can offer unique insight that can be integrated into the client's RTW plan. It is important to solicit input from the client, the family, and the potential employer. The plan should be individualized and client-centered.

Client Instruction and Advisement

Client instruction and advisement involves providing the client with information and instruction to assist with conducting a job search and, once employed, use of compensatory strategies at work. Many individuals with TBI will not be able to profit from this office-based intervention because of cognitive impairments.

Selective Placement

Selective placement involves job placement assistance followed by minimal interaction and intervention. This approach assumes that neither intensive on-the-job assistance nor ongoing support is necessary. Ongoing contact with the individual may be maintained more closely than with the employer.

Supported Employment

Supported employment is effective in increasing employment among those with TBI,[22] with a job retention rate of more than 70%.[26] This approach is characterized by individualized employment support, provided and/or facilitated by a vocational rehabilitation specialist sometimes referred to as a job coach. These services are specifically tailored to assist an individual with severe TBI with gaining and maintaining competitive employment. This approach begins with a functional vocational assessment, followed by an immediate job search (in place of prolonged pre-employment training or treatment) that is aligned with the information gathered during client assessment and review of the employer's business needs. Once the job seeker is hired, the job coach facilitates on and off job-site supports. On-the-job training is often provided, including assisting the new hire with developing and learning to use various supports like compensatory memory strategies. The job coach gauges how the new hire is progressing toward meeting the employer's standards and expectations, and adjusts instructional strategies accordingly. Ongoing long-term follow-up or job retention services are also provided throughout the client's tenure. This could include assisting the employee with resolving novel challenges as they arise or new skills training if indicated.[1,8]

Workplace Supports

Common physical, cognitive, and emotional impairments can be addressed with workplace accommodations and supports.

- Challenges due to physical impairments (e.g., seizures, heterotopic ossification, spasticity) can be minimized via the following[27]:
  - Identify a job that will utilize residual strengths versus merely avoiding points of weakness.
  - Select or modify the work environment to ensure safety in the event of the recurrence of a seizure or in the setting of balance dysfunction and dizziness; teach the client to recognize symptoms and take steps to "be safe"; educate the employer on reaction to occurrence, if appropriate.
  - Rearrange the workspace to help accommodate decreased range of motion and strength.
  - Consider ergonomic modifications.
  - Consider how pattern or sequencing of activities impacts speed and accuracy, endurance and fatigue; make modifications where feasible.
  - Utilize assistive technology and/or adaptive equipment if necessary.

■ Cognitive and neurobehavioral impairments (e.g., memory deficits, impaired attention/concentration, lack of self-awareness, disinhibited behaviors). Some ways to help ameliorate cognitive, emotional, and behavioral dysfunction at work include:
  ● Cognitive rehabilitation[8]
  ● Cognitive behavioral therapy that focuses on developing mechanisms for emotional and behavioral self-regulation and for developing self-awareness[8]
  ● Employment supports[27]
  ● Assistive technology
  ● Procedural modifications or process reorganization (e.g., changing sequence of tasks)
  ● Compensatory strategies; for example, creating associations and utilizing verbal rehearsing, check lists, flow charts, reference manuals, and so on
  ● Identify/avoid factors associated with triggering behaviors
  ● Model positive interactions
  ● Provide counseling to address emotional distress and difficulty adjusting to the effects of injury

Additional Considerations

With the advent of supported employment and assistive technology, virtually no one should be considered too disabled to work. Workshop settings, a place where individuals with disabilities congregate together to perform contract work or to receive training, are not acceptable, nor are group models sometimes referred to as enclaves or mobile work crews. Even individuals with very severe injuries have been assisted to RTW through a supported approach.[1,2,8,13] Awareness of the distinctions among these vocational rehabilitation approaches is key, as TBI providers may need to take a leadership role in ensuring that the TBI survivor is directed toward services that will lead to real work for real pay/competitive employment in every appropriate circumstance.

KEY POINTS

■ RTW remains a significant challenge for individuals with moderate to severe TBI, with RTW rates across studies at approximately 40%.

■ Individuals who experience an MTBI and who have impairments significant enough to warrant time away from work have higher RTW rates and regain employment more quickly than individuals with moderate to severe brain injuries.

■ Vocational rehabilitation interventions fall under three broad categories: program-based rehabilitation, supported employment, and case coordination. All have advantages and disadvantages, and the evidence regarding best practices is inconclusive. Nevertheless, research shows that early and any vocational rehabilitation intervention/support increases chances of RTW.

STUDY QUESTIONS

1. Although it is difficult to predict RTW outcomes due to the complex interaction between premorbid characteristics, injury factors, post-injury impairments, and personal and environmental factors, which factor has been shown to be associated with successful RTW?

    a. Pre-injury employment as a manual laborer
    b. Lack of awareness
    c. Age <40 at the time of injury
    d. Poor social support network

2. Which model of vocational rehabilitation intervention has been demonstrated to improve outcomes for individuals with severe TBI?
    a. Supported employment
    b. Selective placement
    c. Workplace support
    d. Client instruction and advisement

3. Common physical, cognitive, and emotional impairments can be addressed with workplace accommodations. What is considered an appropriate way of ameliorating problems in these areas?
    a. Only work on the days the client is feeling well
    b. Have a job coach do the job
    c. Educate the employer and staff so they can ignore inappropriate behaviors
    d. Assistive technology

4. Despite the fact that RTW remains a significant challenge for individuals with moderate to severe TBI, with vocational support, they are able to return to work if they were employed prior to the injury. What is the average percentage of survivors who are able to RTW?
    a. 20%
    b. 30%
    c. 40%
    d. 50%

ADDITIONAL READING

Virginia Commonwealth University's Rehabilitation Research and Training Center on training and employment services www.vcurrtc.org

DiSanto D, Kumar RG, Juengst SB, et al. Employment stability in the first 5 years after moderate-to-severe traumatic brain injury. *Arch Phys Med Rehabil*. 2019;100(3):412–421. doi:10.1016/j.apmr.2018.06.022

Dornonville de la Cour FL, Rasmussen MA, Foged EM, et al. Vocational rehabilitation in mild traumatic brain injury: supporting return to work and daily life functioning. *Front Neurol*. 2019;10:103. doi:10.3389/fneur.2019.00103

Hart T, Ketchum JM, O'Neil-Pirozzi TM, et al. Neurocognitive status and return to work after moderate to severe traumatic brain injury. *Rehabil Psychol*. 2019;64(4):435–444. doi:10.1037/rep0000290

Weber E, Spirou A, Chiaravalloti N, Lengenfelder J. Impact of frontal neurobehavioral symptoms on employment in individuals with TBI. *Rehabil Psychol*. 2018;63(3):383–391. doi:10.1037/rep0000208

ANSWERS TO STUDY QUESTIONS

1. Correct Answer: c
Younger age at the time of injury has been found to contribute to successful employment outcomes.

Further Reading:
Mitrushina M, Tomaszewski R. Factors associated with return to work in patients with long-term disabilities due to neurological and neuropsychiatric disorders. *Neuropsychol Rehabil*. 2019;29(9):1313–1331.

2. Correct Answer: a
Supported employment is effective in increasing employment among those with severe TBI.

Further Reading:
Wehman P, Targett P, West M, Kregel J. Productive work and employment for persons with traumatic brain injury: what have we learned after 20 years? *J Head Trauma Rehabil*. 2005;20(2):115–127.

3. Correct Answer: d
Assistive technology can help address a client's cognitive impairments. It can range from low-tech, such as a notebook/calendar or voice recorder, to sophisticated technology, such as an electronic tablet, to help with organization and memory.
West M, Targett P, Crockatt S, Wehman P. Return to work following traumatic brain injury. In: Zasler N, Katz D, Zafonte R, Arciniegas D, Bullock MR, Kreutzer J, ed. *Brain Injury Medicine*. 2nd ed. Demos Medical Publishing; 2013:1349–1359.

4. Correct Answer: c
Approximately 40% of survivors with moderate to severe TBI who were employed preinjury RTW.

Further Reading:
Cuthbert JP, Harrison-Felix C, Corrigan JD, et al. Unemployment in the United States after traumatic brain injury for working-age individuals: prevalence and associated factors 2 years postinjury. *J Head Trauma Rehabil*. 2015;30(3):160–174.

REFERENCES

The full reference list appears in the digital product found on http://connect.springer-pub.com/content/book/978-0-8261-4768-4/part/part05/chapter/ch70

RESOURCES FOR TRAUMATIC BRAIN INJURY SURVIVORS AND CAREGIVERS

SARAH TAYLOR

BACKGROUND

Need for Transitional Support

Many brain injury survivors and their families will require significant support as they transition from hospital or rehabilitation to home and community. While many will need support throughout their lifetimes, the type and amount of support needed is likely to change over time.[1,2] Because the residual effects of each brain injury will have a unique impact on the existing family unit, individualized transitional planning is important for successful community reintegration,[3] an important aspect of quality of life.[1] As transitional plans are developed, it is useful to consider the general domains of living: (a) activities of daily living, (b) vocational/school reentry, and (c) leisure/social/wellness. Consideration also needs to be given to available community resources. Although it is widely acknowledged that many traumatic brain injury (TBI) survivors and their families need transitional support services following hospitalization, many do not receive services due to the lack of availability (or because barriers exist to accessing those services).[4,5] Electronic databases with resources for patients and caregivers can help to fill the gap when services cannot be directly accessed.

Barriers to Resource Access

Lack of Knowledgeable Providers

When developing a community support network for the survivor and the family, it is important to find reputable, experienced, and knowledgeable service providers. Most community programs simply do not employ staff educated in brain injury. Medical professionals, psychologists, and even rehabilitation professionals may not have had experience with the TBI population or their needs. However, knowledgeable staff can be found, and an effort should be made to identify them. For example, many large park districts have programming for those with varying abilities; community mental health programs may have individuals who have worked with the TBI population, and some counties may have special community case management services available. In addition, advocacy groups often have experience working with TBI survivors and their families.

Financial/Funding Considerations

TBI affects not just the financial status of the survivor, but of the entire family.[6,7] Lost wages are a consideration for the survivor, but may affect the spouse or parent as well. Parents or spouses may become primary caregivers of the TBI survivors, impacting their employment status and the family's financial well-being. The cost to provide in-home care, outpatient rehabilitation, day care, and transportation services can be quite high.[8] Equipment and medications can be costly as well. Since these or other services may be required over a

---

The full reference list appears in the digital product found on http://connect.springerpub.com/content/book/978-0-8261-4768-4/part/part05/chapter/ch71

lifetime, the costs can become significant. Historically, community services for TBI survivors and their families have not been well funded in the public sector. However, financial support opportunities for eligible families are available. See, for example, www.traumaticbraininjury.com/funding-resources/

Limited Local or Regional Resource Availability

The specific state or area in which the survivor/family reside may hinder service access. Some rural areas do not have the resources of larger urban centers. Also, states vary widely in the financial support made available to survivors/families or to the providers who offer services to persons with traumatic brain injuries. However, the development of telemedicine and web-based education programs can fill a gap in providing access to resources for persons in rural areas.[9,10]

RESOURCES

Although most resources for the TBI survivor and the family are accessed at a local level, they are usually first identified through national information sources. This resource list will therefore focus on general categories of support needs and national resources, which can, in turn, lead to local resource information. The Internet can be a valuable medium through which information about the management of cognitive issues resulting from TBI can be accessed.[11]

Traumatic Brain Injury Education

The following organizations and centers provide web-based access to TBI educational materials of value to both consumers and professionals:

- Brain Injury Association of America (BIAA): www.biausa.org
- Brain Injury Resource Center: www.headinjury.com
- BrainLine: www.brainline.org
- Centers for Disease Control and Prevention: www.cdc.gov/TraumaticBrainInjury/index.html
- Center for Neuro Skills: www.neuroskills.com
- National Institute of Neurological Disorders and Stroke: https://www.ninds.nih.gov/Topic-Areas/traumatic-brain-injury
- National Resource Center for Traumatic Brain Injury: www.tbinrc.com
- The Brain Injury Guide & Resources: http://braininjuryeducation.com
- The Center of Excellence for Medical Multimedia Traumatic Brain Injury Website: https://tbi.cemmlibrary.org
- Traumatic Brain Injury Survival Guide: www.tbiguide.com
- U.S. Department of Veterans Affairs Traumatic Brain Injury: https://www.publichealth.va.gov/exposures/traumatic-brain-injury.asp

Medical

Ongoing medical management is important for most brain injury survivors. Physicians who specialize in TBI may be identified through selected professional organizations:

- American Academy of Physical Medicine and Rehabilitation: www.aapmr.org
- American Academy of Neurology: https://www.aan.com
- American Board of Psychiatry and Neurology (search for Brain Injury Medicine certified doctors): https://application.abpn.com/verifycert/verifyCert.asp?a=4

- Brainline.org: www.brainline.org provides a resource page describing how to choose a high-quality medical rehabilitation program.
- Local academic medical centers may be able to assist in identifying physicians who have specialty expertise in managing TBI.
- There are currently 16 civilian and 5 Veteran's Affairs facility TBI Model System Centers located throughout the United States (see www.tbindsc.org/Centers.aspx). These centers are recognized providers of expert care for TBI. To learn more about the TBI Model systems program, visit the Model Systems Knowledge Translation Center: www.msktc.org/tbi

Neuropsychological/Psychological

Neuropsychological assessments should be conducted and interpreted by those who have experience working with individuals with TBI. Neuropsychologists can significantly enhance understanding of the effects of the brain injury. In addition, psychologists who understand the effects of sudden loss or change on family systems can also be helpful to survivors and families trying to cope with the effects of brain injury. See:

- The American Psychological Association: www.apa.org (Search by city/state—does not provide information by subspecialty.)
- BIAA: www.biausa.org (Local offices often maintain lists of psychologists/neuropsychologists with TBI experience.)

Neurorehabilitation

The ongoing rehabilitation needs of each survivor will vary according to the residual effects of the brain injury. Home health services, long-term care/skilled nursing/subacute programs, day treatment, and outpatient programs are the usual categories of programs that may be recommended for a survivor. One means of locating services available in your area is through your state Brain Injury Association of America (BIAA) chapter.

- Home Care Association of America: www.hcaoa.org to find a provider by city & state, ZIP code, or company.

Survivor and Caregiver Support/Resources

Caregiver burden and the impact that caregivers can have on the recovery process for persons with TBIs are widely discussed in the literature.[12,13] The burden experienced by a caregiver of a TBI survivor—generally a family member—may be particularly difficult given the lengthy recovery process and the altered abilities and personality of the survivor. Often, the caregivers' wellness is sacrificed when their needs for support are not understood and prioritized. Wellness, respite, and spiritual and social networking can be important components of a caregiver support plan. Support groups for the caregiver, as well as for the survivor, can be found throughout most states and are often important sources of caregiver wellness information. Your state BIAA chapter/affiliate is one helpful resource for locating these groups. The following are also useful caregiver resources:

- Brainline.org Caregiving & Brain Injury: https://www.brainline.org/caregivers
- Bridging the Gap: www.tbibridge.org
- Family Caregiver Alliance: https://www.caregiver.org/health-issues/brain-injury
- HelpGuide.org Caregiver support guide: https://www.helpguide.org/home-pages/family-caregiving.htm
- Henry B. Betts LIFE Center at the Shirley Ryan Ability Lab: https://www.sralab.org/lifecenter

- Traumatic Brain Injury Resource for Survivors and Caregivers: www.northeastern. edu/nutraumaticbraininjury

Advocacy/Legal

In seeking out and obtaining needed services, advocacy is often necessary at some juncture. The advocacy role is generally played by the spouse, parent, or caregiver.

- Every state and territory in the United States has a Protection and Advocacy Agency. All of these agencies are part of a network known as the National Disability Rights Network. To search for your local agency go to: www.ndrn.org/index.php and select your state.
- For assistance with independent living, consider contacting Centers for Independent Living at www.virtualcil.net/cils which provides links to independent living centers throughout the country, as does the National Council on Independent Living: www.ncil.org
- For legal information/resources see: www.ada.gov/cguide.htm or Council for Disability Rights: https://thedrlc.org

Vocational

Supported employment interventions improve job placement and retention for TBI survivors.[6] Vocational counselors and job coaches experienced in working with TBI survivors can be an invaluable resource, advocating with employers, recommending job modifications, and providing individualized retraining. Every state has a Department or Division of Rehabilitation Services that may help with vocational support. The following websites may also be helpful:

- Brain Injury Resource Center: www.headinjury.com/jobs.htm#funds and resources
- National Organization on Disability: http://nod.org/disability_resources
- U.S. Department of Education www2.ed.gov/about/contacts/state/index.html?src=ln
- Unites States Department of Labor Office of Disability Employment Policy: www.dol. gov

Recreation, Leisure, and Social Networking for Survivors

Leisure and social relationships are often adversely affected by a TBI.[14] Support groups, special "clubhouses" for survivors, and local park districts can become core aspects of community re-entry and social interaction. In additional to undertaking a website search under "Special Recreation Associations TBI" or "Parks & Recreation TBI," the following resources can provide assistance:

- International Brain Injury Clubhouse Alliance: www.braininjuryclubhouses.net (Choose "Find a Clubhouse Near You")
- BIAA: www.biausa.org
- National Center on Health, Physical Activity and Disability (NCHPAD) is a public health practice and resource center on health promotion for people with disability: www.nchpad.org

Research

- Sixteen "model systems" across the nation have been funded by the National Institute on Disability, Independent Living, and Rehabilitation Research (NIDILRR) to

conduct ongoing TBI research. Their studies can be accessed at: www.msktc.org/tbi/model-system-centers
- To locate current clinical trials, go to: http://clinicaltrials.gov (search TBI)
- National Institute of Neurological Disorders and Stroke (NINDS): www.ninds.nih.gov/index.htm
- The Brain Trauma Foundation: www.braintrauma.org

SPECIALIZED NEEDS

Military

Approximately 413,858 military persons worldwide have sustained a TBI.[15] Those who have served in the military and their families have access to support through:

- Military Health System Traumatic Brain Injury Center of Excellence: https://health.mil/About-MHS/OASDHA/Defense-Health-Agency/Research-and-Development/Traumatic-Brain-Injury-Center-of-Excellence
- Department of Veterans Affairs: www.va.gov
- Military healthcare (Tricare) benefit information: www.military.com/benefits/tricare
- Feds Hire Vets: www.dol.gov/vets
- National Organization on Disability: http://nod.org/research_publications/wwc_vets
- U.S. Department of Veterans Affairs Veterans Health Library: https://www.veteranshealthlibrary.va.gov/livingwith/traumaticbraininjury/
- Hines Fisher House provides temporary housing for families of injured and ill soldiers: www.fisherhouse.org
- Wounded Warrior Project provides information to plan for changes in income, special compensation, estimation of disability ratings, and more: www.woundedwarriorproject.org
- My Army Benefits: http://myarmybenefits.us.army.mil
- National Resource Directory for Veterans and Military: www.nrd.gov

Pediatrics/Adolescents

For children and adolescents, the major focus of community re-entry will be return to school. Issues related to pediatric TBI and education have been widely discussed.[16,17] Individualized accommodations may be in place as per federal and local laws. Neuropsychologists with expertise in pediatric neuropsychological testing are good resources to ensure appropriate placement and support, especially for those children with cognitive issues. Families/caregivers should seek support to ensure that an appropriate *Individualized Education Plan* (IEP) is in place and is reviewed regularly as required by local law.

- Brainline.org: Students with TBI: www.brainline.org/content/2010/06/students-with-tbi-learn-about-the-iep504-.html
- National Information for Children and Youth with Disabilities: www.parentcenterhub.org/nichcy-resources
- Family Voices provides resources and support for children and youth to receive family-centered care: www.familyvoices.org/about?id=0003
- Family Resource Center on Disabilities provides information, training, and assistance: www.frcd.org
- Brain Injury Association of America (BIAA): www.biausa.org/brain-injury-children.htmTBI.org; www.tbi.org/category/pediatric-tbi

Mild Traumatic Brain Injury

Because mild TBI (MTBI) deficits are often subtle, individuals with MTBI may not be easily identified and may be misunderstood by community agency personnel. The following resource may be of use:

- Centers for Disease Control and Prevention: www.cdc.gov/concussion/signs_symptoms.html

---

KEY POINTS

- TBI impacts quality of life for patients, families, and caregivers. Information and resources are necessary to support living life to its fullest.
- Resources provide knowledge and information so that persons with TBI, their families, and/or caregivers can make informed decisions about their care.
- A multi-prong approach to accessing resources is often necessary to aid in reintegrating persons with TBI into the community after this life-changing event.

STUDY QUESTIONS

1. What are the general domains of daily living?
   a. Activities of daily living
   b. Vocational/school re-entry
   c. Leisure/social/wellness
   d. All of the above

2. What is a valuable medium to increase access to information about the management of cognitive issues resulting from TBI?
   a. Word of mouth
   b. Internet
   c. Old text books
   d. Pamphlets

3. How many TBI Model Systems are there?
   a. 16
   b. 15
   c. 20
   d. 17

4. Why is the burden on a caregiver of a TBI survivor particularly difficult?
   a. Quick recovery process
   b. Lengthy recovery process
   c. Altered abilities and personality of the survivor
   d. b and c

5. What is the major focus of community re-entry for children and adolescents who have experienced a TBI?
   a. Return to work
   b. Return to school
   c. Return to driving
   d. b and b

ANSWERS TO STUDY QUESTIONS

1. Correct Answer: d
   The general domains of living: (a) activities of daily living, (b) vocational/school re-entry, and (c) leisure/social/wellness.

   Further Reading:
   Hammel J, Magasi S, Heinemann A, et al. Environmental barriers and supports to everyday participation: a qualitative insider perspective from people with disabilities. *Arch Phys Med Rehabil*. 2015;96(4):578–588. doi:10.1016/j.apmr.2014.12.008.
   Heffernan DS, Vera RM, Monaghan SF, et al. Socio-ethnic factors on outcomes following traumatic brain injury. *J Trauma Inj Infect Crit Care*. 2011;70(3):527–534. doi:10.1097/TA.0b013e31820d0ed7.

2. Correct Answer: b
   Although all of these resources may come in handy, a valuable tool to increase access to information is the Internet. This chapter included many websites to provide easy access to several important resources.

   Further Reading:
   Poulin V, Dawson DR, Bottari C, et al. Managing cognitive difficulties after traumatic brain injury: a review of online resources for families. *Disabil Rehabil*. 2019; 41:16, 1955–1965. doi:10.1080/09638288.2018.1451560

3. Correct Answer: a
   The Traumatic Brain Injury Model System consists of 16 established civilian rehabilitation centers, each national leaders in patient care and clinical research.

   Further Reading:
   Model Systems Knowledge Translation Center: www.msktc.org/tbi

4. Correct Answer: d
   The burden experienced by a caregiver of a TBI survivor—generally a family member—may be particularly difficult given the lengthy recovery process and the altered abilities and personality of the survivor.

   Further Reading:
   Vangel SJ, Rapport LJ, Hanks RA. Effects of family and caregiver psychological functioning on outcomes in persons with traumatic brain injury. *J Head Trauma Rehabil*. 2011;26(1):20–29. doi:10.1097/HTR.0b013e318204a70d

Lefebrvre H, Levert MJ. The close relatives of people who have had a traumatic brain injury and their special needs. *Brain Inj*. 2012;26(6):1084–1097. doi:10.3109/02699052.2012.666364

5. Correct Answer: b
For children and adolescents, the major focus of community re-entry will be return to school. Families/caregivers should seek support to ensure that an appropriate *Individualized Education Plan* (IEP) is in place and is reviewed regularly as required by local law.

Further Reading:
Zonfrillo MR, Durbin DR, Winston FK, et al. Residual cognitive disability after completion of inpatient rehabilitation among injured children. *J Pediatr*. 2014;164(1):130–135. doi:10.1016/j.jpeds.2013.09.022
Anderson V, Godfrey JV, Catroppa C. Effects of traumatic brain injury linger 10 years later. *Pediatrics*. 2012;129(2):254–261. doi:10.1542/peds.2011-0311

REFERENCES

The full reference list appears in the digital product found on http://connect.springer-pub.com/content/book/978-0-8261-4768-4/part/part05/chapter/ch71

LIVING WITH TRAUMATIC BRAIN INJURY: FROM A SURVIVOR'S PERSPECTIVE

JENNIFER FIELD

I was 17 years old. From the age of six, I had been a competitive rider on the equestrian show circuit and was now at the Grand Prix level of show jumping. I was champion in the Junior Jumpers at the Washington International Horse Show in Landover, Maryland, and fresh off a third place win at the Maclay Equitation Finals at the Madison Square Garden horse show. My plan was to graduate early from high school and compete in Europe with an eye to the Olympics.

But on a snowy Friday in November, I wasn't thinking about any of that. The year had ended in the competitive show world, I was back in school, and I could finally take time for myself. My mother was leaving for the weekend and my boyfriend Matt was coming up from Connecticut College; we had schemed this secret rendezvous since our last time together at the Garden.

I skipped my last class to go home, change clothes, and make it back to school to meet Matt. I couldn't be late. Queen's Under Pressure blasted through my Black Saab 900 as I sped 55 mph down a winding country road. A severe, early-winter storm was predicted and it was just beginning to snow. I had lived in New Hampshire long enough to know that these conditions were the deadliest—but I was not deterred. I could only think of Matt.

Without warning, I hit black ice, skidded uncontrollably into the other lane, and collided with a tractor–trailer barreling toward me. The bumper of the truck, towering above me, smashed the passenger-side rear window. The impact was so severe, my seat collapsed and my head ricocheted back through the driver side rear window. Glass was embedded in my skull. My neck was twisted, the airway was blocked, and I had stopped breathing.

I'm not sure how long I lay there, unconscious, unable to breathe, but I was later told that a volunteer firefighter was in the area and arrived on the scene after hearing about the accident on his CB radio. He knew from the position of my head that I wasn't breathing, and although a fire crew was trying frantically to get me out of the car, the volunteer firefighter found the strength to open the door and reposition my head so that I could breathe again. The ambulance took me to the local community hospital, where the emergency team quickly assessed the severity of my injury and made arrangements for me to be transported to a regional hospital.

Life as I had known it was over. From then on, I would become consumed with the search for a complete healing. At first, I wanted the old me, to regain my old life. Now, almost 30 years later, I realize on that day I was reborn.

> *I picked up the phone and a voice said, "This is the Monadnock Community Hospital calling. Your daughter has been in an accident." So I asked how Jennifer was and the woman on the phone said, "I should really get the doctor," and I just went nuts. I just screamed and screamed and I guess the doctor came on and I asked "Is she alive?" and he said, "Yes." And then I don't think I could talk anymore.*
> —Joanne Field, Jennifer's mom

The doctors at the regional hospital had little hope for my survival. Tubes were coming out of my body, wires were attached to monitors, and I had a pressure gauge in my head. A renowned neurosurgeon from Chicago had been flown to New Hampshire to see if there was something more that could be done. After reading my computed tomography (CT) scan, he concluded that I could not be moved, that I would survive, but I might never speak again.

I lay in a coma for 3 weeks; I was on a respirator, my left arm and leg pumped continuously, of their own volition, and because of severe tone, my right arm curled inward and remained frozen for months. My vitals had begun to stabilize and the pressure gauge measuring swelling had been removed from my head.

Brain injured patients are evaluated on the Rancho Los Amigos scale, indicating the severity of the condition and the likelihood that the patient would respond to, and benefit from, treatment. Using this one-to-ten scale, I was ranked a "three." Given that a "one" indicates a vegetative state, I wasn't doing very well.

I was being fed through a tube, and was nonresponsive, so doctors suggested to my mom that she decorate my room with personal effects to stimulate a response. My mom brought photos, a saddle, some of my horse's mane, and even some manure. None of it created the response everyone was hoping for. I have no memory from this time in the coma, and even the early months after, so my mother has filled in the blanks for me.

> One morning, nurses were washing her face and I saw Jennifer's left eye open. Stunned, I told the nurse her eye had opened, but the nurse said "Oh, Joanne, I know how badly you want this to happen ..." and just at that moment, "bing!" her eye opened again. I went tearing down the hallway of the hospital and told everyone in the waiting room—and this hoard of family and friends came thundering down the ICU, which was completely against the rules. Of course, both eyes were closed by the time we arrived in her room and remained closed for three days. And then, Jen opened her left eye and this time, it remained opened.
> —Joanne Field

Some say you emerge from a coma in stages, like a butterfly coming out of a cocoon. Truly, it's not that beautiful, but maybe just as miraculous. My first memory of waking up from my coma was being on the floor of a blue padded room, looking up at my best friend Kristin and an unfamiliar male face. It was Matt; someone had to tell me he was my boyfriend. To this day, I think it is the first memory I have of being conscious after the accident. I was put in that padded room as a safety precaution because as you come out of a coma you can get really violent and either hurt yourself, or someone else. It can be difficult for family members to watch a loved one coming out of a coma, and I'm sure that it's difficult, too, for families to muster patience in the face of just how slow recovery can be: weeks, months, even, as in my case, years.

I had sustained a diffuse, closed-head injury. Although the truck hit the right side of my head, the whiplash was so severe that the left side of my brain received the brunt of the trauma. The human body works in diagonals. The left part of the brain controls the right side of the body; the right controls the left. So when I eventually awoke, the right side of my body was completely paralyzed. I couldn't walk, talk, or use my right arm. And my right eye was completely closed.

During this time, I wasn't troubled by the severity of my condition. I remember being calm and tranquil. My moment-by-moment experiences were all I knew. My whole world was a blue padded room.

The rehabilitation schedule that followed my coming out of the coma was a series of good and bad days, each one including numerous doctors, specialists, therapists, exercises, tests, and evaluations. The good days were filled with small hard-won victories and the bad days were filled with insurmountable, soul-destroying, and energy-sapping impossibilities. Some of the tests should have been so simple, such as clipping clothes pegs to an upright ruler, and yet I found this almost impossible to do. When I achieved that task with my right arm, which had been a cement block of severe tone, it was a tremendous victory.

I was starting my life over again as if I were a toddler, joined at the hip to my mother. I was learning how to wipe my face, dress and feed myself, brush my hair, and blow my nose, from the same woman who had taught me those basic skills the first time around.

Meanwhile my speech was hardly audible: My voice was whispery and my words were slurred and halting because of the cognitive challenge of trying to track what I had just said at the same time as I was trying to recall the word that meant what I hoped to say next. Suffice it to say, it wasn't easy for others to understand me.

At the culmination of long months of intensive rehabilitation, doctors told my mother, "Your daughter will make most of her improvements in the first year and very few after that," and "Don't you realize the severity of your daughter's injury? She will never get any better, this is it." On the verge of tears, my mother said nothing, but inside she thought, "No, this will not be it."

Back home in Peterborough, New Hampshire, as my mother lay in bed one night, a voice came into her head with the message, "Go downstairs and get your alternative medicine books, and search for another way."

Thus began a 2-year odyssey across the United States, to Mexico, Canada, and Europe in search of therapies that could address the cognitive and physical constraints that my mom and I were determined I would overcome. Standard medical rehabilitation techniques had helped me to regain a measure of function, but I was far from achieving even a semblance of physical independence. During this next period of my journey, I regained significant functionality from a combination of alternative therapies, including craniosacral therapy, soft-tissue manipulation, osteopathy, acupuncture, neuro-optometric rehabilitation, electroencephalography (EEG) neurofeedback, nutrition, hyperbaric oxygen, various healers, and Continuum Movement.

Experimenting with these modalities, and adjusting the degree of emphasis on each practice in my rehabilitation regimen, I began to increase my physical capacity and confidence—in my balance, in my ability to move and walk, in my capability to coordinate different functions, in my reasoning and thought process and, finally, in my speech.

Finding, practicing, and testing the many therapies became a full-time job for my mom and me. It wasn't easy, it wasn't always fun, and it was often tiring for both of us, even with significant support from family and friends. Fortunately for me, diligence and unwavering determination were qualities that my mom had in abundance.

Years later, I would overhear her saying to her friends, "When I look back on my life, what gives me the most pride is Jennifer's recovery."

After 2 years of pursuing alternative therapies, I wanted more out of life. I wanted to go to college, to be "normal." I applied to Wheaton College, was accepted, and began my freshman classes in 1995. It wasn't always easy to fit in socially. Academically, college required long hours of dedicated study on my part, extra help from others, and unlimited time on exams, but the result was an important personal victory: I graduated Magna Cum Laude in Art History in 2000. I was ready for my next challenge.

I left New England and moved to my own apartment in Santa Monica, California. It was a big step to live on my own. I immersed myself in Continuum Movement practices, which I have found to be a vital tool for me to experience the fullness of what it means to be alive. Over time I have found that combining the slow, and graceful work of Continuum with balance and strength training is ultimately where I find the most benefit today. When I practice Continuum I get lost in myself. This is my meditation.

At this time, my speech was still slow and halting—and word retrieval remained difficult. New people I encountered often thought I was drunk—or high—when I spoke. Not all of the therapies I had engaged in were centered around my physical recovery. Some were about finding ways to express my "inner experience" of dealing with the day-to-day grind and how long my recovery was taking. Sometimes I became very frustrated with life. When you lose your physical independence and have to start relying on other people for everything, you can feel helpless, "locked out," and forgotten. So, while searching for ways to express what was going on inside, I began to write and paint.

Prior to my injury, I had never considered taking up a creative practice. I was totally focused on my riding. I had absolutely no idea if I was even capable of producing anything worth looking at or reading, but I did it anyway and it was a tremendous help. The first writing I did was poetry, then my writing became more autobiographical. I have discovered that to write about or speak about my journey has been very powerful in my recovery. The colors I used in my paintings were expressive. Given my struggle with impaired speech, engaging in creative expression was a welcome change of pace.

From 2003 to 2006, I complemented writing, painting, and Continuum Movement work with acting classes. Acting was difficult for me at first, not only because of the damage to my vocal chords, but because I struggled to memorize my lines. When a friend suggested, "Why don't you turn what you're writing into a one-woman play about your life?" I just laughed, but ultimately that's exactly what I did.

I have performed my one-woman show, "A Distant Memory," in theaters and at colleges, high schools, hospitals, rehab centers, and conferences since 2006. The act of performing and repeating my story has strengthened my verbal skills, which continue to improve to this day. And it has helped me to build my confidence. Coming offstage after my very first performance of the show, I remember saying to John Ruskin, the director of the theater, "I found it again! I found the feeling I had when entering the ring on my horse to compete."

As John Lennon wrote, "Life is what happens while you're busy making other plans." I had my goal of riding and show jumping, but during my years of recovery, I started to realize that in my pursuit to become "normal," to get back to my "old self" and the life I had before the accident, I was actually living my life. As I grew to appreciate the meaning of this, it became easier to welcome new challenges and improve upon the life I was building. And I think that is the basis of a pretty "normal" and satisfying life.

When it first happened, everyone thought of my accident as a horrific tragedy from which I would never really recover. Well, I have recovered, and the more time passes, the more I don't want to use the words accident and tragedy to describe what happened to me. In rising to overcome difficulties, our lives become enriched and we grow.

I think angels come into our lives in many different forms. Even in the forms of tragedies and accidents. Not to punish, but to teach us. Maybe hitting that truck was a harsh and dramatic way to learn a lesson. I can't know what my life would have been like, or what kind of person I would be, if I had never had this challenge to overcome, but I am completely certain that this experience has helped me to develop a rich spiritual and emotional life. I doubt I would have achieved this on the course I was originally headed. And part of my path now is to communicate the lessons I've learned to others.

Years after the accident, I believe that a key to my healing was a conviction that both my mother and I developed: There is always an alternative. It may not be immediately apparent. You may have to search for it. But it's there.

You see, my own road to recovery began after someone else, who had been in this same situation, reached out to help me. My mother received a phone call 2 days after my accident from a woman whose daughter had suffered a similar brain injury in a fall from a horse. This daughter's mother said to my mother, "Don't listen to everything the doctors say. Stay with your daughter. DO NOT leave her. She will get better."

That woman was right. No one with a traumatic brain injury should ever have to accept someone saying, "You can't," "That's not going to be possible," "That's all that is available to you," or "That's all that can be done, you must learn to live with it."

My position, borne of experience, persistence, and hard work, is that you don't have to just live with the devastation of traumatic brain injury. There are always options. There is always hope. There is always possibility.

What is a new normal for me in 2020? In the early days after the injury, a new normal was giving up my identity as an equestrian. In the course of my healing, I did literally do the proverbial "get back on the horse." I fell off. I got on again. And I fell off again. The moment I hit the ground that second time, I realized I would never ride again. With all the advances I had made in my therapies and all the healing I had experienced, it wasn't worth it to risk further brain injury. So, now I faced the unknown. Who was I?

For many years my accident and subsequent therapies defined me. Then as I took acting classes and honed my one-woman show, I found a new path: giving others inspiration and guidance by sharing my experiences. I never imagined I could stand up in front of people and talk. I had never felt like I was good enough or wise enough. But like riding, I guess I do like being in the spotlight. There is something inside of me that compels me to perform. With each of my performances, a bit of the trauma drops away. I'm not, and do not want to be, that person people feel sorry for. I want to be the person from whom others can learn. This is my new normal.

In my new normal, I can't drive or bike or go out running. (A boyfriend once took me roller-blading in Santa Monica, and that was a short-lived romance.) But I have so many things in my life to be thankful for. And my focus is now elsewhere: writing, speaking, and helping others through my foundation.

Some might call my car wreck an accident, but I feel I was caught up in destiny. I believe it was my destiny to inspire people to believe that anything is possible by staying focused and determined. I feel my healing will never stop. It's been almost 30 years since my TBI and my brain is still constantly improving.

One thing that always seemed to help my healing process was changing my direction and focus and trying something new. You can always go back to what you were doing before, but what really encourages the brain to continue healing is to create new neural pathways, a new therapy, a new hobby, begin swimming, water aerobics, or start running a little and skipping, instead of just walking. Each day something happens to me to promote growth, improvement, and acceptance. I am constantly amazed that, almost every time I am reconnected with a friend who I haven't seen for a while, this may be a few weeks, months, or years, they almost always make a point of commenting on how much better my speech has gotten, my balance, or my speed and flow of movements. I don't believe there is ever an end to the healing process.

I once heard a quote that was something along the lines of, "Live life for what tomorrow can bring and not what yesterday has taken away from you. Every day is a gift." Try to be grateful for even the smallest gifts: a sunny morning, a beautiful sunset, a special song on the radio that brings back great memories, a cup of tea with the person you love. These are only a few small gifts in my daily life that I am extremely grateful for.

When I was about to turn 40, a milestone age, I wondered if my "normal" would ever include a husband. I had come to terms that maybe it wouldn't happen for me. But sometimes when you accept your fate, that's when the change happens.

Now, 5 years later I am with a man who is in love with me, the new me. I did not think that could ever be possible. I have learned that receiving unconditional love can be the best healer. He makes me feel beautiful and special, just the way I am. Is there any gift better than that?

I was about to give my one woman show at the La Grua Center in Stonington, Connecticut, when my producer and editor invited me to go with her on a dog walk at nearby Charleston, Rhode Island. People on the walk that afternoon were reuniting rescue dogs that had been littermates. I was nervous I would be knocked over surrounded by so many large and excited dogs rough-housing around me.

Scared for my balance, all of a sudden I heard, "Do you know Jennifer Field?" I was being introduced to a very kind and gentle looking man. Bruce and I began walking and talked until the park closed for the day. Along the way, I just decided I was going to tell him about my car accident, struggles, and ongoing recovery. Either he would still be standing next to me at the end of our walk, or he wouldn't. I had had many disappointments in my life when people left after they learned about my brain injury. I didn't blame some people for getting scared, because I got scared at times myself.

A few days later Bruce did show up at my talk, then he joined us for dinner after. That evening was capped off with a Hallmark movie appropriately called, "Boyfriends and Dogs," and our first kiss. Little did I know that this was just the beginning of the next chapter of my life.

Four years later, we were sitting under lemon trees in a restaurant called Paulino, in Capri, Italy. This was our first trip to Europe, and without my knowledge, when Bruce had asked my father for his permission to marry me, Dad recommended that Bruce propose to me at Paulino. The ceiling was made of entwined lemon branches with lemons everywhere. After a wonderful dinner, Bruce ordered a lemoncello for dessert, and I had continued with my never-ending espresso. We asked the waiter to call a taxi, and I noticed Bruce getting increasingly nervous, ordering one lemoncello, after another... Finally they told us the taxi was here, and as we were going out Bruce motioned me over to a side area. I said, "What are you doing, the taxi is waiting?" "Just humor me, this is so beautiful," he said. He got down on one knee and asked me to marry him. I was overcome with happiness, and said yes. We kissed as clapping began all around us and I heard the repeated click of a camera with lights flashing. Bruce had arranged for the island photographer to capture his proposal!

We had a beautiful ceremony at our family summer house above a small lake in New Hampshire. Family and friends surrounded us as we took our wedding vows. It was truly one of the best days of my life.

I could not believe it. Twenty-six years after my traumatic brain injury, I was about to be married to an amazing man. This was a day that I never could have imagined happening to me! I never would have believed that anyone would want to marry this damaged woman. The feeling I had inside as I walked down the grassy path with my father was of complete pride and happiness! I had done it. I had become a woman who had fought her way back and was now a bride. Another important new chapter in my life was about to begin.

We had loved being in Italy so much on our first trip, that we decided to return to Capri for our honeymoon. My new husband patiently helped me to navigate the steep and windy cliffs of the Amalfi coast, which I could never have climbed by myself. The tremor in my left arm became very dramatic from the intense Italian caffeine!! We loved just sitting out under the late afternoon sunset, sipping our espresso.

I think everyone who undergoes a trauma is faced with becoming a new person, whether they want to accept that or not. Discovering the "new you" can be a very exciting process, but it is also very daunting and frightening. This process of discovery only happens if there is true acceptance of the trauma. Usually there is simply no choice, and how you learn to deal with the "new you" can be what defines how much healing you will ultimately experience.

Even though my accident was more than 25 years ago, I am still making strides forward. Recovery is a constant struggle, which encourages me to continue working so that

I keep making improvements. I think this applies to all brain injury survivors, or really anyone with a challenge. The drive to get better pushes one forward.

As you have read on previous pages, my prognosis was dismal after my accident. But with each passing year, I know how mistaken some of the experts were. I am very grateful that my life's work is to encourage others to never give up. One of my biggest surprises is that I've not only learned to play bridge, but I really like it. It is a competitive card game that requires memory and skill. And I feel that using my brain in such a way will ultimately cause new neural pathways to form. Bridge awakens that competitive side of me that has always been there. I would never have thought I could find something that is so competitive without being physical. Yes, I miss horseback riding and running, but I have learned you can find fulfillment in other areas if you keep looking and trying new things.

I continue to be a new person in a new world, and I don't think I could have gotten there without going through the process of working hard and healing every day. I treasure and accept what I have learned, what I have been given, and what has been taken away. I try to write a monthly inspirational newsletter for my website and have developed the J. Field Foundation, Inc., which provides hope and healing for brain-injured children. I want so desperately to give back to those who are suffering, who believe that they may never recover. I want everyone to be excited about achieving and accepting their new normal.

INDEX

Note: Page references followed by "*f*" and "*t*" denote figures and tables, respectively.